Nursing Pharmacology

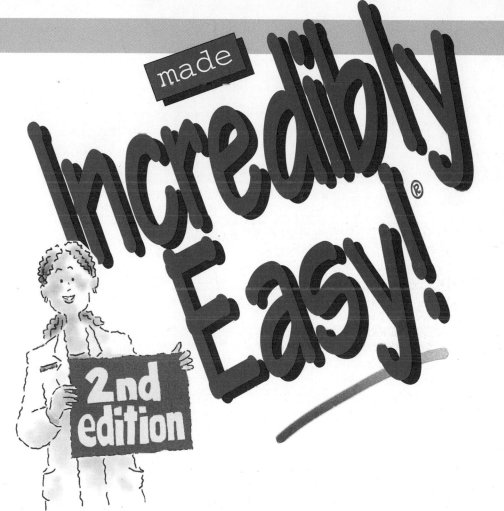

made **Incredibly Easy!** ®

2nd edition

 Wolters Kluwer | Lippincott Williams & Wilkins
Health

Philadelphia · Baltimore · New York · London
Buenos Aires · Hong Kong · Sydney · Tokyo

Staff

Executive Publisher
Judith A. Schilling McCann, RN, MSN

Editorial Director
David Moreau

Clinical Director
Joan M. Robinson, RN, MSN

Art Director
Mary Ludwicki

Electronic Project Manager
John Macalino

Senior Managing Editor
Jaime Stockslager Buss, MSPH, ELS

Clinical Project Manager
Jennifer Meyering, RN, BSN, MS, CCRN

Editors
Margaret Eckman, Diane Labus, Gale Thompson

Clinical Editor
Anita Lockhart, RNC, MSN

Copy Editors
Kimberly Bilotta (supervisor), Jane Bradford,
Heather Ditch, Jeannine Fielding, Shana
Harrington, Dorothy P. Terry, Pamela Wingrod

Designer
Georg W. Purvis IV

Illustrator
Bot Roda

Digital Composition Services
Diane Paluba (manager), Joyce Rossi Biletz,
Donna Morris

Associate Manufacturing Manager
Beth J. Welsh

Editorial Assistants
Karen J. Kirk, Jeri O'Shea, Linda K. Ruhf

Indexer
Barbara Hodgson

Library of Congress Cataloging-in-Publication Data
Nursing pharmacology made incredibly easy. — 2nd ed.
   p. ; cm.
   Includes bibliographical references and index.
   1. Pharmacology. 2. Nurses. I. Lippincott Williams &
Wilkins.
   [DNLM: 1. Drug Therapy — nursing — Handbooks.
   2. Pharmacology — Handbooks. WY 49 N97499 2009]
   RM125.N846 2009
   615'.1 — dc22
   ISBN-13: 978-0-7817-9289-9 (alk. paper)
   ISBN-10: 0-7817-9289-4 (alk. paper)   2008015160

Contents

Contributors and consultants

Katrina D. Allen, RN, MSN, CCRN
Nursing Instructor
Faulkner State Community College
Bay Minette, AL

Judith D. Brock, RN, BA, BSN, MPH
Assistant Professor of Nursing
Mesa State College
Grand Junction, CO

Marsha L. Conroy, RN, MSN, APN
Nurse Educator
Cuyahoga Community College
Cleveland, OH

Margaret Covington, MS, RN, CNS
Nurse Educator
Gateway Community College
Phoenix, AZ

Christine Frazer, DNSC, CNS, RN
Nursing Instructor
Penn State University
Hershey, PA

Stephen Gilliam, PHD, RN, FNP, APRN-BC
Assistant Professor
Medical College of Georgia
School of Nursing
Athens, GA

Margaret M. Gingrich, RN, MSN
Professor
Harrisburg Area Community College
Harrisburg, PA

Jaclynn A. Johnson, RNC, MSN
Lead Nursing Instructor
Otero Junior College
La Junta, CO

Ronnette C. Langhorne, RN, MS
Assistant Professor
Thomas Nelson Community College
Hampton, VA

Darlene Rainwater, MSN, RN
Associate Professor
St. Elizabeth School of Nursing
Lafayette, IN
Instructor
St. Joseph's College Consortium
Rensselear, IN

Wynona Wiggins, MSN, RN, CCRN
Assistant Professor of Nursing
Arkansas State University
State University, AR

Margaret A. Wilson, RN, MSN, EDD
Professor of Nursing
Cypress College
Cypress, CA
California State University
Fullerton, CA

Not another boring foreword

If you're like me, you're too busy caring for your patients to have the time to wade through a foreword that uses pretentious terms and umpteen dull paragraphs to get to the point. So let's cut right to the chase! Here's why this book is so terrific:

 It will teach you all the important things you need to know about nursing pharmacology. (And it will leave out all the fluff that wastes your time.)

It will help you remember what you've learned.

It will make you smile as it enhances your knowledge and skills.

Don't believe me? Try these recurring logos on for size:

 Prototype pro—details actions, indications, and nursing considerations for common prototype drugs.

 Pharm function—explains and illustrates the way drugs act in the body.

 Before you give that drug—alerts you to drug warnings that should be considered before administration.

 Education edge—provides important information you should share with your patient.

See? I told you! And that's not all. Look for me and my friends in the margins throughout this book. We'll be there to explain key concepts, provide important care reminders, and offer reassurance. Oh, and if you don't mind, we'll be spicing up the pages with a bit of humor along the way, to teach and entertain in a way that no other resource can.

I hope you find this book helpful. Best of luck throughout your career!

Joy

Fundamentals of nursing pharmacology

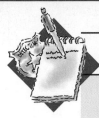

Just the facts

In this chapter, you'll learn:

♦ pharmacology basics

♦ key concepts of pharmacokinetics, pharmacodynamics, and pharmacotherapeutics

♦ key types of drug interactions and adverse reactions

♦ the nursing process.

Pharmacology basics

Pharmacology is the scientific study of the origin, nature, chemistry, effects, and uses of drugs. This knowledge is essential to providing safe and accurate medication administration to your patients.

The big three

This chapter reviews the three basic concepts of pharmacology:

   pharmacokinetics—the absorption, distribution, metabolism, and excretion of drugs by the body

   pharmacodynamics—the biochemical and physical effects of drugs and the mechanisms of drug actions

   pharmacotherapeutics—the use of drugs to prevent and treat diseases.

In addition, it discusses other important aspects of pharmacology, including:

• how drugs are named and classified
• how drugs are derived
• how drugs are administered
• how new drugs are developed.

Naming and classifying drugs

Drugs have a specific kind of nomenclature—that is, a drug can go by three different names:
- The *chemical name* is a scientific name that precisely describes the drug's atomic and molecular structure.
- The *generic*, or *nonproprietary*, *name* is an abbreviation of the chemical name.
- The *trade name* (also known as the *brand name* or *proprietary name*) is selected by the drug company selling the product. Trade names are protected by copyright. The symbol ® after a trade name indicates that the name is registered by and restricted to the drug manufacturer.

To avoid confusion, it's best to use a drug's generic name because any one drug can have a number of trade names.

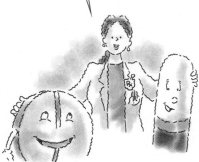

Drugs may have many different trade names. To avoid confusion, refer to a drug by its generic name.

Making it official

In 1962, the federal government mandated the use of official names so that only one official name would represent each drug. The official names are listed in the *United States Pharmacopeia* and *National Formulary*.

Class act

Drugs that share similar characteristics are grouped together as a *pharmacologic class* (or family). Beta-adrenergic blockers are an example of a pharmacologic class.

A second type of drug grouping is the *therapeutic class*, which categorizes drugs by therapeutic use. Antihypertensives are an example of a therapeutic class.

A pharmacologic class groups drugs by their shared characteristics. A therapeutic class groups drugs by their therapeutic use.

Where drugs come from

Traditionally, drugs were derived from *natural* sources, such as:
- plants
- animals
- minerals.

Today, however, laboratory researchers have used traditional knowledge, along with chemical science, to develop *synthetic* drug sources. One advantage of chemically developed drugs is that they're free from the impurities found in natural substances. Also, re-

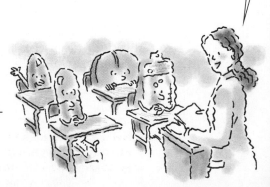

searchers and drug developers can manipulate the molecular structure of substances such as antibiotics so that a slight change in the chemical structure makes the drug effective against different organisms. The first-, second-, third-, and fourth-generation cephalosporins are an example.

Sowing the seeds of drugs

The earliest drug concoctions from plants used everything: the leaves, roots, bulb, stem, seeds, buds, and blossoms. As a result, harmful substances often found their way into the mixture.

Reaping the rewards of research

As the understanding of plants as drug sources became more sophisticated, researchers sought to isolate and intensify *active components* while avoiding harmful ones. The active components of plants vary in character and effect:

- *Alkaloids*, the most active component in plants, react with acids to form a salt that's able to dissolve more readily in body fluids. The names of alkaloids and their salts usually end in "-ine"; examples include atropine, caffeine, and nicotine.
- *Glycosides* are naturally occurring active components that are found in plants and have both beneficial and toxic effects. They usually have names that end in "-in," such as digoxin.
- *Gums* give products the ability to attract and hold water. Examples include seaweed extractions and seeds with starch.
- *Resins*, of which the chief source is pine tree sap, commonly act as local irritants or as laxatives and caustic agents.
- *Oils*, thick and sometimes greasy liquids, are classified as volatile or fixed. Examples of volatile oils, which readily evaporate, include peppermint, spearmint, and juniper. Fixed oils, which aren't easily evaporated, include castor oil and olive oil.

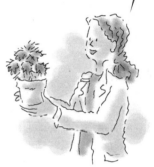

Active components of plant sources include alkaloids, glycosides, gums, resins, and oils.

Aid from animals

The body fluids or glands of animals are also natural drug sources. The drugs obtained from animal sources include:

- *hormones*, such as insulin
- *oils* and *fats* (usually fixed), such as cod-liver oil
- *enzymes*, which are produced by living cells and act as catalysts, such as pancreatin and pepsin
- *vaccines*, which are suspensions of killed, modified, or attenuated microorganisms.

Many minerals

Metallic and nonmetallic minerals provide various inorganic materials not available from plants or animals. Mineral sources are used as they occur in nature or they're combined with other ingredients. Examples of drugs that contain minerals are iron, iodine, and Epsom salts.

Lab report

Today, most drugs are produced in laboratories. Examples of such drugs include thyroid hormone (from natural sources) and cimetidine (from synthetic sources).

DNA paving the way

Recombinant deoxyribonucleic acid (DNA) research has led to another chemical source of organic compounds. For example, the reordering of genetic information enables scientists to develop bacteria that produce insulin for humans.

How drugs are administered

A drug's administration route influences the quantity given and the rate at which the drug is absorbed and distributed. These variables affect the drug's action and the patient's response.

Buccal, sublingual, and translingual

Certain drugs, such as nitroglycerin, are given buccally (in the pouch between the cheek and teeth), sublingually (under the tongue), or translingually (on the tongue) to prevent their destruction or transformation in the stomach or small intestine.

Gastric

The gastric route allows direct administration of a drug into the GI system. This route is used when patients can't ingest the drug orally.

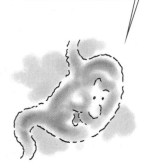

Looks like I need to get involved here. The gastric route is used when a patient can't ingest a drug orally.

Intradermal

In intradermal administration, drugs are injected into the skin. A needle is inserted at a 10- to 15-degree angle so that it punctures only the skin's surface. This form of administration is used mainly for diagnostic purposes, such as testing for allergies or tuberculosis.

Intramuscular

The I.M. route allows drugs to be injected directly into various muscle groups at varying tissue depths. This form of administration provides rapid systemic action and allows for absorption of relatively large doses (up to 5 ml). Aqueous suspensions and solutions in oil as well as drugs that aren't available in oral forms are given I.M.

Intravenous

The I.V. route allows injection of drugs and other substances directly into the bloodstream through a vein. Appropriate substances to administer I.V. include drugs, fluids, blood or blood products, and diagnostic contrast agents. Administration can range from a single dose to an ongoing infusion that's delivered with great precision.

Oral

Oral administration is usually the safest, most convenient, and least expensive route. Oral drugs are administered to patients who are conscious and able to swallow.

Rectal and vaginal

Suppositories, ointments, creams, or gels may be instilled into the rectum or vagina to treat local irritation or infection. Some drugs applied to the mucosa of the rectum or vagina can also be absorbed systemically.

Respiratory

Drugs that are available as gases can be administered into the respiratory system through inhalation. These drugs are rapidly absorbed. In addition, some of these drugs can be self-administered by devices such as the metered-dose inhaler. The respiratory route is also used in emergencies—for example, to administer some injectable drugs directly into the lungs via an endotracheal tube.

Subcutaneous

In subcutaneous (subQ) administration, small amounts of a drug are injected beneath the dermis and into the subcutaneous tissue, usually in the patient's upper arm, thigh, or abdomen. This allows the drug to move into the bloodstream more rapidly than if given by mouth. Drugs given by the subQ route include nonirritating aqueous solutions and suspensions contained in 0.5 to 2 ml of fluid, such as heparin and insulin.

Topical

The topical route is used to deliver a drug via the skin or a mucous membrane. This route is used for most dermatologic, ophthalmic, otic, and nasal preparations.

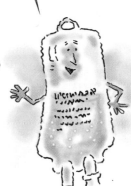

Talk about going with the flow! I.V. administration puts substances right into the bloodstream.

Specialized infusions

Drugs may also be given as specialized infusions. They're given directly to a specific site in the patient's body. Specific types of infusions include:

- epidural—injected into the epidural space
- intrapleural—injected into the pleural cavity
- intraperitoneal—injected into the peritoneal cavity
- intraosseous—injected into the rich vascular network of a long bone
- intra-articular—injected into a joint.

New drug development

In the past, drugs were found by trial and error. Now, they're developed primarily by systematic scientific research. The Food and Drug Administration (FDA) carefully monitors new drug development, which can take many years to complete.

Only after reviewing extensive animal studies and data on the safety and effectiveness of the proposed drug does the FDA approve an application for an Investigational New Drug (IND). (See *Phases of new drug development.*)

> The FDA can expedite approval of certain investigational drugs if they show promise in treating a significant public health threat.

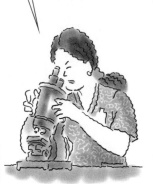

Phases of new drug development

When the Food and Drug Administration (FDA) approves an application for an investigational new drug, the drug must undergo clinical evaluation involving human subjects. This clinical evaluation is divided into four phases.

Phase I
In phase I, the drug is tested on healthy volunteers to make sure the drug can be given safely to people.

Phase II
Phase II involves trials with human subjects who have the disease for which the drug is thought to be effective.

Phase III
Large numbers of patients in medical research centers receive the drug in phase III. This larger sampling provides information about infrequent or rare adverse effects. The FDA approves a new drug application if phase III studies are satisfactory.

Phase IV
Phase IV is voluntary and involves postmarket surveillance of the drug's therapeutic effects at the completion of phase III. The pharmaceutical company receives reports from doctors and other health care professionals about the therapeutic results and adverse effects of the drug. Some drugs, for example, have been found to be toxic and have been removed from the market after their initial release.

On the FDA fast track

Although most INDs undergo all four phases of clinical evaluation mandated by the FDA, a few can receive expedited approval. For example, because of the public health threat posed by acquired immunodeficiency syndrome (AIDS), the FDA and drug companies have agreed to shorten the IND approval process for drugs to treat the disease. This allows doctors to give qualified AIDS patients "Treatment INDs" that aren't yet approved by the FDA.

Sponsors of drugs that reach phase II or III clinical trials can apply for FDA approval of Treatment IND status. When the IND is approved, the sponsor supplies the drug to doctors whose patients meet appropriate criteria. (See *Cheaper and easier.*)

Pharmacokinetics

The term *kinetics* refers to movement. Pharmacokinetics deals with a drug's actions as it moves through the body. Therefore, pharmacokinetics discusses how a drug is:
- absorbed (taken into the body)
- distributed (moved into various tissues)
- metabolized (changed into a form that can be excreted)
- excreted (removed from the body).

This branch of pharmacology is also concerned with a drug's onset of action, peak concentration level, and duration of action.

Absorption

Drug absorption covers the progress of a drug from the time it's administered, through the time it passes to the tissues, until it becomes available for use by the body.

How drugs are absorbed

On a cellular level, drugs are absorbed by several means—primarily through active or passive transport.

No energy required

Passive transport requires no cellular energy because the drug moves from an area of higher concentration to one of lower concentration (diffusion). It occurs when small molecules diffuse across membranes. Diffusion stops when the drug concentrations on both sides of the membrane are equal. Oral drugs use passive

---

Cheaper and easier

In the past, only a few drugs for acute conditions (such as headaches and colds) were available without prescription. Now, however, the Food and Drug Administration approves more drugs for over-the-counter use, making the drugs more easily accessible and much less expensive to consumers. Some examples include GI medications (such as ranitidine and cimetidine) and antihistamines (such as loratadine).

Drugs are absorbed through active or passive transport. I prefer my transport to be active!

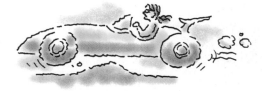

transport; they move from higher concentrations in the GI tract to lower concentrations in the bloodstream.

Get active

Active transport requires cellular energy to move the drug from an area of lower concentration to one of higher concentration. Active transport is used to absorb electrolytes, such as sodium and potassium, as well as some drugs, such as levodopa.

Taking a bite out of particles

Pinocytosis is a unique form of active transport that occurs when a cell engulfs a drug particle. Pinocytosis is commonly employed to transport the fat-soluble vitamins (A, D, E, and K).

> We're fat soluble, which means we're absorbed through pinocytosis.

Factors affecting absorption

Various factors—such as the route of administration, the amount of blood flow, and the form of the drug—can affect the rate of a drug's absorption.

Fast and furious

If only a few cells separate the active drug from systemic circulation, absorption occurs rapidly and the drug quickly reaches therapeutic levels in the body. Typically, drug absorption occurs within seconds or minutes when administered sublingually, I.V., or by inhalation.

Slow but steady

Absorption occurs at slower rates when drugs are administered by the oral, I.M., or subQ routes because the complex membrane systems of GI mucosal layers, muscle, and skin delay drug passage.

> Sublingual, I.V., or inhaled drugs are usually absorbed much faster than rectally administered or sustained-release drugs.

At a snail's pace

At the slowest absorption rates, drugs can take several hours or days to reach peak concentration levels. A slow rate usually occurs with rectally administered or sustained-release drugs.

Intestinal interference

Several other factors can affect absorption of a drug. For example, most absorption of oral drugs occurs in the small intestine. If a patient has had large sections of the small intestine surgically removed, drug absorption decreases because of the reduced surface area and the reduced time the drug is in the intestine.

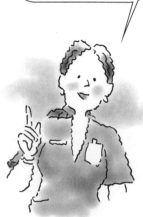

Liver-lowered levels

Drugs absorbed by the small intestine are transported to the liver before being circulated to the rest of the body. The liver may metabolize much of the drug before it enters circulation. This mechanism is referred to as the *first-pass effect*. Liver metabolism may inactivate the drug; if so, the first-pass effect lowers the amount of active drug released into the systemic circulation. Therefore, higher drug dosages must be administered to achieve the desired effect.

Watch out for my first-pass effect! It lowers the amount of active drug released into the systemic circulation.

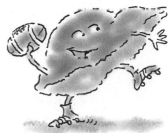

More blood, more absorption

Increased blood flow to an absorption site improves drug absorption, whereas reduced blood flow decreases absorption. More rapid absorption leads to a quicker onset of drug action.

For example, the muscle area selected for I.M. administration can make a difference in the drug absorption rate. Blood flows faster through the deltoid muscle (in the upper arm) than through the gluteal muscle (in the buttocks). The gluteal muscle, however, can accommodate a larger volume of drug than the deltoid muscle.

More pain, more stress, less drug

Pain and stress can also decrease the amount of drug absorbed. This may be due to a change in blood flow, reduced movement through the GI tract, or gastric retention triggered by the autonomic nervous system's response to pain.

Watch what your patient eats. High-fat meals and solid food can delay intestinal absorption of a drug.

Whatcha eatin'?

High-fat meals and solid foods slow the rate at which contents leave the stomach and enter the intestines, delaying intestinal absorption of a drug.

Form factors

Drug formulation (such as tablets, capsules, liquids, sustained-release formulas, inactive ingredients, and coatings) affects the drug absorption rate and the time needed to reach peak blood concentration levels. For example, enteric-coated drugs are specifically formulated so that they don't dissolve immediately in the stomach. Rather, they release in the small intestine. Liquid forms, however, are readily absorbed in the stomach and at the beginning of the small intestine.

Combo considerations

Combining one drug with another drug or with food can cause interactions that increase or decrease drug absorption, depending on the substances involved.

Distribution

Drug distribution is the process by which the drug is delivered to the tissues and fluids of the body. Distribution of an absorbed drug within the body depends on several factors, including:
• blood flow
• solubility
• protein binding.

Go with the flow

After a drug has reached the bloodstream, its distribution in the body depends on blood flow. The drug is distributed quickly to those organs with a large supply of blood, including the heart, liver, and kidneys. Distribution to other internal organs, skin, fat, and muscle is slower.

Breaching the barrier

The ability of a drug to cross a cell membrane depends on whether the drug is water- or lipid- (fat-) soluble. Lipid-soluble drugs easily cross through cell membranes, whereas water-soluble drugs can't. Lipid-soluble drugs can also cross the blood-brain barrier and enter the brain.

In a bind

As a drug travels through the body, it comes in contact with proteins, such as the plasma protein albumin. The drug can remain free or bind to the protein. The portion of a drug that's bound to a protein is inactive and can't exert a therapeutic effect. Only the free, or unbound, portion remains active. A drug is said to be *highly protein-bound* if more than 80% of it binds to protein.

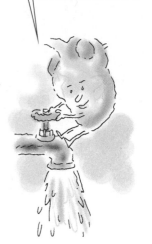

Having a large blood supply, like I do, means drugs flow quickly toward me. Let's keep that flow going!

Metabolism

Drug metabolism, or *biotransformation*, refers to the body's ability to change a drug from its dosage form to a more water-soluble form that can then be excreted. Drugs can be metabolized in several ways:
• Most commonly, a drug is metabolized into inactive metabolites (products of metabolism), which are then excreted.

- Some drugs can be converted to active metabolites, meaning they're capable of exerting their own pharmacologic action. These metabolites may undergo further metabolism or may be excreted from the body unchanged.
- Other drugs can be administered as inactive drugs, called *pro-drugs*, and don't become active until they're metabolized.

Where the magic happens

Most drugs are metabolized by enzymes in the liver; however, metabolism can also occur in the plasma, kidneys, and membranes of the intestines. Some drugs inhibit or compete for enzyme metabolism, which can cause the accumulation of drugs when they're given together. This accumulation increases the potential for an adverse reaction or drug toxicity.

Metabolism busters

Certain diseases can reduce metabolism. These include liver disease, such as cirrhosis, and heart failure, which reduces circulation to the liver.

In the genes

Genetics allow some people to be able to metabolize drugs rapidly, whereas others metabolize them more slowly.

Environmental effects

Environment, too, can alter drug metabolism. For example, if a person is surrounded by cigarette smoke, the rate of metabolism of some drugs may be affected. A stressful environment, such as one involving prolonged illness or surgery, can also change how a person metabolizes drugs.

Age alterations

Developmental changes can also affect drug metabolism. For example, infants have immature livers that reduce the rate of metabolism, and elderly patients experience a decline in liver size, blood flow, and enzyme production that also slows metabolism.

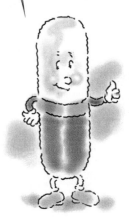

Although most drugs are metabolized in the liver, metabolism can also occur in the plasma, kidneys, and intestines.

Excretion

Drug excretion refers to the elimination of drugs from the body. Most drugs are excreted by the kidneys and leave the body through urine. Drugs can also be excreted through the lungs, exocrine glands (sweat, salivary, or mammary glands), skin, and intestinal tract.

Half in and half out

The half-life of a drug is the time it takes for the plasma concentration of a drug to fall to half its original value—in other words, the time it takes for one-half of the drug to be eliminated by the body. Factors that affect a drug's half-life include its rates of absorption, metabolism, and excretion. Knowing how long a drug remains in the body helps determine how frequently a drug should be taken.

A drug that's given only once is eliminated from the body almost completely after four or five half-lives. A drug that's administered at regular intervals, however, reaches a steady concentration (or *steady state*) after about four or five half-lives. Steady state occurs when the rate of drug administration equals the rate of drug excretion.

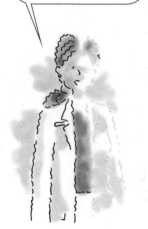

A drug's half-life is the time it takes for its plasma concentration to drop to half its original value. I must say, I feel like I'm only half here myself today...

Onset, peak, and duration

In addition to absorption, distribution, metabolism, and excretion, three other factors play important roles in a drug's pharmacokinetics:
- onset of action
- peak concentration
- duration of action.

How long 'til we see some action?

Onset of action refers to the time interval that starts when the drug is administered and ends when the therapeutic effect actually begins. Rate of onset varies depending on the route of administration and other pharmacokinetic properties.

When will it reach peak performance?

As the body absorbs more drug, blood concentration levels rise. The peak concentration level is reached when the absorption rate equals the elimination rate. However, the time of peak concentration isn't always the time of peak response.

How long will it last?

The duration of action is the length of time the drug produces its therapeutic effect.

Pharmacodynamics

Pharmacodynamics is the study of the drug mechanisms that produce biochemical or physiologic changes in the body. The interaction at the cellular level between a drug and cellular components, such as the complex proteins that make up the cell membrane, enzymes, or target receptors, represents drug action. The response resulting from this drug action is called the *drug effect*.

Fooling with function

A drug can modify cell function or the rate of function, but a drug can't impart a new function to a cell or target tissue. Therefore, the drug effect depends on what the cell is capable of accomplishing.

A drug can alter the target cell's function by:
• modifying the cell's physical or chemical environment
• interacting with a receptor (a specialized location on a cell membrane or inside a cell).

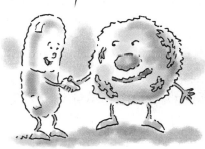

A drug's action refers to the interaction between the drug and the body's cellular components. Pleased to meet you!

Stimulating response

An *agonist* is an example of a drug that interacts with receptors. An agonist drug has an attraction, or affinity, for a receptor and stimulates it. The drug then binds with the receptor to produce its effect. The drug's ability to initiate a response after binding with the receptor is referred to as *intrinsic activity*.

Preventing response

If a drug has an affinity for a receptor but displays little or no intrinsic activity, it's called an *antagonist*. The antagonist prevents a response from occurring.

Antagonists can be competitive or noncompetitive:
• A *competitive antagonist* competes with the agonist for receptor sites. Because this type of drug binds reversibly to the receptor site, administering large doses of an agonist can overcome the antagonist's effects.
• A *noncompetitive antagonist* binds to receptor sites and blocks the effects of the agonist. Administering large doses of the agonist can't reverse its action.

I find you very attractive. Care to engage in some intrinsic activity?

Not so choosy

If a drug acts on a variety of receptors, it's said to be *nonselective* and can cause multiple and widespread effects.

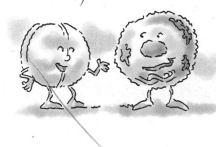

Potent quotient

Drug potency refers to the relative amount of a drug required to produce a desired response. Drug potency is also used to compare two drugs. If drug X produces the same response as drug Y but at a lower dose, then drug X is more potent than drug Y.

Observe the curve

As its name implies, a dose-response curve is used to graphically represent the relationship between the dose of a drug and the response it produces. (See *Dose-response curve.*)

On the dose-response curve, a low dose usually corresponds with a low response. At a low dose, an increase in dose produces only a slight increase in response. With further increases in dose, there's a marked rise in drug response. After a certain point, an increase in dose yields little or no increase in response. At this point, the drug is said to have reached *maximum effectiveness.*

From desired effect to dangerous dose

Most drugs produce multiple effects. The relationship between a drug's desired therapeutic effects and its adverse effects is called the drug's *therapeutic index.* It's also referred to as its *margin of safety.*

The therapeutic index usually measures the difference between:
- an effective dose for 50% of the patients treated
- the minimal dose at which adverse reactions occur.

Dose-response curve

This graph shows the dose-response curve for two different drugs. As you can see, at low doses of each drug, a dosage increase results in only a small increase in drug response (for example, from point A to point B). At higher doses, an increase in dosage produces a much greater response (from point B to point C). As the dosage continues to climb, an increase in dose produces very little increase in response (from point C to point D).

This graph also shows that drug X is more potent than drug Y because it results in the same response, but at a lower dose (compare point A to point E).

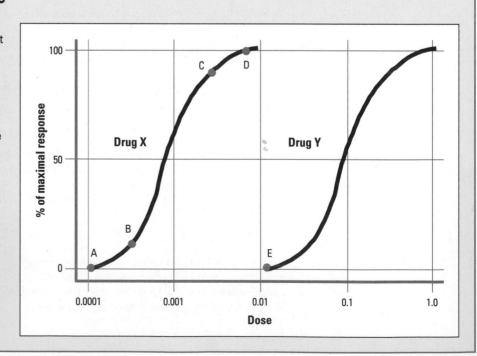

The lowdown on a low index

A drug with a low or narrow therapeutic index has a narrow range of safety between an effective dose and a lethal one. On the other hand, a drug with a high therapeutic index has a wide range of safety and less risk of toxic effects.

Pharmacotherapeutics

Pharmacotherapeutics is the use of drugs to treat disease. When choosing a drug to treat a particular condition, health care providers consider the drug's effectiveness as well as such factors as the type of therapy the patient will receive.

Pick your therapy

The type of therapy prescribed depends on the severity, urgency, and prognosis of the patient's condition. Therapy types include:
* *acute therapy*, if the patient is critically ill and requires acute intensive therapy
* *empiric therapy*, based on practical experience rather than on pure scientific data
* *maintenance therapy*, for patients with chronic conditions that don't resolve
* *supplemental* or *replacement therapy*, to replenish or substitute for missing substances in the body
* *supportive therapy*, which doesn't treat the cause of the disease but maintains other threatened body systems until the patient's condition resolves
* *palliative therapy*, used for end-stage or terminal diseases to make the patient as comfortable as possible.

It's all personal

A patient's overall health as well as other individual factors can alter his response to a drug. Coinciding medical conditions and personal lifestyle characteristics must also be considered when selecting drug therapy. (See *Factors affecting patient response to a drug.*)

Decreased response...

Certain drugs have a tendency to create drug tolerance and drug dependence in patients. *Drug tolerance* occurs when a patient has a decreased response to a drug over time. The patient then requires larger doses to produce the same response.

Keep the patient's coinciding medical conditions and lifestyle in mind when selecting drug therapy.

...and increased desire

Tolerance differs from *drug dependence*, in which a patient displays a physical or psychological need for the drug. Physical dependence produces withdrawal symptoms when the drug is stopped, whereas psychological dependence is based on a desire to continue taking the drug to relieve tension and avoid discomfort.

Drug interactions

Drug interactions can occur between drugs or between drugs and foods. They can interfere with the results of a laboratory test or produce physical or chemical incompatibilities. The more drugs a patient receives, the greater the chances are that a drug interaction will occur.

Potential drug interactions include:
- additive effects
- potentiation
- antagonistic effects
- decreased or increased absorption
- decreased or increased metabolism and excretion.

When it all adds up

An *additive* effect can occur when two drugs with similar actions are administered to a patient. The effects are equivalent to the sum of the effects of either drug administered alone in higher doses. Giving two drugs together, such as two analgesics (pain relievers), has these potential advantages:
- Lower doses of each drug can be administered, which can decrease the probability of adverse reactions because higher doses increase the risk of adverse reactions.
- Greater pain control can be achieved than from administration of one drug alone (most likely because of different mechanisms of action).

Empowering effects

A synergistic effect, also called *potentiation*, occurs when two drugs that produce the same effect are given together and one drug potentiates (enhances the effect) of the other drug. This produces greater effects than either drug taken alone.

When two isn't better than one

An *antagonistic* drug interaction occurs when the combined response of two drugs is less than the response produced by either drug alone.

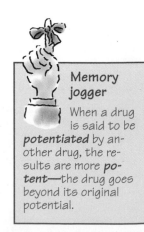

Memory jogger

When a drug is said to be **potentiated** by another drug, the results are more **potent**—the drug goes beyond its original potential.

Altering absorption

Two drugs given together can change the absorption of one or both of the drugs. For example, drugs that change the acidity of the stomach can affect the ability of another drug to dissolve in the stomach. Other drugs can interact and form an insoluble compound that can't be absorbed. Sometimes, an absorption interaction can be avoided by separating drug administration by at least 2 hours.

> For some drugs, you can avoid absorption interactions by separating their administration times by at least 2 hours.

Binding battles

After a drug is absorbed, blood distributes it throughout the body as a free drug or one that's bound to plasma protein. When two drugs are given together, they can compete for protein-binding sites, leading to an increase in the effects of one drug as that drug is displaced from the protein and becomes a free, unbound drug.

Turning toxic

Toxic drug levels can occur when a drug's metabolism and excretion are inhibited by another drug. Some drug interactions affect excretion only.

Tampering with tests

Drug interactions can also alter laboratory tests and can produce changes seen on a patient's electrocardiogram.

Factor in food

Food can alter the therapeutic effects of a drug as well as the rate and amount of drug absorbed from the GI tract, affecting bioavailability (the amount of a drug dose available to the systemic circulation). Dangerous interactions can also occur. For example, when food that contains tyramine (such as aged cheddar cheese) is eaten by a person taking a monoamine oxidase inhibitor, hypertensive crisis can occur. Also, grapefruit can inhibit the metabolism of certain drugs and result in toxic blood levels; examples include fexofenadine and albendazole.

> Patients may need to avoid certain foods when taking drugs. For example, grapefruit can inhibit the metabolism of certain drugs and result in toxic blood levels. Here, have some orange juice instead!

Elevating enzymes

Some drugs stimulate enzyme production, increasing metabolic rates and the demand for vitamins that are enzyme cofactors (which must unite with the enzyme in order for the enzyme to function). Drugs can also impair vitamin and mineral absorption.

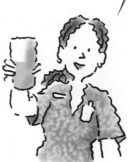

Adverse drug reactions

A drug's desired effect is called the *expected therapeutic response*. An adverse drug reaction, on the other hand (also called a *side effect* or *adverse effect*), is a harmful, undesirable response. Adverse drug reactions can range from mild reactions that disappear when the drug is stopped to debilitating diseases that become chronic. Adverse reactions can appear shortly after starting a new drug but may become less severe with time.

Due to the dose or the patient?

Adverse drug reactions can be classified as dose-related or patient sensitivity–related. Most adverse drug reactions result from the known pharmacologic effects of a drug and are typically dose-related. These types of reactions can be predicted in most cases.

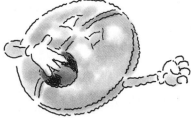

Sedation is an example of a secondary effect.

Dose-related reactions

Dose-related reactions include:
- secondary effects
- hypersusceptibility
- overdose
- iatrogenic effects.

Secondary effects

A drug typically produces a major therapeutic effect as well as secondary effects that can be beneficial or adverse. For example, morphine used for pain control can lead to two undesirable secondary effects: constipation and respiratory depression. Diphenhydramine used as an antihistamine is accompanied by the secondary effect of sedation, which is why the drug is also sometimes used as a sleep aid.

Hypersusceptibility

A patient can be hypersusceptible to the pharmacologic actions of a drug. Even when given a usual therapeutic dose, a hypersusceptible patient can experience an excessive therapeutic response.

Hypersusceptibility typically results from altered pharmacokinetics (absorption, metabolism, and excretion), which lead to higher-than-expected blood concentration levels. Increased receptor sensitivity can also increase the patient's response to therapeutic or adverse effects.

Overdose

A toxic drug reaction can occur when an excessive dose is taken, either intentionally or accidentally. The result is an exaggerated response to the drug that can lead to transient changes or more serious reactions, such as respiratory depression, cardiovascular collapse, and even death. To avoid toxic reactions, chronically ill or elderly patients commonly receive low drug doses.

Iatrogenic effects

Some adverse drug reactions, known as *iatrogenic effects,* can mimic pathologic disorders. For example, such drugs as antineoplastics, aspirin, corticosteroids, and indomethacin commonly cause GI irritation and bleeding. Other examples of iatrogenic effects include induced asthma with propranolol and induced deafness with gentamicin.

Patient sensitivity–related adverse reactions

Patient sensitivity–related adverse reactions aren't as common as dose-related reactions. Sensitivity-related reactions result from a patient's unusual and extreme sensitivity to a drug. These adverse reactions arise from a unique tissue response rather than from an exaggerated pharmacologic action. Extreme patient sensitivity can occur as a drug allergy or an idiosyncratic response.

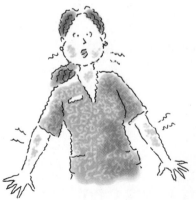

Allergic reactions to drugs can range from a mild rash to life-threatening anaphylaxis. Get some help! Stat!

Allergic reaction

A *drug allergy* occurs when a patient's immune system identifies a drug, a drug metabolite, or a drug contaminant as a dangerous foreign substance that must be neutralized or destroyed. Previous exposure to the drug or to one with similar chemical characteristics sensitizes the patient's immune system, and subsequent exposure causes an allergic reaction (hypersensitivity).

A shock to the system

An allergic reaction not only directly injures cells and tissues but also produces broader systemic damage by initiating cellular release of vasoactive and inflammatory substances. The allergic reaction can vary in intensity from a mild reaction with a rash and itching to an immediate, lifethreatening anaphylactic reaction with circulatory collapse and swelling of the larynx and bronchioles.

Idiosyncratic response

Some sensitivity-related adverse reactions don't result from the pharmacologic properties of a drug or from an allergy but are specific to the individual patient. These are called *idiosyncratic responses*. A patient's idiosyncratic response sometimes has a genetic cause.

The nursing process

One of the most significant advances in nursing has been the development of the nursing process. This problem-solving approach to nursing care provides a systematic method of determining the patient's health problems, developing a care plan to address those problems, implementing the plan, and evaluating the plan's effectiveness. The nursing process guides nursing decisions about drug administration to ensure the patient's safety and to meet medical and legal standards.

The five steps of the nursing process are dynamic, flexible, and interrelated. They include:
- assessment
- nursing diagnosis
- planning
- implementation
- evaluation.

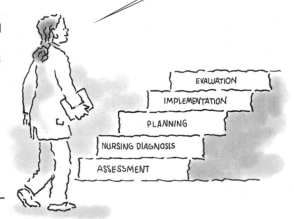

The nursing process guides decisions about drug administration to ensure patient safety and to meet medical and legal standards.

EVALUATION
IMPLEMENTATION
PLANNING
NURSING DIAGNOSIS
ASSESSMENT

Assessment

Assessment involves collecting data that are used to identify the patient's actual and potential health needs. You can obtain data by taking a health history, performing a physical examination, and reviewing pertinent laboratory and diagnostic information. The health history includes documenting drugs and herbal preparations that the patient is taking as well as any allergies.

Nursing diagnosis

NANDA International defines the nursing diagnosis as a "clinical judgment about individual, family, or community responses to actual or potential health problems or life processes." It goes on to say that "Nursing diagnoses provide the basis for the selection of nursing interventions to achieve outcomes for which the nurse is accountable." Nursing diagnoses need to be individualized for each patient, based on the patient's medical condition and the drugs he's receiving.

Planning

After you establish a nursing diagnosis, you'll develop a written care plan. A written care plan serves as a communication tool among health care team members that helps ensure continuity of care. The plan consists of two parts.

☞ patient outcomes, or expected outcomes, which describe behaviors or results to be achieved within a specific time

✌ nursing interventions needed to achieve those outcomes.

Implementation

The implementation phase is when you put your care plan into action. Implementation encompasses all nursing interventions, including drug therapy, that are directed toward meeting the patient's health care needs. While you coordinate implementation, you collaborate with the patient and the patient's family and consult with other caregivers. Implementation can involve a multidisciplinary approach depending on the needs of the patient and his family.

Evaluation

The final step in the nursing process is evaluation. During evaluation, you must determine if the interventions carried out have enabled the patient to achieve the desired outcomes. If you stated the outcome criteria in measurable terms, then you can easily evaluate the extent to which the outcomes were met. This includes evaluating the effectiveness of drug interventions, such as pain relief after the patient received an analgesic. Evaluation is an ongoing process, and reassessment leads to the development of new nursing diagnoses and nursing interventions based on the patient's response to treatment.

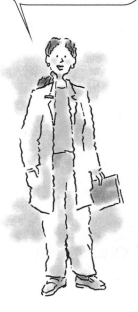

Your care plan should include expected outcomes and the nursing interventions needed to achieve those outcomes.

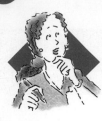

Quick quiz

1. How a drug is absorbed or excreted is called:

 A. pharmacodynamics.

 B. pharmacotherapeutics.

 C. pharmacokinetics.

 D. drug interactions.

Answer: C. Pharmacokinetics involves the absorption, distribution, metabolism, and excretion of a drug.

2. What type of drug interaction occurs when two drugs that produce the same effect are given together?

 A. Additive effect

 B. Potentiation

 C. Increased absorption

 D. Decreased effect

Answer: B. Potentiation occurs when two drugs that produce the same effect are given together. One drug enhances the effect of the other drug, resulting in greater effects of both drugs.

3. Expected outcomes are defined as:

 A. goals the patient and family ask you to accomplish.

 B. goals that are above the level the patient can realistically reach.

 C. goals that were met by the patient in the past.

 D. goals the patient should reach as a result of planned nursing interventions.

Answer: D. Expected outcomes are realistic, measurable goals for the patient.

Scoring

☆☆☆ If you answered all three questions correctly, fantastic! You obviously know your fundamental pharm facts.

☆☆ If you answered two questions correctly, terrific! You can clearly interact well with this material.

☆ If you answered fewer than two questions correctly, don't have an adverse reaction. You can improve your absorption of this chapter with a quick review.

Autonomic nervous system drugs

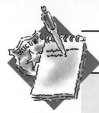

Just the facts

In this chapter, you'll learn:

♦ classes of drugs that affect the autonomic nervous system

♦ uses and actions of these drugs

♦ absorption, distribution, metabolization, and excretion of these drugs

♦ drug interactions and adverse reactions to these drugs.

Drugs and the autonomic nervous system

The autonomic nervous system regulates the body's involuntary functions, including heart rate, respiratory rate, and digestion. It works through a balance of its two main components, the sympathetic and parasympathetic nervous systems. Types of drugs used to treat disorders of the autonomic nervous sytem include:
• cholinergic drugs
• anticholinergic drugs
• adrenergic drugs
• adrenergic blocking drugs.

Cholinergic drugs

Cholinergic drugs promote the action of the neurotransmitter acetylcholine. These drugs are also called *parasympathomimetic drugs* because they produce effects that imitate parasympathetic nerve stimulation.

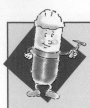

Pharm function

How cholinergic drugs work

Cholinergic drugs fall into one of two major classes: cholinergic agonists and anticholinesterase drugs. Here's how these drugs achieve their effects.

Cholinergic agonists

When a neuron in the parasympathetic nervous system is stimulated, the neurotransmitter acetylcholine is released. Acetylcholine crosses the synapse and interacts with receptors in an adjacent neuron. Cholinergic agonist drugs work by stimulating cholinergic receptors, mimicking the action of acetylcholine.

Anticholinesterase drugs

After acetylcholine stimulates the cholinergic receptor, it's destroyed by the enzyme acetylcholinesterase. Anticholinesterase drugs produce their effects by inhibiting acetylcholinesterase. As a result, acetylcholine isn't broken down and begins to accumulate; therefore, the effects of acetylcholine are prolonged.

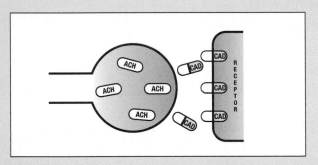

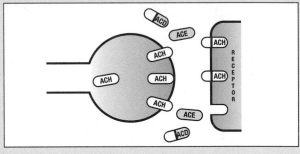

Key:

ACH Acetylcholine   CAD Cholinergic agonist drug   ACE Acetylcholinesterase   ACD Anticholinesterase drug

Mimic or inhibit

There are two major classes of cholinergic drugs:
• *Cholinergic agonists* mimic the action of the neurotransmitter acetylcholine.
• *Anticholinesterase drugs* work by inhibiting the destruction of acetylcholine at cholinergic receptor sites. (See *How cholinergic drugs work.*)

Cholinergic agonists

By directly stimulating cholinergic receptors, cholinergic agonists mimic the action of the neurotransmitter acetylcholine. They include such drugs as:
• acetylcholine (not to be confused with the neurotransmitter)
• bethanechol

> Simon says, act like an acetylcholine neurotransmitter!

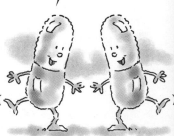

- carbachol
- cevimeline
- pilocarpine.

Pharmacokinetics (how drugs circulate)

The action and metabolism of cholinergic agonists vary widely and depend on the affinity of the individual drug for muscarinic or nicotinic receptors. For example, the drug acetylcholine poorly penetrates the central nervous system (CNS), and its effects are primarily peripheral, with a widespread parasympathetic action. The drug is rapidly destroyed in the body. Pilocarpine, on the other hand, binds to muscarinic receptors and stimulates smooth muscles in the urinary tract, bronchi, and biliary and intestinal tracts.

The "eyes" (and the mouth, and the skin) have it!

Cholinergic agonists are usually administered:
- topically, with eyedrops
- orally
- by subcutaneous (subQ) injection.
    SubQ injections begin to work more rapidly than oral doses.

N-O to I.M. or I.V.

The cholinergic agonists rarely are administered by I.M. or I.V. injection because they're almost immediately broken down by cholinesterase in the interstitial spaces between tissues and inside the blood vessels. Moreover, they begin to work rapidly and can cause a cholinergic crisis (a drug overdose resulting in extreme muscle weakness and possible paralysis of the muscles used in respiration).

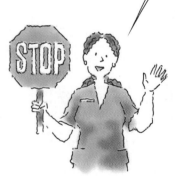

Giving cholinergic agonists I.M. or I.V. can cause cholinergic crisis.

Fast operators

Cholinergic agonists are absorbed rapidly and reach peak levels within 2 hours. Food decreases their absorption. Less than 20% of a cholinergic agonist is protein bound.
    All cholinergic agonists are metabolized by cholinesterase:
- at the muscarinic and nicotinic receptor sites
- in the plasma (the liquid portion of the blood)
- in the liver.
    These drugs are excreted by the kidneys.

Pharmacodynamics (how drugs act)

Cholinergic agonists work by mimicking the action of acetylcholine on the neurons in certain organs of the body, called *target or-*

gans. When they combine with receptors on the cell membranes of target organs, they stimulate the muscle and produce:
- salivation
- bradycardia (a slow heart rate)
- dilation of blood vessels
- constriction of the pulmonary bronchioles
- increased activity of the GI tract
- increased tone and contraction of the muscles of the bladder
- constriction of the pupils.

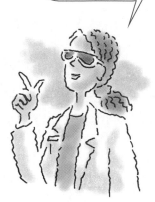

Cholinergic agonists stimulate the muscles of target organs, causing such effects as pupil constriction. Is it getting darker in here, or is it just me?

Pharmacotherapeutics (how drugs are used)

Cholinergic agonists are used to:
- treat atonic (weak) bladder conditions and postoperative and postpartum urine retention
- treat GI disorders, such as postoperative abdominal distention and GI atony
- reduce eye pressure in patients with glaucoma and during eye surgery
- treat salivary gland hypofunction caused by radiation therapy and Sjögren's syndrome.

Drug interactions

Cholinergic agonists have specific interactions with other drugs. Here are some examples:
- Other cholinergic drugs, particularly anticholinesterase drugs (such as ambenonium, edrophonium, neostigmine, physostigmine, and pyridostigmine) boost the effects of cholinergic agonists and increase the risk of toxicity.
- Anticholinergic drugs (such as atropine, belladonna, homatropine, methscopolamine, propantheline, and scopolamine) reduce the effects of cholinergic drugs.
- Quinidine reduces the effectiveness of cholinergic agonists.

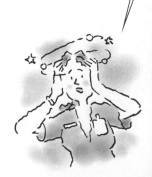

Adverse effects of cholinergic agonists include nausea and vomiting, cramps and diarrhea, and blurred vision. It makes me dizzy just to think about it!

Adverse reactions

Because they bind with receptors in the parasympathetic nervous system, cholinergic agonists can produce adverse effects in any organ innervated by the parasympathetic nerves.

I'm not feeling well...

Adverse effects of cholinergic agonists can include:
- nausea and vomiting
- cramps and diarrhea
- blurred vision
- decreased heart rate and low blood pressure
- shortness of breath

- urinary frequency
- increased salivation and sweating.

Nursing process

These nursing process steps are appropriate for patients undergoing treatment with cholinergic agonists.

Assessment

- Assess for disorders in which cholinergic agonists are used, such as myasthenia gravis.
- Assess for urine retention and bladder distention; determine the patient's fluid intake and time and amount of last urination.
- Assess for possible paralytic ileus (paralysis of the small intestine) by checking for bowel sounds and abdominal distention and determining the patient's elimination patterns.
- Assess for disorders that may be aggravated by cholinergic agonists, such as Alzheimer's disease.

Key nursing diagnoses

- Impaired gas exchange related to increased secretions, bronchospasm, or respiratory paralysis
- Ineffective airway clearance related to increased respiratory secretions
- Impaired urinary elimination related to cholinergic drug action

Planning outcome goals

- The patient will maintain effective oxygenation of tissues.
- The patient will regain usual patterns of urinary and bowel elimination.
- Therapeutic effects of cholinergic drugs will be observed.
- The patient will demonstrate correct drug administration.

Implementation

- Administer cholinergic drugs as prescribed. Be aware that some drugs, such as bethanechol, should be given before meals.
- Monitor for effects of cholinergic drugs and report adverse reactions.

Now, just breathe easy...

- Assess for signs of respiratory adequacy, and perform measures to promote adequate gas exchange, such as deep breathing and coughing, suctioning, and proper positioning of the patient.
- Assess for urinary adequacy and signs of urine retention.

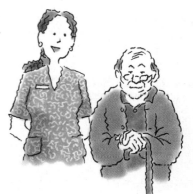

Before giving cholinergic agonists, check for disorders such as Alzheimer's disease that may be aggravated by these drugs.

Education edge

Teaching about cholinergic drugs

If cholinergic drugs are prescribed, review these points with the patient and his caregivers:
• Take the drug as directed on a regular schedule to maintain consistent blood levels of the drug and symptom control.
• Don't chew or crush sustained-release tablets or capsules.
• Take oral cholinergics on an empty stomach to lessen nausea and vomiting and increase the drug's absorption.
• If diarrhea or vomiting occurs, ensure adequate fluid intake.
• Cholinergic drugs for urine retention act within 60 minutes of taking them. Make sure bathroom facilities are available.
• If taking a cholinergic drug long term, such as for myasthenia gravis, bladder problems, or Alzheimer's disease, wear or carry medical alert identification.
• If indicated, record symptoms of myasthenia gravis and the effects of the drug in a journal, especially if the dosage is adjusted.

• Report abdominal cramping, diarrhea, or excesive salivation to the prescriber.
• If taking cholinergic drugs for myasthenia gravis, plan rest periods between activities and space activities throughout the day. The goal of therapy is to obtain optimal benefit from the drug using the lowest possible dose with fewest adverse effects. If activity increases, the dosage may need to be increased. Report increased muscle weakness, difficulty breathing, recurrence of myasthenia gravis symptoms, and other adverse reactions to the prescriber.
• If dizziness or syncope occurs, lie down and rest, then get up gradually. Ambulation should be supervised.
• Don't take over-the-counter drugs or herbal preparations without first consulting with the prescriber because interactions may occur. For example, remedies such as St. John's wort alter the blood levels of donepezil.

• Assist the patient in establishing a drug administration schedule that meets his needs.
• Provide patient teaching. (See *Teaching about cholinergic drugs.*)

Evaluation
• Patient's underlying condition improves.
• Patient maintains a normal respiratory rate.
• Patient maintains a normal voiding pattern.
• Patient regains normal bowel patterns.
• Patient and his family demonstrate an understanding of drug therapy.

Anticholinesterase drugs

Anticholinesterase drugs block the action of the enzyme acetylcholinesterase at cholinergic receptor sites, preventing the breakdown of the neurotransmitter acetylcholine. As acetylcholine builds up, it continues to stimulate the cholinergic receptors.

Anticholinesterase drugs are divided into two categories—reversible and irreversible.

The short...

Reversible anticholinesterase drugs have a short duration of action and include:

- ambenonium
- donepezil
- edrophonium
- galantamine
- guanidine
- neostigmine
- physostigmine
- pyridostigmine
- rivastigmine
- tacrine.

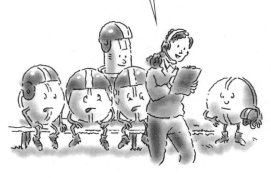

Now, I want you anticholinesterase drugs to go out there and block the acetylcholinesterase enzymes from breaking down the neurotransmitter acetylcholine. Got it?

...and the long of it

Irreversible anticholinesterase drugs have long-lasting effects and are used primarily as toxic insecticides and pesticides or as nerve gas agents in chemical warfare. (Pyridostigmine enhances the effects of antidotes used to counteract nerve agents.) Only one has therapeutic usefulness: echothiophate.

Pharmacokinetics

Here's a brief rundown of how anticholinesterase drugs move through the body.

Ready to be readily absorbed

Many of the anticholinesterase drugs are readily absorbed from the GI tract, subcutaneous tissue, and mucous membranes.

Poorly absorbed but packs some action

Because neostigmine is poorly absorbed from the GI tract, the patient needs a higher dose when taking this drug orally. The duration of action for an oral dose is longer, however, so the patient doesn't need to take it as frequently.

Need it now?

When a rapid effect is needed, the drug should be given by the I.M. or I.V. route.

Diverse delivery

The distribution of anticholinesterase drugs varies. For example, physostigmine is able to cross the blood-brain barrier (a protective barrier between the capillaries and brain tissue that prevents harmful substances from entering the brain). Donepezil is highly

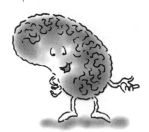

Physostigmine is an anticholinesterase drug that can cross the blood-brain barrier.

bound to plasma proteins, whereas tacrine is about 55% bound to plasma proteins, rivastigmine is 40% bound, and galantamine is 18% bound.

Most anticholinesterase drugs are metabolized in the body by enzymes in the plasma and excreted in the urine. Donepezil, galantamine, rivastigmine, and tacrine, however, are metabolized in the liver but still excreted in urine.

Pharmacodynamics

Anticholinesterase drugs, like cholinergic agonists, promote the action of acetylcholine at receptor sites. Depending on the site and the drug's dose and duration of action, they can produce a stimulant or depressant effect on cholinergic receptors.

How long do the effects go on?

Reversible anticholinesterase drugs block the breakdown of acetylcholine for minutes to hours. The blocking effect of irreversible anticholinesterase drugs can last for days or weeks.

Pharmacotherapeutics

Anticholinesterase drugs have various therapeutic uses. They're used:
• to reduce eye pressure in patients with glaucoma and during eye surgery
• to increase bladder tone
• to improve tone and peristalsis (movement) through the GI tract in patients with reduced motility and paralytic ileus
• to promote muscular contraction in patients with myasthenia gravis
• to diagnose myasthenia gravis (neostigmine and edrophonium)
• as antidotes to anticholinergic drugs, tricyclic antidepressants, belladonna alkaloids, and opioids
• to treat mild to moderate dementia and enhance cognition in patients with Alzheimer's disease (donepezil, galantamine, rivastigmine, and tacrine).

Drug interactions

These interactions can occur with anticholinesterase drugs:
• Other cholinergic drugs, particularly cholinergic agonists (such as bethanechol, carbachol, and pilocarpine), increase the risk of toxic effects when taken with anticholinesterase drugs.
• Carbamazepine, dexamethasone, rifampin, phenytoin, and phenobarbital may increase the elimination rate of donepezil.

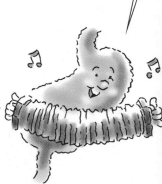

Anitcholinesterase drugs improve tone and peristalsis through the GI tract. I'd say my tone is improving already!

Covering up a cholinergic crisis

• Aminoglycoside antibiotics, anesthetics, anticholinergic drugs (such as atropine, belladonna, propantheline, and scopolamine), magnesium, corticosteroids, and antiarrhythmic drugs (such as procainamide and quinidine) can reduce the effects of anticholinesterase drugs and can mask early signs of a cholinergic crisis.

• Other drugs with cholinergic-blocking properties, such as tricyclic antidepressants, bladder relaxants, and antipsychotics, can counteract the effects of anticholinesterase drugs.

• The effects of tacrine, donepezil, and galantamine may be increased when combined with known inhibitors of cytochrome P-450 (CYP450), such as cimetidine and erythromycin.

• Cigarette use increases the clearance (how quickly the drug is excreted from the body) of rivastigmine.

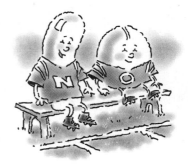

Giving cholinergic agonists with anticholinesterase drugs increases the risk of toxic effects. I guess together, we spell N-O!

Adverse reactions

Most of the adverse reactions to anticholinesterase drugs result from increased action of acetylcholine at receptor sites. Adverse reactions associated with these drugs include:

• cardiac arrhythmias
• nausea and vomiting
• diarrhea
• seizures
• headache
• anorexia
• insomnia
• pruritus
• urinary frequency and nocturia
• shortness of breath, wheezing, or tightness in the chest. (See *Recognizing a toxic response.*)

Recognizing a toxic response

It's difficult to predict adverse reactions to anticholinesterase drugs in a patient with myasthenia gravis because the therapeutic dose varies from day to day. Increased muscle weakness can result from:

• resistance to the drug
• receiving too little anticholinesterase drug
• receiving too much anticholinesterase drug.

Enter edrophonium

Deciding whether a patient is experiencing a toxic drug response (too much drug) or a myasthenic crisis (extreme muscle weakness and severe respiratory difficulties) can be difficult. Edrophonium can be used to distinguish between a toxic drug effect and myasthenic crisis. If a test dose of edrophonium improves the patient's symptoms, the patient is experiencing a myasthenic crisis.

When edrophonium is used, suction equipment, oxygen, mechanical ventilation, and emergency drugs (such as atropine) must be readily available in case a cholinergic crisis occurs.

Nursing process

These nursing process steps are appropriate for patients undergoing treatment with anticholinesterase drugs.

Assessment

• Assess for disorders in which anticholinesterase drugs are used, such as myasthenia gravis, Alzheimer's disease, glaucoma, and altered bladder function.

Fluid fundamentals

• Assess for urine retention and bladder distention, determine the patient's fluid intake, and find out the time and amount of his last urination.
• Assess for possible paralytic ileus by checking for bowel sounds and abdominal distention and determining the patient's elimination patterns.

Key nursing diagnoses

• Impaired gas exchange related to bronchospasm or respiratory paralysis
• Impaired tissue integrity related to effects of anticholinergic drugs
• Impaired urinary elimination related to anticholinergic drug action

Planning outcome goals

• The patient wil maintain effective oxygenation of tissues.
• The patient will regain normal patterns of urinary and bowel elimination.
• Therapeutic effects of anticholinesterase drugs will be observed.
• The patient will demonstrate correct drug administration.

Implementation

• Administer anticholinesterase drugs as prescribed. Give these drugs before meals unless otherwise directed.
• Monitor for effects of anticholinesterase drugs and report adverse reactions.
• Assess for signs of respiratory adequacy and perform measures to promote adequate gas exchange, such as deep breathing and coughing, suctioning, and proper positioning of the patient.
• Assess for urinary adequacy and signs of urine retention.
• Assist the patient in establishing a drug administration schedule that meets his needs.
• Provide patient teaching. (See *Teaching about anticholinesterase drugs.*)

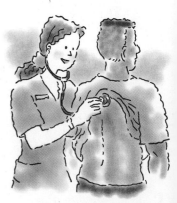

Assess for signs of respiratory adequacy and perform measures to promote adequate gas exchange.

Education edge

Teaching about anticholinesterase drugs

If anticholinesterase drugs are prescribed, review these points with the patient and his caregivers:

• The drug doesn't alter underlying degenerative disease but can alleviate symptoms.

• Memory improvement may be subtle. A more likely result of therapy is a slower decline in memory loss.

• When used for myasthenia gravis, these drugs relieve ptosis, double vision, difficulty chewing and swallowing, and trunk and limb weakness.

• Take the drug exactly as ordered. The drug may have to be taken for life.

• If you have myasthenia gravis, wear or carry medical alert identification.

• Immediately report significant adverse effects or changes in overall health status.

• Report the use of anticholinesterase drugs to the health care team before receiving anesthesia.

• Report episodes of nausea, vomiting, or diarrhea.

• Consult the prescriber before taking over-the-counter drugs or herbal preparations because they may interact with the anticholinesterase drug.

• If you're taking tacrine, your liver aminotransferase levels will be monitored weekly for 18 weeks at the start of therapy and then weekly for 6 weeks if the dosage is increased.

Evaluation

• Patient's underlying condition improves.
• Patient maintains a normal respiratory rate.
• Patient maintains a normal voiding pattern.
• Patient regains normal bowel patterns.
• Patient and his family state an understanding of drug therapy.

Anticholinergic drugs

Anticholinergic drugs (also called *cholinergic blockers*) interrupt parasympathetic nerve impulses in the CNS and autonomic nervous system. They also prevent acetylcholine from stimulating cholinergic receptors.

For muscarinic sites only

Anticholinergic drugs don't block all cholinergic receptors, just the muscarinic receptor sites. Muscarinic receptors are cholinergic receptors that are stimulated by the alkaloid muscarine and blocked by atropine.

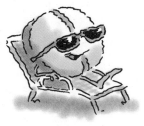

I prefer muscarinic receptor sites to other receptor sites. I'm really quite selective, you know.

Belladonna alkaloids and other derivatives

The major anticholinergic drugs are the belladonna alkaloids:
- atropine (see *Anticholinergic drugs: Atropine*)
- belladonna
- homatropine
- hyoscyamine
- ipratropium
- scopolamine.

Synthetic string

Synthetic derivatives of belladonna alkaloids (the quaternary ammonium drugs) include:
- glycopyrrolate
- methscopolamine
- propantheline.

Third string

The tertiary amines are newer synthetic drugs. They're centrally acting and more selective. They also have fewer adverse effects. Examples of tertiary amines include:
- benztropine
- dicyclomine
- oxybutynin

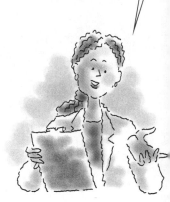

Each type of drug has its own benefits. For example, the belladonna alkaloids are absorbed more readily through the GI tract and distribute widely, but tertiary amines have fewer adverse effects.

Prototype pro

Anticholinergic drugs: Atropine

Actions
- Competitively antagonizes the actions of acetylcholine and other cholinergic agonists at the muscarinic receptors

Indications
- Symptomatic bradycardia
- Preoperative reduction of secretions and blockage of cardiac vagal reflexes
- Adjunct treatment of peptic ulcer disease
- Functional GI disorders

Nursing considerations
- Monitor for adverse reactions, such as headache, tachycardia, restlessness, dizziness, blurred vision, dry mouth, urinary hesitancy, and constipation.
- Monitor vital signs, cardiac rhythm, urine output, and vision for signs of impending toxicity.
- Provide stool softeners or bulk laxatives as ordered for constipation.

- tolterodine
- trihexyphenidyl.

Pharmacokinetics

The belladonna alkaloids are absorbed from the eyes, GI tract, mucous membranes, and skin.

GI reliant

The quaternary ammonium drugs and tertiary amines are absorbed primarily through the GI tract, although not as readily as the belladonna alkaloids.

Instant gratification

When administered I.V., anticholinergic drugs such as atropine begin to work immediately. The belladonna alkaloids are distributed more widely throughout the body than the quaternary ammonium derivatives or tertiary amines. The alkaloids readily cross the blood-brain barrier; the other drugs in this class don't.

Ready and able

The belladonna alkaloids have low to moderate binding with serum proteins and are only slightly to moderately protein bound. This means that a moderate to high amount of the drug is active and available to produce a therapeutic response. They're metabolized in the liver and excreted by the kidneys as unchanged drug and metabolites.

Metabolism of the tertiary amines is unknown, but excretion is usually through the kidneys and in feces.

Complicated quaternary kinetics

The quaternary ammonium drugs are a bit more complicated. Hydrolysis occurs in the GI tract and the liver; excretion is in feces and urine. Dicyclomine's metabolism is unknown, but it's excreted equally in feces and urine.

Pharmacodynamics

Anticholinergic drugs can have paradoxical effects on the body, depending on the dosage, the condition being treated, and the target organ. For example, anticholinergic drugs can produce a stimulating or depressing effect. In the brain, they do both—low drug levels stimulate and high drug levels depress.

Disorder-related dynamics

A patient's disorder can also impact the effects of a drug. Parkinson's disease, for example, is characterized by low dopamine levels that intensify the stimulating effects of acetylcholine. Cholinergic blockers, however, depress this effect. In other disorders, these same drugs stimulate the CNS.

Pharmacotherapeutics

Here's how anticholinergic drugs are used in various GI situations:
• All anticholinergic drugs are used to treat spastic or hyperactive conditions of the GI and urinary tracts because they relax muscles and decrease GI secretions. However, for bladder relaxation and urinary incontinence, the quaternary ammonium compounds, such as propantheline, are the drugs of choice because they cause fewer adverse reactions than the belladonna alkaloids.
• The belladonna alkaloids are used with morphine to treat biliary colic (pain caused by stones in the bile duct).
• Anticholinergic drugs are given by injection before some diagnostic procedures, such as endoscopy or sigmoidoscopy, to relax the GI smooth muscle.

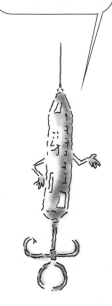

Giving anticholinergics by injection before diagnostic procedures relaxes GI smooth muscle.

Preop purposes

Anticholinergic drugs such as atropine are given before surgery to:
• reduce oral, gastric, and respiratory secretions
• prevent a drop in heart rate caused by vagal nerve stimulation during anesthesia.

Brain games

The belladonna alkaloids can affect the brain. For example, when given with the pain medications morphine or meperidine, scopolamine causes drowsiness and amnesia. It's also used to treat motion sickness.

Heart matters

The belladonna alkaloids also have therapeutic effects on the heart. Atropine is the drug of choice to treat:
• symptomatic sinus bradycardia—when the heart beats too slowly, causing low blood pressure or dizziness (See *How atropine speeds heart rate.*)
• arrhythmias resulting from anesthetics, choline esters, or succinylcholine.

Belladonna alkaloids have therapeutic effects on the heart.

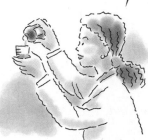

In your eyes

Anticholinergic drugs are also used as cycloplegics, which means they paralyze the ciliary muscles of the eye (used for fine focusing) and alter the shape of the lens of the eye. Furthermore, anticholinergic drugs act as mydriatics to dilate the pupils of the eye, making it easier to measure refractive

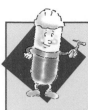

Pharm function

How atropine speeds heart rate

To understand how atropine affects the heart, first consider how the heart's electrical conduction system functions.

Without the drug

When the neurotransmitter acetylcholine is released, the vagus nerve stimulates the sinoatrial (SA) node (the heart's pacemaker) and atrioventricular (AV) node, which controls conduction between the atria and ventricles of the heart. This inhibits electrical conduction and causes the heart rate to slow down.

With the drug

When a patient receives atropine, a cholinergic blocking drug, it competes with acetylcholine for binding with the cholinergic receptors on the SA and AV nodes. By blocking acetylcholine, atropine speeds up the heart rate.

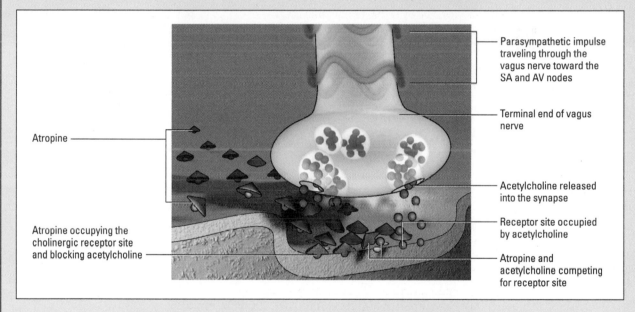

Parasympathetic impulse traveling through the vagus nerve toward the SA and AV nodes

Terminal end of vagus nerve

Atropine

Acetylcholine released into the synapse

Receptor site occupied by acetylcholine

Atropine occupying the cholinergic receptor site and blocking acetylcholine

Atropine and acetylcholine competing for receptor site

errors during an eye examination or to perform surgery on the eye.

Antidote-i-ful

The belladonna alkaloids, particularly atropine and hyoscyamine, are effective antidotes to cholinergic and anticholinesterase drugs. Atropine is the drug of choice to treat poisoning from organophosphate pesticides. Atropine and hyoscyamine also counteract the effects of the neuromuscular blocking drugs by competing for the same receptor sites.

Drug interactions

Because anticholinergic drugs slow the passage of food and drugs through the stomach, drugs remain in prolonged contact with the mucous membranes of the GI tract. This increases the amount of the drug that's absorbed and, therefore, increases the risk of adverse effects.

Effect boosters

Drugs that increase the effects of anticholinergic drugs include:
• antidyskinetics (such as amantadine)
• antiemetics and antivertigo drugs (such as buclizine, cyclizine, meclizine, and diphenhydramine)
• antipsychotics (such as haloperidol, phenothiazines, and thioxanthenes)
• cyclobenzaprine
• disopyramide
• orphenadrine
• tricyclic and tetracyclic antidepressants.

Effect busters

Drugs that decrease the effects of anticholinergic drugs include:
• anticholinesterase drugs (such as neostigmine and pyridostigmine)
• cholinergic agonists (such as bethanechol).

And there's more

Here are other drug interactions that can occur:
• The risk of digoxin toxicity increases when digoxin is taken with an anticholinergic drug.
• Opiate-like analgesics further enhance the slow movement of food and drugs through the GI tract when taken with cholinergic blockers.
• The absorption of nitroglycerin tablets placed under the tongue is reduced when taken with a cholinergic blocker.

Adverse reactions

Adverse reactions of anticholinergic drugs are closely related to drug dose. The difference between a therapeutic and a toxic dosage is small with these drugs.
   Adverse reactions may include:
• dry mouth
• reduced bronchial secretions
• increased heart rate
• blurred vision
• decreased sweating.

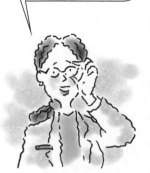

You can clearly see you'll need to monitor vital signs, cardiac rhythm, urine output, and vision for potential drug toxicity.

Nursing process

These nursing process steps are appropriate for patients undergoing treatment with anticholinergic drugs.

Assessment

• Assess for conditions in which anticholinergic drugs would be used, such as bradycardia, heart block (a delay or interruption in the conduction of electrical impulses between the atria and ventricles), diarrhea, and peptic ulcer disease.

When to be anti-anticholinergics

• Assess for conditions in which anticholinergic drugs would be contraindicated, such as glaucoma, myasthenia gravis, prostatic hyperplasia, reflux esophagitis, or GI obstructive disease.

Key nursing diagnoses

• Urinary retention related to adverse effects on the bladder
• Constipation related to adverse effects on the GI tract
• Risk for injury related to adverse drug effects

Planning outcome goals

• The patient will experience relief of symptoms.
• The patient will remain free from adverse reactions.

Implementation

• Follow dosage recommendations. Some drugs should be given with meals.
• Monitor vital signs, cardiac rhythm, urine output, and vision for potential drug toxicity.
• Monitor for adverse reactions, such as dry mouth, increased heart rate, and blurred vision.
• Have emergency equipment available to treat new cardiac arrhythmias.
• Help alleviate symptoms if adverse effects occur. For example, provide lozenges and frequent mouth care for patients experiencing dry mouth.
• Provide patient teaching. (See *Teaching about anticholinergic drugs.*)

Evaluation

• Patient's underlying condition improves.
• Patient maintains a normal heart rate.
• Patient maintains a normal voiding pattern.
• Patient regains normal bowel patterns.
• Patient and his family demonstrate an understanding of drug therapy.

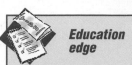

Education edge

Teaching about anticholinergic drugs

If anticholinergic drugs are prescribed, review these points with the patient and his caregivers:
• Take the drug as prescribed; don't take other drugs with the anticholinergic unless prescribed.
• Avoid hazardous tasks if dizziness, drowsiness, or blurred vision occurs.
• The drug may increase sensitivity to high temperatures, resulting in dizziness.
• Avoid alcohol because it may have additive central nervous system effects.
• Drink plenty of fluids and eat a high-fiber diet to prevent constipation.
• Notify the prescriber promptly if confusion, rapid or pounding heartbeat, dry mouth, blurred vision, rash, eye pain, a significant change in urine volume, pain on urination, or difficulty urinating occur.
• Women should report planned or known pregnancy.

Adrenergic drugs

Adrenergic drugs are also called *sympathomimetic drugs* because they produce effects similar to those produced by the sympathetic nervous system.

Sort by chemical...

Adrenergic drugs are classified into two groups based on their chemical structure: catecholamines (both naturally occurring as well as synthetic) and noncatecholamines.

...or by action

Adrenergic drugs are also divided by how they act. They can be:
• *direct-acting*, in which the drug acts directly on the organ or tissue innervated (supplied with nerves or nerve impulses) by the sympathetic nervous system
• *indirect-acting*, in which the drug triggers the release of a neurotransmitter, usually norepinephrine
• *dual-acting*, in which the drug has direct and indirect actions.
(See *How adrenergics work.*)

Catecholamines

Because of their common basic chemical structure, catecholamines share certain properties—they stimulate the nervous system, constrict peripheral blood vessels, increase heart rate, and dilate the bronchi. They can be manufactured in the body or in a laboratory. Common catecholamines include:
• dobutamine
• dopamine
• epinephrine, epinephrine bitartrate, and epinephrine hydrochloride
• norepinephrine (levarterenol)
• isoproterenol hydrochloride and isoproterenol sulfate.

Pharmacokinetics

Here's an overview of how catecholamines move through the body.

No P.O.

Catecholamines can't be taken orally because they're destroyed by digestive enzymes. In contrast, when these drugs are given sublingually (under the tongue), they're rapidly absorbed through the mucous membranes. Any sublingual drug not completely absorbed is rapidly metabolized by swallowed saliva.

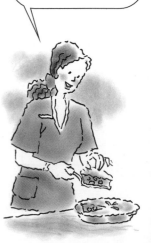

Catecholamines can't be taken orally because they're destroyed by digestive enzymes. I'll let those digestive enzymes work on this pie instead!

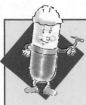

Pharm function

How adrenergics work

Adrenergic drugs are distinguished by how they achieve their effect. The illustrations below show the action of direct-, indirect-, and dual-acting adrenergics.

Direct-acting adrenergic action
Direct-acting adrenergic drugs directly stimulate adrenergic receptors.

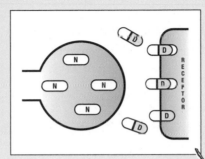

Adrenergic drugs can be direct-acting, indirect-acting, or both.

Indirect-acting adrenergic action
Indirect-acting adrenergic drugs stimulate the release of norepinephrine from nerve endings into the synapse.

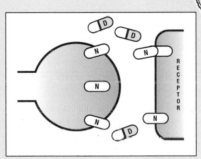
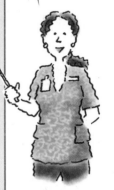

Dual-acting adrenergic action
Dual-acting adrenergic drugs stimulate both adrenergic receptor sites and the release of norepinephrine from nerve endings.

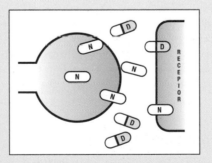

Key:
 Norepinephrine   ⬭D Adrenergic drug

SubQ vs. I.M.

Absorption by the subQ route is slowed because catecholamines cause the blood vessels around the injection site to constrict. I.M. absorption is more rapid because less constriction of local blood vessels occurs.

Catecholamines are widely distributed in the body. They're metabolized and inactivated predominantly in the liver but can also be metabolized in the GI tract, lungs, kidneys, plasma, and tissues.

On the way out

Catecholamines are excreted primarily in urine; however, a small amount of isoproterenol is excreted in feces and some epinephrine is excreted in breast milk.

Pharmacodynamics

Catecholamines are primarily direct-acting. When catecholamines combine with alpha-adrenergic receptors or beta-adrenergic receptors, they cause either an excitatory or inhibitory effect. Typically, activation of alpha-adrenergic receptors generates an excitatory response except for intestinal relaxation. Activation of the beta-adrenergic receptors mostly produces an inhibitory response except in the cells of the heart, where norepinephrine produces excitatory effects.

Workin' the heart

The clinical effects of catecholamines depend on the dosage and the route of administration. Catecholamines are potent inotropes—they make the heart contract more forcefully. As a result, the ventricles of the heart empty more completely with each heartbeat, increasing the workload of the heart and the amount of oxygen it needs to do this harder work.

Kickin' up the beat

Catecholamines also produce a positive chronotropic effect, which means they cause the heart to beat faster. That's because pacemaker cells in the sinoatrial (SA) node of the heart depolarize at a faster rate. As catecholamines cause blood vessels to constrict and blood pressure to rise, heart rate can fall as the body tries to compensate and prevent an excessive rise in blood pressure.

All fired up

Catecholamines can cause the Purkinje fibers (an intricate web of fibers that carry electrical impulses into the ventricles of the heart) to fire spontaneously, possibly producing abnormal heart rhythms, such as premature ventricular contractions and fibrillation. Epinephrine is more likely than norepinephrine to produce this spontaneous firing.

Memory jogger

To help you remember the effects of catecholamines on alpha and beta receptors, remember that **A** stands for **a**lpha (and **a**ctivation, suggesting an excitatory response), and **B** stands for **b**eta (or **b**anished, which suggests an inhibitory effect).

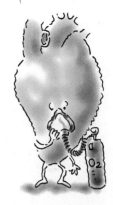

Catecholamines make me need more oxygen.

Pharmacotherapeutics

How adrenergic drugs are used depends on which receptors they stimulate and to what degree. Adrenergic drugs can affect:

- alpha-adrenergic receptors
- beta-adrenergic receptors
- dopamine receptors.

Most adrenergics produce their effects by stimulating alpha-adrenergic receptors and beta-adrenergic receptors. These drugs mimic the action of norepinephrine and epinephrine.

Of the catecholamines:

- norepinephrine has the most nearly pure alpha activity
- dobutamine and isoproterenol have only beta-related therapeutic uses
- epinephrine stimulates alpha-adrenergic receptors and beta-adrenergic receptors
- dopamine primarily exhibits dopaminergic activity (it acts on sympathetic nervous system receptors that are stimulated by dopamine).

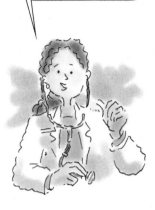

Catecholamines that stimulate alpha-adrenergic receptors are used to treat hypotension.

Helping hypotension

Catecholamines that stimulate alpha-adrenergic receptors are used to treat low blood pressure (hypotension). As a rule, catecholamines work best when used to treat hypotension caused by:

- relaxation of the blood vessels (also called a *loss of vasomotor tone*)
- blood loss (such as from hemorrhage).

Rhythm makers

Catecholamines that stimulate $beta_1$-adrenergic receptors are used to treat:

- bradycardia
- heart block
- low cardiac output.

Increasing response

Because they're believed to make the heart more responsive to defibrillation (using an electrical current to terminate a deadly arrhythmia), $beta_1$-adrenergic drugs are used to treat:

- ventricular fibrillation (quivering of the ventricles resulting in no pulse)
- asystole (no electrical activity in the heart)
- cardiac arrest.

Breathing better with $beta_2$ activity

Catecholamines that exert $beta_2$-adrenergic activity are used to treat:

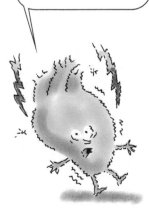

$Beta_1$-adrenergic drugs make the heart more responsive to defibrillation. Yikes! I'm responding already!

- acute and chronic bronchial asthma
- emphysema
- bronchitis
- acute hypersensitivity (allergic) reactions to drugs.

More blood for the kidneys

Dopamine, which stimulates dopaminergic receptors, is used in low doses to improve blood flow to the kidneys because it dilates the renal blood vessels.

Home grown vs. manufactured

The effects of catecholamines produced by the body differ somewhat from the effects of manufactured catecholamines. Manufactured catecholamines have a short duration of action, which can limit their therapeutic usefulness.

Drug interactions

Drug interactions involving catecholamines can be serious:
- Alpha-adrenergic blockers, such as phentolamine, used with catecholamines can produce hypotension.
- Because the catecholamine epinephrine may cause hyperglycemia, diabetic patients receiving epinephrine may require an increased dose of insulin or oral antidiabetics.
- Beta-adrenergic blockers, such as propranolol, used with catecholamines can lead to bronchial constriction, especially in patients with asthma.

Adding it all up

- Other adrenergic drugs can produce additive effects, such as hypertension (high blood pressure) and arrhythmias, and enhance adverse effects.
- Tricyclic antidepressants used with catecholamines can lead to hypertension.

Adverse reactions

Adverse reactions to catecholamines include:
- restlessness
- anxiety
- dizziness
- headache
- palpitations
- cardiac arrhythmias
- hypotension
- hypertension and hypertensive crisis
- stroke

- angina
- increased glucose levels
- tissue necrosis and sloughing (if a catecholamine given I.V. leaks into the surrounding tissue).

Nursing process

These nursing process steps are appropriate for patients undergoing treatment with catecholamines.

Assessment

- Assess the patient's condition before therapy and regularly thereafter.

Keeping an eye on the ECG

- Continuously monitor electrocardiogram (ECG), blood pressure, pulmonary artery wedge pressure, cardiac condition, and urine output.
- Monitor electrolyte levels.
- Throughout therapy, assess for adverse reactions, drug interactions, and acidosis, which decreases effectiveness of dopamine.
- After dopamine is stopped, watch closely for a sudden drop in blood pressure.
- Assess the patient's and family's knowledge of drug therapy.

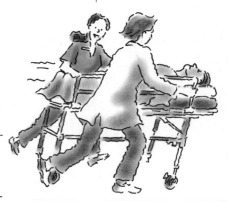

Catecholamines can cause a number of adverse reactions including hypertensive crisis and stroke.

Key nursing diagnoses

- Decreased cardiac output related to underlying condition
- Ineffective tissue perfusion (cerebral, cardiopulmonary, and renal) related to underlying condition
- Risk for injury related to drug-induced adverse reactions
- Acute pain related to headache
- Deficient knowledge related to drug therapy

Planning outcome goals

- The patient will maintain cardiac output.
- The patient will maintain effective tissue perfusion.
- The risk for injury will be minimized.
- The patient's pain will decrease.
- The patient will demonstrate an understanding of the purpose and intended effect of therapy.

Implementation

- Before starting catecholamines, correct hypovolemia with plasma volume expanders.

• Give cardiac glycosides before catecholamines; cardiac glycosides increase atrioventricular (AV) node conduction and patients with atrial fibrillation may develop rapid ventricular rate.

• Administer drug using a central venous catheter or large peripheral vein. Adjust the infusion according to the prescriber's order and the patient's condition. Use an infusion pump.

• Dilute the concentrate for injection before administration, according to pharmacy guidelines.

• Watch for irritation and infiltration; extravasation can cause an inflammatory response.

• Don't give catecholamines in the same I.V. line as other drugs; be aware of incompatibilities. For example, dobutamine is incompatible with heparin, hydrocortisone sodium succinate, cefazolin, cefamandole, cephalothin, penicillin, and ethacrynate sodium.

• Don't mix dobutamine or dopamine with sodium bicarbonate injection or phenytoin because the drug is incompatible with alkaline solutions.

• Change I.V. sites regularly to avoid phlebitis.

• Provide patient teaching.

> Sometimes the order of drug administration matters. For example, cardiac glycosides should be given before catecholamines.

Evaluation

• Patient regains adequate cardiac output (evidenced by stable vital signs, normal urine output, and clear mental status).

• Patient regains adequate cerebral, cardiopulmonary, and renal tissue perfusion.

• Patient doesn't experience injury as a result of drug-induced adverse reactions.

• Patient's headache is relieved with analgesic administration.

• Patient and his family state an understanding of drug therapy.

> Don't mix me up! Catecholamines shouldn't be administered in the same I.V. line as other drugs.

Noncatecholamines

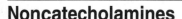

Noncatecholamine adrenergic drugs have many therapeutic uses because of the various effects these drugs can have on the body, including:

• local or systemic constriction of blood vessels (phenylephrine)

• nasal and eye decongestion and dilation of the bronchioles (albuterol, bitolterol, ephedrine, formoterol, isoetharine hydrochloride, isoproterenol, levalbuterol, metaproterenol, pirbuterol, salmeterol, and terbutaline)

• smooth-muscle relaxation (terbutaline).

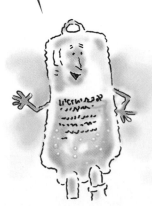

Pharmacokinetics

Absorption of noncatecholamines depends on the route of administration:

Breathe deep...

• Inhaled drugs, such as albuterol, are gradually absorbed from the bronchi of the lungs and result in lower drug levels in the body.

Open wide...

• Oral drugs are absorbed well from the GI tract and are distributed widely in the body fluids and tissues.
• Some noncatecholamine drugs (such as ephedrine) cross the blood-brain barrier and can be found in high concentrations in the brain and cerebrospinal fluid (fluid that moves through and protects the brain and spinal cord).

Metabolism and inactivation of noncatecholamines occur primarily in the liver but can also occur in the lungs, GI tract, and other tissues.

Exit time varies

These drugs and their metabolites are excreted primarily in urine. Some, such as inhaled albuterol, are excreted within 24 hours; others, such as oral albuterol, within 3 days. Acidic urine increases excretion of many noncatecholamines; alkaline urine slows excretion.

Pharmacodynamics

Noncatecholamines can be direct-acting, indirect-acting, or dual-acting (unlike catecholamines, which are primarily direct-acting).
• Direct-acting noncatecholamines that stimulate alpha activity receptors include phenylephrine. Those that selectively stimulate $beta_2$ activity receptors include albuterol, isoetharine, metaproterenol, and terbutaline.
• Indirect-acting noncatecholamines exert their effect by indirect action on adrenergic receptors.
• Dual-acting noncatecholamines include ephedrine.

Pharmacotherapeutics

Noncatecholamines stimulate the sympathetic nervous system and produce various effects on the body. For example, terbutaline is used to stop preterm labor. It's important to become familiar with each individual drug, including its indication, route, dose, and administration technique. Monitor the patient closely for therapeutic effect and tolerance.

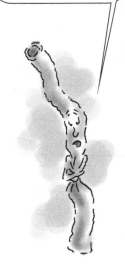

Noncatecholamines have several therapeutic effects, including local or systemic constriction of blood vessels. I must say, this doesn't feel terribly therapeutic!

Drug interactions

Here are a few examples of how other drugs may interact with noncatecholamines:

• Anesthetics (general), cyclopropane, and halogenated hydrocarbons can cause arrhythmias. Hypotension can also occur if these drugs are taken with noncatecholamines that have predominantly beta$_2$ activity, such as ritodrine and terbutaline.

A deadly combo

• Monoamine oxidase inhibitors taken with noncatecholamines can cause severe hypertension and even death.
• Oxytocic drugs that stimulate the uterus to contract can be inhibited when taken with terbutaline. When taken with other noncatecholamines, oxytocic drugs can cause hypertensive crisis or a stroke.
• Tricyclic antidepressants can cause hypertension and arrhythmias.
• Urine alkalizers, such as acetazolamide and sodium bicarbonate, slow excretion of noncatecholamine drugs, prolonging their action.

Adverse reactions

Adverse reactions to noncatecholamines may include:
• headache
• restlessness
• anxiety or euphoria
• irritability
• trembling
• drowsiness or insomnia
• light-headedness
• incoherence
• seizures
• hypertension or hypotension
• palpitations
• bradycardia or tachycardia
• irregular heart rhythm
• cardiac arrest
• cerebral hemorrhage
• tingling or coldness in the arms or legs
• pallor or flushing
• angina
• changes in heart rate and blood pressure in a pregnant woman and her fetus.

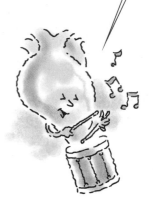

Keep in mind that using noncatecholamines with tricyclic antidepressants can cause arrhythmias. Gotta make sure I maintain my steady beat!

Nursing process

These nursing process steps are appropriate for patients undergoing treatment with noncatecholamines.

Assessment

• Obtain a baseline assessment of the patient's respiratory status, and assess it frequently throughout therapy.
• Assess for adverse reactions and drug interactions.
• Assess the patient's and family's knowledge of drug therapy.

Key nursing diagnoses

• Impaired gas exchange related to underlying respiratory condition
• Risk for injury related to drug-induced adverse reactions
• Deficient knowledge related to drug therapy

Planning outcome goals

• The patient will maintain adequate gas exchange.
• The risk of injury will be minimized.
• The patient will demonstrate understanding of the purpose and intended effect of drug therapy.

Implementation

• If using the inhalation route, wait at least 2 minutes between doses if more than one dose is ordered. If a corticosteroid inhaler also is used, first have the patient use the bronchodilator, wait 5 minutes, and then have the patient use the corticosteroid inhaler. This permits the bronchodilator to open air passages for maximum corticosteroid effectiveness.
• Give the injectable form (terbutaline) in the lateral deltoid area. Protect the injection from light. Don't use the drug if it's discolored.
• Notify the prescriber immediately if bronchospasms develop during therapy.
• Instruct the patient to use the aerosol form 15 minutes before exercise to prevent exercise-induced bronchospasm as indicated.
• Provide patient teaching. (See *Teaching about noncatecholamines*, page 50.)

Evaluation

• Patient's respiratory signs and symptoms improve.
• Patient has no injury from adverse drug reactions.
• Patient and his family demonstrate an understanding of drug therapy.

Keep in mind that noncatecholamines can change heart rate and blood pressure in a pregnant woman and her fetus.

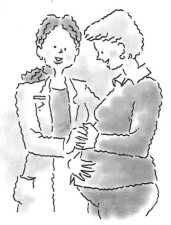

Education edge

Teaching about noncatecholamines

If noncatecholamines are prescribed, review these points with the patient and his caregivers:
• Stop the drug immediately if paradoxical bronchospasm occurs.
• Follow these instructions for using a metered-dose inhaler:
 – Clear the nasal passages and throat.
 – Breathe out, expelling as much air from the lungs as possible.
 – Place the mouthpiece well into the mouth and inhale deeply as the dose is released.
 – Hold your breath for several seconds, remove the mouthpiece, and exhale slowly.
 – Wait at least 2 minutes before repeating the procedure if more than one inhalation is ordered.
• Avoid accidentally spraying the inhalant form into the eyes; doing so may temporarily blur vision.
• Reduce intake of foods and herbs containing caffeine, such as coffee, cola, and chocolate, when using a bronchodilator.
• Check pulse rate before and after using the bronchodilator. Call the prescriber if pulse rate increases more than 20 to 30 beats/minute.

Adrenergic blocking drugs

Adrenergic blocking drugs, also called *sympatholytic drugs*, are used to disrupt sympathetic nervous system function. These drugs work by blocking impulse transmission (and thus sympathetic nervous system stimulation) at adrenergic neurons or adrenergic receptor sites. Their action at these sites can be exerted by:
• interrupting the action of adrenergic drugs
• reducing available norepinephrine
• preventing the action of cholinergic drugs.

Classified information

Adrenergic blocking drugs are classified according to their site of action as:
• alpha-adrenergic blockers (also called *alpha blockers*)
• beta-adrenergic blockers (also called *beta blockers*).

Alpha-adrenergic blockers

Alpha-adrenergic blockers work by interrupting the actions of the catecholamines epinephrine and norepinephrine at alpha receptors. This results in:

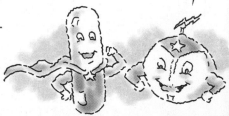

We're adrenergic blocking drugs. We block impulse transmissions from adrenergic neurons and receptor sites. It's quite a job, but we're up to it!

Prototype pro

Alpha-adrenergic blockers: Prazosin

Actions
• Inhibits alpha-adrenergic receptors, causing arterial and venous dilation that reduces peripheral vascular resistance

Indications
• Mild to moderate hypertension

Nursing considerations
• Monitor for adverse reactions, such as dizziness, first-dose syncope, palpitations, or nausea.
• Monitor pulse rate and blood pressure frequently.
• Advise the patient to rise slowly and to avoid abrupt position changes.

• relaxation of the smooth muscle in the blood vessels
• increased dilation of blood vessels
• decreased blood pressure.
    Drugs in this class include:
• ergoloid mesylates
• ergotamine
• phenoxybenzamine
• phentolamine
• terazosin
• doxazosin
• prazosin (see *Alpha-adrenergic blockers: Prazosin*).

Two actions in one

Ergotamine is a mixed alpha agonist and antagonist; at high doses, it acts as an alpha-adrenergic blocker.

Pharmacokinetics

Most alpha-adrenergic blockers are absorbed erratically when given orally and more rapidly and completely when given sublingually. Alpha-adrenergic blockers vary considerably in their onset of action, peak concentration levels, and duration of action.

Pharmacodynamics

Alpha-adrenergic blockers work in one of two ways:
• They interfere with or block the synthesis, storage, release, and reuptake of norepinephrine by neurons.

• They antagonize epinephrine, norepinephrine, or adrenergic drugs at alpha-receptor sites.

Alpha-adrenergic blockers include drugs that block stimulation of alpha$_1$ receptors and drugs that may block alpha$_2$ stimulation.

More flow, less pressure

Alpha-adrenergic blockers occupy alpha-receptor sites on the smooth muscle of blood vessels. (See *How alpha-adrenergic blockers affect peripheral blood vessels.*) This prevents catecholamines from occupying and stimulating the receptor sites. As a result, blood vessels dilate, increasing local blood flow to the skin and other organs. The decreased peripheral vascular resistance (resistance to blood flow) helps to decrease blood pressure.

Watch your patient's tone

The therapeutic effect of an alpha-adrenergic blocker depends on the sympathetic tone (the state of partial constriction of blood vessels) in the body before the drug is administered. For instance, when the drug is given with the patient lying down, only a small change in blood pressure occurs. In this position, the sympathetic nerves release very little norepinephrine.

On the other hand, when a patient stands up, norepinephrine is released to constrict the veins and shoot blood back up to the heart. If the patient receives an alpha-adrenergic blocker, however, the veins can't constrict and blood pools in the legs. Because blood return to the heart is reduced, blood pressure drops. This drop in blood pressure that occurs when a person stands up is called *orthostatic hypotension.*

Pharmacotherapeutics

Because alpha-adrenergic blockers cause smooth muscles to relax and blood vessels to dilate, they increase local blood flow to the skin and other organs and reduce blood pressure. As a result, they're used to treat:

• hypertension
• peripheral vascular disorders (disease of the blood vessels of the extremities), especially those in which spasm of the blood vessels causes poor local blood flow, such as Raynaud's disease (characterized by intermittent pallor, cyanosis, or redness of the fingers), acrocyanosis (characterized by symmetrical mottled cyanosis [bluish color] of the hands and feet), and frostbite
• pheochromocytoma (a catecholamine-secreting tumor causing severe hypertension)

My job is to block alpha receptor sites so that catecholamines can't occupy them. Sorry, catecholamine. This seat is taken.

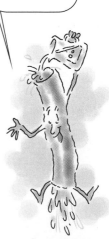

Thanks alpha-adrenergic blockers for helping me dilate!

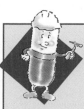

Pharm function

How alpha-adrenergic blockers affect peripheral blood vessels

By occupying alpha-receptor sites, alpha-adrenergic blocking drugs cause blood vessel walls to relax. This leads to dilation of blood vessels and reduced peripheral vascular resistance (the pressure that blood must overcome as it flows in a vessel).

One result: Orthostatic hypotension
These effects can cause orthostatic hypotension, a drop in blood pressure that occurs when changing position from lying down to standing. Redistribution of blood to the dilated blood vessels of the legs causes hypotension.

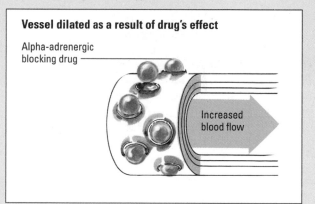

Vessel before drug's effect

Alpha-adrenergic blocking drug

Alpha receptor site

Blood flow

Vessel dilated as a result of drug's effect

Alpha-adrenergic blocking drug

Increased blood flow

• vascular headaches (treated with ergoloid mesylates, ergotamine).

Drug interactions

Many drugs interact with alpha-adrenergic blockers, producing a synergistic or exaggerated effect that may lead to such conditions as severe hypotension or vascular collapse.

Here are some examples of interactions that can occur:
• Prazosin taken with diuretics, propranolol, or other beta-adrenergic blockers results in increased frequency of syncope with loss of consciousness.
• Doxazosin or terazosin taken with clonidine results in decreased clonidine effects.
• Terazosin taken with antihypertensives may cause excessive hypotension.

These effects are specific to ergoloid mesylates and ergotamine:
• Caffeine and macrolide antibiotics can increase the effects of ergotamine.
• Dopamine increases the pressor (rise in blood pressure) effect.

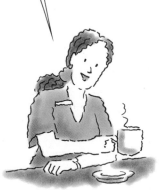

Taking caffeine with ergotamine can increase ergotamine's effects. I'll stick with decaf!

• Nitroglycerin can produce hypotension due to excessive dilation of blood vessels.
• Adrenergic drugs, including many over-the-counter drugs, can increase the stimulating effects on the heart. Hypotension with rebound hypertension can occur.

Adverse reactions

Most adverse reactions associated with alpha-adrenergic blockers are caused primarily by dilation of the blood vessels. They include:
• orthostatic hypotension or severe hypertension
• bradycardia or tachycardia
• edema
• difficulty breathing
• light-headedness
• flushing
• arrhythmias
• angina or heart attack
• spasm of the blood vessels in the brain
• a shocklike state.

Nursing process

These nursing process steps are appropriate for patients undergoing treatment with alpha-adrenergic blockers.

Assessment
• Obtain vital signs, especially blood pressure.
• Assess the patient for adverse reactions.
• Assess the patient's and family's knowledge of drug therapy.

Key nursing diagnoses
• Decreased cardiac output related to hypotension
• Ineffective (peripheral) tissue perfusion related to vasoconstriction
• Acute pain related to headache
• Excess fluid volume related to fluid retention
• Deficient knowledge related to drug therapy

Planning outcome goals
• Adequate cardiac output will be demonstrated.
• Peripheral tissue perfusion will improve, as evidenced by adequate circulatory checks and pulses.
• The patient will state that pain is decreased.
• Fluid volume status will remain adequate, as demonstrated by adequate blood pressure, urine output, and cardiac parameters.

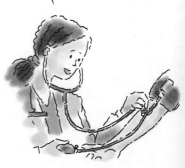

The patient's blood pressure indicates whether his fluid volume is adequate.

Education edge

Teaching about alpha-adrenergic blockers

If alpha-adrenergic blockers are prescribed, review these points with the patient and his caregivers:
• Don't rise suddenly from a lying or sitting position.
• Avoid hazardous tasks that require mental alertness until the full effects of the drug are known.
• Keep in mind that alcohol, excessive exercise, prolonged standing, and heat exposure intensify adverse effects.
• Report dizziness or irregular heartbeat.

• Don't eat, drink, or smoke while the sublingual tablet is dissolving.
• Don't increase the drug dosage without first consulting the prescriber.
• Avoid prolonged exposure to cold weather whenever possible. Cold may increase adverse reactions to ergotamine.
• If receiving long-term ergotamine therapy, check for and report coldness in the limbs or tingling in the fingers or toes. Severe vasoconstriction may result in tissue damage.

Implementation
• Give drugs at bedtime to minimize dizziness or light-headedness.
• Begin therapy with a small dose to avoid syncope with the first dose.
• Give ergotamine during the prodromal stage of a headache or as soon as possible after onset.
• Don't give sublingual tablets with food or drink.
• Provide patient teaching.

Evaluation
• Patient maintains adequate cardiac output.
• Patient maintains adequate tissue perfusion to limbs throughout therapy.
• Patient's headache is relieved.
• Patient has no edema.
• Patient and his family demonstrate an understanding of drug therapy. (See *Teaching about alpha-adrenergic blockers.*)

Beta-adrenergic blockers

Beta-adrenergic blockers, the most widely used adrenergic blockers, prevent stimulation of the sympathetic nervous system by inhibiting the action of catecholamines at beta-adrenergic receptors.

Some are picky, others aren't

Beta-adrenergic blockers are selective or nonselective. Nonselective beta-adrenergic blockers affect:
• beta$_1$ receptor sites (located mainly in the heart)

• beta$_2$ receptor sites (located in the bronchi, blood vessels, and uterus).

Nonselective beta-adrenergic blocking drugs include carvedilol, labetalol, levobunolol, nadolol, penbutolol, pindolol, propranolol, sotalol, and timolol. (Carvedilol and labetalol also block alpha$_1$ receptors.)

Selective beta-adrenergic blockers primarily affect just the beta$_1$-adrenergic sites. They include acebutolol, atenolol, betaxolol, bisoprolol, esmolol, and metoprolol tartrate.

Part blocker, part stimulator

Some beta-adrenergic blockers, such as pindolol and acebutolol, also have intrinsic sympathetic activity. This means that instead of attaching to beta receptors and blocking them, these beta-adrenergic blockers attach to beta receptors and stimulate them. These drugs are sometimes classified as *partial agonists*.

Pharmacokinetics

Beta-adrenergic blockers are usually absorbed rapidly from the GI tract. They are protein-bound to some extent. Some beta-adrenergic blockers are absorbed more completely than others.

When it comes to beta-adrenergic blockers, you can't beat me to peak levels!

Reach the peak faster: Go I.V.

The onset of action of beta-adrenergic blockers is primarily dose- and drug-dependent. The time it takes to reach peak concentration levels depends on the route of administration. Beta-adrenergic blockers given I.V. reach peak levels much more rapidly than when given by mouth.

Beta-adrenergic blockers are distributed widely in body tissues, with the highest concentrations found in the heart, liver, lungs, and saliva.

The liver delivers

With the exception of nadolol and atenolol, beta-adrenergic blockers are metabolized in the liver. They're excreted primarily in urine, as metabolites or in unchanged form, but can also be excreted in feces and bile, with some secretion in breast milk.

Pharmacodynamics

Beta-adrenergic blockers have widespread effects in the body because they produce their blocking action not only at adrenergic nerve endings but also in the adrenal medulla.

Happenings in the heart

Effects on the heart include increased peripheral vascular resistance, decreased blood pressure, decreased force of heart contractions, decreased oxygen consumption by the heart, slowed conduction of impulses between the atria and ventricles of the heart, and decreased cardiac output (the amount of blood pumped by the heart each minute). (See *How beta-adrenergic blockers work*.)

Choosy blockers choose beta₁ receptors...

Some of the effects of beta-adrenergic blocking drugs depend on whether the drug is classified as selective or nonselective. Selective beta-adrenergic blockers, which preferentially block beta₁ re-

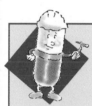

Pharm function

How beta-adrenergic blockers work

By occupying beta-receptor sites, beta-adrenergic blockers prevent catecholamines (norepinephrine and epinephrine) from occupying these sites and exerting their stimulating effects. This illustration shows the effects of beta-adrenergic blockers on the heart, lungs, and blood vessels.

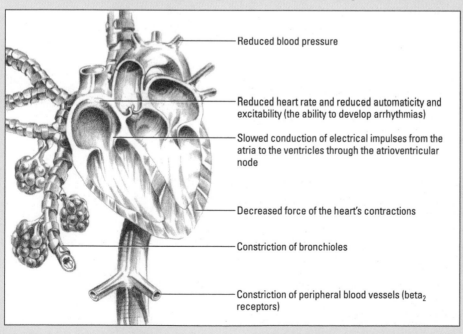

Reduced blood pressure

Reduced heart rate and reduced automaticity and excitability (the ability to develop arrhythmias)

Slowed conduction of electrical impulses from the atria to the ventricles through the atrioventricular node

Decreased force of the heart's contractions

Constriction of bronchioles

Constriction of peripheral blood vessels (beta₂ receptors)

ceptor sites, reduce stimulation of the heart. They're commonly referred to as *cardioselective beta-adrenergic blockers*.

Nonselective beta-adrenergic blockers, which block both beta$_1$ and beta$_2$ receptor sites, not only reduce stimulation of the heart but also cause the bronchioles of the lungs to constrict. Therefore, nonselective beta-adrenergic blockers can cause bronchospasm in patients with chronic obstructive lung disorders. This adverse effect isn't seen when nonselective beta-adrenergic blockers are given at lower doses.

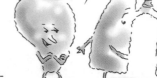

The most selective beta-adrenergic blockers have the good taste to choose me over you!

Pharmacotherapeutics

Beta-adrenergic blockers are used to treat many conditions and are under investigation for use in many more. As mentioned earlier, their clinical usefulness is based largely (but not exclusively) on how they affect the heart. (See *Are beta-adrenergic blockers underused in elderly patients?*)

Taken to heart

Beta-adrenergic blockers can be prescribed after a heart attack to prevent another heart attack or to treat:
- angina (chest pain)
- hypertension
- hypertrophic cardiomyopathy (a disease of the heart muscle)
- supraventricular arrhythmias (irregular heartbeats that originate in the atria, SA node, or AV node).

Are beta-adrenergic blockers underused in elderly patients?

Research has clearly shown that using a beta-adrenergic blocker after a heart attack reduces the risk of death and another heart attack. Even so, these drugs aren't being prescribed for elderly patients.

What one study found
One study found that only 34% of patients were prescribed a beta-adrenergic blocker after discharge from the hospital following a heart attack. The least likely patients to receive beta-adrenergic blockers included blacks and very sick and elderly patients.

Why?
The chief investigator of a study that looked at the use of beta-adrenergic blockers in elderly patients believes that many doctors fear the adverse effects of these drugs on older patients. The study suggested that a beta-adrenergic blocker can be given safely to an elderly patient after a heart attack if the lowest effective dose of a selective beta-adrenergic blocker is prescribed.

Very versatile

Beta-adrenergic blockers are also used to treat:
• anxiety
• cardiovascular symptoms associated with thyrotoxicosis (over-production of thyroid hormones)
• essential tremor
• migraine headaches
• open-angle glaucoma
• pheochromocytoma.

Drug interactions

Many drugs can interact with beta-adrenergic blocking drugs to cause potentially dangerous effects. Some of the most serious effects include cardiac depression, arrhythmias, respiratory depression, severe bronchospasm, and severe hypotension that can lead to vascular collapse. Here are some others:
• Increased effects or toxicity can occur when digoxin, calcium channel blockers (primarily verapamil), and cimetidine are taken with beta-adrenergic blockers.
• Decreased effects can occur when antacids, calcium salts, barbiturates, anti-inflammatories (such as indomethacin and salicylates), and rifampin are taken with beta-adrenergic blockers.
• The requirements for insulin and oral antidiabetic drugs can be altered when taken with beta-adrenergic blockers.
• Potential lidocaine toxicity can occur when it's taken with beta-adrenergic blockers.
• The ability of theophylline to produce bronchodilation is impaired by nonselective beta-adrenergic blockers.
• Clonidine taken with a nonselective beta-adrenergic blocker can result in life-threatening hypertension during clonidine withdrawal.
• Sympathomimetics and nonselective beta-adrenergic blockers can cause hypertension and reflex bradycardia.

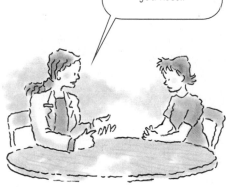

Beta-adrenergic blockers may affect how much antidiabetic drug you need.

Adverse reactions

Beta-adrenergic blockers generally cause few adverse reactions; the adverse reactions that do occur are drug- or dose-dependent and include:
• hypotension
• bradycardia
• peripheral vascular insufficiency
• AV block
• heart failure

- bronchospasm
- diarrhea or constipation
- nausea
- vomiting
- abdominal discomfort
- anorexia
- flatulence
- rash
- fever with sore throat
- spasm of the larynx
- respiratory distress (allergic response).

Nursing process

These nursing process steps are appropriate for patients undergoing treatment with beta-adrenergic blockers.

Assessment

- Assess the patient's condition before therapy and regularly thereafter.
- Assess respiratory status, especially in a patient with chronic obstructive pulmonary disease or asthma because of the potential risk of bronchospasm.

Rating the pulse rate

- Check apical pulse rate daily; alert the prescriber about extremes, such as a pulse rate below 60 beats/minute.
- Monitor blood pressure, ECG, and heart rate and rhythm frequently; be alert for progression of AV block or bradycardia.
- If the patient has heart failure, weigh him regularly and watch for weight gain of more than 5 lb (2.3 kg) per week.
- Observe the diabetic patient for sweating, fatigue, and hunger. Signs of hypoglycemic shock are masked.
- Be alert for adverse reactions and drug interactions.
- Assess the patient's and family's knowledge of drug therapy.

Key nursing diagnoses

- Risk for injury related to adverse CNS effects
- Excess fluid volume related to edema
- Decreased cardiac output related to bradycardia or hypotension
- Deficient knowledge related to drug therapy

Planning outcome goals

- The patient's chances for injury will be diminished.
- The patient will experience normal fluid volume as shown by adequate urine output and blood pressure.

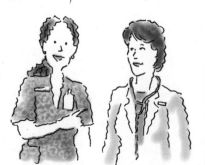

If your patient is undergoing surgery, make sure you tell the anesthesiologist that he's taking a beta-adrenergic blocker.

Implementation

- Before any surgical procedure, notify the anesthesiologist that the patient is taking a beta-adrenergic blocker.
- Keep glucagon nearby in case it's prescribed to reverse beta-adrenergic blocker overdose.
- Check the apical pulse before giving drug; if it's slower than 60 beats/minute, withhold the drug and call the prescriber immediately.
- Give the drug with meals because food may increase absorption.
- For I.V. use, give the drug undiluted and by direct injection, unless recommended otherwise by a pharmacy.

Evaluation

- Patient remains free from injury.
- Patient has no signs of edema.
- Patient maintains normal blood pressure and heart rate.
- Patient and his family demonstrate an understanding of drug therapy. (See *Teaching about beta-adrenergic blockers.*)

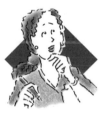

Quick quiz

1. Which effect is expected when using cholinergic agonists?
   - A. Dry mouth
   - B. Tachycardia
   - C. Pupil dilation
   - D. Increased bladder tone

Answer: D. Effects of cholinergic agonists include increased tone and contraction of bladder muscles, salivation, bradycardia, dilated blood vessels, constricted pulmonary bronchioles, increased activity of the GI tract, and constricted pupils.

2. Which drug would the nurse give to a patient experiencing symptomatic sinus bradycardia?
   - A. Atropine
   - B. Belladonna
   - C. Digoxin
   - D. Propranolol

Answer: A. Atropine is the drug of choice to treat symptomatic sinus bradycardia.

Education edge

Teaching about beta-adrenergic blockers

If beta-adrenergic blocking drugs are prescribed, review these points with the patient and his caregivers:

- Take the drug exactly as prescribed, even if signs or symptoms are relieved.
- Don't stop the drug suddenly. This can worsen angina or precipitate myocardial infarction.
- Take the oral form of the drug with meals to enhance absorption.
- Don't take over-the-counter drugs or herbal remedies without medical consent.
- Be aware of potential adverse reactions and report unusual effects of the drug.
- Avoid performing hazardous activities until central nervous system effects of the drug are known.

3.   Which finding indicates that a patient is having an adverse re-
action to catecholamines?
 A.   Nausea and vomiting
 B.   Diarrhea
 C.   Decreased glucose levels
 D.   Palpitations

Answer: D. Adverse reactions to catecholamines include palpitations, restlessness, anxiety, dizziness, headache, cardiac arrhythmias, hypotension, hypertension and hypertensive crisis, stroke,
angina, and increased glucose levels.

4.   Which drug is a catecholamine?
 A.   Dopamine
 B.   Albuterol
 C.   Prazosin
 D.   Labetalol

Answer: A. Dopamine is a catecholamine.

5.   Which noncatecholamine is dual-acting?
 A.   Albuterol
 B.   Isoetharine
 C.   Ephedrine
 D.   Terbutaline

Answer: C. Ephedrine is a dual-acting noncatecholamine.

6.   Which drug causes toxicity in a patient taking a beta-adrenergic
blocker?
 A.   An antacid
 B.   Rifampin
 C.   A nonsteroidal anti-inflammatory drug
 D.   Digoxin

Answer: D. Increased effects or toxicity can occur when digoxin, calcium channel blockers (primarily verapamil), and cimetidine are taken with beta-adrenergic blockers.

Scoring

☆☆☆ If you answered all six questions correctly, super! Your receptors
      must really be stimulated by this information.

☆☆ If you answered four or five questions correctly, good work! You
      have no reason to be nervous about working with autonomic
      nervous system drugs.

☆ If you answered fewer than four questions correctly, no need to
      agonize over it. Assess your trouble spots and plan some
      time for review.

Neurologic and neuromuscular drugs

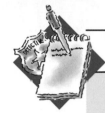

Just the facts

In this chapter, you'll learn:

♦ classes of drugs used to treat neurologic and neuromuscular disorders

♦ uses and actions of these drugs

♦ absorption, distribution, metabolization, and excretion of these drugs

♦ drug interactions and adverse reactions to these drugs.

Drugs and the neurologic and neuromuscular systems

The neurologic or nervous system includes the central nervous system (brain and spinal cord) and the peripheral nervous system (somatic and autonomic nervous systems). The neuromuscular system consists of the muscles of the body and the nerves that supply them. Several types of drugs are used to treat disorders of these two major systems, including:

• skeletal muscle relaxants
• neuromuscular blocking drugs
• antiparkinsonian drugs
• anticonvulsant drugs
• antimigraine drugs.

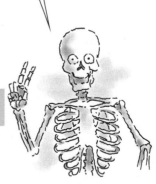

This chapter reviews drugs that are used to treat two major body systems—the neurologic and the neuromuscular.

Skeletal muscle relaxants

Skeletal muscle relaxants relieve musculoskeletal pain or spasms and severe musculoskeletal spasticity (stiff, awkward movements). They're used to treat acute, painful musculoskeletal conditions and muscle spasticity associated with multiple sclerosis

(MS), a progressive demyelination of the white matter of the brain and spinal cord that causes widespread neurologic dysfunction; cerebral palsy, a motor function disorder caused by neurologic damage; stroke, the death of brain cells caused by a reduced supply of oxygen to the brain that can result in neurologic deficits; and spinal cord injuries, which can result in paralysis or death. This section discusses centrally acting, direct-acting, and other skeletal muscle relaxants.

> Skeletal muscle relaxants like me can help control your spasticity.

Centrally acting agents

Centrally acting skeletal muscle relaxants are used to treat acute muscle spasms caused by such conditions as anxiety, inflammation, pain, and trauma. They also treat spasticity from such conditions as MS and cerebral palsy.
    Examples of these drugs include:
- carisoprodol
- chlorphenesin
- chlorzoxazone
- cyclobenzaprine
- metaxalone
- methocarbamol
- orphenadrine
- tizanidine.

Pharmacokinetics (how drugs circulate)

Much is still unknown about how centrally acting skeletal muscle relaxants circulate within the body. In general, these drugs are absorbed from the GI tract, widely distributed in the body, metabolized in the liver, and excreted by the kidneys.

> I'm an agent of the CAA: Centrally Acting Agency.

Cyclobenzaprine sticks around

When administered orally, these drugs can take from 30 minutes to 1 hour to be effective. Although the duration of action of most of these drugs varies from 4 to 6 hours, cyclobenzaprine has the longest duration of action at 12 to 25 hours.

Pharmacodynamics (how drugs act)

Although their precise mechanism of action is unknown, the centrally acting drugs don't relax skeletal muscles directly or depress neuronal conduction, neuromuscular transmission, or muscle excitability. Rather, centrally acting drugs are known to be central nervous system (CNS) depressants. The skeletal muscle relaxant effects that they cause are likely related to their sedative effects.

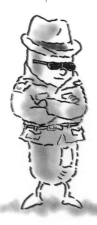

Pharmacotherapeutics (how drugs are used)

Patients receive centrally acting skeletal muscle relaxants to treat acute, painful musculoskeletal conditions. They're usually prescribed along with rest and physical therapy.

Drug interactions

Centrally acting skeletal muscle relaxants interact with other CNS depressants (including alcohol, opioids, barbiturates, anticonvulsants, tricyclic antidepressants, and antianxiety drugs), causing increased sedation, impaired motor function, and respiratory depression. In addition, some of these drugs have other interactions, such as those listed here:
• Cyclobenzaprine interacts with monoamine oxidase (MAO) inhibitors and can result in a high body temperature, excitation, and seizures.
• Cyclobenzaprine can decrease the antihypertensive effects of the blood pressure–lowering drugs clonidine and guanethidine.
• Orphenadrine and cyclobenzaprine sometimes enhance the effects of cholinergic blocking drugs.
• Orphenadrine can reduce the effects of phenothiazines.

Add it up!

• Taking orphenadrine and propoxyphene together can cause additive CNS effects, including mental confusion, anxiety, and tremors.
• Methocarbamol can antagonize the cholinergic effects of the anticholinesterase drugs used to treat myasthenia gravis.
• Tizanidine combined with diuretics, central alpha-adrenergic agonists, or antihypertensives may increase hypotensive drug effects.
• Concurrent use of tizanidine with other CNS depressants may cause additive CNS depression.
• Hormonal contraception agents may reduce the clearance of tizanidine, necessitating a dose reduction.

Adverse reactions

Long-term use of centrally acting muscle relaxants can result in physical and psychological dependence. Abrupt cessation of these drugs can cause severe withdrawal symptoms.

Adverse reactions can also occur when a patient is taking these drugs. Common reactions include dizziness and drowsiness. Severe reactions include allergic reactions, arrhythmias, and bradycardia. Less common reactions include abdominal distress, ataxia, constipation, diarrhea, heartburn, nausea, and vomiting.

Nursing process

These nursing process steps are appropriate for patients undergoing treatment with centrally acting skeletal muscle relaxants.

Assessment

- Obtain a history of the patient's pain and muscle spasms and reassess regularly thereafter.
- Monitor the patient for hypersensitivity reactions.
- Assess the degree of relief obtained to help the prescriber determine when the dosage can be reduced.
- Closely monitor complete blood count (CBC) results.
- In a patient receiving cyclobenzaprine, monitor platelet counts.

That fainting feeling

- Watch for orthostatic hypotension in a patient receiving methocarbamol.
- In a patient receiving long-term chlorzoxazone therapy, monitor hepatic function and urinalysis results.
- Assess compliance of a patient receiving long-term therapy.
- Evaluate the patient's and family's understanding of drug therapy.

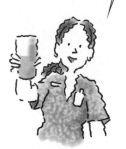

Give oral forms of centrally acting agents with meals or milk to prevent GI distress. Bottoms up!

Key nursing diagnoses

- Risk for injury related to drug-induced adverse reactions
- Risk for falls related to underlying diagnosis and drug-induced adverse reactions
- Acute pain related to underlying disorder
- Deficient knowledge related to drug therapy

Planning outcome goals

- The patient's risk of injury will be minimized.
- The patient's risk for falls will be minimized.
- The patient will acknowledge decreased discomfort after administration of medication.
- The patient and his family will verbalize an understanding of the medication's purpose and intended effect.

Implementation

- After long-term therapy (unless the patient has severe adverse reactions), avoid stopping carisoprodol abruptly to prevent withdrawal symptoms, such as insomnia, headache, nausea, and abdominal pain.
- Institute safety precautions as needed.
- Give oral forms of these drugs with meals or milk to prevent GI distress.

Education edge

Teaching about skeletal muscle relaxants

If skeletal muscle relaxants are perscribed, review these points with the patient and his caregivers:
• Take the drug exactly as prescribed. Don't stop baclofen or carisoprodol suddenly after long-term therapy to avoid withdrawal symptoms.
• Avoid hazardous activities that require mental alertness until the central nervous system effects of the drug are known. Drowsiness is usually transient.
• Avoid alcohol or other depressants during therapy.
• Follow the prescriber's advice regarding rest and physical therapy.
• Try to spread out activities throughout the day and allow rest periods to avoid fatigue, weakness, and drowsiness. If adverse effects become too severe, consult with the prescriber.
• Change positions slowly to help avoid dizzy spells. If dizziness occurs, avoid driving, operating dangerous machinery, or performing delicate tasks.
• Take the drug with food or milk to prevent GI distress.
• Report urinary hesitancy with cyclobenzaprine or baclofen therapy.
• Be aware that urine may be discolored when taking methocarbamol or chlorzoxazone.
• Make sure you keep regular medical follow-up appointments to evaluate the effects of this drug.

• Obtain an order for mild analgesics to relieve drug-induced headache.
• Avoid abrupt discontinuation to reduce withdrawal symptoms, such as returning spasticity, hypotension, paresthesia, and muscle rigidity.

Evaluation

• Patient doesn't experience injury as a result of drug-induced drowsiness.
• Patient doesn't experience a fall as a result of drug-induced drowsiness.
• Patient reports that pain and muscle spasms have ceased with drug therapy.
• Patient complies with therapy, as evidenced by pain relief or improvement of spasticity.
• Patient and his family state an understanding of drug therapy.
(See *Teaching about skeletal muscle relaxants.*)

Direct-acting agents

Dantrolene sodium is the only direct-acting skeletal muscle relaxant. Although dantrolene has therapeutic effects similar to those of the centrally acting drugs, it works through a different mechanism of action.

Head case

Dantrolene is most effective for spasticity of cerebral origin. Because the drug produces muscle weakness, the benefits of dantrolene administration in a patient with borderline strength are questionable.

Pharmacokinetics

Although the peak drug concentration of dantrolene occurs within about 5 hours of ingestion, the patient may not notice any therapeutic benefit for a week or more. Dantrolene is absorbed slowly and incompletely (but consistently) from the GI tract and is highly plasma protein–bound. This means that only a small portion of the drug is available to produce a therapeutic effect.

Hiking up the half-life

Dantrolene is metabolized by the liver and excreted in urine. Its elimination half-life in a healthy adult is about 9 hours. Because dantrolene is metabolized in the liver, its half-life can be prolonged in a patient with impaired liver function.

Pharmacodynamics

Dantrolene is chemically and pharmacologically unrelated to other skeletal muscle relaxants. It acts directly on muscle to interfere with calcium ion release from the sarcoplasmic reticulum and weaken the force of contractions. At therapeutic concentrations, dantrolene has little effect on cardiac or intestinal smooth muscle.

Pharmacotherapeutics

Dantrolene can be used to help manage several types of spasticity but is most effective in patients with:
• cerebral palsy
• MS
• spinal cord injury
• stroke.

Anesthesia antidote

Dantrolene is also used to treat and prevent malignant hyperthermia. This rare but potentially fatal complication of anesthesia is characterized by skeletal muscle rigidity and high fever. (See *How dantrolene reduces muscle rigidity*.)

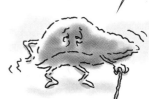

Dantrolene has a half-life of about 9 hours in a healthy adult, but impaired liver function can prolong that half-life. I think I'll need a little extra time to metabolize...

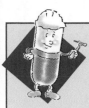

Pharm function

How dantrolene reduces muscle rigidity

Dantrolene appears to decrease the number of calcium ions released from the sarcoplasmic reticulum (a structure in muscle cells that controls muscle contraction and relaxation by releasing and storing calcium). The lower the calcium level in the muscle plasma or myoplasm, the less energy produced when calcium prompts interaction of the muscle's actin and myosin filaments (responsible for muscle contraction). Less energy means a weaker muscle contraction.

Reducing rigidity, halting hyperthermia
By promoting muscle relaxation, dantrolene prevents or reduces the rigidity that contributes to the life-threatening body temperatures of malignant hyperthermia.

Drug interactions

CNS depressants can increase the depressive effects of dantrolene and result in sedation, lack of coordination, and respiratory depression. In addition, dantrolene may have other drug interactions:

• Estrogens, when given with dantrolene, can increase the risk of liver toxicity.
• I.V. verapamil shouldn't be administered if giving dantrolene because it may result in cardiovascular collapse.
• Alcohol may increase CNS depression when taken with dantrolene.

Adverse reactions

Because its major effect is on the muscles, dantrolene has a lower incidence of adverse CNS reactions. However, high therapeutic doses are toxic to the liver. Common adverse effects of dantrolene include drowsiness, dizziness, malaise, and muscle weakness. More serious adverse effects include bleeding, seizures, and hepatitis.

Nursing process

These nursing process steps are appropriate for patients undergoing treatment with dantrolene.

Assessment
• Obtain a history of the patient's pain and muscle spasms before therapy and reassess regularly thereafter.
• Monitor the patient for hypersensitivity reactions.

• Assess the degree of relief obtained to help the prescriber determine when the dosage can be reduced.
• Monitor CBC results closely and monitor liver function tests.
• Assess compliance of a patient receiving long-term therapy.
• Evaluate the patient's and family's understanding of drug therapy.

Key nursing diagnoses
• Risk for injury related to drug-induced adverse reactions
• Acute pain related to underlying disorder
• Deficient knowledge related to drug therapy

Planning outcome goals
• The patient's risk of injury will be minimized.
• The patient will acknowledge decreased discomfort after administration of medication.
• The patient and his family will verbalize an understanding of the medication's purpose and intended effect.

Implementation
• Institute safety precautions as needed.
• If hepatitis, severe diarrhea, severe weakness, or sensitivity reactions occur, withhold the dose and notify the prescriber.
• Give the oral form of the drug with meals or milk to prevent GI distress.
• Obtain an order for a mild analgesic to relieve drug-induced headache.
• Avoid abrupt discontinuation to prevent the return of symptoms, such as spasticity, paresthesia, and muscle rigidity.

Evaluation
• Patient doesn't experience injury as a result of drug-induced drowsiness.
• Patient reports that pain and muscle spasms have ceased with drug therapy.
• Patient complies with therapy, as evidenced by pain relief or improvement of spasticity.
• Patient and his family state an understanding of drug therapy.
(See *Teaching about skeletal muscle relaxants*, page 67.)

Other skeletal muscle relaxants

Two additional drugs used as skeletal muscle relaxants are diazepam and baclofen. Because diazepam is primarily used as an antianxiety drug, this section discusses only baclofen. (See *Diazepam as a skeletal muscle relaxant*.)

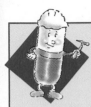

Pharm function

Diazepam as a skeletal muscle relaxant

Diazepam is a benzodiazepine drug that's used to treat acute muscle spasms as well as spasticity caused by chronic disorders. It seems to work by promoting the inhibitory effect of the neurotransmitter gamma-aminobutyric acid on muscle contraction. Other uses of diazepam include treating anxiety, alcohol withdrawal, and seizures.

The negatives: Sedation and tolerance
Diazepam can be used alone or in conjunction with other drugs to treat spasticity, especially in patients with spinal cord lesions and, occasionally, in patients with cerebral palsy. It's also helpful in patients with painful, continuous muscle spasms who aren't too susceptible to the drug's sedative effects. Unfortunately, diazepam's use is limited by its central nervous system effects and the tolerance that develops with prolonged use.

Pharmacokinetics

Baclofen is absorbed rapidly from the GI tract. It's distributed widely (with only small amounts crossing the blood-brain barrier), undergoes minimal liver metabolism, and is excreted primarily unchanged in urine.

A long wait

It can take hours to weeks before the patient notices beneficial effects of baclofen. The elimination half-life of baclofen is 2½ to 4 hours.

Pharmacodynamics

It isn't known exactly how baclofen works. Chemically similar to the neurotransmitter gamma-aminobutyric acid (GABA), baclofen probably acts in the spinal cord. It reduces nerve impulses from the spinal cord to skeletal muscle, decreasing the number and severity of muscle spasms and the associated pain.

A choice drug

Because baclofen produces less sedation than diazepam and less peripheral muscle weakness than dantrolene, it's the drug of choice to treat spasticity.

Pharmacotherapeutics

Baclofen's major clinical use is for paraplegic or quadriplegic patients with spinal cord lesions, most commonly caused by MS or

Prototype pro

Skeletal muscle relaxants: Baclofen

Actions
• Unknown
• Appears to reduce the transmission of impulses from the spinal cord to skeletal muscle
• Relieves muscle spasms

Indications
• Spasticity in multiple sclerosis and spinal cord injury
• Management of severe spasticity in the patient who doesn't respond to or can't tolerate oral baclofen therapy (intrathecal baclofen)

Nursing considerations
• Give oral baclofen with meals or milk to prevent GI distress.
• Avoid abrupt discontinuation of intrathecal baclofen because this can result in high fever, altered mental status, exaggerated rebound spasticity, and muscle rigidity that, in rare cases, may progress to rhabdomyolysis, multiple organ system failure, and death.
• If intrathecal baclofen is delayed, treatment with a gamma-aminobutyric acid agonist or I.V. benzodiazepines may prevent potentially fatal sequelae.

trauma. For these patients, baclofen significantly reduces the number and severity of painful flexor spasms. Unfortunately, however, baclofen doesn't improve stiff gait, manual dexterity, or residual muscle function.

Baclofen can be administered intrathecally for patients who are unresponsive to oral baclofen or who experience intolerable adverse effects. After a positive response to a bolus dose, an implantable port for chronic therapy can be placed. Extreme caution should be taken to avoid abrupt discontinuation of intrathecal baclofen.

No abrupt endings

Abrupt withdrawal of intrathecal baclofen has resulted in high fever, altered mental status, exaggerated rebound spasticity, and muscle rigidity that—in rare cases—has progressed to rhabdomyolysis, multiple organ system failure, and death. (See *Skeletal muscle relaxants: Baclofen*.)

Drug interactions

Baclofen has few drug interactions:
• The most significant drug interaction is an increase in CNS depression when baclofen is administered with other CNS depressants, including alcohol.

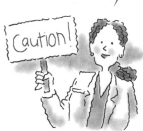

Avoid abrupt discontinuation of intrathecal baclofen treatment.

• Analgesia can be prolonged when fentanyl and baclofen are administered together.
• Lithium carbonate and baclofen taken together can aggravate hyperkinesia (an abnormal increase in motor function or activity).
• Tricyclic antidepressants and baclofen taken together can increase muscle relaxation.

Adverse reactions

The most common adverse reaction to baclofen is transient drowsiness. Some less common effects include nausea, fatigue, vertigo, hypotonia, muscle weakness, depression, and headache.

Nursing process

These nursing process steps are appropriate for patients undergoing treatment with the skeletal muscle relaxant baclofen.

Assessment

• Obtain a history of the patient's pain and muscle spasms before therapy and reassess regularly thereafter.
• Monitor the patient for hypersensitivity reactions.
• Assess the degree of relief obtained to help the prescriber determine when the dosage can be reduced.
• Monitor CBC results closely.
• Assess compliance of a patient receiving long-term therapy.
• Evaluate the patient's and family's understanding of drug therapy.

Key nursing diagnoses

• Risk for injury related to drug-induced adverse reactions
• Acute pain related to underlying disorder
• Deficient knowledge related to drug therapy

Planning outcome goals

• The patient's risk of injury will be minimized.
• The patient will acknowledge decreased discomfort after administration of the medication.
• The patient and his family will verbalize an understanding of the medication's purpose and intended effect.

Implementation

• Institute safety precautions as needed. Watch for an increased risk of seizures in the patient with a seizure disorder. Seizures have been reported during overdose and withdrawal of intrathecal baclofen as well as in patients maintained on therapeutic doses. Monitor the patient carefully and institute seizure precautions.

• Give the oral forms of the drug with meals or milk to prevent GI distress.
• Obtain an order for a mild analgesic to relieve drug-induced headache.

Warning! Wrong way

• Don't administer an intrathecal injection by the I.V., I.M., subcutaneous, or epidural route.
• Avoid an abrupt discontinuation of intrathecal baclofen. Early symptoms of baclofen withdrawal include return of baseline spasticity, pruritus, hypotension, and paresthesia. Symptoms that have occurred include high fever, altered mental status, exaggerated rebound spasticity, and muscle rigidity that—in rare cases—has advanced to rhabdomyolysis, multiple organ system failure, and death.

Evaluation

• Patient doesn't experience injury as a result of drug-induced drowsiness.
• Patient reports that pain and muscle spasms have ceased with drug therapy.
• Patient and his family state an understanding of drug therapy. (See *Teaching about skeletal muscle relaxants*, page 67.)

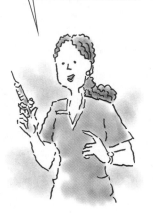

Make sure you don't administer intrathecal baclofen by the I.V., I.M., subcutaneous, or epidural route.

Neuromuscular blocking drugs

Neuromuscular blocking drugs relax skeletal muscles by disrupting the transmission of nerve impulses at the motor end plate (the branching terminals of a motor nerve axon). (See *How neuromuscular blocking drugs work.*)

Relax, reduce, and manage

Neuromuscular blockers have three major clinical indications:
• to relax skeletal muscles during surgery
• to reduce the intensity of muscle spasms in drug-induced or electrically induced seizures
• to manage patients who are fighting the use of a ventilator to help with breathing.

Polar opposites

There are two main classes of natural and synthetic drugs used as neuromuscular blockers—nondepolarizing and depolarizing.

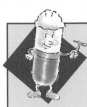

Pharm function

How neuromuscular blocking drugs work

The motor nerve axon divides to form branching terminals called *motor end plates*. These are enfolded in muscle fibers, but separated from the fibers by the synaptic cleft.

Competing with contraction
A stimulus to the nerve causes the release of acetylcholine into the synaptic cleft. There, acetylcholine occupies receptor sites on the muscle cell membrane, depolarizing the membrane and causing muscle contraction. Neuromuscular blocking agents act at the motor end plate by competing with acetylcholine for the receptor sites or by blocking depolarization.

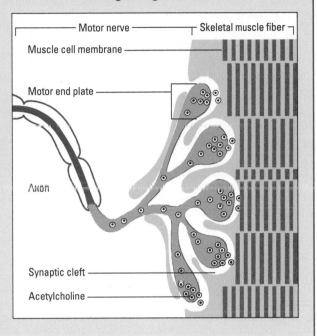

Nondepolarizing blocking drugs

Nondepolarizing blocking drugs, also called *competitive* or *stabilizing* drugs, are derived from curare alkaloids and synthetically similar compounds. They include:
- atracurium
- cisatracurium
- doxacurium
- mivacurium
- pancuronium
- rocuronium
- vecuronium.

Pharmacokinetics

Because nondepolarizing blockers are poorly absorbed from the GI tract, they're administered parenterally. The I.V. route is preferred because the action is more predictable.

Fast movers

Nondepolarizing blockers are distributed rapidly throughout the body. Some drugs, such as pancuronium, rocuronium, and vecuronium, are partially metabolized in the liver. After I.V. administration, atracurium undergoes rapid metabolism by a physiologic process known as *Hofmann elimination* and by enzymatic hydrolysis; it's also partially metabolized in the liver. Mivacurium is hydrolyzed by plasma pseudocholinesterase. It isn't known how doxacurium is metabolized.

These drugs are excreted primarily in urine, and some, such as cisatracurium, doxacurium, and vecuronium, are also excreted in feces.

Pharmacodynamics

Nondepolarizing blockers compete with acetylcholine at the cholinergic receptor sites of the skeletal muscle membrane. This blocks acetylcholine's neurotransmitter action, preventing the muscle from contracting.

The effect can be counteracted by anticholinesterase drugs, such as neostigmine or pyridostigmine, which inhibit the action of acetylcholinesterase, the enzyme that destroys acetylcholine.

Paralysis pattern

The initial muscle weakness produced by these drugs quickly changes to a flaccid (loss of muscle tone) paralysis that affects the muscles in a specific sequence. The first muscles to exhibit flaccid paralysis are those of the eyes, face, and neck. Next, the limb, abdomen, and trunk muscles become flaccid. Finally, the intercostal muscles (between the ribs) and diaphragm (the breathing muscle) are paralyzed. Recovery from the paralysis usually occurs in the reverse order.

Conscious—and anxious

Because these drugs don't cross the blood-brain barrier, the patient remains conscious and able to feel pain. Although the patient is paralyzed, he's aware of what's happening to him and can experience extreme anxiety. However, he can't communicate his feelings. For this reason, an analgesic or antianxiety drug should be administered along with a neuromuscular blocker.

Pharmacotherapeutics

Nondepolarizing blockers are used for intermediate or prolonged muscle relaxation to:
• ease the passage of an endotracheal (ET) tube (a tube placed in the trachea)

Nondepolarizing blockers provide intermediate or prolonged muscle relaxation for several procedures. I find that *this* procedure also provides quite a bit of muscle relaxation!

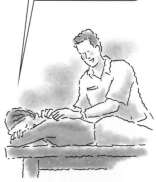

• decrease the amount of anesthetic required during surgery
• facilitate realigning broken bones and dislocated joints
• paralyze the patient who needs ventilatory support, but who resists the ET tube and mechanical ventilation due to agitation and restlessness
• prevent muscle injury during electroconvulsive therapy (ECT) (passage of an electric current through the brain to treat depression) by reducing the intensity of muscle spasms.

Drug interactions

Several drugs alter the effects of nondepolarizing neuromuscular blockers:
• Aminoglycoside antibiotics and anesthetics potentiate or exaggerate the neuromuscular blockade.

That's so intense...

• Drugs that alter serum levels of the electrolytes calcium, magnesium, or potassium also alter the effects of nondepolarizing blockers.
• Anticholinesterases (neostigmine, pyridostigmine, and edrophonium) antagonize nondepolarizing blockers and are used as antidotes.
• Drugs that can increase the intensity and duration of paralysis when taken with a nondepolarizing blocking drug include inhalation anesthetics, aminoglycosides, clindamycin, polymyxin, verapamil, quinine derivatives, ketamine, lithium, nitrates, thiazide diuretics, tetracyclines, and magnesium salts.
• Drugs that can cause decreased neuromuscular blockade when taken with a nondepolarizing blocking drug include carbamazepine, hydantoins, ranitidine, and theophylline. Corticosteroids may result in prolonged muscle weakness.

Adverse reactions

A patient taking nondepolarizing drugs may experience these adverse reactions:
• apnea
• hypotension
• skin reactions
• bronchospasm
• excessive bronchial and salivary secretions.
    A patient taking pancuronium may also experience tachycardia, cardiac arrhythmias, and hypertension.

Nursing process

These nursing process steps are appropriate for patients undergoing treatment with nondepolarizing muscle relaxants.

Assessment

• Assess the patient's condition before therapy and regularly thereafter.
• Monitor the patient's baseline electrolyte levels (electrolyte imbalance can increase neuromuscular effects) and vital signs.
• Measure the patient's fluid intake and output; renal dysfunction may prolong the duration of action because 25% of the drug is unchanged before excretion.
• As ordered, provide nerve stimulator and train-of-four monitoring (a procedure in which electrodes are applied to the skin and electrical stimulation is delivered to measure the degree of neuromuscular blockade) to confirm the antagonism of neuromuscular blockade and recovery of muscle strength. Before attempting pharmacologic reversal with neostigmine, you should see some evidence of spontaneous recovery.
• Monitor the patient's respirations closely until he fully recovers from the neuromuscular blockade, as evidenced by tests of muscle strength (hand grip, head lift, and ability to cough).
• Assess the patient's skin for pressure areas and breakdown.
• Assess for incomplete closure of the eyelids (neuromuscular blockade results in loss of corneal reflex and blocks the action of eye muscles).
• Be alert for adverse reactions and drug interactions.
• Evaluate the patient's and family's knowledge of drug therapy.

Key nursing diagnoses

• Ineffective health maintenance related to condition
• Ineffective breathing pattern related to the drug's effect on respiratory muscles
• Deficient knowledge related to drug therapy

Planning outcome goals

• The patient's vital signs will remain within normal parameters while he's on drug therapy.
• The patient will maintain respiratory function as evidenced by adequate arterial blood gas (ABG) values and ventilatory parameters.
• The patient and his family will verbalize an understanding of the medication's purpose and intended effect.

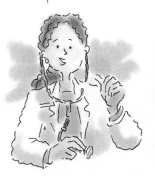

The patient's vital signs should remain normal while he's on drug therapy.

Education edge

Teaching about neuromuscular blocking drugs

If neuromuscular blocking drugs are prescribed, make sure to tell the patient what you're going to do before administering care. Review these points with the patient and his caregivers:

• The drug causes complete paralysis; therefore, expect to be unable to move or speak while receiving the drug. This experience can be very frightening.

• Expect to be unable to breathe (assistance will be provided).

• Expect to be aware of what's going on. The drug doesn't affect level of consciousness.

A reassuring word

The patient will be able to see, hear, and feel, and will be aware of his surroundings. Make sure to explain all events, and reassure the patient and his family.

• Tell the patient that someone will be with him at all times to try to anticipate his needs and explain what's going on.

• Assure the patient that he'll be monitored at all times.

• Tell the patient that pain and antianxiety medication will be provided, if appropriate.

• Tell the patient that eyedrops will be administered or his eyes may be covered to prevent drying of the cornea.

Implementation

• Administer sedatives or general anesthetics before neuromuscular blockers. Neuromuscular blockers don't reduce consciousness or alter the pain threshold. Give analgesics for pain. Note that general anesthetics should only be administered by qualified personnel, such as nurse-anesthetists or anesthesiologists.

• Keep in mind that neuromuscular blockers should be used only by personnel skilled in airway management.

• Mix the drug only with fresh solutions; precipitates form if alkaline solutions, such as barbiturate solutions, are used. Vecuronium may be given by rapid I.V. injection or diluted to be titrated in a drip form. Store reconstituted solutions in the refrigerator.

• Allow succinylcholine effects to subside before giving pancuronium.

• Store the drug in a refrigerator. Don't store it in plastic containers or syringes, although plastic syringes may be used for administration.

• Have emergency respiratory support equipment (ET equipment, ventilator, oxygen, atropine, edrophonium, epinephrine, and neostigmine) immediately available.

• Provide skin care and turning to prevent skin breakdown.

• Provide eye care, such as administering lubricating eyedrops and patching and taping eyelids, during neuromuscular blockade.

• When spontaneous recovery starts, drug-induced neuromuscular blockade may be reversed with an anticholinesterase (such as neostigmine or edrophonium), usually given with an anticholinergic such as atropine.

Evaluation

- Patient's condition improves.
- Patient maintains adequate ventilation with mechanical assistance.
- Patient and his family state an understanding of drug therapy.

(See *Teaching about neuromuscular blocking drugs*, page 79.)

Depolarizing blocking drugs

Succinylcholine is the only therapeutic depolarizing blocking drug. Although it's similar to the nondepolarizing blockers in its therapeutic effect, its mechanism of action differs. Succinylcholine acts like acetylcholine, but it isn't inactivated by cholinesterase. It's the drug of choice when short-term muscle relaxation is needed.

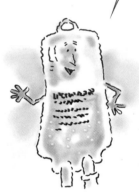

Because succinylcholine is absorbed poorly from the GI tract, the I.V. route is used most often.

Pharmacokinetics

Because succinylcholine is absorbed poorly from the GI tract, the I.V. route is the preferred administration method; the I.M. route can also be used if necessary.

Succinylcholine is hydrolyzed in the liver and plasma by the enzyme pseudocholinesterase, producing a metabolite with a nondepolarizing blocking action. It's excreted by the kidneys; a small amount is excreted unchanged.

Pharmacodynamics

After administration, succinylcholine is rapidly metabolized, although at a slower rate than acetylcholine. As a result, succinylcholine remains attached to receptor sites on the skeletal muscle membrane for a longer period. This prevents repolarization of the motor end plate and results in muscle paralysis.

Pharmacotherapeutics

Succinylcholine is the drug of choice for short-term muscle relaxation such as that needed during intubation and ECT.

Drug interactions

The action of succinylcholine is potentiated by a number of anesthetics and antibiotics. In contrast to their interaction with nondepolarizing blockers, anticholinesterases increase succinylcholine blockade.

Adverse reactions

The primary adverse reactions to succinylcholine are prolonged apnea, and hypotension.

Genetics: Raising the risk

The risk associated with succinylcholine is increased with certain genetic predispositions, such as a low pseudocholinesterase level and the tendency to develop malignant hyperthermia.

Nursing process

These nursing process steps are appropriate for patients receiving treatment with a depolarizing muscle relaxant.

Assessment

• Assess the patient's condition before therapy and regularly thereafter.
• Monitor the patient's baseline electrolyte determinations (electrolyte imbalance can increase neuromuscular effects) and vital signs.
• Measure the patient's fluid intake and output; renal dysfunction may prolong the duration of action because 25% of the drug is unchanged before excretion.
• As ordered, provide nerve stimulator and train-of-four monitoring are recommended to confirm the antagonism of the neuromuscular blockade and recovery of muscle strength.

Testing, testing...

• Monitor the patient's respirations closely until he fully recovers from the neuromuscular blockade, as evidenced by tests of muscle strength (handgrip, head lift, and ability to cough).
• Be alert for adverse reactions and drug interactions.
• Evaluate the patient's and family's knowledge of drug therapy.

Key nursing diagnoses

• Ineffective health maintenance related to the patient's condition
• Ineffective breathing pattern related to the drug's effect on respiratory muscles
• Deficient knowledge related to drug therapy

Planning outcome goals

• The patient's vital signs will remain within normal parameters while he's on drug therapy.
• The patient's will maintain respiratory function as evidenced by adequate ABG values and ventilatory parameters.

• The patient's family will verbalize an understanding of the medication's purpose and intended effect.

Implementation

• Succinylcholine is the drug of choice for short procedures (less than 3 minutes) and for orthopedic manipulations; use caution in the treatment of fractures or dislocations.
• Administer sedatives or general anesthetics before neuromuscular blockers. Neuromuscular blockers don't reduce consciousness or alter pain threshold. Give analgesics for pain. Note that general anesthesia and succinylcholine should only be administered by personnel skilled in airway management, such as nurse-anesthetists and anesthesiologists.
• Allow succinylcholine effects to subside before giving pancuronium.
• Have emergency respiratory support equipment (ET equipment, ventilator, oxygen, atropine, epinephrine) available for immediate use.
• For I.V. use, to evaluate the patient's ability to metabolize succinylcholine, give a test dose after he has been anesthetized. A normal response (no respiratory depression or transient depression for up to 5 minutes) indicates that the drug may be given. Don't give subsequent doses if the patient develops respiratory paralysis sufficient to permit ET intubation.
• For I.M. use, give deep I.M., preferably high into the deltoid.

The storage situation

• Store the injectable form in a refrigerator. Store the powder form at room temperature in a tightly closed container and use it immediately after reconstitution. Don't mix with alkaline solutions (thiopental sodium, sodium bicarbonate, or barbiturates).
• Reversing drugs shouldn't be used. Unlike what happens with nondepolarizing drugs, giving neostigmine or edrophonium with succinylcholine may worsen neuromuscular blockade.
• Continuous infusions of succinylcholine are not advised; this may reduce response or prolong muscle relaxation and apnea.

Evaluation

• Patient's condition improves.
• Patient maintains adequate ventilation with mechanical assistance.
• Patient and his family state an understanding of drug therapy. (See *Teaching about neuromuscular blocking drugs*, page 79.)

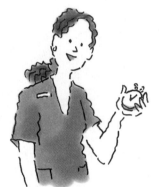

Succinylcholine is the drug of choice for short procedures— less than 3 minutes.

Antiparkinsonian drugs

Drug therapy is an important part of the treatment of Parkinson's disease, a progressive neurologic disorder characterized by four cardinal features:
- muscle rigidity (inflexibility)
- akinesia (loss of voluntary muscle movement)
- tremors at rest
- disturbances of posture and balance.

Upsetting the balance

Reduction of dopamine in the corpus striatum disturbs the normal balance between two neurotransmitters, acetylcholine and dopamine. When nerve cells in the brain become impaired, they can no longer produce dopamine. This results in a relative excess of acetylcholine. The excessive excitation caused by cholinergic activity creates the movement disorders of Parkinson's disease.

Defect in the dopamine pathway

Parkinson's disease affects the extrapyramidal system, which influences movement. The extrapyramidal system includes the corpus striatum, globus pallidus, and substantia nigra of the brain. In Parkinson's disease, dopamine deficiency occurs in the basal ganglia, the dopamine-releasing pathway that connects the substantia nigra to the corpus striatum.

Other culprits

Parkinsonism can also result from drugs, encephalitis, neurotoxins, trauma, arteriosclerosis, or other neurologic disorders and environmental factors.

Bringing back balance

The goal of drug therapy is to provide symptom relief and maintain the patient's independence and mobility. This can be achieved by correcting the imbalance of neurotransmitters in one of several ways, including:
- inhibiting cholinergic effects (with anticholinergic drugs)
- enhancing the effects of dopamine (with dopaminergic drugs)
- inhibiting catechol-O-methyltransferase (COMT) with COMT-inhibiting drugs.

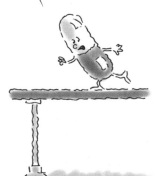

Drug therapy to correct the imbalance of neurotransmitters in patients with Parkinson's disease can help maintain mobility.

Anticholinergic drugs

Anticholinergic drugs are sometimes called *parasympatholytic drugs* because they inhibit the action of acetylcholine at special receptors in the parasympathetic nervous system. Anticholinergics used to treat Parkinson's disease include synthetic tertiary amines, such as benztropine, biperiden hydrochloride, biperiden lactate, procyclidine, and trihexyphenidyl.

Pharmacokinetics

Typically, anticholinergic drugs are well absorbed from the GI tract and cross the blood-brain barrier to their action site in the brain. Most are metabolized in the liver, at least partially, and are excreted by the kidneys as metabolites or unchanged drug. The exact distribution of these drugs is unknown.

Benztropine is a long-acting drug with a duration of action of up to 24 hours in some patients. For most anticholinergics, half-life is undetermined.

Pharmacodynamics

High acetylcholine levels produce an excitatory effect on the CNS, which can cause parkinsonian tremors. Patients with Parkinson's disease take anticholinergic drugs to inhibit the action of acetylcholine at receptor sites in the central and autonomic nervous systems, thus reducing tremors.

Pharmacotherapeutics

Anticholinergics are used to treat all forms of parkinsonism. They're most commonly used in the early stages of Parkinson's disease, when symptoms are mild and don't have a major impact on the patient's lifestyle.

Playing the percentages

These drugs effectively control sialorrhea (excessive flow of saliva) and are about 20% effective in reducing the incidence and severity of akinesia and rigidity.

Anticholinergics can be used alone or with amantadine in the early stages of Parkinson's disease. Anticholinergics can be given with levodopa during the later stages of Parkinson's disease to further relieve symptoms.

Drug interactions

Interactions can occur when certain medications are taken with anticholinergics:
• Amantadine can cause increased anticholinergic adverse effects.
• The absorption of levodopa can be decreased, which can lead to worsening of parkinsonian signs and symptoms.

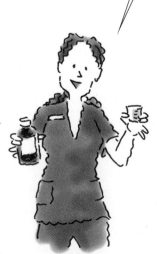

Over-the-counter cough and cold preparations, diet aids, and analeptics—which, unfortunately, includes caffeine—increase anticholinergic effects.

• Antipsychotics (such as phenothiazines, thiothixene, haloperidol, and loxapine) and anticholinergics taken together decrease the effectiveness of both drugs. The incidence of anticholinergic adverse effects can also increase.

• Over-the-counter cough and cold preparations, diet aids, and analeptics (drugs used to stay awake) increase anticholinergic effects.

• Alcohol increases CNS depression.

Adverse reactions

Mild, dose-related adverse reactions to anticholinergics are seen in 30% to 50% of patients. Dry mouth may be a dose-related reaction to trihexyphenidyl.

Cataloging common complaints

Some common adverse reactions to anticholinergic drugs include:
• confusion
• restlessness
• agitation and excitement
• drowsiness or insomnia
• tachycardia
• palpitations
• constipation
• nausea and vomiting
• urine retention
• increased intraocular pressure (IOP), blurred vision, pupil dilation, and photophobia.

Sensitivity-related reactions to anticholinergics can include hives and allergic rashes.

Senior sensitivity

Among elderly patients, increased sensitivity to anticholinergic drugs may occur. Signs and symptoms include mental confusion, agitation and, possibly, psychotic symptoms such as hallucinations.

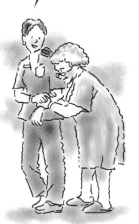

Elderly patients may have an increased sensitivity to anticholinergic drugs.

Nursing process

These nursing process steps are appropriate for patients undergoing treatment with anticholinergic drugs.

Assessment

• Obtain a baseline assessment of the patient's impairment.

• Monitor drug effectiveness by regularly checking body movements for signs of improvement; keep in mind that the full effect of the drug may take several days.

• Monitor the patient for adverse reactions and be alert for drug interactions. Some adverse reactions may result from atropine-like toxicity and are dose related.
• Monitor the patient's vital signs, especially during dosage adjustments.
• Evaluate the patient's and family's understanding of drug therapy.

Key nursing diagnoses
• Impaired physical mobility related to dyskinetic movements
• Risk for injury related to adverse CNS effects
• Urinary retention related to anticholinergic effects on the bladder
• Deficient knowledge related to drug therapy

Planning outcome goals
• The patient will exhibit improved mobility with a reduction in muscle rigidity, akinesia, and tremors.
• The patient's risk of injury will be reduced.
• The patient's voiding pattern won't change.
• The patient and his family will state an understanding of drug therapy.

Implementation
• Administer the drug with food to prevent GI irritation.
• Adjust the dosage according to the patient's response and tolerance.
• Never withdraw the drug abruptly; reduce the dosage gradually.
• Institute safety precautions.

Care for a drink? Candy? Gum?
• Provide ice chips, drinks, or sugarless hard candy or gum to relieve dry mouth. Increase fluid and fiber intake to prevent constipation as appropriate.
• Notify the prescriber about urine retention and be prepared to catheterize the patient if necessary.
• Give the drug at bedtime if the patient receives a single daily dose.

Evaluation
• Patient achieves highest mobility level possible.
• Patient remains free from injury.
• Patient has no change in voiding pattern.
• Patient and his family state an understanding of drug therapy.
(See *Teaching about antiparkinsonian drugs*.)

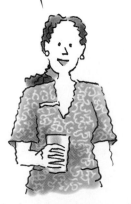

Providing ice chips, drinks, or sugarless hard candy or gum can help relieve dry mouth.

Education edge

Teaching about antiparkinsonian drugs

If antiparkinsonian drugs are prescribed, review these points with the patient and his caregivers:
• Take the drug exactly as prescribed and don't stop the drug suddenly.
• Take the drug with food to prevent GI upset. Don't crush or break tablets, especially catechol-O-methyltransferase (COMT) inhibitors, and take them at the same time as carbidopa-levodopa.
• To relieve dry mouth, suck on ice chips, take sips of water, suck on sugarless candy, or chew sugarless gum.
• Avoid hazardous tasks if adverse central nervous system effects occur. Also avoid alcohol use during therapy.
• Use caution when standing after a prolonged period of sitting or lying down because dizziness may occur, especially early in therapy.

• Report severe or persistent adverse reactions. Also report any uncontrolled movements of the body, chest pain, palpitations, depression or mood changes, difficulty voiding, or severe or persistent nausea or vomiting. With COMT inhibitors, hallucinations, increased dyskinesia, nausea, and diarrhea may occur.
• Don't take vitamins, herbal products, or over-the-counter preparations without consulting a health care provider.
• Be aware that COMT inhibitors may cause urine to turn brownish-orange.
• Tell all health care providers about the drug therapy.
• Schedule frequent rest periods to prevent overexertion and fatigue.
• Obtain regular medical follow-up, which is necessary to evaluate the effects of this drug.

Dopaminergic drugs

Dopaminergics include drugs that are chemically unrelated. These drugs increase the effects of dopamine at receptor sites and are useful in treating symptoms of Parkinson's disease. Examples include:
• levodopa, the metabolic precursor to dopamine
• carbidopa-levodopa, a combination drug composed of carbidopa and levodopa
• amantadine, an antiviral drug with dopamine activity
• bromocriptine, an ergot-type dopamine agonist
• ropinirole and pramipexole, two non-ergot-type dopamine agonists
• selegiline, a type B MAO inhibitor.

Pharmacokinetics

Like anticholinergic drugs, dopaminergic drugs are absorbed from the GI tract into the bloodstream and delivered to their action site in the brain. The body absorbs most levodopa, carbidopa-levodopa, pramipexole, or amantadine from the GI tract after oral administration, but only about 28% of bromocriptine is absorbed. Absorption of levodopa is slowed and reduced when it's ingested with food. In some patients, levodopa can significantly interact with foods. Dietary amino acids can decrease levodopa's effectiveness by competing with it for absorption from the intestine and slowing its transport to the brain. About 73% of an oral dose of selegiline is absorbed.

Levodopa is widely distributed in body tissues, including those in the GI tract, liver, pancreas, kidneys, salivary glands, and skin. Carbidopa-levodopa and pramipexole are also widely distributed. Amantadine is distributed in saliva, nasal secretions, and breast milk. Bromocriptine is highly protein bound. The distribution of selegiline is unknown.

Would you prefer the liver or the kidneys?

Dopaminergic drugs are metabolized extensively in various areas of the body and are eliminated by the liver, the kidneys, or both. Here are more specifics about the metabolism and excretion of dopaminergic drugs:
• Large amounts of levodopa are metabolized in the stomach and during the first pass through the liver. It's metabolized extensively and excreted by the kidneys.
• Carbidopa isn't metabolized extensively. The kidneys excrete approximately one-third of it unchanged within 24 hours. (See *Antiparkinsonian drugs: Carbidopa and levodopa.*)
• Amantadine, ropinirole, and pramipexole are excreted by the kidneys largely unchanged.
• Almost all of a bromocriptine dose is metabolized by the liver to pharmacologically inactive compounds and primarily eliminated in feces; only a small amount is excreted in urine.
• Selegiline is metabolized to amphetamine, methamphetamine, and N-desmethylselegiline (the major metabolite), which are eliminated in urine.

Pharmacodynamics

Dopaminergic drugs act in the brain to improve motor function in one of two ways: by increasing the dopamine concentration or by enhancing the neurotransmission of dopamine.

Two is better than one

Levodopa is inactive until it crosses the blood-brain barrier and is converted to dopamine by enzymes in the brain, increasing dopamine concentrations in the basal ganglia. Carbidopa enhances levodopa's effectiveness by blocking the peripheral conversion of L-dopa, thus permitting more levodopa to be transported to the brain.

The other dopaminergic drugs have various mechanisms of action:

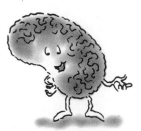

Dopaminergic drugs act in the brain to improve motor function by increasing dopamine concentration or enhancing the neurotransmission of dopamine. I'm feeling better already!

Prototype pro

Antiparkinsonian drugs: Carbidopa and levodopa

Actions
- Improves voluntary movement

Levodopa
- Chemical effect of levodopa unknown; thought to be carboxylated to dopamine, countering depletion of striatal dopamine in extrapyramidal centers

Carbidopa
- Inhibits peripheral decarboxylation of levodopa without affecting levodopa's metabolism within the central nervous system, making more levodopa available to be decarboxylated to dopamine in the brain

Indications
- Idiopathic Parkinson's disease
- Postencephalitic parkinsonism
- Symptomatic parkinsonism resulting from carbon monoxide or manganese intoxication

Nursing considerations
- If the patient is being treated with levodopa, discontinue the drug at least 8 hours before starting carbidopa-levodopa.
- The dosage should be adjusted according to the patient's response and tolerance.
- Withhold the dose and notify the prescriber if the patient's vital signs or mental status change significantly. A reduced dosage or discontinuation may be necessary.
- Monitor the patient for adverse effects, such as choreiform, dystonic, dyskinetic movements; involuntary grimacing; head movements; myoclonic jerks; ataxia; suicidal tendencies; hypotension; dry mouth; nausea and vomiting; signs and symptoms of hematologic disorders; and hepatoxicity.
- A patient on long-term therapy should be tested for acromegaly and diabetes.

- Amantadine's mechanism of action isn't clear. It's thought to release dopamine from intact neurons, but it may also have non-dopaminergic mechanisms.
- Bromocriptine, ropinirole, and pramipexole stimulate dopamine receptors in the brain, producing effects similar to those of dopamine.
- Selegiline can increase dopaminergic activity by inhibiting type B MAO activity or by other mechanisms.

Pharmacotherapeutics

The choice of therapy is highly individualized and is determined by the patient's symptoms and level of disability. A patient with mild Parkinson's disease with predominantly symptoms of tremor is commonly given anticholinergics or amantadine. Selegiline is indicated for extending the duration of levodopa by blocking its breakdown; it has also been used in early Parkinson's disorder because of its neuroprotective properties and potential to slow the progression of parkinsonism. Usually, dopaminergic drugs are used to treat the patient with severe Parkinson's disease or the patient who doesn't respond to anticholinergics alone.

Levodopa is the most effective drug used to treat Parkinson's disease. When fluctuations in response to levodopa occur, dosage adjustments and increased frequency of administration may be tried. Alternatively, adjunctive therapy, such as dopamine agonists, selegiline, amantadine, or a COMT inhibitor may be added. Controlled-release formulations of carbidopa-levodopa may be helpful in managing the wearing-off effect or delayed-onset motor fluctuations.

Add carbidopa, reduce levodopa

When carbidopa is given with levodopa, the dosage of levodopa can be reduced, decreasing the risk of GI and cardiovascular adverse effects. Levodopa is almost exclusively combined with carbidopa as the standard therapy for Parkinson's disease.

Tapered treatment

Some dopaminergic drugs, such as amantadine, levodopa, pramipexole, and bromocriptine, must be gradually tapered to avoid precipitating parkinsonian crisis (sudden marked clinical deterioration) and possible life-threatening complications (including a syndrome with muscle rigidity, elevated body temperature, tachycardia, mental changes, and increased serum creatine kinase [CK] resembling neuroleptic malignant syndrome).

Drug interactions

Dopaminergic drugs can interfere with many other drugs, causing potentially fatal reactions. Here are some examples:
• The effectiveness of levodopa can be reduced when taking pyridoxine (vitamin B_6), phenytoin, benzodiazepines, reserpine, and papaverine.
• Concomitant use with a type A MAO inhibitor, such as tranylcypromine, increases the risk of hypertensive crisis.
• Antipsychotics, such as phenothiazines, thiothixene, haloperidol, and loxapine, can reduce the effectiveness of levodopa.
• Amantadine may potentiate anticholinergic adverse effects of anticholinergic drugs, such as confusion and hallucinations, and can reduce the absorption of levodopa.
• Meperidine taken with selegiline at higher than recommended doses can cause a fatal reaction.

Adverse reactions

Adverse reactions to dopaminergic drugs vary with the drug prescribed.

Levodopa

Adverse effects of levodopa include:
- nausea and vomiting
- orthostatic hypotension
- anorexia
- neuroleptic malignant syndrome
- arrhythmias
- irritability
- confusion.

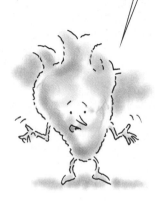

Levodopa can cause arrhythmias. Why me?

Amantadine

Adverse effects of amantadine include orthostatic hypotension and constipation.

Bromocriptine

Adverse effects of bromocriptine include:
- persistent orthostatic hypotension
- ventricular tachycardia
- bradycardia
- worsening angina.

Selegiline

Adverse effects of selegiline include:
- headache
- insomnia
- dizziness
- nausea
- arrhythmias.

Ropinirole and pramipexole

Adverse effects of ropinirole and pramipexole include:
- orthostatic hypotension
- dizziness
- confusion
- insomnia.

Nursing process

These nursing process steps are appropriate for patients undergoing treatment with dopaminergic drugs.

Assessment

- Assess the patient's underlying condition before therapy and regularly thereafter; therapeutic response usually follows each dose and disappears within 5 hours but may vary considerably.
- Monitor drug effectiveness by regularly checking body movements for signs of improvement; the full effect of the drug may take several days.

The telltale twitch

- Monitor the patient for adverse reactions and be alert for drug interactions. Some adverse reactions may result from atropine-like toxicity and are dose-related. Immediately report muscle twitching and blepharospasm (twitching of the eyelids), which may be early signs of drug overdose.
- Monitor the patient's vital signs, especially during dosage adjustments.
- Evaluate the patient's and family's understanding of drug therapy.

Key nursing diagnoses

- Impaired physical mobility related to dyskinetic movements
- Risk for injury related to adverse CNS effects
- Disturbed thought processes related to drug-induced CNS adverse reactions
- Deficient knowledge related to drug therapy

Planning outcome goals

- The patient will exhibit improved mobility with reduction in muscle rigidity, akinesia, and tremors.
- The patient's risk of injury will be reduced.
- The patient's voiding pattern won't change.
- The patient and his family will state an understanding of drug therapy.

Implementation

- Administer the drug (except levodopa) with food to prevent GI irritation.
- The dosage should be adjusted by the prescriber according to the patient's response and tolerance.
- Never withdraw the drug abruptly; reduce the dosage gradually.
- Withhold the dose and notify the prescriber if the patient's vital signs or mental status change significantly. A reduced dosage or discontinuation may be necessary.
- Institute safety precautions.

• Provide ice chips, drinks, or sugarless hard candy or gum to relieve dry mouth. Increase fluid and fiber intake to prevent constipation as appropriate.

Better at bedtime

• Give the drug at bedtime if the patient receives a single daily dose.
• If the patient is being treated with levodopa, discontinue the drug at least 8 hours before starting carbidopa-levodopa.
• Treat a patient with open-angle glaucoma with caution. Monitor him closely, watch for a change in intraocular pressure, and arrange for periodic eye exams.
• A patient receiving long-term therapy should be tested regularly for diabetes and acromegaly and should have periodic tests of liver, renal, and hematopoietic function.

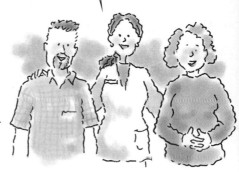

Patient and family understanding is important with any type of drug therapy.

Evaluation

• Patient exhibits improved mobility with a reduction of muscular rigidity and tremor.
• Patient remains free from injury.
• Patient remains mentally alert.
• Patient and his family state an understanding of drug therapy.
(See *Teaching about antiparkinsonian drugs*, page 87.)

COMT inhibitors

COMT inhibitors are used as adjunctive treatments to carbidopa-levodopa in the management of a patient with Parkinson's disease who experiences "wearing off" at the end of the dosing interval.

Choice of two

Two COMT inhibitors are currently available:
• tolcapone
• entacapone.

Pharmacokinetics

Tolcapone and entacapone are rapidly absorbed by the GI tract, and absolute bioavailability of each agent is 65% and 35%, respectively. Both drugs are highly bound to albumin and, therefore, have limited distribution to the tissues. They're almost completely metabolized in the liver to inactive metabolites and are excreted in urine.

Pharmacodynamics

Tolcapone and entacapone are selective and reversible inhibitors of COMT, the major metabolizing enzyme for levodopa in the presence of a decarboxylase inhibitor such as carbidopa. Inhibition of COMT alters the pharmacokinetics for levodopa, leading to sustained plasma levels of levodopa. This results in more sustained dopaminergic stimulation in the brain and improvement in the signs and symptoms of Parkinson's disease.

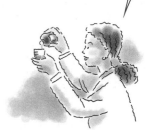

Combining COMT inhibitors with carbidopa-levodopa may reduce wearing-off effects at the end of a dosing interval.

Pharmacotherapeutics

Tolcapone or entacapone may be added to carbidopa-levodopa in a patient who experiences a wearing-off effect at the end of a dosing interval or random on-off fluctuations in response to carbidopa-levodopa. COMT inhibitors have no antiparkinsonian effect when used alone and should always be combined with carbidopa-levodopa. Addition of a COMT inhibitor commonly necessitates a decrease in the dose of carbidopa-levodopa, particularly in the patient receiving a levodopa dose of more than 800 mg.

Not so fast!

Rapid withdrawal of COMT inhibitors may lead to parkinsonian crisis and may cause a syndrome of muscle rigidity, high fever, tachycardia, confusion, and elevated serum CK similar to neuroleptic malignant syndrome. A slow tapering of the dosage is suggested to avoid rapid withdrawal.

Drug interactions

COMT inhibitors can interfere with many drugs. Here are some examples:
• COMT inhibitors shouldn't be used concurrently with type A MAO inhibitors, but may be used with selegiline.
• Significant arrhythmias may result when COMT inhibitors are combined with catecholamine drugs (such as dopamine, dobutamine, epinephrine, methyldopa, and norepinephrine).
• The use of COMT inhibitors with CNS depressants (benzodiazepines, tricyclic antidepressants, antipsychotics, ethanol, opioid analgesics, and other sedative hypnotics) may cause additive CNS effects.
• Entacapone chelates iron and, therefore, iron absorption may be decreased.
• Because of MAO inhibition, COMT inhibitors shouldn't be taken concomitantly with linezolid.
• Fibrotic complications have been associated with the use of entacapone and bromocriptine.

• Drugs that interfere with glucuronidation (erythromycin, rifampin, cholestyramine, and probenecid) may decrease entacapone elimination.
• When using COMT inhibitors for a patient on dopaminergic therapy, the potential for orthostatic hypotension may be increased.

Adverse reactions

Common adverse reactions to COMT inhibitors include:
• nausea
• dyskinesia
• diarrhea
• brown orange urine discoloration (entacapone)
• hyperkinesia or hypokinesia.
    Less common adverse reactions include:
• orthostatic hypotension
• syncope
• dizziness
• fatigue
• abdominal pain
• constipation
• vomiting
• dry mouth
• back pain
• diaphoresis.

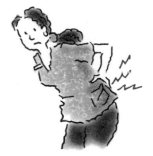

Thank goodness back pain is one of the less common adverse reactions to COMT inhibitors!

You bet your life!

Life-threatening reactions to COMT inhibitors include acute liver failure. Because of this risk, tolcapone should be used only in a patient with Parkinson's disease who experiences fluctuations in levodopa response and doesn't respond to or isn't an appropriate candidate for other adjunctive therapies. The patient should be advised of the risks of liver injury, and written informed consent should be obtained before drug administration. Liver function tests should be obtained at baseline and every 2 weeks for the first year, every 4 weeks for the next 3 months, and every 8 weeks thereafter.

Nursing process

These nursing process steps are appropriate for patients undergoing treatment with COMT inhibitors.

Assessment

• Assess the patient's hepatic and biliary function before starting therapy.

• Monitor the patient's blood pressure closely. Watch for orthostatic hypotension.
• Monitor the patient for hallucinations.
• Evaluate the patient's and family's knowledge of drug therapy.

Key nursing diagnoses

• Impaired physical mobility related to presence of parkinsonism
• Disturbed thought processes related to drug-induced adverse reactions
• Deficient knowledge related to drug therapy

Planning outcome goals

• The patient's physical mobility will improve.
• The patient will be alert and able to verbalize orientation adequately.
• The patient and his family will verbalize an understanding of drug therapy.

Implementation

• Give the drug with immediate or sustained-release carbidopa-levodopa as ordered, with or without food.
• Check to see that the drug is used only with carbidopa-levodopa; no antiparkinsonian effects will occur when the drug is given as monotherapy.
• Keep in mind that carbidopa-levodopa dosage requirements are usually lower when given with entacapone; the carbidopa-levodopa dosage should be lowered or the dosing interval should be increased to avoid adverse effects.
• Keep in mind that the drug may cause or worsen dyskinesia despite a reduced levodopa dosage.
• Watch the patient for onset of diarrhea, which usually begins 4 to 12 weeks after therapy starts but may begin as early as the first week or as late as many months.
• Keep in mind that rapid withdrawal or abrupt reduction in the dosage could lead to signs and symptoms of Parkinson's disease; it may also lead to hyperpyrexia and confusion, a symptom complex resembling neuroleptic malignant syndrome. Discontinue the drug slowly and monitor the patient closely. Adjust other dopaminergic treatments.
• Observe for urine discoloration.
• Watch for signs of rhabdomyolysis, which can rarely occur with drug use.

Evaluation

• Patient exhibits improved physical mobility.
• Patient maintains normal thought processes.

• Patient and his family state an understanding of drug therapy. (See *Teaching about antiparkinsonian drugs*, page 87.)

Anticonvulsant drugs

Anticonvulsant drugs inhibit neuromuscular transmission. They can be prescribed for:
• long-term management of chronic epilepsy (recurrent seizures)
• short-term management of acute isolated seizures not caused by epilepsy such as seizures after trauma or brain surgery.

In addition, some anticonvulsants are used in the emergency treatment of status epilepticus (a continuous seizure state).

Try one, then another, before together

Treatment of epilepsy should begin with a single drug, increasing the dosage until seizures are controlled or adverse effects become problematic. Generally, a second alternative should be tried as monotherapy before considering combination therapy. Choice of drug treatment depends on the seizure type, the drug's characteristics, and the patient's preferences.

Class discussion

Anticonvulsants can be categorized into several major classes:
• hydantoins
• barbiturates
• iminostilbenes
• benzodiazepines
• carboxylic acid derivatives
• 1 (aminomethyl) cyclohexane acetic acid
• phenyltriazine
• carboxamide
• sulfamate-substituted monosaccharides
• succinimides
• sulfonamides.

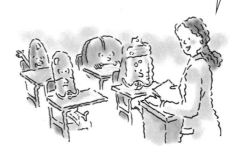

Anticonvulsants can be categorized into several major classes.

Hydantoins

The two most commonly prescribed anticonvulsant drugs—phenytoin and phenytoin sodium—belong to the hydantoin class. Other hydantoins include fosphenytoin and ethotoin.

Pharmacokinetics

The pharmacokinetics of hydantoins varies from drug to drug.

Phenytoin: Slow start, fast finish

Phenytoin is absorbed slowly after oral and I.M. administration. It's distributed rapidly to all tissues and is highly (90%) protein bound. Phenytoin is metabolized in the liver. Inactive metabolites are excreted in bile and then reabsorbed from the GI tract. Eventually, however, they're excreted in urine.

Ethotoin: Moves out as metabolites

Ethotoin is metabolized by the liver. Extensively protein bound, ethotoin is excreted in urine, primarily as metabolites.

Fosphenytoin: A short-term solution

Fosphenytoin is indicated for short-term I.M. or I.V. administration. It's widely distributed throughout the body, is highly (90%) protein bound, and is metabolized by the liver and excreted in urine.

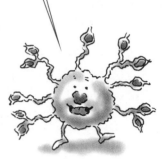

Hydantoins stabilize us nerve cells to keep us from getting overexcited!!! Okay, calming down, now...

Pharmacodynamics

In most cases, the hydantoin anticonvulsants stabilize nerve cells to keep them from getting overexcited. Phenytoin appears to work in the motor cortex of the brain, where it stops the spread of seizure activity. The pharmacodynamics of fosphenytoin and ethotoin are thought to mimic those of phenytoin.

Pharmacotherapeutics

Because of its effectiveness and relatively low toxicity, phenytoin is the most commonly prescribed anticonvulsant and one of the drugs of choice to treat:
• complex partial seizures (also called *psychomotor* or *temporal lobe seizures*)
• tonic-clonic seizures.

The enzyme system responsible for the metabolism of phenytoin is saturable. A change in dose can result in disproportional changes in serum concentration. (See *Anticonvulsants: Phenytoin.*)

Resistance is futile

Health care providers sometimes prescribe ethotoin in combination with other anticonvulsants for partial and tonic-clonic seizures in patients who are resistant to or intolerant of other anticonvulsants. Phenytoin and fosphenytoin are the long-acting anticonvulsants of choice to treat status epilepticus after initial I.V. benzodiazepines.

Prototype pro

Anticonvulsants: Phenytoin

Actions
• Stabilizes neuronal membranes and limits seizure activity by either increasing efflux or decreasing influx of sodium ions across cell membranes in the motor cortex during generation of nerve impulses

Indications
• Control of tonic-clonic and complex partial seizures
• Status epilepticus
• Prevention of and treatment for seizures during neurosurgery

Nursing considerations
• Monitor the patient for adverse effects, such as ataxia, slurred speech, mental confusion, nystagmus, blurred vision, gingival hyperplasia, nausea, vomiting, hematologic disorders, hepatitis, Stevens-Johnson syndrome, and hirsutism.
• Don't withdraw the drug suddenly; seizures may occur.
• Monitor drug levels as ordered; therapeutic levels range from 10 to 20 mcg/ml.

Drug interactions

Hydantoins interact with several drugs. Here are some drug interactions of major to moderate clinical significance:
• The effect of phenytoin is reduced when taken with phenobarbital, diazoxide, theophylline, carbamazepine, rifampin, antacids, and sucralfate.

Oral interference

• Enteral tube feedings may interfere with the absorption of oral phenytoin. Stop feedings for 2 hours before and after phenytoin administration.
• The effect of phenytoin is increased and the risk of toxicity increases when phenytoin is taken with allopurinol, cimetidine, disulfiram, fluconazole, isoniazid, omeprazole, sulfonamides, oral anticoagulants, chloramphenicol, valproic acid, and amiodarone.
• The effect of the following drugs is reduced when taken with a hydantoin anticonvulsant: oral anticoagulants, levodopa, amiodarone, corticosteroids, doxycycline, methadone, metyrapone, quinidine, theophylline, thyroid hormone, hormonal contraceptives, valproic acid, cyclosporine, and carbamazepine.

Adverse reactions

Adverse reactions to hydantoins include:
• drowsiness

- ataxia
- irritability and restlessness
- headache
- nystagmus
- dizziness and vertigo
- dysarthria
- nausea and vomiting
- abdominal pain
- anorexia
- depressed atrial and ventricular conduction
- ventricular fibrillation (in toxic states)
- bradycardia, hypotension, and cardiac arrest (with I.V. administration)
- hypersensitivity reactions.

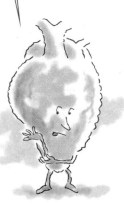

Bradycardia, hypotension, and cardiac arrest can occur with I.V. administration of hydantoins.

Nursing process

These nursing process steps are appropriate for patients undergoing treatment with hydantoin anticonvulsant drugs.

Assessment

- Monitor the patient's response to the prescribed drug and serum levels as indicated.
- Assess the patient's condition before therapy and regularly thereafter.
- Monitor the patient's blood levels; the therapeutic level for phenytoin is 10 to 20 mcg/ml.
- Monitor CBC and calcium level every 6 months.
- Periodically monitor hepatic function.
- Check the patient's vital signs, blood pressure, and electrocardiography (ECG) during I.V. administration.
- Monitor the patient for adverse reactions.
- Assess the patient's compliance with therapy at each follow-up visit.
- Monitor the patient for increased seizure activity; mononucleosis may decrease the phenytoin level.
- Evaluate the patient's and family's knowledge of drug therapy.

Key nursing diagnoses

- Risk for injury related to adverse reactions
- Impaired physical mobility related to sedation
- Deficient knowledge related to drug therapy
- Noncompliance related to long-term therapy

Planning outcome goals

- Risk of injury to the patient will be minimized.

• The patient will be able to perform activities of daily living (ADLs).
• The patient and his family will verbalize an understanding of drug therapy.
• The patient will use support systems to help modify noncompliant behavior.

Implementation

• Administer oral forms with food to reduce GI irritation.
• Phenytoin binds with tube feedings, thus decreasing the absorption of the drug. Turn off tube feedings for 2 hours before and after giving phenytoin, according to your facility's policy.

Forecast: Chance of precipitation

• If using as an infusion, don't mix the drug with dextrose 5% in water (D_5W) because phenytoin will precipitate. Clear I.V. tubing first with normal saline solution. Mix with normal saline solution if necessary and infuse over 30 to 60 minutes with an in-line filter.
• Avoid giving phenytoin by I.V. push into veins on the back of the hand to avoid discoloration known as *purple glove syndrome.* Inject into larger veins or a central venous catheter, if available.
• Discard any unused drug 4 hours after preparation for I.V. administration.
• Don't give phenytoin I.M. unless dosage adjustments are made. The drug may precipitate at the site, cause pain, and be erratically absorbed.
• Expect to adjust the dosage according to the patient's response.
• Administer safety precautions if the patient has an adverse CNS reaction.

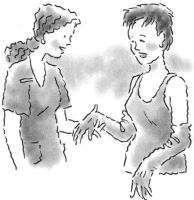

No, I don't think this is what is meant by a case of purple glove syndrome...

Evaluation

• Patient sustains no injury from adverse reactions.
• Patient is free from seizure activity.
• Patient maintains physical mobility.
• Patient complies with therapy and has no seizures.
• Patient and his family state an understanding of drug therapy.
(See *Teaching about anticonvulsants,* page 102.)

Education edge

Teaching about anticonvulsants

If anticonvulsants are prescribed, review these points with the patient and his caregivers:
• Take the drug exactly as prescribed and don't stop the drug without medical supervision. The drug must be taken regularly to be effective.
• Take the drug with food to reduce GI upset and loss of appetite. Eating small, frequent meals can help.
• Don't change brands or dosage forms.
• Avoid hazardous activities that require mental alertness if adverse central nervous system reactions occur.
• Wear or carry medical identification at all times.
• Record and report any seizure activity while taking the drug.
• Don't stop the drug abruptly. If for some reason you can't continue taking the drug, notify the health care provider at once; the drug must be slowly withdrawn when it's discontinued.

• Try to space activities throughout the day and allow rest periods to avoid fatigue, weakness, and drowsiness. Take safety precautions and avoid driving or operating dangerous machinery if these conditions occur.
• Report persistent or bothersome adverse effects to the health care provider.
• Perform oral hygiene and see a dentist for regular examinations, especially if taking phenytoin or its derivatives.
• Be aware that phenytoin may discolor urine pink, red, or red-brown.
• Don't take over-the-counter medications or herbal preparations without first consulting your health care provider.
• Be aware that heavy alcohol use may diminish the drug's benefit.
• Make sure you have regular medical follow-up, possibly including blood tests, to help evaluate the effects of the drug.

Barbiturates

Formerly one of the most widely used anticonvulsants, the long-acting barbiturate phenobarbital is now used less frequently because of its sedative effects. Phenobarbital is sometimes used for long-term treatment of epilepsy and is prescribed selectively for treatment of status epilepticus if hydantoins aren't effective.

Other options

Mephobarbital, also a long-acting barbiturate, is sometimes used as an anticonvulsant. Primidone, a structural analog of phenobarbital that's closely related chemically to the barbiturate-derivative anticonvulsants, is also used in the chronic treatment of epilepsy.

Pharmacokinetics

Each barbiturate has a slightly different set of pharmacokinetic properties.

Phenobarbital for the long haul

Although absorbed slowly, phenobarbital is well absorbed from the GI tract. Peak plasma concentration levels occur 8 to 12 hours after a single dose. The drug is 20% to 45% bound to serum proteins and to a similar extent to other tissues, including the brain. The liver metabolizes about 75% of a phenobarbital dose, and 25% is excreted unchanged in urine.

Mephobarbital: A master metabolizer

Almost half of a mephobarbital dose is absorbed from the GI tract, and it's well distributed in body tissues. The drug is bound to tissue and plasma proteins. Mephobarbital undergoes extensive metabolism by the liver; only 1% to 2% is excreted unchanged in urine.

Primidone evens out

Approximately 60% to 80% of a primidone dose is absorbed from the GI tract, and it's distributed evenly among body tissues. The drug is protein bound to a small extent in the plasma. Primidone is metabolized by the liver to two active metabolites, phenobarbital and phenylethylmalonamide (PEMA). From 15% to 25% of primidone is excreted unchanged in urine, 15% to 25% is metabolized to phenobarbital, and 50% to 70% is excreted in urine as PEMA.

Pharmacodynamics

Barbiturates exhibit anticonvulsant action at doses below those that produce hypnotic effects. For this reason, the barbiturates usually don't produce addiction when used to treat epilepsy. Barbiturates elevate the seizure threshold by decreasing postsynaptic excitation.

Pharmacotherapeutics

The barbiturate anticonvulsants are effective alternative therapy for:
- partial seizures
- tonic-clonic seizures
- febrile seizures.

Barbiturates can be used alone or with other anticonvulsants. I.V. phenobarbital is also used to treat status epilepticus. The major disadvantage of using phenobarbital for status epilepticus is a delayed onset of action when an immediate response is needed. Barbiturate anticonvulsants are ineffective in treating absence seizures.

"Ph" before "pr"

Mephobarbital has no advantage over phenobarbital and is used when the patient can't tolerate phenobarbital's adverse effects. In general, because of monitoring, costs, and dosing frequency, phenobarbital is tried before primidone. Primidone may be effective in a patient who doesn't respond to phenobarbital.

Drug interactions

Here are some drug interactions of barbiturates:
• The effects of barbiturates can be reduced when taken with rifampin.
• The risk of toxicity increases when phenobarbital is taken with CNS depressants, valproic acid, chloramphenicol, felbamate, cimetidine, or phenytoin.
• The metabolism of corticosteroids, cimetidine, or phenytoin can be enhanced with phenobarbital therapy, leading to decreased effects. Evening primrose oil may increase anticonvulsant dosage requirements.

Reduced rates

In addition, the effects of many drugs can be reduced when taken with a barbiturate, including such drugs as beta-adrenergic blockers, corticosteroids, digoxin, estrogens, doxycycline, oral anticoagulants, hormonal contraceptives, quinidine, phenothiazine, metronidazole, tricyclic antidepressants, theophylline, cyclosporine, carbamazepine, felodipine, and verapamil.

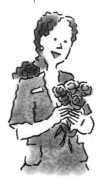

Evening primrose oil may increase anticonvulsant dosage requirements.

Adverse reactions

Adverse reactions to phenobarbital and mephobarbital include:
• drowsiness
• lethargy
• dizziness
• nystagmus, confusion, and ataxia (with large doses)
• laryngospasm, respiratory depression, and hypotension (when administered I.V.).

And then some

Primidone can cause the same CNS and GI adverse reactions as phenobarbital. It can also cause acute psychoses, hair loss, impotence, and osteomalacia.

As a group

All three barbiturate anticonvulsants can produce hypersensitivity rashes and other rashes, lupuslike syndrome (an inflammatory disorder), and enlarged lymph nodes.

Nursing process

These nursing process steps are appropriate for patients undergoing treatment with barbiturate anticonvulsant drugs.

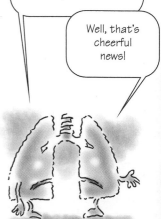

When given I.V., phenobarbital and mephobarbital can sometimes cause respiratory depression.

Well, that's cheerful news!

Assessment
• Monitor the patient's response to the prescribed drug and serum levels, as indicated.
• Assess the patient's condition before therapy and regularly thereafter.
• Monitor the patient's blood level closely as indicated.
• Monitor the patient for adverse reactions.
• Assess the patient's compliance with therapy at each follow-up visit.

Key nursing diagnoses
• Risk for injury related to adverse reactions
• Impaired physical mobility related to sedation
• Noncompliance related to long-term therapy

Planning outcome goals
• Risk of injury to the patient will be minimized.
• The patient will be able to perform ADLs.
• The patient will verbalize factors that contribute to noncompliance.

Implementation
• Administer oral forms of the drug with food to reduce GI irritation.
• I.V. phenobarbital is reserved for emergency treatment; monitor the patient's respirations closely and don't give more than 60 mg/minute. Have resuscitation equipment available.
• Don't stop the drug abruptly because seizures may worsen. Call the prescriber immediately if adverse reactions occur.

Nothing superficial about it
• Give the I.M. injection deeply. Superficial injection may cause pain, sterile abscess, and tissue sloughing.
• Expect to adjust the dosage according to the patient's response.
• Administer safety precautions if the patient has adverse CNS reactions.

Evaluation
• Patient sustains no trauma from adverse reactions.
• Patient maintains physical mobility.
• Patient complies with therapy and has no seizures.

Iminostilbenes

Carbamazepine is the most commonly used iminostilbene anticonvulsant. It effectively treats:
- partial and generalized tonic-clonic seizures
- mixed seizure types
- complex partial seizures (first choice of treatment).

Pharmacokinetics

Carbamazepine is absorbed slowly from the GI tract, is metabolized in the liver by the cytochrome P-450 isoform 3A4 (CYP3A4), and is excreted in urine. Carbamazepine is distributed rapidly to all tissues; 75% to 90% is bound to plasma proteins. The half-life varies greatly.

Pharmacodynamics

Carbamazepine's anticonvulsant effect is similar to that of phenytoin. The anticonvulsant action of the drug can occur because of its ability to inhibit the spread of seizure activity or neuromuscular transmission in general.

Pharmacotherapeutics

Carbamazepine is the drug of choice, in adults and children, for treating:
- generalized tonic-clonic seizures
- simple and complex partial seizures.

Neutralizes neuralgia, benefits bipolar

Carbamazepine also relieves pain when used to treat trigeminal neuralgia (tic douloureux, characterized by excruciating facial pain along the trigeminal nerve) and may be useful in some psychiatric disorders, such as bipolar affective disorder and intermittent explosive disorder. Carbamazepine may increase absence or myoclonic seizures and isn't recommended for treatment for these types of seizures.

Drug interactions

Carbamazepine can reduce the effects of several drugs, including oral anticoagulants, haloperidol, bupropion, lamotrigine, tricyclic antidepressants, hormonal contraceptives, doxycycline, felbamate, theophylline, and valproic acid.

Other drug interactions can also occur:
- Increased carbamazepine levels and toxicity can occur with cimetidine, danazol, diltiazem, erythromycin, isoniazid, selective

serotonin reuptake inhibitors (SSRIs), propoxyphene, troleandomycin, ketoconazole, valproic acid, and verapamil.
• Lithium and carbamazepine taken together increase the risk of
toxic neurologic effects.
• Carbamazepine levels can decrease when taken with barbiturates, felbamate, or phenytoin.
• Plantain may inhibit GI absorption.

Adverse reactions

Occasionally, serious hematologic toxicity occurs. Because
carbamazepine is related structurally to the tricyclic antidepressants, it can cause similar toxicities and affect behaviors and emotions. Hives and Stevens-Johnson syndrome (a
potentially fatal inflammatory disease) can occur. Rashes
are the most common hypersensitivity response.

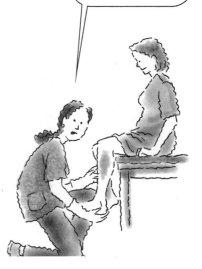

Rashes are the
most common
hypersensitivity
response to
carbamazepine.

Nursing process

These nursing process steps are appropriate for patients
undergoing treatment with iminostilbene anticonvulsant
drugs.

Assessment
• Assess the patient's seizure disorder or trigeminal neuralgia be-
fore therapy and regularly thereafter.
• Obtain baseline determinations of urinalysis, blood urea nitrogen level, liver function, CBC, platelet and reticulocyte counts,
and iron level. Reassess regularly.
• Monitor drug level and drug effects closely; the therapeutic level ranges from 4 to 12 mcg/ml.
• Monitor the patient's response to the prescribed drug and serum
levels, as indicated.
• Monitor the patient for adverse reactions.
• Assess the patient's compliance with therapy at each follow-up
visit.

Key nursing diagnoses
• Risk for injury related to adverse reactions
• Impaired physical mobility related to sedation
• Noncompliance related to long-term therapy

Planning outcome goals
• Risk of injury to the patient will be minimized.
• The patient will be able to perform ADLs.
• The patient will exhibit behaviors that comply with the health
care regimen.

Implementation

- Administer oral forms with food to reduce GI irritation. Give the drug in divided doses when possible to maintain a consistent blood level.

Shake it up!

- Shake an oral suspension well before measuring the dose.
- When giving the drug by nasogastric tube, mix the dose with an equal volume of water, normal saline solution, or D_5W. Flush the tube with 100 ml of diluent after administering the dose.
- Expect to adjust the dosage according to the patient's response.
- Administer safety precautions if the patient has adverse CNS reactions.
- Never suddenly discontinue the drug when treating seizures or status epilepticus.
- Notify the prescriber immediately if adverse reactions occur.

Evaluation

- Patient sustains no injury from adverse reactions.
- Patient maintains physical mobility.
- Patient complies with therapy and has no seizures.

Benzodiazepines

The four benzodiazepine drugs that provide anticonvulsant effects are:
- diazepam (in the parenteral form)
- clonazepam
- clorazepate
- lorazepam.

Only one for ongoing treatment

Only clonazepam is recommended for long-term treatment of epilepsy. Diazepam is restricted to acute treatment of status epilepticus and rectally for repetitive seizures. I.V. lorazepam is considered the drug of choice for acute management of status epilepticus. Clorazepate is prescribed as an adjunct in treating partial seizures.

Pharmacokinetics

The patient can receive benzodiazepines orally, parenterally or, in special situations, rectally. These drugs are absorbed rapidly and almost completely from the GI tract but are distributed at different rates. Protein binding of benzodiazepines ranges from 85% to 90%.

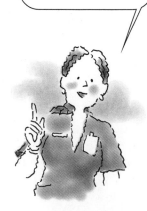

There's only one benzodiazepine recommended for the long-term treatment of epilepsy—clonazepam.

Benzodiazepines are metabolized in the liver to multiple metabolites and are then excreted in urine. The benzodiazepines readily cross the placenta and are excreted in breast milk.

Pharmacodynamics

Benzodiazepines act as:
- anticonvulsants
- antianxiety agents
- sedative-hypnotics
- muscle relaxants.

Their mechanism of action is poorly understood.

Pharmacotherapeutics

Each of the benzodiazepines can be used in slightly different ways:
- Clonazepam is used to treat absence (petit mal), atypical absence (Lennox-Gastaut syndrome), atonic, and myoclonic seizures.
- I.V. lorazepam is currently considered the benzodiazepine of choice for status epilepticus.
- I.V. diazepam is used to control status epilepticus. Because diazepam provides only short-term effects of less than 1 hour, the patient must also be given a long-acting anticonvulsant, such as phenytoin or phenobarbital, during diazepam therapy.

Reining in repetitive seizures

- Diazepam rectal gel is approved for the treatment of repetitive seizures and has reduced the incidence of recurrent seizures in children.
- Diazepam isn't recommended for long-term treatment because of its potential for addiction and the high serum concentrations required to control seizures.
- Clorazepate is used with other drugs to treat partial seizures.

Drug interactions

When benzodiazepines are taken with CNS depressants, sedative and other depressant effects become enhanced. This can cause motor skill impairment, respiratory depression, and even death at high doses.

Cimetidine and hormonal contraceptives taken with a benzodiazepine drug can also cause excessive sedation and CNS depression.

Adverse reactions

The most common adverse reactions to benzodiazepines include:
- drowsiness
- confusion
- ataxia
- weakness
- dizziness
- nystagmus
- vertigo
- fainting
- dysarthria
- headache
- tremor
- glassy-eyed appearance.

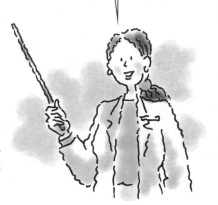

These are the most common adverse reactions to benzodiazepines.

Comin' round the less common bend

Less common adverse reactions include respiratory depression and decreased heart rate (with high doses and with I.V. diazepam) as well as rash and acute hypersensitivity reactions.

Nursing process

These nursing process steps are appropriate for patients undergoing treatment with benzodiazepine anticonvulsant drugs.

Assessment
- Obtain a history of the patient's underlying condition before therapy and reassess regularly thereafter.
- Monitor the patient's respiratory rate every 5 to 15 minutes and before each repeated I.V. dose.
- Periodically monitor liver, kidney, and hematopoietic function studies in a patient receiving repeated or prolonged therapy.
- Monitor the patient's response to prescribed drug and serum levels as indicated.
- Monitor the patient for adverse reactions.
- Assess the patient's compliance with therapy at each follow-up visit.

Key nursing diagnoses
- Risk for injury related to adverse reactions
- Impaired physical mobility related to sedation
- Noncompliance related to long-term therapy
- Deficient knowledge related to drug therapy

Planning outcome goals

• Risk of injury to the patient will be minimized.
• The patient will be able to perform ADLs.
• The patient will verbalize factors that contribute to noncompliance.
• The patient and his family will verbalize an understanding of drug therapy.

Implementation

• Administer oral forms of the drug with food to reduce GI irritation. If an oral concentrate solution is used, dilute the dose immediately before administering. Use water, juice, or carbonated beverages, or mix with semisolid foods, such as applesauce or pudding.
• Avoid use of diazepam rectal gel for more than five episodes per month or one episode every 5 days.
• If giving the I.V. form of diazepam, administer no more than 5 mg/minute and inject directly into a vein or watch the insertion site closely.
• Have emergency resuscitation equipment and oxygen at the bedside when giving these drugs I.V.
• Use I.M. forms only when the I.V. and oral routes aren't applicable; I.M. forms aren't recommended because absorption is variable and injection is painful.
• Don't store parenteral diazepam solutions in plastic syringes.
• Expect to adjust the dosage according to the patient's response.
• Administer safety precautions if the patient has adverse CNS reactions.

Evaluation

• Patient sustains no trauma from adverse reactions.
• Patient maintains physical mobility.
• Patient complies with therapy and has no seizures.
• Patient and his family state an understanding of drug therapy.

Parenteral diazepam solutions shouldn't be stored in plastic syringes. Got it?

Got it.

Carboxylic acid derivatives

The drugs in this class are:
• valproate
• valproic acid
• divalproex.

Pharmacokinetics

Valproate is converted rapidly to valproic acid in the stomach. Divalproex is a precursor of valproic acid that separates into valproic acid in the GI tract. Valproic acid is a hepatic enzyme inhibitor. It's absorbed well, strongly protein bound, and metabolized in the liver. Metabolites and unchanged drug are excreted in urine.

Valproic acid readily crosses the placental barrier and also appears in breast milk.

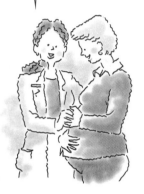

Keep in mind that valproic acid crosses the placental barrier and appears in breast milk.

Pharmacodynamics

The mechanism of action for valproic acid remains unknown. It's thought to increase levels of GABA, an inhibitory neurotransmitter, as well as having a direct-membrane stabilizing effect. (See *Happy accident.*)

Pharmacotherapeutics

Valproic acid is prescribed for long-term treatment of:
• absence seizures
• myoclonic seizures
• tonic-clonic seizures
• partial seizures.

Baby blues

Valproic acid may also be useful for neonatal seizures. However, it must be used cautiously in children younger than 2 years old, particularly those receiving multiple anticonvulsants, those with congenital metabolic disorders or hepatic disease, those with severe seizures and mental retardation, and those with organic brain disease. For these patients, the drug carries a risk of potentially fatal liver toxicity (usually within the first 6 months of treatment). This risk limits the use of valproic acid as a drug of choice for seizure disorders.

Drug interactions

Here are the most significant drug interactions associated with valproic acid:
• Cimetidine, aspirin, erythromycin, and felbamate may increase levels of valproic acid.
• Carbamazepine, lamotrigine, phenobarbital, primidone, phenytoin, and rifampin may decrease levels of valproic acid.
• Valproic acid may decrease the effects of lamotrigine, phenobarbital, primidone, benzodiazepines, CNS depressants, warfarin, and zidovudine.

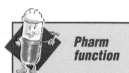

Pharm function

Happy accident

The anticonvulsant properties of valproic acid were actually discovered when it was being used as a vehicle for other compounds being tested for anticonvulsant properties. Structurally, valproic acid is unlike other anticonvulsants. Its mechanism of action isn't completely understood.

Adverse reactions

Rare, but deadly, liver toxicity has occurred with valproic acid use. The drug should be used with caution in the patient who has a history of liver disease. Pediatric patients younger than 2 years old are at considerable risk for developing hepatotoxicity. Most other adverse reactions to valproic acid are tolerable and dose-related. These include:

* nausea and vomiting
* diarrhea or constipation
* sedation
* dizziness
* ataxia
* headache
* muscle weakness
* increased blood ammonia.

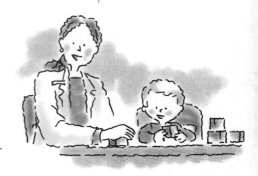

The use of valproic acid for seizures in children age 2 and younger should be limited due to the risk of potentially fatal liver toxicity.

Nursing process

These nursing process steps are appropriate for patients undergoing treatment with carboxylic acid derivative anticonvulsant drugs.

Assessment
* Assess the patient's condition before therapy and regularly thereafter.
* Monitor the level of the drug in the blood (therapeutic level is 50 to 100 mcg/ml).
* Monitor liver function studies, platelet counts, and prothrombin time before starting the drug and periodically thereafter.
* Monitor the patient's response to the drug, especially for adverse reactions.
* Be aware that the drug may produce false-positive test results for ketones in urine.
* Assess the patient's compliance with therapy at each follow-up visit.

Key nursing diagnoses
* Risk for injury related to adverse reactions
* Impaired physical mobility related to sedation
* Noncompliance related to long-term therapy

Planning outcome goals
* The risk of injury to the patient will be minimized.
* The patient will be able to perform ADLs.
* The patient will verbalize factors that contribute to noncompliance.

Implementation

• Administer oral forms of the drug with food to reduce GI irritation. Don't give the syrup form to a patient who needs sodium restriction. Check with the prescriber.
• Dilute the drug with at least 50 ml of a compatible diluent (D_5W, saline solution, lactated Ringer's solution) if injecting I.V. and give over 1 hour. Don't exceed 20 mg/minute.
• Avoid sudden withdrawal, which may worsen seizures.
• Expect to adjust the dosage according to the patient's response. In elderly patients, a reduced starting dose is suggested, with slower dosage increases.
• Administer safety precautions if the patient has adverse CNS reactions to the drug.
• Monitor closely for hepatotoxicity because it may follow nonspecific symptoms, such as malaise, fever, and lethargy.

Evaluation

• Patient sustains no injury from adverse reactions.
• Patient maintains physical mobility.
• Patient complies with therapy and has no seizures.

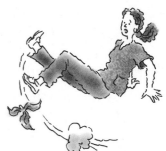

Reducing the patient's risk of injury is an important planning goal. In fact, I think I'll make that one of my *own* planning goals! Yikes!

1 (aminomethyl) cyclohexane acetic acid

The 1 (aminomethyl) cyclohexane acetic acid drug class includes the drug gabapentin. This drug was designed to be a GABA agonist, but its exact mechanism of action is unknown. It's approved as adjunctive therapy for partial seizures in adults with epilepsy and in children age 3 and older. Gabapentin has also been used for the treatment of pain from diabetic neuropathy and postherpetic neuralgia, tremors associated with MS, bipolar disorder, migraine prophylaxis, and Parkinson's disease.

Pharmacokinetics

Gabapentin is readily absorbed in the GI tract. Bioavailability isn't dose-proportional; as the dose increases, the bioavailability decreases.

An exclusive deal

Gabapentin isn't metabolized and is excreted exclusively by the kidneys. The patient with renal impairment requires dosage reduction.

Pharmacodynamics

The exact mechanism of action of gabapentin isn't known.

Gabbing on about GABA

Originally designed as a GABA agonist, gabapentin doesn't appear to act at the GABA receptor, affect GABA uptake, or interfere with GABA transaminase. Rather, it appears to bind to a carrier protein and act at a unique receptor, resulting in elevated GABA in the brain.

Pharmacotherapeutics

Gabapentin is used as adjunctive therapy in adults and children age 3 and older with partial and secondarily generalized seizures. Although not approved by the Food and Drug Administration (FDA), gabapentin also appears effective as monotherapy. Like carbamazepine, gabapentin may worsen myoclonic seizures.

Drug interactions

Antacids and cimetidine may affect gabapentin concentration.

Adverse reactions

Adverse reactions to gabapentin commonly include:
- fatigue
- somnolence
- dizziness
- ataxia
- leukopenia.
    Some less common reactions include:
- edema
- weight gain
- hostility
- emotional lability
- nausea and vomiting
- bronchitis
- viral infection
- fever
- nystagmus
- rhinitis
- diplopia
- tremor.

Nursing process

These nursing process steps are appropriate for patients undergoing treatment with 1 (aminomethyl) cyclohexane acetic acid anticonvulsant drugs.

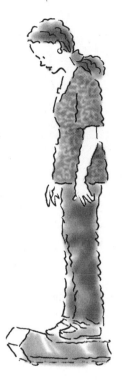

Weight gain is one of the less common adverse effects of gabapentin.

Assessment

- Assess the patient's disorder before therapy and regularly thereafter.
- Monitor the patient's serum levels and response to the prescribed drug, as indicated.
- Monitor the patient for adverse reactions.
- Assess the patient's compliance with therapy at each follow-up visit.

Key nursing diagnoses

- Risk for injury related to adverse reactions
- Impaired physical mobility related to sedation
- Noncompliance related to long-term therapy

Planning outcome goals

- The risk to the patient will be minimized.
- The patient will be able to perform ADLs.
- The patient will verbalize factors that contribute to noncompliance.

Implementation

- Administer oral forms of the drug with food to reduce GI irritation.
- Expect to adjust the drug dosage according to the patient's response.
- Administer safety precautions if the patient has adverse CNS reactions to the drug. Administer the first dose at bedtime to minimize the effect of drowsiness, dizziness, fatigue, and ataxia.
- Withdraw the drug gradually over 1 week to minimize seizure risk. Don't suddenly withdraw other anticonvulsants in the patient starting gabapentin therapy.

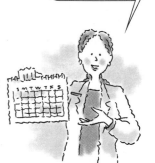

Withdraw gabapentin gradually over 1 week to minimize seizure risk.

Evaluation

- Patient sustains no injury from adverse reactions.
- Patient maintains physical mobility.
- Patient complies with therapy and has no seizures.

Phenyltriazine

Lamotrigine belongs to the phenyltriazine drug class and is chemically unrelated to other anticonvulsants.

Stamp of approval

Lamotrigine is FDA approved for adjunctive therapy in adults with partial seizures and in children older than age 2 with generalized seizures or Lennox-Gastaut syndrome.

Pharmacokinetics

Lamotrigine is well absorbed by the body at a rapid rate. It's metabolized by the liver and excreted by the kidneys. Clearance increases in the presence of other enzyme-inducing anticonvulsant drugs. The drug isn't significantly bound to plasma proteins.

Pharmacodynamics

The precise mechanism of action of lamotrigine is unknown, but it is thought to involve a use-dependent blocking effect on sodium channels, resulting in inhibition of the release of excitatory neurotransmitters, glutamate, and aspartate.

Pharmacotherapeutics

Lamotrigine is approved for adjunctive therapy in adults and children older than age 2 with generalized seizures or Lennox-Gastaut syndrome. It may also be used for conversion to mono therapy in adults. Lamotrigine appears effective for many types of generalized seizures, but can worsen myoclonic seizures. Lamotrigine may also lead to improvement in the patient's mood.

Drug interactions

• Carbamazepine, phenytoin, phenobarbital, primidone, and acetaminophen may result in decreased lamotrigine effects.
• Valproic acid may decrease the clearance of lamotrigine and the steady-state level of lamotrigine.
• Lamotrigine may produce additive effects when combined with folate inhibitors.

Adverse reactions

Adverse reactions to lamotrigine commonly include:
• dizziness
• ataxia
• somnolence
• headache
• diplopia
• nausea
• vomiting
• rash.

Don't be rash

Several types of rash may occur with lamotrigine use, including Stevens-Johnson syndrome. This generalized, erythematous, morbilliform rash usually appears in the first 3 to 4 weeks of therapy and is usually mild to moderate but may be severe. The drug now carries a "black box" warning regarding the rash, and the manufacturer recommends discontinuing the drug at the first sign of a rash. The risk of rash may be increased by starting at high doses, by rapidly increasing doses, or by using the drug with valproate.

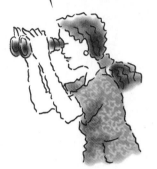

Discontinue lamotrigine at the first sight of a rash.

Nursing process

These nursing process steps are appropriate for patients undergoing treatment with phenyltriazine anticonvulsant drugs.

Assessment
• Obtain a history of the patient's seizure disorder before therapy.
• Evaluate the patient for reduction in seizure frequency and duration after therapy begins. Check the adjunct anticonvulsant's level periodically.
• Monitor the patient's serum levels and response to the prescribed drug as indicated.
• Monitor the patient for adverse reactions.
• Assess the patient's compliance with therapy at each follow-up visit.

Key nursing diagnoses
• Risk for injury related to adverse reactions
• Impaired physical mobility related to sedation
• Noncompliance related to long-term therapy

Planning outcome goals
• Risk to the patient will be minimized.
• The patient will be able to perform ADLs.
• The patient will exhibit behaviors that comply with long-term therapy.

Implementation
• Administer oral forms of the drug with food to reduce GI irritation.
• Expect the dosage to be lowered if the drug is added to a multidrug regimen that includes valproic acid.
• Expect that a lowered maintenance dosage will be used in a patient with severe renal impairment.

Come to a slow, steady stop

- Don't stop the drug abruptly. Abrupt withdrawal increases the risk of seizures. Instead, drug withdrawal should be tapered over at least 2 weeks.
- A rash may be life threatening. Stop the drug and notify the prescriber at the first sign of a rash.
- Administer safety precautions if the patient has adverse CNS reactions.

Evaluation

- Patient sustains no injury from adverse reactions.
- Patient maintains physical mobility.
- Patient complies with therapy and has no seizures.

Carboxamide

Oxcarbazepine, a carboxamide, is chemically similar to carbamazepine but causes less induction of liver enzymes. Oxcarbazepine is useful as adjunctive therapy or monotherapy in adults for partial seizures and in children as adjunctive therapy for partial seizures.

Pharmacokinetics

Oxcarbazepine is completely absorbed and extensively metabolized via liver enzymes to the 10-monohydroxy metabolite (MHD) that's responsible for its pharmacologic activity. It's excreted primarily by the kidneys. The half-life of MHD is about 9 hours. Unlike carbamazepine, oxcarbazepine doesn't induce its own metabolism.

Pharmacodynamics

The precise mechanism of oxcarbazepine and MHD is unknown, but antiseizure activity is thought to occur through blockade of sodium-sensitive channels, which prevents seizure spread in the brain.

Pharmacotherapeutics

Oxcarbazepine is FDA approved for adjunctive therapy of partial seizures in adults and children older than age 4 and as monotherapy in adults. As with carbamazepine, it's also effective for generalized seizures but may worsen myoclonic and absence seizures.

Drug interactions

Carbamazepine, phenytoin, phenobarbital, valproic acid, and verapamil may decrease the levels of active MHD. Oxcarbazepine may decrease the effectiveness of hormonal contraceptives and felodipine.

A dip in the dosage

Reduced dosages are necessary in the patient with renal impairment (clearance less than 30 ml/minute) and in the patient at risk for renal impairment (such as an elderly patient).

Adverse reactions

Adverse reactions to oxcarbazepine commonly include:
- somnolence
- dizziness
- diplopia
- ataxia
- nausea
- vomiting
- abnormal gait
- tremor
- aggravated seizures
- abdominal pain.
    Some less common reactions include:
- agitation
- confusion
- hypotension
- hyponatremia
- rhinitis
- speech disorder
- back pain
- upper respiratory tract infection.
    About 20% to 30% of patients who have had an allergic reaction to carbamazepine will experience a hypersensitivity reaction to oxcarbazepine.

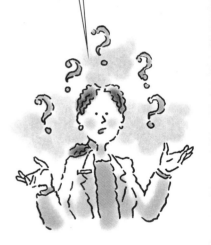

Quiz the patient about a history of hypersensitivity to carbamazepine.

Nursing process

These nursing process steps are appropriate for patients undergoing treatment with carboxamide anticonvulsant drugs.

Assessment
- Question the patient about a history of hypersensitivity reactions to carbamazepine.
- Obtain a history of the patient's underlying condition before therapy and reassess it regularly thereafter.

- Monitor the patient's serum levels and response to the prescribed drug as indicated.
- Monitor the patient for adverse reactions.
- Assess the patient's compliance with therapy at each follow-up visit.

Key nursing diagnoses

- Risk for injury related to adverse reactions
- Impaired physical mobility related to sedation
- Noncompliance related to long-term therapy

Planning outcome goals

- Risk to the patient will be minimized.
- The patient will be able to perform ADLs.
- The patient will exhibit behaviors that comply with long-term therapy.

Implementation

- Withdraw the drug gradually to minimize the risk of increased seizure frequency.
- Correct hyponatremia as needed.

A "shaky" situation

- For an oral suspension, shake well before administration. It can be mixed with water or may be swallowed directly from the syringe. It can be taken without regard to food. Oral suspensions and tablets may be interchanged at equal doses.
- Expect to adjust the dosage according to the patient's response.
- Administer safety precautions if the patient has adverse CNS reactions.

Evaluation

- Patient sustains no injury from adverse reactions.
- Patient maintains physical mobility.
- Patient complies with therapy and has no seizures.

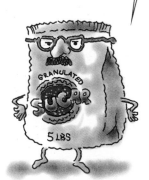

These sulfamate-substituted monosaccharides may be derived from the natural monosaccharide D-fructose, but I bet I taste sweeter.

Sulfamate-substituted monosaccharides

Sulfamate-substituted monosaccharides are structurally distinct from other anticonvulsant drug classes. The effect is to block the spread of seizures rather than to raise the threshold (like other anticonvulsant drugs). This class of drugs is derived from the natural monosaccharide D-fructose. Topiramate is an anticonvulsant drug in this class.

Pharmacokinetics

Topiramate is rapidly absorbed by the body. It's partially metabolized in the liver and excreted mostly unchanged in urine. For the patient with renal impairment (creatinine clearance less than 70 ml/minute), the dosage of topiramate is reduced.

Pharmacodynamics

Topiramate is believed to act by blocking voltage-dependent sodium channels, enhancing the activity of GABA receptors and antagonizing glutamate receptors.

Pharmacotherapeutics

Topiramate is approved as adjunctive therapy for partial and primary generalized tonic-clonic seizures in adults and children older than age 2 and for children with Lennox-Gastaut syndrome. The drug may also prove beneficial for other types of seizures and as monotherapy.

Drug interactions

Carbamazepine, phenytoin, and valproic acid may cause decreased topiramate levels. Topiramate may decrease the efficacy of hormonal contraceptives and may decrease valproic acid levels. CNS depressants may be potentiated when combined with topiramate.

Adverse reactions

Psychomotor slowing, difficulty finding words, impaired concentration, and memory impairment are common and may require stopping the drug. Low starting doses and slow titration may minimize these effects.

Other common adverse reactions to topiramate include:
- drowsiness
- dizziness
- headache
- ataxia
- nervousness
- confusion
- paresthesia
- weight gain
- diplopia.

Serious but uncommon adverse reactions include:
- secondary angle-closure glaucoma
- liver failure

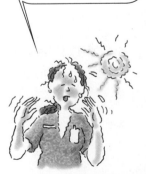

Serious but uncommon adverse reactions to topiramate include hyperthermia and heat stroke. Whew! Is it getting hotter, or is it just me?

- hypohidrosis
- hyperthermia
- heat stroke
- renal calculi.

Nursing process

These nursing process steps are appropriate for patients undergoing treatment with sulfamate-substituted monosaccharide anticonvulsant drugs.

Assessment

- Assess the patient's seizure disorder before therapy and regularly thereafter.
- Carefully monitor the patient taking topiramate in conjunction with other antiepileptic drugs; dosage adjustments may be needed to achieve an optimal response.
- Monitor the patient's serum levels and response to the prescribed drug as indicated.
- Monitor the patient for adverse reactions.
- Assess the patient's compliance with therapy at each follow-up visit.

Key nursing diagnoses

- Risk for injury related to adverse reactions
- Impaired physical mobility related to sedation
- Noncompliance related to long-term therapy

Planning outcome goals

- Risk to the patient will be minimized.
- The patient will be able to perform ADLs.
- The patient will exhibit behaviors that comply with long-term drug therapy.

Implementation

- Administer oral forms of the drug with food to reduce GI irritation.
- Expect to adjust the dosage according to the patient's response.
- Administer safety precautions if the patient has adverse CNS reactions.

Dial up the dose for hemodialysis

- The patient with renal insufficiency requires a reduced dosage. For the patient on hemodialysis, supplemental doses may be needed to avoid rapid drops in drug levels during prolonged treatment.

• Discontinue the drug if an ocular adverse event occurs, characterized by acute myopia and secondary angle-closure glaucoma.

Evaluation
• Patient sustains no injury from adverse reactions.
• Patient maintains physical mobility.
• Patient complies with therapy and has no seizures.

Succinimides

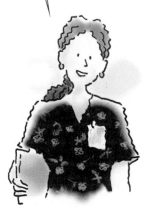

Ethosuximide is considered the drug of choice for absence seizures.

The succinimides, ethosuximide and methsuximide, are used for the management of absence seizures. Because ethosuximide is considered the drug of choice for this indication, the remainder of this section will focus on that drug.

Pharmacokinetics
The succinimides are readily absorbed from the GI tract, metabolized in the liver, and excreted in urine. Metabolites are believed to be inactive. The elimination half-life of ethosuximide is about 60 hours in adults and 30 hours in children.

Pharmacodynamics
Ethosuximide raises the seizure threshold; it suppresses the characteristic spike-and-wave pattern by depressing neuronal transmission in the motor cortex and basal ganglia. It's indicated for absence seizures.

Pharmacotherapeutics
The only indication for ethosuximide is the treatment of absence seizures. It's the treatment of choice for this type of seizure disorder, but may be used in combination with valproic acid for difficult-to-control absence seizures.

Drug interactions
Ethosuximide may interact with concurrently administered anticonvulsant drugs. It can also elevate serum phenytoin levels. Carbamazepine may induce the metabolism of ethosuximide. Valproic acid may increase or decrease levels of ethosuximide.

Adverse reactions
Ethosuximide is generally well tolerated and causes few adverse reactions. The most common effects include anorexia, nausea,

and vomiting (in up to 40% of cases). Other common adverse effects include:

- drowsiness and fatigue
- lethargy
- dizziness
- hiccups
- headaches
- mood changes.

Rarely, blood dyscrasias, rashes (including Stevens-Johnson syndrome, erythema multiforme, and lupuslike syndrome), and psychotic behavior can occur.

Nursing process

These nursing process steps are appropriate for patients undergoing treatment with succinimide anticonvulsant drugs.

Assessment

- Monitor the patient's serum levels and response to the prescribed drug as indicated.
- Monitor the patient for adverse reactions.
- Assess the patient's compliance with therapy at each follow-up visit.

Key nursing diagnoses

- Risk for injury related to adverse reactions
- Impaired physical mobility related to sedation
- Noncompliance related to long-term therapy

Planning outcome goals

- The risk to the patient will be minimized.
- The patient will be able to perform ADLs.
- The patient will exhibit behaviors that comply with long-term therapy.

Implementation

- Administer oral forms of the drug with food to reduce GI irritation.
- Expect to adjust the dosage according to the patient's response.
- Administer safety precautions if the patient has adverse CNS reactions.

Evaluation

- Patient sustains no injury from adverse reactions.
- Patient maintains physical mobility.
- Patient complies with therapy and has no seizures.

Sulfonamides

Sulfonamides are a group of compounds consisting of amides of sulfanilic acid. They're known for their bacteriostatic effects; they interfere with the functioning of the enzyme necessary for bacteria metabolism, growth, and multiplication. Zonisamide, a sulfonamide, is approved for the adjunctive treatment of partial seizure in adults.

Pharmacokinetics

Peak concentrations of zonisamide occur within 2 to 6 hours of administration. The drug is widely distributed and is extensively bound to erythrocytes. Zonisamide is metabolized by the CYP3A4 enzyme in the liver and is excreted in urine, primarily as the parent drug and the glucuronide metabolite. Low doses should be initiated in elderly patients because of the possibility of renal impairment.

Pharmacodynamics

The precise mechanism of zonisamide is unknown, but it's believed to involve stabilization of neuronal membranes and suppression of neuronal hypersensitivity.

Pharmacotherapeutics

Zonisamide is approved only as adjunctive therapy for partial seizures in adults. Despite its limited indication, it has demonstrated usefulness in other types of seizure activity (infantile spasms and myoclonic, generalized, and atypical absence seizures).

Drug interactions

Drugs that induce liver enzymes (such as phenytoin, carbamazepine, or phenobarbital) increase the metabolism and decrease the half-life of zonisamide. Concurrent use of zonisamide with drugs that inhibit or induce CYP3A4 can be expected to increase or decrease the serum concentration of zonisamide. Zonisamide isn't an inducer of CYP3A4, so it's unlikely to affect other drugs metabolized by the CYP3A4 system.

Adverse reactions

Common adverse reactions to zonisamide include:
- somnolence
- dizziness
- confusion

- anorexia
- nausea
- diarrhea
- weight loss
- rash.

Slow she goes

Slow titration of the dosage and administration with meals may decrease the incidence of adverse reactions.

Serious sides

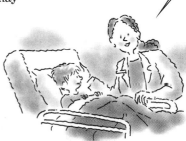

The safety and effectiveness of zonisamide in children younger than age 16 hasn't been established.

More serious adverse reactions that have been associated with zonisamide include:
- Stevens-Johnson syndrome
- toxic epidermal necrolysis
- psychosis
- aplastic anemia
- agranulocytosis
- oligohidrosis, hyperthermia, and heatstroke (in children).

Zonisamide is contraindicated in patients with allergies to sulfonamides. Zonisamide is in category C for pregnancy, and its disposition in breast milk is unknown. The safety and effectiveness of the drug in children younger than age 16 hasn't been established. The use of zonisamide in patients with renal clearances of less than 50 ml/minute isn't recommended.

Nursing process

These nursing process steps are appropriate for patients undergoing treatment with sulfonamide anticonvulsant drugs.

Assessment

- Obtain a history of the patient's underlying condition before therapy and reassess it regularly thereafter.
- Monitor the patient's body temperature, especially during the summer, because decreased sweating may occur (especially in children ages 17 and younger) resulting in heat stroke and dehydration.
- Monitor the patient's renal function periodically.
- Monitor the patient's serum levels and response to the prescribed drug as indicated.
- Monitor the patient for hypersensitivity or adverse reactions.
- Assess the patient's compliance with therapy at each follow-up visit.

Key nursing diagnoses

- Risk for injury related to adverse reactions

• Impaired physical mobility related to sedation
• Noncompliance related to long-term therapy

Planning outcome goals

• Risk to the patient will be minimized.
• The patient will be able to perform ADLs.
• The patient will exhibit behavior that complies with drug therapy.

Implementation

• The drug may be taken with or without food. Tell the patient not to bite or break the capsule.
• Use cautiously in the patient with hepatic or renal disease; he may need slower adjustments and more frequent monitoring. If the patient's glomerular filtration rate is less than 50 ml/minute, don't use the drug.
• Reduce the dosage or discontinue the drug gradually; abrupt withdrawal of the drug may cause increased frequency of seizures or status epilepticus.
• Increase the patient's fluid intake to help increase urine output and help prevent renal calculi, especially if he has predisposing factors.
• Expect to adjust the drug dosage according to the patient's response.
• Administer safety precautions if the patient has adverse CNS reactions.

Evaluation

• Patient sustains no injury from adverse reactions.
• Patient maintains physical mobility.
• Patient complies with therapy and has no seizures.

Antimigraine drugs

A migraine, an episodic headache disorder, is one of the most common primary headache disorders, affecting an estimated 24 million people in the United States. A migraine is usually described as a unilateral headache pain that's pounding, pulsating, or throbbing. It may be preceded by an aura. Other symptoms typically associated with a migraine are sensitivity to light or sound, nausea, vomiting, and constipation or diarrhea.

Current theories suggest that the symptoms of migraines are due to vasodilation or to the release of vasoactive and proinflammatory substances from nerves in an activated trigeminal system.

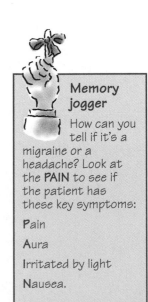

Memory jogger

How can you tell if it's a migraine or a headache? Look at the **PAIN** to see if the patient has these key symptoms:

Pain

Aura

Irritated by light

Nausea.

So many choices

Treatment for migraines is targeted at altering an attack after it's under way (abortive and symptomatic treatment) or preventing the attack before it begins. The choice of therapy depends upon the severity, duration, frequency, and degree of disability the headache creates as well as the patient's characteristics. Abortive treatments may include analgesics (aspirin and acetaminophen), nonsteroidal anti-inflammatory drugs (NSAIDs), ergotamine, 5-HT agonists, and other miscellaneous agents (such as isometheptene combinations, intranasal butorphanol, metoclopramide, and corticosteroids). Prophylactic therapy includes beta-adrenergic blockers, tricyclic antidepressants, valproic acid, and NSAIDs, to name a few.

5-HT agonists

The 5-HT agonists, commonly known as the *triptans*, are the treatment of choice for moderate to severe migraine. Drugs in this class include:
- almotriptan
- eletriptan
- frovatriptan
- naratriptan
- rizatriptan
- sumatriptan
- zolmitriptan.

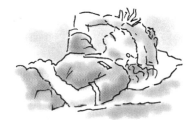

This chapter is giving me a migraine!

Pharmacokinetics

When comparing the triptans, key pharmacokinetic features are onset of effect and duration of action. Most triptans have a half-life of approximately 2 hours; almotriptan and eletriptan have half-lives of 3 to 4 hours, naratriptan has a half-life of about 6 hours, and frovatriptan has the longest half-life (25 hours) and the most delayed onset of action.

Freedom of choice

All of the triptans are available in an oral formulation. Rizatriptan is available in a rapid-dissolve tablet, and sumatriptan is also available in an injectable and intranasal formulation. The injectable form of sumatriptan has the most rapid onset of action.

Pharmacodynamics

Triptans are specific serotonin 5-HT$_1$ receptor agonists that result in cranial vessel constriction as well as inhibition and reduction of the inflammatory process along the trigeminal nerve pathway. These actions may abort or provide symptomatic relief for a migraine. Triptans are effective in controlling the pain, nausea, and vomiting associated with migraines.

Pharmacotherapeutics

The choice of a triptan depends on patient preferences for dosage form (if nausea and vomiting are present), presence of recurrent migraine, and formulary restrictions. A patient experiencing nausea and vomiting may prefer injectable or intranasal sumatriptan. Recurrent migraines may respond better to triptans with longer half-lives, such as frovatriptan and naratriptan; however, these drugs have delayed onset of effects. Two newer triptans, almotriptan and eletriptan, have rapid onset and an intermediate half-life.

Triptans have many contraindications and should not be used in patients with certain conditions. (See *Contra-triptans*.)

More than 3 in 30

The safety of treating an average of more than three migraine attacks in a 30-day period hasn't been established.

Drug interactions

These drug interactions are possible when taking triptans:
• The administration of a triptan within 24 hours of treatment with another 5-HT_1 agonist ergotamine-containing or ergot-type medication (such as dihydroergotamine) may cause prolonged vaso spastic reactions. The use of ergot-containing medications and 5-HT agonists within 24 hours of each other should be avoided.

A timely warning

• Eletriptan shouldn't be used within at least 72 hours of treatment with the following potent CYP3A4 inhibitors: ketoconazole, itraconazole, nefazodone, clarithromycin, ritonavir, and nelfinavir or other drugs that have demonstrated potent CYP3A4 inhibition.
• Almotriptan, rizatriptan, sumatriptan, and zolmitriptan shouldn't be used with or within 2 weeks of discontinuing an MAO inhibitor.
• Although rare, SSRIs, such as citalopram, fluoxetine, fluvoxamine, paroxetine, and sertraline, have been reported to cause weakness, hyperreflexia, and incoordination when coadministered with 5-HT_1 agonists. Monitor the patient closely if concomitant treatment with a triptan and an SSRI is clinically warranted. This reaction has also been reported with coadministration of a triptan and sibutramine.

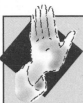

Before you give that drug

Contra-triptans

Before administering triptans to a patient, be aware of these contraindications.

A hearty no

Triptans are contraindicated in patients with ischemic heart disease (such as angina pectoris, history of myocardial infarction, or documented silent ischemia) and in patients who have symptoms or findings consistent with ischemic heart disease, coronary artery vasospasm (including Prinzmetal's variant angina), or other significant underlying cardiovascular conditions.

No strokes allowed

Triptans shouldn't be prescribed for patients with cerebrovascular syndromes (such as strokes of any type or transient ischemic attacks) or for patients with peripheral vascular disease, including, but not limited to, ischemic bowel disease. Triptans also shouldn't be given to patients with uncontrolled hypertension or to patients with hemiplegic or basilar migraines.

Not for the faint of heart

Triptans aren't recommended for use in the patient who has coronary artery disease (CAD) or risk factors for CAD (such as hypertension, hypercholesterolemia, smoking, obesity, diabetes, a strong family history of CAD, or a surgically or physiologically menopausal woman, or a male over age 40) unless a cardiovascular evaluation provides satisfactory evidence that the patient is reasonably free from underlying cardiovascular disease. If a triptan is used for a patient who has any of these risk factors, it's strongly recommended that the first dose be administered in a physician's office or other medically staffed and equipped facility.

It's further suggested that intermittent, long-term users of 5-HT agonists or those who have or acquire risk factors undergo periodic cardiac evaluation.

• The bioavailability of frovatriptan is 30% higher in a patient taking oral forms of hormonal contraceptives.
• Propranolol increases the bioavailability of zolmitriptan, rizatriptan, frovatriptan, and eletriptan.

Adverse reactions

Adverse reactions to triptans include:
• tingling
• warm or hot sensations or flushing
• nasal and throat discomfort
• visual disturbances
• paresthesia
• dizziness
• weakness and fatigue

> That's quite a list of adverse reactions...

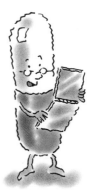

- somnolence
- chest pain or pressure
- neck or throat pain
- jaw pain or pressure
- dry mouth
- dyspepsia
- nausea
- sweating
- injection site reaction (subcutaneous sumatriptan)
- taste disturbances (intranasal sumatriptan).

The heart takes part

Serious cardiac events, including acute myocardial infarction, arrhythmias, and death, have been reported within a few hours after taking triptans. However, the incidence of these events is considered extremely low.

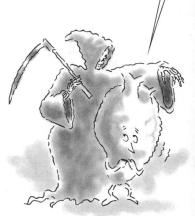

I don't like the sound of these "serious cardiac events" triptans may trigger. Thank goodness they're very rare!

Nursing process

These nursing process steps are appropriate for patients undergoing treatment with triptans.

Assessment
- Assess the patient's condition before and during drug therapy. These drugs aren't intended for the patient with ischemic heart disease or hemiplegic or basilar migraines.
- Obtain a list of the patient's medication intake within 24 hours to prevent drug interactions. Use caution when giving the drug to a patient who's taking an MAO inhibitor or a CYP-450 3A4 or 2D6 inhibitor. Don't give the drug with other serotonin agonist or ergotamine derivatives.
- Be alert for adverse reactions.
- Monitor the ECG in a patient with risk factors for coronary artery disease (CAD) or with symptoms similar to those of CAD, such as chest or throat tightness, pain, and heaviness.
- Evaluate the patient's and family's knowledge of drug therapy.

Key nursing diagnoses
- Acute pain related to the presence of an acute migraine attack
- Risk for injury related to drug-induced interactions
- Deficient knowledge related to drug therapy

Planning outcome goals
- The patient will state that pain is decreased.
- Risk of injury to the patient will be reduced.
- The patient and his family will verbalize an understanding of drug therapy.

Education edge

Teaching about migraine drugs

If migraine drugs are prescribed, review these points with the patient and his caregivers:
• Take the drug exactly as prescribed, such as only when you're having a migraine, and repeat the dosage as per the prescriber's orders. Don't exceed the prescribed dosage.
• Avoid possible migraine triggers, such as cheese, chocolate, citrus fruits, caffeine, and alcohol.
• Don't take other medicines, over-the-counter preparations, or herbal preparations without first consulting with your prescriber. Drug interactions can occur.
• Immediately report adverse reactions (chest, throat, jaw, or neck tightness, pain, or heaviness) to the prescriber and discontinue use of the drug until further notice.
• Use caution when driving or operating machinery while taking migraine drugs.

Implementation
• Give the dose as soon as the patient complains of migraine symptoms.
• Reduce the dosage in a patient with poor renal or hepatic function.
• Repeat the dose as ordered and as needed, and monitor the patient for effect.
• Don't give more than two doses within 24 hours.

Evaluation
• Patient's symptoms are alleviated and the patient is free from pain.
• Patient doesn't develop serious complications from drug interactions.
• Patient and his family state an understanding of drug therapy. (See *Teaching about migraine drugs*.)

Ergotamine preparations

Ergotamine and its derivatives may be used as abortive or symptomatic therapy for migraines.

Common preparations used for migraines include:

- ergotamine—sublingual or oral tablet or suppository (combined with caffeine)
- dihydroergotamine—injectable or intranasal.

Pharmacokinetics

Ergotamine is incompletely absorbed from the GI tract. The intranasal form of dihydroergotamine is rapidly absorbed. Peak plasma concentrations, following subcutaneous injection, occur within 45 minutes, and 90% of the dose is plasma protein bound. Ergotamine is metabolized in the liver, and 90% of the metabolites are excreted in bile; traces of unchanged drug are excreted in urine.

Pharmacodynamics

Ergotamine derivative antimigraine effects are believed to be due to a blockade of neurogenic inflammation. They also act as partial agonists or antagonists at serotonin, dopaminergic, and alpha-adrenergic receptors, depending on their site. Ergotamine preparations commonly need to be prescribed with antiemetic preparations when used for migraines.

Dihydroergotamine, a hydrogenated form of ergotamine, differs mainly in the degree of activity. It has less vasoconstrictive action than ergotamine and much less emetic potential.

Pharmacotherapeutics

Ergotamine preparations are used to prevent or treat vascular headaches, such as migraines, migraine variants, and cluster headaches. Dihydroergotamine is used when rapid control of migraines is desired or when other routes are undesirable.

Drug interactions

These drug interactions can occur in a patient taking ergotamine preparations:

Getting cold feet

- Propranolol and other beta-adrenergic blockers close the natural pathway for vasodilation in the patient receiving ergotamine preparations, resulting in excessive vasoconstriction and cold extremities.
- The patient may be at increased risk for weakness, hyperflexion, and incoordination when ergotamine preparations are used with SSRIs.

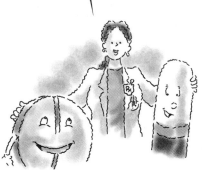

When prescribed for migraines, an ergotamine preparation is commonly accompanied by an antiemetic.

- Sumatriptan may cause an additive effect when taken with ergotamine derivatives, increasing the risk of coronary vasospasm. An ergotamine preparation shouldn't be given within 24 hours of administeration of a triptan.
- Drugs inhibiting CYP3A4 enzymes (such as erythromycin, clarithromycin, troleandomycin, ritonavir, nelfinavir, indinavir, and azole-derivative antifungal agents) may alter the metabolism of ergotamine, resulting in increased serum concentrations of ergotamine. This increases the risk of vasospasm and cerebral or peripheral ischemia. These drugs shouldn't be used together.
- Vasoconstrictors may cause an additive effect when given with ergotamine preparations, increasing the risk of high blood pressure.

Adverse reactions

Adverse reactions to ergotamine derivatives include:
- nausea
- vomiting
- numbness
- tingling
- muscle pain
- leg weakness
- itching.

Prolonged administration of ergotamine derivatives may result in ergotism, gangrene, and rebound headaches.

Nursing process

These nursing process steps are appropriate for patients undergoing treatment with ergotamine preparations.

Assessment

- Assess the patient for coronary, cerebral, or peripheral vascular disease; hypertension; and liver or kidney disease. These are contraindications to the use of ergotamine preparations.
- Assess the patient's condition before and during drug therapy.
- Be alert for adverse reactions and drug interactions.

On the rebound

- Be alert for ergotamine rebound or an increase in the frequency and duration of headaches, which may occur if the drug is discontinued suddenly.
- Monitor the ECG in a patient with risk factors for CAD or with symptoms similar to those of CAD, such as chest or throat tightness, pain, and heaviness.
- Evaluate the patient's and family's knowledge of drug therapy.

Key nursing diagnoses
• Acute pain related to the presence of an acute migraine attack
• Risk for injury related to drug-induced interactions
• Deficient knowledge related to drug therapy

Planning outcome goals
• The patient will acknowledge a decrease in pain.
• Risk of injury to the patient will be reduced.
• The patient and his family will verbalize an understanding of drug therapy.

Implementation
• Give the dose as soon as the patient complains of migraine symptoms.
• Avoid prolonged administration and don't exceed the recommended dosage.
• Don't give sublingual tablets with food or drink while tablets are dissolving. Sublingual tablets are preferred during the early stage of an attack because of their rapid absorption.
• Monitor the patient for signs of vasoconstriction and report them to the prescriber.

Evaluation
• Patient's symptoms are alleviated, and the patient is free from pain.
• Patient doesn't develop serious complications from drug interactions.
• Patient and his family state an understanding of drug therapy.

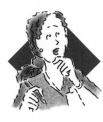

Quick quiz

1. A 15-year-old patient has a tonic-clonic seizure disorder and is prescribed phenytoin. Which term best describes the absorption rate of oral phenytoin?

    A.   Rapid
    B.   Slow
    C.   Erratic
    D.   Moderate

Answer: B. Phenytoin is absorbed slowly through the GI tract. It's absorbed much more rapidly when administered I.V.

2. An 11-year-old patient develops myoclonic seizures. Which potential adverse reaction makes it unlikely that valproate will be prescribed for this patient?

    A. Liver toxicity
    B. CNS sedation
    C. Respiratory depression
    D. Hyperthermia

Answer: A. When administered to children and patients taking other anticonvulsants, valproate carries a risk of potentially fatal liver toxicity.

3. Anticonvulsants fall into several major classes, including:

    A. anticholinergics.
    B. fluoroquinolones.
    C. succinimides.
    D. dopaminergics.

Answer: C. Major classes of anticonvulsants include succinimides, hydantoins, barbiturates, benzodiazepines, and sulfonamides.

4. A 48-year-old patient has been prescribed trihexyphenidyl for her Parkinson's disease. Which adverse reaction to this drug can be dose-related?

    A. Excessive salivation
    B. Dryness of mouth
    C. Bradycardia
    D. Constipation

Answer: B. Dry mouth may be a dose-related adverse effect of trihexyphenidyl therapy.

5. The effectiveness of levodopa can be reduced when taking:

    A. pyridoxine.
    B. amantadine.
    C. bromocriptine.
    D. topiramate.

Answer: A. Levodopa's effectiveness can be reduced when taking pyridoxine (vitamin B_6), phenytoin, benzodiazepines, reserpine, and papaverine.

6. Barbiturate anticonvulsants are effective in treating all of these seizure types *except:*

    A. partial seizures.
    B. tonic-clonic seizures.
    C. febrile seizures.
    D. absence seizures.

Answer: D. Barbiturate anticonvulsants are effective in treating partial, tonic-clonic, and febrile seizures. They're an ineffective treatment for absence seizures.

Scoring

☆☆☆ If you answered all six questions correctly, marvelous! Your knowledge has a rapid onset and long duration.

☆☆ If you answered four or five questions correctly, congrats! You obviously answered these questions about neurologic drugs logically.

☆ If you answered fewer than four questions correctly, don't worry. Just give yourself another dose of this chapter and recheck the results.

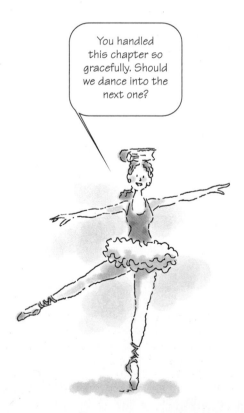

You handled this chapter so gracefully. Should we dance into the next one?

4

Pain medications

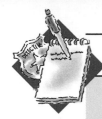

Just the facts

In this chapter, you'll learn:

♦ classes of drugs used to control pain

♦ uses and actions of these drugs

♦ absorption, distribution, metabolization, and excretion of these drugs

♦ drug interactions and adverse reactions to these drugs.

Drugs and pain control

Drugs used to control pain range from mild, over-the-counter (OTC) preparations, such as acetaminophen, to potent general anesthetics. Drug classes in this category include:
• nonopioid analgesics, antipyretics, and nonsteroidal anti-inflammatory drugs (NSAIDs)
• opioid agonist and antagonist drugs
• anesthetic drugs.

Nonopioid analgesics, antipyretics, and NSAIDs

Nonopioid analgesics, antipyretics, and NSAIDs are a broad group of pain medications. In addition to pain control, they also produce antipyretic (fever control) and anti-inflammatory effects. They can be used alone or as adjuvant medications. These drugs have a ceiling effect, and no physical dependence is associated with them.

The drug classes included in this group are:
• salicylates (especially aspirin), which are widely used
• acetaminophen, a para-aminophenol derivative acetaminophen
• NSAIDs (nonselective and selective)

• phenazopyridine hydrochloride, a urinary tract analgesic.

Salicylates

Salicylates are among the most commonly used pain medications. They're used to control pain and reduce fever and inflammation.

Cheap, easy, and reliable

Salicylates usually cost less than other analgesics and are readily available without a prescription. Aspirin is the most commonly used salicylate for anti-inflammatory drug therapy.

Other salicylates include:
• choline magnesium trisalicylate
• choline salicylate
• diflunisal
• salsalate
• sodium salicylate.

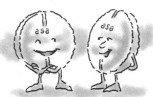

We salicylates are among the most commonly used medications.

Pharmacokinetics (how drugs circulate)

Taken orally, salicylates are partially absorbed in the stomach but are primarily absorbed in the upper part of the small intestine. The pure and buffered forms of aspirin reabsorb readily, but sustained-release and enteric-coated salicylate preparations or food or antacids in the stomach delay absorption. Enteric-coated products are slowly absorbed and not suitable for acute effects. They cause less GI bleeding and may be better suited for long-term therapy such as for arthritis. Absorption after rectal administration is slow and variable, depending on how long the suppository is retained.

Dynamite distribution, marvelous metabolism

Salicylates are distributed widely throughout body tissues and fluids, including breast milk. In addition, they easily cross the placenta. The liver metabolizes salicylates extensively into several metabolites. The kidneys excrete the metabolites and some unchanged drug.

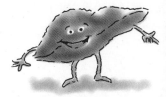

I'm great at metabolizing salicylates into metabolites!

Pharmacodynamics (how drugs act)

The different effects of salicylates stem from their separate mechanisms of action. They relieve pain primarily by inhibiting the synthesis of prostaglandin. (Recall that prostaglandin is a chemical mediator that sensitizes nerve cells to pain.) In addition, they may reduce inflammation by inhibiting prostaglandin synthesis and release that occurs during inflammation.

Sweating goes up, temperature goes down

Salicylates reduce fever by stimulating the hypothalamus and producing peripheral blood vessel dilation and increased sweating. This promotes heat loss through the skin and cooling by evaporation. Also, because prostaglandin E increases body temperature, inhibiting its production lowers fever.

Bonus effect

One salicylate, aspirin, inhibits platelet aggregation (the clumping of platelets to form a clot) by interfering with the production of thromboxane A_2, a substance necessary for platelet aggregation. Unlike aspirin, NSAIDs' effects on platelet aggregation are temporary. As a result, aspirin can be used to enhance blood flow during myocardial infarction (MI) and to prevent an event such as recurrent MI.

Pharmacotherapeutics (how drugs are used)

Salicylates are primarily used to relieve pain and reduce fever. However, they don't effectively relieve visceral pain (pain from the organs and smooth muscle) or severe pain from trauma. They can also be used to reduce an elevated body temperature in conjunction with relieving headache and muscle ache. When used to reduce inflammation in rheumatic fever, rheumatoid arthritis, and osteoarthritis, salicylates can provide considerable relief within 24 hours.

How low can you go?

No matter what the clinical indication, the main guideline of salicylate therapy is to use the lowest dose that provides relief. This reduces the likelihood of adverse reactions. (See *Salicylate warning.*)

Drug interactions

Because salicylates are highly protein bound, they can interact with many other protein-bound drugs by displacing those drugs from sites to which they normally bind. This increases the serum concentration of the unbound active drug, causing increased pharmacologic effects (the unbound drug is said to be *potentiated*). Here are some drug interactions that may occur:
• Oral anticoagulants, heparin, methotrexate, oral antidiabetic agents, and insulin are among the drugs that have increased effects or risk of toxicity when taken with salicylates.
• Probenecid, sulfinpyrazone, and spironolactone may have decreased effects when taken with salicylates.

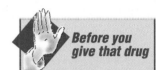

Before you give that drug

Salicylate warning

Before administering salicylates to a patient, be aware of its risks to special populations:
• *Children and teenagers:* Avoid the use of aspirin and salicylates to treat flulike symptoms or chickenpox because Reye's syndrome may develop.
• *Surgical patients:* If possible, discontinue aspirin 1 week before surgery because of the risk of postoperative bleeding.
• *Asthmatics:* Be aware that these patients are more likely to develop bronchospasm, urticaria, angioedema, or shock when salicylates are administered.

• Corticosteroids may decrease plasma salicylate levels and increase the risk of ulcers.
• Alkalinizing drugs and antacids may reduce salicylate levels.
• The antihypertensive effects of angiotensin-converting enzyme (ACE) inhibitors and beta-adrenergic blockers (commonly called *beta blockers*) may be reduced when these drugs are taken concomitantly with salicylates.
• NSAIDs may have reduced therapeutic effects and an increased risk of GI effects when taken with salicylates.

Adverse reactions

The most common adverse reactions to salicylates include gastric distress, nausea, vomiting, and bleeding tendencies. (Choline magnesium is a salicylate that doesn't increase bleeding time.) Other adverse reactions include:
• hearing loss (when taken for prolonged periods)
• diarrhea
• thirst
• sweating
• tinnitus
• confusion
• dizziness
• impaired vision
• hyperventilation (rapid breathing)
• Reye's syndrome (when given to children with chickenpox or flulike symptoms).

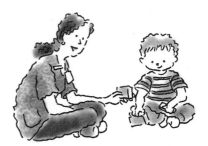

Children with chickenpox or flulike symptoms shouldn't take salicylates because of the risk of Reye's syndrome.

Nursing process

These nursing process steps are appropriate for patients undergoing treatment with salicylates.

Assessment

• Assess the patient's level of pain and inflammation before therapy begins and evaluate drug effectiveness after administration.
• Monitor the patient for signs and symptoms of bleeding. Assess bleeding time if he's scheduled to undergo surgery.
• Monitor the patient's ophthalmic and auditory function before drug therapy and periodically thereafter to detect toxicity.
• Periodically monitor complete blood count (CBC), platelet count, prothrombin time (PT), and hepatic and renal function to detect abnormalities.
• Be alert for adverse reactions and drug interactions. Watch for bronchospasm in the patient with aspirin hypersensitivity, rhinitis or nasal polyps, or asthma.

• During long-term therapy, monitor serum salicylate levels. A therapeutic level in a patient with arthritis is 10 to 30 mg/dl.
• Evaluate the patient's and family's knowledge of drug therapy.

Key nursing diagnoses
• Acute pain related to the underlying process
• Risk for injury related to adverse reactions
• Deficient knowledge related to drug therapy

Planning outcome goals
• The patient will acknowledge a reduction in pain.
• No serious complications will occur while the patient is on drug therapy.
• The patient and his family will verbalize an understanding of the purpose and intended effect of drug therapy.

Implementation
• Give aspirin with food, milk, antacids, or a large glass of water to reduce GI reactions.

A hard pill to swallow
• If the patient has trouble swallowing the drug, crush tablets or mix them with food or fluid. Don't crush enteric-coated aspirin.

Education edge

Teaching about salicylates

If salicylates are prescribed, review these points with the patient and his caregivers:
• If receiving high-dose prolonged treatment, maintain adequate fluid intake and watch for petechiae, bleeding gums, and signs of GI bleeding. Use a soft toothbrush.
• Be aware that various over-the-counter (OTC) preparations contain aspirin. Because numerous drug interactions are possible when taking aspirin, check with the prescriber or pharmacist before taking herbal preparations or OTC medications containing aspirin.
• Avoid alcohol consumption during drug therapy.
• Restrict caffeine intake during drug therapy.
• Take the drug as directed to achieve the desired effect. Know that the benefits of drug therapy may not be noticeable for 2 to 4 weeks.

• Take the drug with food or milk to prevent GI upset.
• Don't chew enteric-coated products.
• Notify the prescriber about severe or persistent adverse reactions.
• Be sure to safely store medications in the home. Aspirin is a leading cause of poisoning in children. Keep aspirin and other drugs out of children's reach. Use child-resistant containers in households with children.
• If salicylate therapy will be long-term, be sure to follow the prescriber's orders for monitoring laboratory values, especially blood urea nitrogen and creatinine levels, liver function, and complete blood count.

- Withhold the dose and notify the prescriber if bleeding, salicylism (salicylate poisoning, characterized by tinnitus or hearing loss), or adverse GI reactions occur.
- Stop aspirin 5 to 7 days before elective surgery as ordered.

Evaluation

- Patient states that pain is relieved.
- Patient remains free from adverse GI effects throughout drug therapy.
- Patient and his family state an understanding of drug therapy. (See *Teaching about salicylates*, page 143.)

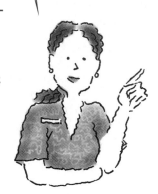

> Be sure not to crush enteric-coated aspirin because these drugs are made to protect the lining of the stomach.

Acetaminophen

Although the class of para-aminophenol derivatives includes two drugs — phenacetin and acetaminophen — only acetaminophen is available in the United States. Acetaminophen is an OTC drug that produces analgesic and antipyretic effects. It appears in many products designed to relieve pain and symptoms associated with colds and influenza.

Pharmacokinetics

Acetaminophen is absorbed rapidly and completely from the GI tract. It's also absorbed well from the mucous membranes of the rectum. It's widely distributed in body fluids and readily crosses the placenta. After the liver metabolizes acetaminophen, it's excreted by the kidneys and, in small amounts, in breast milk.

Pharmacodynamics

Acetaminophen reduces pain and fever but, unlike salicylates, it doesn't affect inflammation or platelet function. It may potentiate the effects of warfarin and increase international normalized ratio values.

Mystery theater

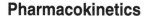

The pain-control effects of acetaminophen aren't well understood. It may work in the central nervous system (CNS) by inhibiting prostaglandin synthesis and in the peripheral nervous system in some unknown way. It reduces fever by acting directly on the heat-regulating center in the hypothalamus.

Pharmacotherapeutics

Acetaminophen is used to reduce fever and relieve headache, muscle ache, and general pain. In addition, the American Arthritis

Association has indicated that acetaminophen is an effective pain reliever for some types of arthritis.

Child's play

Acetaminophen is the drug of choice to treat fever and flulike symptoms in children.

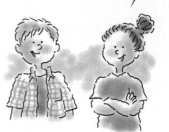

Acetaminophen is commonly used to treat fever and flulike symptoms in children.

Drug interactions

Acetaminophen can produce these drug interactions:
• It may slightly increase the effects of oral anticoagulants, such as warfarin, and thrombolytic drugs.
• The risk of liver toxicity is increased when phenytoin, barbiturates, carbamazepine, and isoniazid are combined with acetaminophen. This risk is also increased with chronic alcohol use.
• The effects of lamotrigine, loop diuretics, and zidovudine may be reduced when taken with acetaminophen.

Adverse reactions

Most patients tolerate acetaminophen well. Unlike the salicylates, acetaminophen rarely causes gastric irritation or bleeding tendencies. However, it may cause liver toxicity, and the total daily dose should be monitored.

Other adverse reactions include:
• skin rash
• hypoglycemia (with overdose)
• neutropenia.

Nursing process

These nursing process steps are appropriate for patients undergoing treatment with acetaminophen.

Assessment

• Assess the patient's level of pain and inflammation before therapy begins, and evaluate drug effectiveness after administration.
• Assess the patient's medication history. Many OTC products and combination prescription pain products contain acetaminophen and must be considered when calculating the total daily dosage.
• Be alert for adverse reactions and drug interactions.
• Evaluate the patient's and family's knowledge of drug therapy.

Key nursing diagnoses

• Acute pain related to underlying process
• Risk for injury related to adverse reactions
• Deficient knowledge related to drug therapy

Planning outcome goals

• The patient will acknowledge a reduction in pain.
• No serious complications will occur while the patient is on drug therapy.
• The patient and his family will verbalize an understanding of the purpose and intended effect of drug therapy.

Implementation

• Administer the liquid form of the drug to children and other patients who have difficulty swallowing.

Deducing the doasge

• When giving oral preparations, calculate the dosage based on the concentration of drug because drops and elixir have different concentrations (for example, 80 mg/ml versus 120 mg/ml).
• Use the rectal route in small children and other patients for whom oral administration isn't feasible.

Evaluation

• Patient states that pain is relieved.
• Patient remains free from adverse effects throughout drug therapy.
• Patient and his family state an understanding of drug therapy. (See *Teaching about acetaminophen*.)

Check your patient's medication history for combination pain products that contain acetaminophen; you'll need to consider that when calculating the total daily acetaminophen dosage. Let's see, divide that by two...

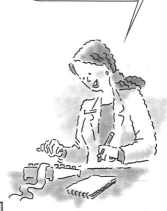

Education edge

Teaching about acetaminophen

If acetaminophen is prescribed, review these points with the patient and his caregivers:
• Consult a prescriber before giving the drug to children younger than age 2.
• Be aware that the drug is for short-term use only. A prescriber should be consulted if the drug is to be administered to children for more than 5 days or to adults for more than 10 days.
• Don't use the drug for marked fever (over 103.1° F [39.5° C]), fever persisting longer than 3 days, or recurrent fever, unless directed by a prescriber.

• Be aware that high doses or unsupervised long-term use can cause liver damage. Excessive ingestion of alcoholic beverages may increase the risk of hepatotoxicity.
• Keep track of daily acetaminophen intake, including over-the-counter and prescription medications. Don't exceed the total recommended dose of acetaminophen per day because of the risk of hepatotoxicity.
• Be aware that the drug is found in breast milk in low levels (less than 1% of the dose). The drug is safe for short-term therapy as long as the recommended dose isn't exceeded.

Nonselective NSAIDs

As their name suggests, nonsteroidal anti-inflammatory drugs, or NSAIDs, are typically used to combat inflammation. Their anti-inflammatory action equals that of aspirin. They also have analgesic and antipyretic effects.

Nonselective NSAIDs inhibit prostaglandin synthesis by blocking two enzymes know as cyclooxygenase-1 (COX-1) and cyclooxygenase-2 (COX-2). These drugs (called *COX-1* and *COX-2 inhibitors*) include indomethacin, ibuprofen, diclofenac, etodolac, fenoprofen, flurbiprofen, ketoprofen, ketorolac, mefenamic acid, meloxicam, nabumetone, naproxen, oxaprozin, piroxicam, and sulindac.

Selective NSAIDs selectively block COX-2 enzymes, thereby inhibiting prostaglandin synthesis. This selective inhibition of COX-2 produces the analgesic and anti-inflammatory effects without causing the adverse GI effects associated with COX-1 inhibition by nonselective NSAIDS. (See *NSAIDs: Ibuprofen*, page 148.)

Pharmacokinetics

All NSAIDs (nonselective and selective) are absorbed in the GI tract. They're mostly metabolized in the liver and excreted primarily by the kidneys.

Pharmacodynamics

Inflammatory disorders produce and release prostaglandins from cell membranes, resulting in pain. Nonselective NSAIDs produce their effects by inhibiting prostaglandin synthesis and cyclooxygenase activity. NSAIDs inhibit both isoenzymes of cyclooxygenase, COX-1 and COX-2, which convert arachidonic acid into prostaglandins. COX-1 produces prostaglandins that maintain the stomach lining, whereas COX-2 produces prostaglandins that mediate an inflammatory response. Therefore, COX-1 inhibition is associated with NSAID-induced GI toxicity, whereas COX-2 inhibition alleviates pain and inflammation.

Pharmacotherapeutics

NSAIDs are primarily used to decrease inflammation. They're also used to relieve pain but are seldom prescribed to reduce fever. (See *Nonselective NSAIDs warning*.)

All in favor?

The following conditions respond favorably to treatment with NSAIDs:

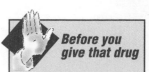

Before you give that drug

Nonselective NSAIDs warning

Before administering a nonsteroidal anti-inflammatory drug (NSAID) to a patient, be aware of its risks to special populations:

• *Children:* Some NSAIDs aren't recommended for use in children.

• *Elderly people:* The risk of ulcers increases with age.

• *Pregnant women:* Ketoprofen, naproxen, flurbiprofen, and diclofenac are category B drugs. Etodolac, ketorolac, meloxicam, nabumetone, oxaprozin, and piroxicam are category C drugs.

• *Nursing mothers:* Most NSAIDs are excreted in breast milk. In general, nonselective NSAIDs shouldn't be administered to nursing mothers.

Prototype pro

NSAIDs: Ibuprofen

Actions
• Interferes with the prostaglandins involved in pain; appears to sensitize pain receptors to mechanical stimulation or to other chemical mediators (such as bradykinin and histamine)
• Inhibits synthesis of prostaglandins peripherally and possibly centrally
• Inhibits prostaglandin synthesis and release during inflammation
• Suppresses prostaglandin synthesis in the central nervous system, causing an antipyretic effect

Indications
• Rheumatoid arthritis
• Osteoarthritis
• Juvenile arthritis
• Mild to moderate pain
• Fever

Nursing considerations
• Monitor the patient for adverse effects, such as bronchospasm, Stevens-Johnson syndrome, hematologic disorders, and aseptic meningitis.
• Keep in mind that it may take 1 to 2 weeks to achieve full anti-inflammatory effects.
• Be aware that the drug may mask the signs and symptoms of infection.

• ankylosing spondylitis (an inflammatory joint disease that first affects the spine)
• moderate to severe rheumatoid arthritis (an inflammatory disease of peripheral joints)
• osteoarthritis (a degenerative joint disease) in the hip, shoulder, or other large joints
• osteoarthritis accompanied by inflammation
• acute gouty arthritis (urate deposits in the joints)
• dysmenorrhea (painful menstruation)
• migraines
• bursitis
• tendonitis
• mild to moderate pain.

Drug interactions
Many drugs can interact with NSAIDs, especially with indomethacin, piroxicam, and sulindac. Because they're highly protein bound, NSAIDs are likely to interact with other protein-bound drugs. Such drugs as fluconazole, phenobarbital, rifampin, ritonavir, and salicylates affect NSAIDs, whereas NSAIDs affect oral anticoagulants, aminoglycosides, ACE inhibitors, beta-adrenergic blockers, digoxin, dilantin, and others.

Adverse reactions

All NSAIDs produce similar adverse reactions, which can include:
- abdominal pain and bleeding
- anorexia
- diarrhea
- nausea
- ulcers
- liver toxicity
- drowsiness
- headache
- dizziness
- confusion
- tinnitus
- vertigo
- depression
- bladder infection
- blood in urine
- kidney necrosis
- hypertension
- heart failure
- pedal edema.

Nursing process

These nursing process steps are appropriate for patients undergoing treatment with nonselective NSAIDs.

Assessment

- Obtain an assessment of the patient's underlying condition before starting drug therapy.
- Assess the patient's level of pain and inflammation before therapy begins and evaluate drug effectiveness after administration.
- Monitor the patient for signs and symptoms of bleeding. Assess bleeding time if he's expected to undergo surgery.
- Monitor the patient's ophthalmic and auditory function before and periodically during therapy to detect toxicity.
- Monitor CBC, platelet count, PT, and hepatic and renal function periodically to detect abnormalities.
- Be alert for adverse reactions and drug interactions. Watch for bronchospasm in the patient with aspirin hypersensitivity, rhinitis or nasal polyps, or asthma.
- Evaluate the patient's and family's knowledge of drug therapy.

Key nursing diagnoses

- Acute pain related to the underlying condition
- Risk for injury related to adverse reactions

Education edge

Teaching about nonselective NSAIDs

If nonselective nonsteroidal anti-inflammatory drugs (NSAIDs) are prescribed, review these points with the patient and his caregivers:

• Take the drug as directed to achieve the desired effect. Be aware that the benefits of some types of therapy may not be achieved for 2 to 4 weeks.

• Take the drug with meals or milk to reduce adverse GI effects.

• Don't exceed the recommended daily dosage, don't give the drug to children younger than age 12, and don't take the drug for extended periods without consulting a prescriber.

• Be aware that using the drug with aspirin, alcohol, or corticosteroids may increase the risk of adverse GI effects.

• Recognize and report signs and symptoms of GI bleeding, such as dark-colored stools, blood in urine, and unusual bleeding (for example, in the gums).

• Use sunblock, wear protective clothing, and avoid prolonged exposure to sunlight during therapy.

• If taking the medication as long-term therapy, check with the prescriber about the need for monitoring of laboratory values, especially blood urea nitrogen and creatinine levels, liver function, and complete blood count.

• Notify the prescriber about severe or persistent adverse reactions.

• Don't take other medications, over-the-counter products, or herbal products without first consulting with the prescriber.

• Deficient knowledge related to drug therapy

Planning outcome goals
• The patient will acknowledge a reduction in pain.
• No serious complications will occur while the patient is on drug therapy.
• The patient and his family will verbalize an understanding of the purpose and intended effect of drug therapy.

Implementation
• Administer oral NSAIDs with 8 oz (240 ml) of water to ensure adequate passage into the stomach. Have the patient sit up for 15 to 30 minutes after taking the drug to prevent it from lodging in the esophagus.
• As needed, crush tablets or mix with food or fluid to aid swallowing.

Stomach soothers
• Give the drug with meals or milk or administer it with antacids to reduce adverse GI reactions.
• Notify the prescriber if the drug is ineffective.

• If renal or hepatic abnormalities occur, stop the drug and notify the prescriber.

Evaluation

• Patient states that pain is relieved.
• Patient remains free from adverse effects throughout drug therapy.
• Patient and his family state an understanding of drug therapy. (See *Teaching about nonselective NSAIDs.*)

Selective NSAIDs

Prostaglandins produced by COX-2 are associated with pain and inflammation. The selective NSAIDs (also called COX-2 inhibitor drugs) are NSAIDs that selectively block COX-2, relieving pain and inflammation. They have fewer adverse effects, such as stomach damage, than nonselective NSAIDs. The only currently available selective NSAID is celecoxib.

Pharmacokinetics

Celecoxib is highly protein bound, primarily to albumin, and is extensively distributed into the tissues. Peak levels occur within 3 hours, and steady plasma states can be expected in 5 days, if given in multiple doses. Celecoxib is metabolized in the liver, with less than 3% unchanged, and excreted in urine and feces.

Pharmacodynamics

Celecoxib produces its effect by selectively blocking the COX-2 enzyme, thereby inhibiting prostaglandin synthesis.

Less than the rest

This selective inhibition of COX-2 produces analgesic and anti-inflammatory effects without the adverse GI effects associated with COX-1 inhibition by nonselective NSAIDs. However, some degree of COX-1 inhibition still occurs.

Pharmacotherapeutics

Celecoxib is primarily used to provide analgesia and to decrease inflammation. It's particularly useful in the treatment of osteoarthritis, rheumatoid arthritis, acute pain, primary dysmenorrhea, and familial adenomatous polyposis.

Drug interactions

Because celecoxib is metabolized by the liver, drug interactions have been identified. For example:
• Celecoxib decreases the clearance of lithium, which can result in lithium toxicity.
• It reduces the antihypertensive effects of ACE inhibitors and diuretics.
• When celecoxib is taken with warfarin, increased PT levels and bleeding complications can occur.
• Celecoxib interacts with herbal preparations that increase the risk of bleeding, such as dong quai, feverfew, garlic, ginger, ginkgo, horse chestnut, and red clover.

Adverse reactions

These adverse reactions may occur with celecoxib:
• dyspepsia
• nausea and vomiting
• GI ulcers (to a lesser degree than with nonselective NSAIDs)
• hypertension
• fluid retention
• peripheral edema
• dizziness
• headache
• rash.

Nursing process

These nursing process steps are appropriate for patients undergoing treatment with selective NSAIDs (COX-2 inhibitors).

Assessment

• Obtain an assessment of the patient's underlying condition before starting drug therapy.
• Obtain an accurate list of the patient's allergies. If he's allergic to or has anaphylactic reactions to sulfonamides, aspirin, or other NSAIDs, he may also be allergic to selective NSAIDs.
• Assess the patient's level of pain and inflammation before therapy begins, and evaluate drug effectiveness after administration.
• Monitor the patient for signs and symptoms of bleeding. Assess bleeding time if he requires surgery.
• Monitor the patient's ophthalmic and auditory function before therapy and periodically thereafter to detect toxicity.
• Periodically monitor CBC, platelet count, PT, and hepatic and renal function to detect abnormalities.
• Closely monitor the patient on celecoxib for signs or symptoms of MI. This drug has been linked to a relatively high risk of heart attacks.

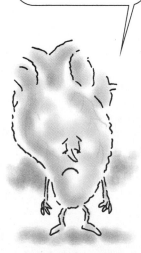

Woe is me! Celecoxib has been linked to a relatively high risk of heart disease.

Education edge

Teaching about selective NSAIDs

If selective nonsteroidal anti-inflammatory drugs (NSAIDs) or cyclooxygenase-2 (COX-2) drugs are prescribed, review these points with the patient and his caregivers:

• Report a history of allergic reactions to sulfonamides, aspirin, or other NSAIDs before starting therapy.

• Immediately report to the prescriber signs of GI bleeding (such as bloody vomitus, blood in urine or stool, and black, tarry stools), rash, and unexplained weight gain or edema.

• Notify the prescriber if you become pregnant or are planning to become pregnant while taking this drug.

• Take the drug with food if stomach upset occurs.

• Be aware that all NSAIDs, including COX-2 inhibitors, may adversely affect the liver. Signs and symptoms of liver toxicity include nausea, fatigue, lethargy, itching, jaundice, right upper quadrant tenderness, and flulike symptoms. Stop therapy and seek immediate medical advice if any of these signs and symptoms develops.

• Be aware that it may take several days to feel consistent pain relief.

• Don't take other medications, over-the-counter products, or herbal remedies unless first approved by the prescriber.

• Inform all health care providers that you're taking this medication.

• Avoid or minimize alcoholic beverages because alcohol increases gastric irritation and the risk of bleeding.

• Evaluate the patient's and family's knowledge of drug therapy.

Key nursing diagnoses

• Acute pain related to the underlying condition
• Risk for injury related to adverse reactions
• Deficient knowledge related to drug therapy

Planning outcome goals

• The patient will acknowledge a reduction in pain.
• No serious complications will occur while the patient is on drug therapy.
• The patient and his family will verbalize an understanding of the purpose and intended effect of drug therapy.

Implementation

• Although the drug can be given without regard to meals, food may decrease GI upset.
• Before starting treatment, be sure to rehydrate the patient.

• Although the drug may be used with low aspirin dosages, the combination may increase the risk of GI bleeding.
• NSAIDs such as celecoxib can cause fluid retention; closely monitor the patient who has hypertension, edema, or heart failure.
• Notify the prescriber if the drug is ineffective.

Evaluation
• Patient states that pain is relieved.
• Patient remains free from adverse effects throughout drug therapy.
• Patient and his family state an understanding of drug therapy. (See *Teaching about selective NSAIDs*, page 153.)

Phenazopyridine hydrochloride

Phenazopyridine hydrochloride, an azo dye used in commercial coloring, produces a local analgesic effect on the urinary tract, usually within 24 to 48 hours after the start of therapy. It's used to relieve the pain, burning, urgency, and frequency associated with urinary tract infections.

Dye job

When taken orally, phenazopyridine is 35% metabolized in the liver, with the remainder excreted unchanged in urine, which may appear orange or red.

Mellow yellow

If the drug accumulates in the body, the skin and sclera of the eye may take on a yellow tinge, and phenazopyridine may need to be stopped.

Pharmacokinetics
The absorption and distribution of phenazopyridine are unknown. The drug is metabolized in the liver and excreted in urine.

Pharmacodynamics
Phenazopyridine hydrochloride has a local anesthetic effect on the urinary mucosa.

Pharmacotherapeutics
Phenazopyridine hydrochloride is used to relieve urinary tract pain.

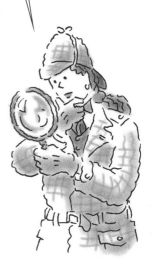

The absorption and distribution of phenazopyridine remain unknown. Perhaps if I examine all the clues again, I can solve this mystery.

Nursing process

These nursing process steps are appropriate for patients undergoing treatment with phenazopyridine.

Assessment
• Obtain an assessment of the patient's underlying condition before starting drug therapy.
• Assess the patient's level of pain and inflammation before therapy begins, and evaluate drug effectiveness after administration.
• Monitor the patient's hydration status if nausea occurs.
• Evaluate the patient's and family's knowledge of drug therapy.

Key nursing diagnoses
• Acute pain related to the underlying condition
• Risk for injury related to adverse reactions
• Deficient knowledge related to drug therapy

Planning outcome goals
• The patient will acknowledge a reduction in pain.
• No serious complications will occur while patient is on drug therapy.
• The patient and his family will verbalize an understanding of the purpose and intended effect of drug therapy.

Implementation
• Administer the drug with food to minimize nausea.
• Advise the patient that the drug colors urine red or orange and may stain fabrics and contact lenses.
• Notify the prescriber if the drug is ineffective and urinary tract pain persists.

Evaluation
• Patient states that pain is relieved.
• Patient remains free from adverse effects throughout drug therapy.
• Patient and his family state an understanding of drug therapy.

Opioid agonists and antagonists

The word *opioid* refers to any derivative of the opium plant or any synthetic drug that imitates natural narcotics. Opioid agonists (also called *narcotic agonists*) include opium derivatives and synthetic drugs with similar properties. They're used to relieve or decrease pain without causing the person to lose consciousness.

Some opioid agonists also have antitussive and antidiarrheal effects.

Some opioid agonists also have...cough, cough...antitussive effects.

Opioid opponent

Opioid antagonists aren't pain medications. They block the effects of opioid agonists and are used to reverse adverse drug reactions, such as respiratory and CNS depression produced by those drugs. Unfortunately, by reversing the analgesic effect, they also cause the patient's pain to recur.

Having it both ways

Some opioid analgesics, called *mixed opioid agonist-antagonists*, have agonist and antagonist properties. The agonist component relieves pain, and the antagonist component decreases the risk of toxicity and drug dependence. These mixed opioid agonist-antagonists reduce the risk of respiratory depression and drug abuse.

Opioid agonists

Opioid agonists include:
- codeine
- fentanyl citrate
- hydrocodone
- hydromorphone hydrochloride
- levorphanol tartrate
- meperidine hydrochloride
- methadone hydrochloride
- morphine sulfate (including morphine sulfate sustained-release tablets and intensified oral solution)
- oxycodone
- oxymorphone
- propoxyphene
- remifentanil.

Gold standard

Morphine sulfate is the standard against which the effectiveness and adverse reactions of other pain medications are measured. (See *Opioid agonists: Morphine.*)

Pharmacokinetics

Opioid agonists can be administered by any route, although inhalation administration is uncommon. Oral doses are absorbed readily from the GI tract. Transmucosal and intrathecal opiates are fast acting. Opioid agonists administered I.V. provide the most

---

Prototype pro

Opioid agonists: Morphine

Actions
- Acts on opiate receptors in the central nervous system

Indications
- Pain

Nursing considerations
- Monitor the patient for adverse effects, such as sedation, euphoria, seizures, dizziness, nightmares, bradycardia, shock, cardiac arrest, nausea, constipation, vomiting, thrombocytopenia, and respiratory depression.
- Keep an opioid antagonist (naloxone) and resuscitation equipment available.

rapid (almost immediate) and reliable pain relief. The subcutaneous and I.M. routes may result in delayed absorption, especially in patients with poor circulation.

Opioid agonists are distributed widely throughout body tissues. They have a relatively low plasma protein-binding capacity (30% to 35%).

Liver lovers

These drugs are metabolized extensively in the liver. For example, meperidine is metabolized to normeperidine, a toxic metabolite with a longer half-life than meperidine. This metabolite accumulates in renal failure and may lead to CNS excitation. Administration of meperidine for more than 48 hours increases the risk of neurotoxicity and seizures from a buildup of normeperidine.

Metabolites are excreted by the kidneys. A small amount is excreted in feces through the biliary tract.

Pharmacodynamics

Opioid agonists reduce pain by binding to opiate receptor sites in the peripheral nervous system and the CNS. When these drugs stimulate the opiate receptors, they mimic the effects of endorphins (naturally occurring opiates that are part of the body's own pain relief system). This receptor-site binding produces the therapeutic effects of analgesia and cough suppression as well as adverse reactions, such as respiratory depression and constipation. (See *How opioid agonists control pain*, page 158.)

Smooth operator

Besides reducing pain, opioid agonists, especially morphine, affect the smooth muscle of the GI and genitourinary tracts (the organs of the reproductive and urinary systems). This causes contraction of the bladder and ureters and slows intestinal peristalsis (rhythmic contractions that move food along the digestive tract), resulting in constipation, a common adverse reaction to opiates.

A fine line

These drugs also cause blood vessels to dilate, especially in the face, head, and neck. In addition, they suppress the cough center in the brain, producing antitussive effects and causing constriction of the bronchial muscles. Any of these effects can become adverse reactions if produced in excess. For example, if the blood vessels dilate too much, hypotension can occur.

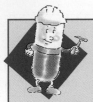

Pharm function

How opioid agonists control pain

Opioid agonists, such as meperidine, inhibit pain transmission by mimicking the body's natural pain control mechanisms.

Where neurons meet
In the dorsal horn of the spinal cord, peripheral pain neurons meet central nervous system (CNS) neurons. At the synapse, the pain neuron releases substance P (a pain neurotransmitter). This agent helps transfer pain impulses to the CNS neurons that carry the impulses to the brain.

Taking up space
In theory, the spinal interneurons respond to stimulation from the descending neurons of the CNS by releasing endogenous opiates. These opiates bind to the peripheral pain neuron to inhibit release of substance P and to retard the transmission of pain impulses.

Stopping substance P
Synthetic opiates supplement this pain-blocking effect by binding with free opiate receptors to inhibit the release of substance P. Opiates also alter consciousness of pain, but how this mechanism works remains unknown.

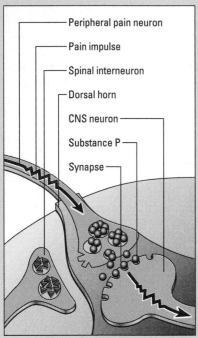

- Peripheral pain neuron
- Pain impulse
- Spinal interneuron
- Dorsal horn
- CNS neuron
- Substance P
- Synapse

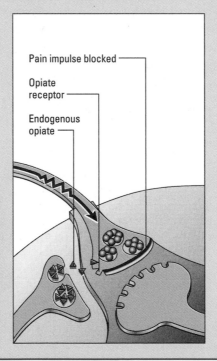

- Pain impulse blocked
- Opiate receptor
- Endogenous opiate

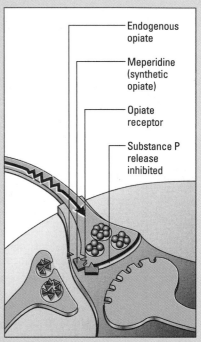

- Endogenous opiate
- Meperidine (synthetic opiate)
- Opiate receptor
- Substance P release inhibited

Pharmacotherapeutics

Opioid agonists are prescribed to relieve severe pain in acute, chronic, and terminal illnesses. They're sometimes prescribed to control diarrhea and suppress coughing. Methadone is used for temporary maintenance of opioid addiction. Opioids such as fentanyl and remifentanil are used for the induction and maintenance of general anesthesia.

Cardio-assistance

Morphine relieves shortness of breath in the patient with pulmonary edema (fluid in the lungs) or left-sided heart failure (inability of the heart to pump enough blood to meet the body's needs). It does this by dilating peripheral blood vessels, keeping more blood in the periphery, and decreasing cardiac preload.

Drug interactions

Drugs that can affect opioid analgesic activity include amitriptyline, protease inhibitors, dilantin, diazepam, and rifampin. Taking tricyclic antidepressants, phenothiazines, or anticholinergics with opioid agonists may cause severe constipation and urine retention. Drugs that may be affected by opioid analgesics include carbamazepine, warfarin, beta-adrenergic blockers, and calcium channel blockers.

The use of opioid agonists with other substances that decrease respiration, such as alcohol, sedatives, hypnotics, and anesthetics, increases the patient's risk of severe respiratory depression. (See *Opioid agonists warning.*)

Adverse reactions

One of the most common adverse reactions to opioid agonists is decreased rate and depth of breathing that worsens as the dose of narcotic is increased. This may cause periodic, irregular breathing or trigger asthmatic attacks in a susceptible patient.

Other adverse reactions include:
• flushing
• orthostatic hypotension
• pupil constriction.

With meperidine administration, these adverse reactions can occur:
• tremors
• palpitations
• tachycardia
• delirium
• neurotoxicity and seizures (if administered for more than 48 hours).

Nursing process

These nursing process steps are appropriate for patients undergoing treatment with opioid agonists.

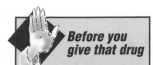

Before you give that drug

Opioid agonists warning

Before administering medications, be aware that morphine sulfate (MSO_4) can be confused with magnesium sulfate ($MgSO_4$). Verify abbreviations, or better yet, spell out the medication to avoid confusion.

Opioid agonists are classified as pregnancy category C, and most appear in breast milk; most doctors recommend waiting 4 to 6 hours after ingestion to breast-feed.

Assessment

• Obtain a baseline assessment of the patient's pain and reassess frequently to determine drug effectiveness.

When beathing easy is hard work

• Evaluate the patient's respiratory status before each dose; watch for a respiratory rate below the patient's baseline level and for restlessness, which may be compensatory signs of hypoxia. Respiratory depression may last longer than the analgesic effect.
• Monitor the patient for other adverse reactions.
• Monitor the patient for tolerance and dependence. The first sign of tolerance to opioids is usually a shortened duration of effect.

Key nursing diagnoses

• Acute pain related to the underlying condition
• Ineffective breathing pattern related to depressive effect on respiratory system
• Deficient knowledge related to drug therapy

Planning outcome goals

• The patient will acknowledge a reduction in pain.
• Throughout therapy, the patient will maintain adequate breathing function.
• The patient and his family will verbalize an understanding of the purpose and intended effect of drug therapy.

Implementation

• Keep resuscitative equipment and a narcotic antagonist (naloxone) available.
• Give the I.V. form of the drug by slow injection, preferably in diluted solution. Rapid I.V. injection increases the risk of adverse effects.
• Give I.M. or subcutaneous (subQ) injections cautiously to a patient with a decreased platelet count and to a patient who's chilled, hypovolemic, or in shock; decreased perfusion may lead to drug accumulation and toxicity. Rotate injection sites to avoid induration.
• Carefully note the strength of the solution when measuring a dose. Oral solutions of varying concentrations are available.
• For maximum effectiveness, give the drug on a regular dosage schedule rather than as needed.
• Institute safety precautions.
• Encourage a postoperative patient to turn, cough, and breathe deeply every 2 hours to avoid atelectasis.
• If GI irritation occurs, give oral forms of the drug with food.

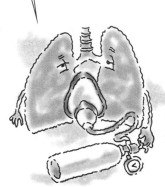

Watch for a respiratory rate below the patient's baseline and for restlessness, possible signs of hypoxia. A little more oxygen, please.

Education edge

Teaching about opioid agonists

If opioid agonists are prescribed, review these points with the patient and his caregivers:
• Take the drug exactly as prescribed. Call the prescriber if you don't experience the desired effect or if you experience significant adverse reactions.
• Be careful when getting out of bed and walking. Avoid hazardous activities until the drug's effects are known.
• Avoid alcohol while taking opioid agonists because it causes additive central nervous system depression.
• To prevent constipation, increase fiber in the diet and use a stool softener.
• Breathe deeply, cough, and change position every 2 hours to avoid respiratory complications.
• Report continued pain.

• Be aware that withdrawal symptoms, including tremors, agitation, nausea, and vomiting, may occur if the drug is stopped abruptly. Monitor the patient with these signs and symptoms carefully and provide supportive therapy.

Evaluation
• Patient states that pain is relieved.
• Patient maintains adequate ventilation, as evidenced by normal respiratory rate and rhythm and pink skin color.
• Patient and his family state an understanding of drug therapy. (See *Teaching about opioid agonists.*)

Mixed opioid agonist-antagonists

Mixed opioid agonist-antagonists are given to relieve pain while reducing toxic effects and dependency. Examples include:
• buprenorphine hydrochloride
• butorphanol tartrate
• nalbuphine hydrochloride
• pentazocine hydrochloride (combined with pentazocine lactate, naloxone hydrochloride, aspirin, or acetaminophen).

A mixed bag

Originally, mixed opioid agonist-antagonists appeared to have less abuse potential than the pure opioid agonists. However, butorphanol and pentazocine have reportedly caused dependence. This class of drugs isn't recommended for use in patients with chronic pain who are taking other opioid agonists.

Pharmacokinetics

Absorption of mixed opioid agonist-antagonists occurs rapidly from parenteral sites. These drugs are distributed to most body tissues and cross the placenta. They're metabolized in the liver and excreted primarily by the kidneys, although more than 10% of a butorphanol dose and a small amount of a pentazocine dose are excreted in stool.

Pharmacodynamics

The exact mechanism of action of mixed opioid agonist-antagonists isn't known. However, researchers believe that these drugs weakly antagonize the effects of morphine, meperidine, and other opiates at one of the opioid receptors. They also exert agonistic effects at other opioid receptors.

In no rush

Buprenorphine binds with receptors in the CNS, altering the perception of and the emotional response to pain through an unknown mechanism. It seems to release slowly from binding sites, producing a longer duration of action than the other drugs in this class.

Don't get emotional

The site of action of butorphanol may be opiate receptors in the limbic system (part of the brain involved in emotion). Like pentazocine, butorphanol also acts on pulmonary circulation, increasing pulmonary vascular resistance (resistance in the blood vessels of the lungs that the right ventricle must pump against). Both drugs also increase blood pressure and the workload of the heart.

Pharmacotherapeutics

Mixed opioid agonist-antagonists are used as analgesia during childbirth as well as postoperatively.

Independence day

Mixed opioid agonist-antagonists are sometimes prescribed in place of opioid agonists because they have a lower risk of drug de-

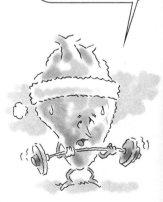

Ack! Pentazocine and butorphanol increase my workload. I'm already doing enough heavy lifting!

pendence. Mixed opioid agonist-antagonists also are less likely to cause respiratory depression and constipation, although they can produce some adverse reactions.

Drug interactions

Increased CNS depression and an additive decrease in respiratory rate and depth may result if mixed opioid agonist-antagonists are administered to a patient taking other CNS depressants, such as barbiturates and alcohol.

Clean and sober?

The patient with a history of opioid abuse shouldn't receive any mixed opioid agonist-antagonists because they can cause withdrawal symptoms.

> A patient with a history of opioid abuse shouldn't receive opioid agonist-antagonists. Withdrawal symptoms may result.

Adverse reactions

The most common adverse reactions to opioid agonist-antagonists include nausea, vomiting, light-headedness, sedation, and euphoria.

Nursing process

These nursing process steps are appropriate for patients undergoing treatment with an opioid agonist-antagonist.

Assessment
• Obtain a baseline assessment of the patient's pain and reassess frequently to determine the drug's effectiveness.
• Evaluate the patient's respiratory status before each dose; watch for a respiratory rate below the baseline level and watch for restlessness, which may be a compensatory sign of hypoxemia. Respiratory depression may last longer than the analgesic effect.
• Monitor the patient for other adverse reactions.
• Monitor the patient for tolerance and dependence. The first sign of tolerance to opioids is usually a shortened duration of effect.

Key nursing diagnoses
• Acute pain related to the underlying condition
• Ineffective breathing pattern related to depressive effect on respiratory system
• Deficient knowledge related to drug therapy

Planning outcome goals
• The patient will acknowledge a reduction in pain.

• Throughout therapy, the patient will maintain an adequate breathing pattern.
• The patient and his family will state an understanding of the purpose and intended effect of drug therapy.

Implementation

• Keep resuscitative equipment and an opioid antagonist (naloxone) available. Naloxone won't completely reverse respiratory depression caused by buprenorphine overdose; mechanical ventilation may be necessary. Doxapram and larger-than-usual doses of naloxone may also be ordered.

Take it slow

• Give the I.V. form of the drug by slow injection, preferably in diluted solution. Rapid I.V. injection increases the risk of adverse effects.
• Institute safety precautions.
• Encourage a postoperative patient to turn, cough, and breathe deeply every 2 hours to avoid atelectasis.

Withdrawal warning

• Be aware that the drug may precipitate withdrawal syndrome in an opioid-dependent patient. Withdrawal symptoms — including tremors, agitation, nausea, and vomiting — may occur if the drug is stopped abruptly. If dependence occurs, withdrawal symptoms may appear up to 14 days after the drug is stopped. Monitor a patient with these symptoms carefully and provide supportive therapy.

Evaluation

• Patient states that pain is relieved.
• Patient maintains adequate ventilation, as evidenced by normal respiratory rate and rhythm and pink skin color.
• Patient and his family state an understanding of drug therapy.

Opioid antagonists

Opioid antagonists attach to opiate receptors, but don't stimulate them, and have a greater attraction for opiate receptors than opioids do. As a result, they prevent opioid drugs, enkephalins, and endorphins from producing their effects.

Opioid antagonists include:
• naloxone hydrochloride
• naltrexone hydrochloride.

Pharmacokinetics

Naloxone is administered I.M., subQ, or I.V. Naltrexone is administered orally in tablet or liquid form. Both drugs are metabolized by the liver and excreted by the kidneys.

Pharmacodynamics

In a process known as *competitive inhibition,* opioid antagonists block the effects of opioids by occupying the opiate receptor sites, displacing opioids attached to opiate receptors and blocking further opioid binding at these sites.

Pharmacotherapeutics

Naloxone is the drug of choice for managing an opioid overdose. It reverses respiratory depression and sedation and helps stabilize the patient's vital signs within seconds after administration.

Because naloxone also reverses the analgesic effects of opioid drugs, a patient who was given an opioid drug for pain relief may complain of pain or even experience withdrawal symptoms.

Kicking the habit

Naltrexone is used along with psychotherapy or counseling to treat drug abuse. It's only given, however, to a patient who has gone through a detoxification program to remove all opioids from the body. A patient who still has opioids in the body may experience acute withdrawal symptoms if given naltrexone.

Drug interactions

Naloxone produces no significant drug interactions. Naltrexone will cause withdrawal symptoms if given to a patient who's receiving an opioid agonist or who's an opioid addict.

Adverse reactions

Naltrexone can cause several adverse reactions, including:
- edema
- hypertension
- palpitations
- phlebitis
- shortness of breath
- anxiety
- depression
- disorientation
- dizziness
- headache

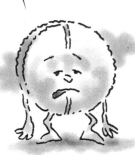

It's tough out there for us opioids. The competitive inhibition of opioid antagonists can keep me from doing my job.

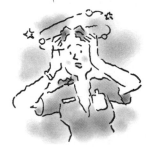

Naltrexone can cause headache, anxiety and—yikes!—dizziness.

- nervousness
- anorexia
- diarrhea or constipation
- nausea and vomiting
- thirst
- urinary frequency
- liver toxicity.

Watch the wake-up

Naloxone may cause nausea, vomiting and, occasionally, hypertension and tachycardia. An unconscious patient returned to consciousness abruptly after naloxone administration may hyperventilate and experience tremors.

Nursing process

These nursing process steps are appropriate for patients undergoing treatment with an opioid antagonist.

Assessment

- Assess the patient's opioid use before therapy.
- Assess the drug's effectiveness regularly throughout therapy.
- Monitor the patient's respiratory depth and rate. The duration of the opioid may exceed that of naloxone, causing relapse into respiratory depression.
- Monitor the patient's hydration status if adverse GI reactions occur.
- Evaluate the patient's and family's knowledge of drug therapy.

Key nursing diagnoses

- Ineffective health maintenance related to opioid use
- Risk for deficient fluid volume related to drug-induced adverse GI reactions
- Deficient knowledge related to drug therapy

Planning outcome goals

- The patient will demonstrate improved health as evidenced by maintenance of vital signs within normal parameters.
- The patient will maintain adequate hydration as evidenced by adequate urine output.
- The patient and his family will verbalize an understanding of the purpose and intended effect of drug therapy.

Implementation

• Provide oxygen, ventilation, and other resuscitation measures when the drug is used in the management of acute opiate overdose and when the patient has severe respiratory depression.
• Keep in mind that these drugs are effective in reversing respiratory depression only when it's caused by opioids. When they're used for this purpose, monitor the patient for tachypnea.
• Be prepared to give continuous I.V. naloxone infusion to control adverse effects of epidural morphine.

Evaluation

• Patient responds well to drug therapy.
• Patient maintains adequate hydration.
• Patient and his family state an understanding of drug therapy.

Anesthetic drugs

Anesthetic drugs can be divided into three groups—general anesthetics, local anesthetics, and topical anesthetics.

Inhale or inject?

General anesthetic drugs are further subdivided into two main types, those given by inhalation and those given I.V.

Inhalation anesthetics

Commonly used general anesthetics given by inhalation include:
• desflurane
• sevoflurane
• enflurane
• isoflurane
• nitrous oxide.

Pharmacokinetics

The absorption and elimination rates of anesthetics are governed by their solubility in blood. Inhalation anesthetics enter the blood from the lungs and are distributed to other tissues. Distribution is most rapid to organs with high blood flow, such as the brain, liver, kidneys, and heart.

Leaving? Try the lungs and liver

Inhalation anesthetics are eliminated primarily by the lungs; enflurane and sevoflurane are also eliminated by the liver. Metabolites are excreted in urine.

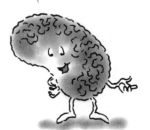

My high blood flow means that anesthetics can make their way to me more quickly.

Pharmacodynamics

Inhalation anesthetics work primarily by depressing the CNS, producing loss of consciousness, loss of responsiveness to sensory stimulation (including pain), and muscle relaxation. They also affect other organ systems.

Pharmacotherapeutics

Inhalation anesthetics are used for surgery because they offer more precise and rapid control of depth of anesthesia than injection anesthetics. These anesthetics, which are liquids at room temperature, require a vaporizer and special delivery system for safe use.

Of the inhalation anesthetics available, desflurane, isoflurane, and nitrous oxide are the most commonly used.

Stop signs

Inhalation anesthetics are contraindicated in a patient with known hypersensitivity to the drug, a liver disorder, or malignant hyperthermia (a potentially fatal complication of anesthesia characterized by skeletal muscle rigidity and high fever). They require cautious use in a pregnant or breast-feeding patient.

Drug interactions

The most important drug interactions involving inhalation anesthetics are with other CNS, cardiac, or respiratory-depressant drugs. These drug combinations can cause CNS depression, cardiac arrhythmias, or respiratory depression, resulting in compromised patient status.

Adverse reactions

The most common adverse reaction to inhalation anesthetics is an exaggerated patient response to a normal dose. Malignant hyperthermia, characterized by a sudden and usually lethal increase in body temperature, is a serious and unexpected reaction to inhalation anesthetics. It occurs in the genetically susceptible patient only and may result from a failure in calcium uptake by muscle cells. The skeletal muscle relaxant dantrolene is used to treat this condition.

Waking up woes

After surgery, a patient may experience reactions similar to those seen with other CNS depressants, including depression of breathing and circulation, confusion, sedation, nausea, vomiting, ataxia, and hypothermia.

> After surgery, a patient may experience reactions similar to those seen with other CNS depressants, including confusion, sedation, and — burr!—hypothermia.

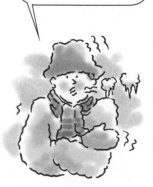

Nursing process

These nursing process steps are appropriate for patients undergoing treatment with anesthetic drugs.

Assessment

- Assess the patient's use of prescription, nonprescription, and herbal remedies, especially within the past 3 days.
- Assess drug allergies and risk factors for complications of anesthesia and surgery (cigarette smoking, obesity, limited exercise or activity, and chronic cardiovascular, respiratory, renal, or other disease processes).
- Assess the patient's vital signs, laboratory data, and physical condition to establish baseline measurements for monitoring changes.

Key nursing diagnoses

- Risk for injury related to impaired sensory perception from anesthetic or sedative drugs
- Risk for ineffective breathing pattern related to respiratory depression
- Deficient knowledge related to drug therapy

Planning outcome goals

- The risk of injury to the patient will be minimized.
- While under anesthesia, the patient will maintain adequate ventilation and breathing pattern.
- The patient and his family will verbalize an understanding of the purpose and intended effect of drug therapy.

Interventions

- Explain the preoperative and expected postoperative phases of the recovery period.
- Review postoperative recovery requirements, such as deep breathing exercises, coughing, leg exercises, early ambulation, maintaining fluid balance, and urine output.
- Monitor the patient's vital signs, level of consciousness (LOC), respiratory and cardiovascular status, and laboratory results, as indicated.
- Monitor the patient's response to pain medication.

Evaluation

- Patient remains free from major complications.
- Patient maintains adequate ventilation.
- Patient and his family state an understanding of anesthetic drug therapy.

I.V. anesthetics

I.V. anesthetics are usually used as general anesthesia when anesthesia is needed for only a short period, such as with outpatient surgery. They're also used to promote rapid induction of anesthesia or to supplement inhalation anesthetics.

A "knockout" bunch

The drugs used as I.V. anesthetics are:
- barbiturates (methohexital, thiopental)
- benzodiazepines (midazolam)
- dissociatives (ketamine)
- hypnotics (etomidate, propofol)
- opiates (fentanyl, sufentanil).

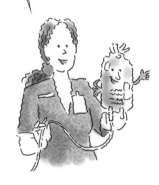

I.V. administration promotes rapid induction of anesthesia.

Pharmacokinetics

I.V. anesthetic agents are lipid soluble and are well distributed throughout the body, crossing the placenta and entering breast milk. These drugs are metabolized in the liver and excreted in urine.

Pharmacodynamics

Opiates work by occupying sites on specialized receptors scattered throughout the CNS and modifying the release of neurotransmitters from sensory nerves entering the CNS. Ketamine appears to induce a profound sense of dissociation from the environment by acting directly on the cortex and limbic system of the brain.

You're getting sleepy

Barbiturates, benzodiazepines, and etomidate seem to enhance responses to the CNS neurotransmitter gamma-aminobutyric acid. This inhibits the brain's response to stimulation of the reticular activating system, the area of the brain stem that controls alertness. Barbiturates also depress the excitability of CNS neurons.

Pharmacotherapeutics

Because of the short duration of action of I.V. anesthetics, they're used in shorter surgical procedures, including outpatient surgery. Barbiturates are used alone in surgery that isn't expected to be painful and as adjuncts to other drugs in more extensive procedures.

Benzodiazepines produce sedation and amnesia, but not pain relief. Etomidate is used to induce anesthesia and to supplement low-potency inhalation anesthetics such as nitrous oxide. The opiates provide pain relief and supplement other anesthetic drugs.

Drug interactions

I.V. anesthetics, particularly ketamine, can produce many drug interactions:
• Verapamil enhances the anesthetic effects of etomidate, producing respiratory depression and apnea.
• Giving ketamine and nondepolarizing drugs together increases neuromuscular effects, resulting in prolonged respiratory depression.

A longer road to recovery

• Using barbiturates or opioids with ketamine may prolong recovery time after anesthesia.
• Ketamine plus theophylline may promote seizures.
• Ketamine and thyroid hormones may cause hypertension and tachycardia (rapid heart rate).

Adverse reactions

Adverse reactions to injection anesthetics vary by drug.

Ketamine

Ketamine can produce these adverse effects:
• prolonged recovery
• irrational behavior
• excitement
• disorientation
• delirium or hallucinations
• increased heart rate
• hypertension
• excess salivation
• tearing
• shivering
• increased cerebrospinal fluid and eye pressure
• seizures.

Propofol

Propofol can cause:
• respiratory depression
• bradycardia
• hiccups
• coughing
• muscle twitching
• hypotension.

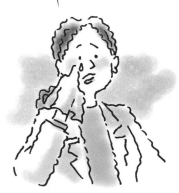

How sad. Ketamine can cause irrational behavior, excessive salivation, and tearing.

Thiopental

Thiopental can cause:
- respiratory depression
- hiccups
- coughing
- muscle twitching
- depressed cardiac function and peripheral dilation.

Etomidate

Etomidate can cause:
- hiccups
- coughing
- muscle twitching
- apnea.

Fentanyl

Fentanyl can cause:
- CNS and respiratory depression
- hypoventilation
- arrhythmias.

Midazolam

Midazolam can cause:
- CNS and respiratory depression
- hypotension
- dizziness
- cardiac arrest.

Nursing process

These nursing process steps are appropriate for patients undergoing treatment with I.V. anesthetics.

Assessment

- Assess the use of prescription, nonprescription, and herbal remedies, especially within the past 3 days.

Recognizing risk factors

- Assess the patient's drug allergies and risk factors for complications of anesthesia and surgery (cigarette smoking, obesity, limited exercise or activity, and chronic cardiovascular, respiratory, renal, or other disease processes).
- Assess the patient's vital signs, laboratory data, and physical condition to establish baseline measurements for monitoring changes.

Key nursing diagnoses
• Risk for injury related to impaired sensory perception from anesthetic or sedative drugs
• Risk for ineffective breathing pattern related to respiratory depression
• Deficient knowledge related to drug therapy

Planning outcome goals
• The risk of injury to the patient will be minimized.
• While under anesthesia, the patient will maintain adequate ventilation and breathing pattern.
• The patient and his family will verbalize an understanding of the purpose and intended effect of drug therapy.

Interventions
• Explain expectations for the preoperative and postoperative phases of the recovery period.
• Review postoperative recovery requirements, such as deep-breathing exercises, coughing, leg exercises, early ambulation, maintaining fluid balance, and urine output.
• Monitor the patient's vital signs, LOC, respiratory and cardiovascular status, and laboratory results, as indicated.
• Monitor the patient's response to pain medication.

Evaluation
• Patient remains free from major complications.
• Patient maintains adequate ventilation.
• Patient and his family state an understanding of drug therapy.

Local anesthetics

Local anesthetics are administered to prevent or relieve pain in a specific area of the body. In addition, these drugs are commonly used as an alternative to general anesthesia for elderly or debilitated patients.

Chain gang

Local anesthetics may be classified as:
• amide drugs (with nitrogen in the molecular chain, such as bupivacaine, ropivacaine, lidocaine, levobupivacaine, mepivacaine, and prilocaine)
• ester drugs (with oxygen in the molecular chain, such as procaine, chloroprocaine, and tetracaine).
(See *Amide and ester examples*, page 174.)

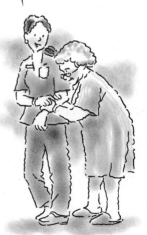

Local anesthetics are typically a safer choice than general anesthesia for elderly patients.

Pharmacokinetics

Absorption of local anesthetics varies widely, but distribution occurs throughout the body. Esters and amides undergo different types of metabolism, but both yield metabolites that are excreted in urine.

Pharmacodynamics

Local anesthetics block nerve impulses at the point of contact in all kinds of nerves. For example, they can accumulate and cause the nerve cell membrane to expand. As the membrane expands, the cell loses its ability to depolarize, which is necessary for impulse transmission.

Pharmacotherapeutics

Local anesthetics are used to prevent and relieve pain caused by medical procedures, diseases, or injuries. They're used for severe pain that topical anesthetics or analgesics can't relieve.

When a general won't do

Local anesthetics are usually preferred to general anesthetics for surgery in elderly or debilitated patients or in patients with disorders that affect respiratory function, such as chronic obstructive pulmonary disease and myasthenia gravis.

Combining and coordinating

For some procedures, a local anesthetic is combined with a drug, such as epinephrine, that constricts blood vessels. Vasoconstriction helps control local bleeding and reduces absorption of the anesthetic. Reduced absorption prolongs the anesthetic's action at the site and limits its distribution and CNS effects.

Drug interactions

Local anesthetics produce few significant interactions with other drugs but can produce adverse reactions.

Adverse reactions

Dose-related CNS reactions include anxiety, apprehension, restlessness, nervousness, disorientation, confusion, dizziness, blurred vision, tremors, twitching, shivering, and seizures. Dose-related cardiovascular reactions may include myocardial depression, bradycardia (slow heart rate), arrhythmias, hypotension, cardiovascular collapse, and cardiac arrest.

Amide and ester examples

Amide anesthetics are local anesthetics that have nitrogen as part of their molecular makeup. They include:
- bupivacaine hydrochloride
- levobupivacaine
- lidocaine hydrochloride
- mepivacaine hydrochloride
- prilocaine hydrochloride
- ropivacaine hydrochloride.

Give them oxygen
Ester anesthetics have oxygen, not nitrogen, as part of their molecular makeup. They include:
- chloroprocaine hydrochloride
- procaine hydrochloride
- tetracaine hydrochloride.

An array of effects

Local anesthetic solutions that contain vasoconstrictors, such as epinephrine, can also produce CNS and cardiovascular reactions, including anxiety, dizziness, headache, restlessness, tremors, palpitations, tachycardia, angina, and hypertension.

Nursing process

These nursing process steps are appropriate for patients undergoing treatment with local anesthetics.

Assessment

• Assess the patient's drug allergies and risk factors for complications of anesthesia and surgery (cigarette smoking, obesity, limited exercise or activity, and chronic cardiovascular, respiratory, renal, or other disease processes).
• Assess the patient's vital signs, laboratory data, and physical condition to establish baseline measurements for monitoring changes.

Key nursing diagnoses

• Risk for injury related to impaired sensory perception from the drug
• Acute pain related to the underlying disorder
• Deficient knowledge related to drug therapy

Planning outcome goals

• The risk of injury to the patient will be minimized.
• The patient will acknowledge a reduction in pain.
• The patient and his family will verbalize an understanding of the purpose and intended effect of drug therapy.

Interventions

• Explain the purpose of therapy and its intended effect.
• Monitor the patient's vital signs, level of pain, respiratory and cardiovascular status, and laboratory results as indicated.
• Monitor the patient's response to medication.

Evaluation

• Patient remains free from major complications.
• Patient has reduced pain.
• Patient and his family state an understanding of drug therapy.

Topical anesthetics

Topical anesthetics are applied directly to intact skin or mucous membranes. All topical anesthetics are used to prevent or relieve minor pain.

All together now

Some injectable local anesthetics, such as lidocaine and tetracaine, also are effective topically. In addition, some topical anesthetics, such as lidocaine, are combined in products.

Other topical anesthetics include:

- dibucaine
- benzocaine
- butacaine
- butamben
- procaine
- dyclonine
- pramoxine
- ethyl chloride
- menthol
- benzyl alcohol.

Pharmacokinetics

Topical anesthetics produce little systemic absorption, except for the application of procaine to mucous membranes. However, systemic absorption may occur if the patient receives frequent or high-dose applications to the eye or large areas of burned or injured skin.

Tetracaine and other esters are metabolized extensively in the blood and to a lesser extent in the liver. Dibucaine, lidocaine, and other amides are metabolized primarily in the liver. Both types of topical anesthetics are excreted in urine.

Pharmacodynamics

Benzocaine, butacaine, butamben, procaine, dyclonine, and pramoxine produce topical anesthesia by blocking nerve impulse transmission. They accumulate in the nerve cell membrane, causing it to expand and lose its ability to depolarize, thus blocking impulse transmission. Dibucaine, lidocaine, and tetracaine may block impulse transmission across nerve cell membranes.

Drowning out input

The aromatic compounds, such as benzyl alcohol and clove oil, appear to stimulate nerve endings. This stimulation causes counterirritation that interferes with pain perception.

Putting on the deep freeze

Ethyl chloride spray superficially freezes the tissue, stimulating the cold sensation receptors and blocking the nerve endings in the frozen area. Menthol selectively stimulates the sensory nerve endings for cold, causing a cool sensation and some local pain relief.

Pharmacotherapeutics

Topical anesthetics are used to:
• relieve or prevent pain, especially minor burn pain
• relieve itching and irritation
• anesthetize an area before an injection is given
• numb mucosal surfaces before a tube, such as a urinary catheter, is inserted
• alleviate sore throat or mouth pain when used in a spray or solution.
    Tetracaine also is used as a topical anesthetic for the eye. Benzocaine is used with other drugs in several ear preparations.

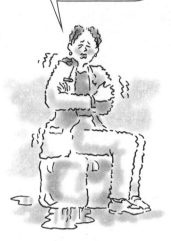

Some topical anesthetics stimulate a c-c-cooling sensation to initiate local pain relief.

Drug interactions

Few interactions with other drugs occur with topical anesthetics because they aren't absorbed well into the systemic circulation.

Adverse reactions

Topical anesthetics can cause several adverse reactions, depending on the specific drug:
• Any topical anesthetic can cause a hypersensitivity reaction, including a rash, itching, hives, swelling of the mouth and throat, and breathing difficulty.
• Benzyl alcohol can cause topical reactions such as skin irritation.
• Refrigerants, such as ethyl chloride, may produce frostbite at the application site.

Nursing process

These nursing process steps are appropriate for patients undergoing treatment with topical anesthetics.

Assessment

• Assess the patient's underlying condition and need for drug therapy.

• Assess the patient's vital signs, laboratory data, level of pain, and physical condition to establish baseline measurements for monitoring changes.

Key nursing diagnoses
• Risk for injury related to impaired sensory perception from drug therapy
• Acute pain related to the underlying process
• Deficient knowledge related to drug therapy

Planning outcome goals
• The risk of injury to the patient will be minimized.
• The patient will acknowledge a reduction in pain.
• The patient and his family will verbalize an understanding of the purpose and intended effect of drug therapy.

Interventions
• Explain the purpose of therapy and its intended effect.
• Monitor the patient's vital signs, level of pain, respiratory and cardiovascular status, and laboratory results, as indicated.
• Monitor the patient's response to pain medication.

Evaluation
• Patient remains free from major complications.
• Patient states pain is lessened with drug therapy.
• Patient and his family state an understanding of drug therapy.
(See *Teaching about topical anesthetics*.)

Education edge

Teaching about topical anesthetics

If topical anesthetics are prescribed, review these points with the patient and his caregivers:
• Use the preparation only on the part of the body for which it was prescribed and the condition for which it was prescribed.
• Apply the topical anesthetic to clean areas.
• Apply the medication only as often as directed to avoid local irritation, rash, or hives.
• If a spray is being used, don't inhale the vapors, spray near food, or store near a heat source.
• Notify the prescriber if the medication isn't effective.
• Inform health care providers of any allergies to medications or local anesthetic drugs.

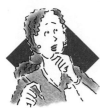

Quick quiz

1. How does the topical anesthetic benzocaine relieve sunburn pain?

    A.   It numbs the skin surface, decreasing the perception of pain.

    B.   It freezes the skin, which prevents nerve impulse transmission.

    C.   It blocks nerve impulse transmission by preventing nerve cell depolarization.

    D.   It occupies sites on specialized receptors, modifying the release of neurotransmitters.

Answer: C. Benzocaine prevents nerve cell depolarization, thus blocking nerve impulse transmission and relieving pain.

2. Which adverse reaction is a patient most likely to experience after receiving general anesthesia for surgery?

    A.   Nausea and vomiting

    B.   Seizures

    C.   Cyanosis

    D.   Increased heart rate

Answer: A. After surgery involving general anesthesia, a patient is most likely to experience adverse reactions similar to those produced by other CNS depressant drugs, including nausea and vomiting.

3. Before administering buprenorphine hydrochloride, the nurse asks a patient if he has used opioids. Administering a mixed opioid agonist-antagonist to a patient dependent on opioid agonists may cause which reaction?

    A.   Hypersensitivity reaction

    B.   Constipation

    C.   Urinary incontinence

    D.   Withdrawal symptoms

Answer: D. Because they can counteract the effects of opioid agonists, mixed opioid agonist-antagonists can cause withdrawal symptoms in the patient who's dependent on opioid agonists.

4. The drug commonly prescribed to treat an opioid overdose is:

    A.   butorphanol.

    B.   naloxone.

    C.   pentazocine.

    D.   nalbuphine.

Answer: B. Naloxone is the drug of choice for managing an opioid overdose.

5. What are the most common adverse reactions to aspirin?
A. Increased rate and depth of respirations
B. Nausea, vomiting, and GI distress
C. Dizziness and vision changes
D. Bladder infection

Answer: B. Aspirin most commonly produces adverse GI reactions, such as nausea, vomiting, and GI distress.

6. Desflurane is which type of anesthetic?
A. General
B. Local
C. Topical
D. I.V.

Answer: A. Desflurane is a commonly used general anesthetic that's administered by inhalation.

7. A topical anesthetic can be used:
A. as an alternative to general anesthesia for an elderly or debilitated patient.
B. to numb a mucosal surface before tube insertion.
C. when anesthesia is needed for only a short period.
D. to prevent or relieve muscle pain in a specific area.

Answer: B. Topical anesthetics are used to numb mucosal surfaces as well as relieve or prevent pain, relieve itching and irritation, anesthetize an area for an injection, and alleviate sore throat or mouth pain.

Scoring

☆☆☆ If you answered all seven questions correctly, bravo! You're a pain medication powerhouse.

☆☆ If you answered five or six questions correctly, fabulous! For you, this chapter was painless.

☆ If you answered fewer than five questions correctly, hey, don't give up! Remember: No pain, no gain.

Cardiovascular drugs

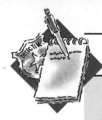

Just the facts

In this chapter, you'll learn:

♦ classes of drugs used to treat cardiovascular disorders

♦ uses and varying actions of these drugs

♦ absorption, distribution, metabolization, and excretion of these drugs

♦ drug interactions and adverse reactions to these drugs.

Drugs and the cardiovascular system

Components of the cardiovascular system include the heart, arteries, veins, and lymphatics. These structures transport life-supporting oxygen and nutrients to cells, remove metabolic waste products, and carry hormones from one part of the body to another. Because this system performs such vital functions, any problem with the heart or blood vessels can seriously affect a person's health.

Types of drugs used to improve cardiovascular function include:
• inotropic drugs
• antiarrhythmic drugs
• antianginal drugs
• antihypertensive drugs
• diuretics (see chapter 8 for a full discussion.)
• antilipemic drugs.

Inotropic drugs

Inotropic drugs influence the strength or contractility of muscular tissue. As a result, they increase the force of the heart's contractions (this is known as a *positive inotropic effect*). Cardiac glycosides and phosphodiesterase (PDE) inhibitors are two types of in-otropic drugs.

In slow motion

Cardiac glycosides also slow the heart rate (a negative chronotropic effect) and slow electrical impulse conduction through the atrioventricular (AV) node (a negative dromotropic effect).

Cardiac glycosides

Cardiac glycosides are a group of drugs derived from digitalis, a substance that occurs naturally in foxglove plants. The most commonly used cardiac glycoside is digoxin. (See *Cardiac glycosides: Digoxin.*)

Pharmacokinetics (how drugs circulate)

The intestinal absorption of digoxin varies greatly. Capsules are absorbed most efficiently, followed by the elixir form, and then tablets. Digoxin is distributed widely throughout the body with highest concentrations in the heart muscle, liver, and kidneys. Digoxin is poorly bound to plasma proteins.

Prototype pro

Cardiac glycosides: Digoxin

Actions
• Inhibits sodium-potassium-activated adenosine triphosphate, an enzyme that regulates the amount of sodium and potassium inside the cell
• Promotes movement of calcium from extracellular to intracellular cytoplasm and strengthens myocardial contraction
• Acts on the central nervous system to enhance vagal tone, slowing contractions through the sinoatrial and atrioventricular nodes and providing an antiarrhythmic effect

Indications
• Heart failure
• Atrial fibrillation and flutter
• Supraventricular tachycardia

Nursing considerations
• Monitor the patient for adverse effects, such as fatigue, agitation, hallucinations, arrhythmias, anorexia, nausea, and diarrhea.
• Withhold the drug if the apical pulse is less than 60 beats/minute, and notify the prescriber.
• Periodically monitor serum potassium and digoxin levels.
• Assess renal function.

Going out the way it came in

In most patients, a small amount of digoxin is metabolized in the liver and gut by bacteria. This effect varies and may be substantial in some people. Most of the drug is excreted by the kidneys unchanged.

Pharmacodynamics (how drugs act)

Digoxin is used to treat heart failure because it boosts intracellular calcium at the cell membrane, enabling stronger heart contractions. Digoxin may also enhance the movement of calcium into the myocardial cells and stimulate the release, or block the reuptake, of norepinephrine at the adrenergic nerve terminal.

What nerve!

Digoxin acts on the central nervous system (CNS) to slow the heart rate, thus making it useful for treating supraventricular arrhythmias (an abnormal heart rhythm that originates above the bundle branches of the heart's conduction system), such as atrial fibrillation and atrial flutter. It also increases the refractory period (the period when the cells of the conduction system can't conduct an impulse).

Pharmacotherapeutics (how drugs are used)

In addition to treating heart failure and supraventricular arrhythmias, digoxin is used to treat paroxysmal atrial tachycardia (an arrhythmia marked by brief periods of tachycardia that alternate with brief periods of sinus rhythm). (See *Load that dose*.)

Drug interactions

Many drugs can interact with digoxin:
• Rifampin, barbiturates, cholestyramine, antacids, kaolin and pectin, sulfasalazine, neomycin, and metoclopramide reduce the therapeutic effects of digoxin.
• Calcium preparations, quinidine, verapamil, cyclosporine, tetracycline, nefazodone, clarithromycin, propafenone, amiodarone, spironolactone, hydroxychloroquine, erythromycin, itraconazole, and omeprazole increase the risk of digoxin toxicity.
• Amphotericin B, potassium-wasting diuretics, and steroids taken with digoxin may cause hypokalemia (low potassium levels) and increase the risk of digoxin toxicity.
• Beta-adrenergic blockers and calcium channel blockers taken with digoxin may cause an excessively slow heart rate and arrhythmias.

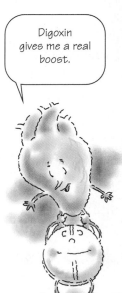

Digoxin gives me a real boost.

Load that dose

Because digoxin has a long half-life, a loading dose must be given to a patient who requires immediate drug effects, as in supraventricular arrhythmia. By giving a larger initial dose, a minimum effective concentration of the drug in the blood may be reached faster. *Note:* Loading doses should be avoided in patients with heart failure to avoid toxicity.

- Neuromuscular-blocking drugs, such as succinylcholine, and thyroid preparations, such as levothyroxine, increase the risk of arrhythmias when taken with digoxin.

When herbs spice things up too much

- The herbal preparations St. John's wort and ginseng can increase levels of digoxin and increase the risk of toxicity.

Adverse reactions

Because cardiac glycosides have a narrow therapeutic index (margin of safety), they may produce digoxin toxicity. To prevent digoxin toxicity, the dosage should be individualized based on the patient's serum digoxin concentration.

Signs and symptoms of digoxin toxicity include:
- nausea and vomiting
- abdominal pain
- diarrhea
- headache
- irritability
- depression
- insomnia
- confusion
- vision changes
- arrhythmias
- complete heart block.

Nursing process

These nursing process steps are appropriate for patients undergoing treatment with cardiac glycosides.

Assessment

- Obtain a history of the underlying condition before therapy.
- Monitor drug effectiveness by taking the patient's apical pulse for 1 minute before each dose. Evaluate the electrocardiogram (ECG) when ordered, and regularly assess the patient's cardiopulmonary status for signs of improvement.
- Monitor digoxin levels (therapeutic blood levels range from 0.5 to 2 ng/ml). Obtain blood for digoxin levels 8 hours after the last dose by mouth (P.O.).
- Closely monitor potassium levels.
- Be alert for adverse reactions and drug interactions.

Key nursing diagnoses

- Decreased cardiac output related to underlying condition

- Risk for injury related to possible adverse reactions and digoxin toxicity
- Deficient knowledge related to drug therapy

Planning outcome goals
- Cardiac output will improve as evidenced by vital signs, urine output, and level of consciousness.
- Risk for digoxin toxicity will be minimized.
- The patient will demonstrate correct drug administration and will verbalize correct symptoms of digoxin toxicity.

Implementation
- Keep in mind that patients with hypothyroidism are extremely sensitive to glycosides and may need lower doses. Reduce the dosage in patients with impaired renal function.
- Before giving a loading dose, obtain baseline data (heart rate and rhythm, blood pressure, and electrolyte levels) and question the patient about recent use of cardiac glycosides (within the previous 3 weeks). The loading dose is always divided over the first 24 hours unless the clinical situation indicates otherwise.

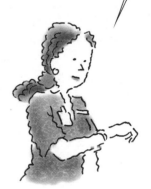

Before giving digoxin, take the patient's apical pulse for 1 full minute.

Pay attention to the pulse
- Before giving the drug, take the patient's apical pulse for 1 full minute. Record and report to the prescriber significant changes (a sudden increase or decrease in pulse rate, pulse deficit, irregular beats, and regularization of a previously irregular rhythm). If these changes occur, check the patient's blood pressure and obtain a 12-lead ECG.
- Withhold the drug and notify the prescriber if the pulse rate slows to 60 beats/minute or less.
- Infuse the I.V. form of the drug slowly over at least 5 minutes.
- Withhold the drug for 1 to 2 days before elective cardioversion. Adjust the dose after cardioversion.
- Remember that colestipol and cholestyramine bind with the drug in the intestine. Treat arrhythmias with phenytoin I.V. or lidocaine I.V., and treat potentially life-threatening toxicity with specific antigen-binding fragments (such as Digoxin Immune Fab).
- Teach the patient about digoxin, including signs and symptoms of digoxin toxicity.

Evaluation
- Patient has adequate cardiac output.
- Patient has no digoxin toxicity.
- Patient and his family demonstrate an understanding of drug therapy. (See *Teaching about digoxin,* page 186.)

Education edge

Teaching about digoxin

If digoxin is prescribed, review these points with the patient and his caregivers:

• Digoxin helps strengthen the heartbeat and relieve ankle swelling, shortness of breath, and fatigue, which can accompany a heart problem.

• Take digoxin and other heart medications as prescribed, usually once daily, at the same time each day.

• Don't miss any doses of the medication.

• Don't take a double dose of the medication if a dose is missed.

• Don't take any over-the-counter medications or herbal remedies without first consulting with your prescriber.

• You will need to have periodic physical examinations, electrocardiograms, and blood tests (for digoxin as well as electrolyte levels) to see whether changes in dosages are needed.

• Report adverse effects, such as changes in heart rate or rhythm, nausea, vomiting, or vision problems, to your prescriber. These signs and symptoms may mean that your dosage needs to be changed.

• Limit salt intake and be sure to get enough potassium. Follow the diet set by your prescriber, and don't take salt substitutes, such as potassium chloride, without first consulting with your prescriber.

• Use the same brand and type of digoxin all the time because forms and concentrations are different and aren't interchangeable.

• Take your pulse as instructed by your prescriber; count your pulse before each dose. If it's less than 60 beats/minute, call your prescriber.

• Don't crush digoxin capsules. Tablets may be crushed and can be taken with or after meals.

• If taking the liquid form of digoxin, measure accurately to prevent overdosage.

PDE inhibitors

PDE inhibitors are typically used for short-term management of heart failure or long-term management in patients awaiting heart transplant surgery. In the United States, two PDE inhibitors (inamrinone and milrinone) have been approved for use.

Pharmacokinetics

Inamrinone is administered I.V., distributed rapidly, metabolized by the liver, and excreted by the kidneys.

Quick and short

Milrinone is also administered I.V. and is distributed rapidly and excreted by the kidneys, primarily as unchanged drug.

Pharmacodynamics

PDE inhibitors improve cardiac output by strengthening contractions. These drugs are thought to help move calcium into the cardiac cells or to increase calcium storage in the sarcoplasmic reticulum. By directly relaxing vascular smooth muscle, they also de-

By decreasing my afterload and preload, PDE inhibitors certainly lighten my load.

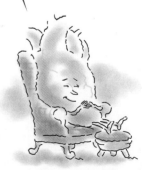

crease peripheral vascular resistance (afterload) and the amount of blood returning to the heart (preload).

Pharmacotherapeutics

Inamrinone and milrinone are used for the management of heart failure in patients who haven't responded adequately to treatment with cardiac glycosides, diuretics, or vasodilators. Prolonged use of these drugs may increase the patient's risk of complications and death. (See *PDE inhibitors warning*.)

Drug interactions

PDE inhibitors may interact with disopyramide, causing hypotension. Because PDE inhibitors reduce serum potassium levels, taking them with a potassium-wasting diuretic may lead to hypokalemia.

Adverse reactions

Adverse reactions to PDE inhibitors are uncommon, but the likelihood increases significantly with prolonged therapy. Adverse reactions may include:
• ventricular arrhythmias
• nausea and vomiting
• headache and fever
• chest pain
• hypokalemia
• thrombocytopenia (especially with inamrinone)
• mild increase in heart rate.
    Inamrinone is rarely used because of its secondary adverse effects (secondary thrombocytopenia).

Nursing process

These nursing process steps are appropriate for patients undergoing treatment with PDE inhibitors.

Assessment

• Assess the patient's heart failure before therapy and regularly thereafter.
• Monitor fluid and electrolyte status, blood pressure, heart rate, and kidney function during therapy.
• Monitor the patient's ECG continuously during therapy.
• Be alert for adverse reactions.
• Evaluate the patient's and family's knowledge of drug therapy.

Key nursing diagnoses

• Impaired gas exchange related to presence of heart failure

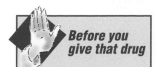

Before you give that drug

PDE inhibitors warning

When giving PDE inhibitors, such as milrinone, remember that improvement of cardiac output may result in enhanced urine output. Expect a dosage reduction in diuretic therapy as heart failure improves. Potassium loss may predispose the patient to digoxin toxicity.

- Decreased cardiac output related to drug-induced cardiac arrhythmias
- Deficient knowledge related to drug therapy

Planning outcome goals

- Adequate gas exchange will be achieved as evidenced by arterial blood gas values.
- Cardiac output will improve as evidenced by blood pressure, vital signs, and cardiac monitoring.
- The patient will state an understanding of drug therapy and the need to report adverse reactions.

Implementation

- Know that milrinone typically is given with digoxin and diuretics.

So aggravating!

- Keep in mind that inotropics may aggravate outflow tract obstruction in hypertrophic cardiomyopathy (also known as *idiopathic hypertrophic subaortic stenosis*).
- Prepare I.V. solutions in dextrose 5% in water (D_5W), normal saline solution, or half-normal saline solution.
- If an excessive decrease in blood pressure occurs, discontinue the drug or infuse it more slowly.
- Provide patient teaching.

Evaluation

- Patient exhibits adequate gas exchange as heart failure resolves.
- Drug-induced arrhythmias don't develop during therapy.
- Patient and his family demonstrate an understanding of drug therapy.

Antiarrhythmic drugs

Antiarrhythmic drugs are used to treat arrhythmias (disturbances in the normal heart rhythm).

For better or worse?

Unfortunately, many antiarrhythmic drugs can also worsen or cause the very arrhythmias they're supposed to treat. Therefore, the benefits of this therapy must always be weighed against its risks.

Antiarrhythmics are categorized into four classes:
- I (which includes classes IA, IB, and IC)
- II

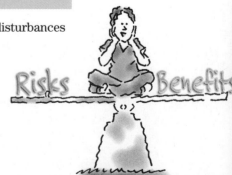

Because many antiarrhythmic drugs can actually worsen the arrhythmias they're supposed to treat, the benefits must always be weighed against the risks.

- III
- IV.

Class I antiarrhythmics, the largest group of antiarrhythmic drugs, consist of sodium channel blockers. Class I agents are usually subdivided into classes IA, IB, and IC. One drug, adenosine (an AV nodal-blocking agent used to treat paroxysmal supraventricular tachycardia [PSVT]), doesn't fall into any of these classes.

The mechanisms of action of antiarrhythmic drugs vary widely, and a few drugs exhibit properties common to more than one class.

Class IA antiarrhythmics

Class IA antiarrhythmics are used to treat a wide variety of atrial and ventricular arrhythmias. Class IA antiarrhythmics include:
- disopyramide phosphate
- procainamide hydrochloride
- quinidine (sulfate, gluconate).

Pharmacokinetics

When administered orally, class IA drugs are rapidly absorbed and metabolized. Because they work so quickly, sustained-release forms of these drugs are available to help maintain therapeutic levels.

The brainy one

These drugs are distributed through all body tissues. Quinidine, however, is the only one that crosses the blood-brain barrier.

All class IA antiarrhythmics are metabolized in the liver and are excreted unchanged by the kidneys. Acidic urine increases the excretion of quinidine.

Pharmacodynamics

Class IA antiarrhythmics control arrhythmias by altering the myocardial cell membrane and interfering with autonomic nervous system control of pacemaker cells. (See *How class I antiarrhythmics work*, page 190.)

No (para)sympathy

Class IA antiarrhythmics also block parasympathetic stimulation of the sinoatrial (SA) and AV nodes. Because stimulation of the parasympathetic nervous system causes the heart rate to slow down, drugs that block the parasympathetic nervous system increase the conduction rate of the AV node.

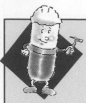

Pharm function

How class I antiarrhythmics work

All class I antiarrhythmics suppress arrhythmias by blocking the sodium channels in the cell membrane during an action potential, thereby interfering with the conduction of impulses along adjacent cardiac cells and producing a more membrane-stabilizing effect. The cardiac action potential, as illustrated below, occurs in five phases (0 through 4). Class I antiarrhythmics exert their effects during different phases of the action potential, binding quickly to sodium channels that are open or inactivated before repolarization occurs in the cell; they're most effective on tachycardia-type rhythms.

Phase 4: This coincides with ventricular diastole and marks the resting membrane potential (between -85 and -95 mV).

Phase 0: During this phase, sodium enters the cell and rapid depolarization takes place. Class IA and IB antiarrhythmics slow this phase of the action potential; class IC antiarrhythmics markedly slow the phase.

Phase 1: During this phase, sodium channels are inactivated.

Phase 2: During this plateau phase, sodium levels are equalized.

Phase 3: This marks when potassium leaves the cell and repolarization occurs. Class IA antiarrhythmics work during this phase to block sodium channels. Active transport via the sodium-potassium pump begins restoring potassium to the inside of the cell and sodium to the outside of the cell.

Phase 4: By this phase, potassium has left the cell, the cell membrane is impermeable to sodium, and the resting potential is restored. Then the cycle begins again.

> Class I antiarrhythmics exert their effects during different phases of the action potential.

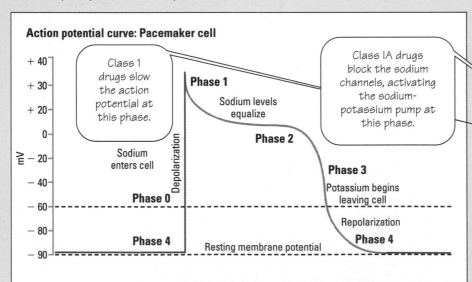

Action potential curve: Pacemaker cell

Class 1 drugs slow the action potential at this phase.

Class IA drugs block the sodium channels, activating the sodium-potassium pump at this phase.

mV: + 40, + 30, + 20, 0, − 20, − 40, − 60, − 80, − 90

Phase 1
Sodium levels equalize
Phase 2
Sodium enters cell
Depolarization
Phase 0
Phase 3
Potassium begins leaving cell
Repolarization
Phase 4
Phase 4
Resting membrane potential

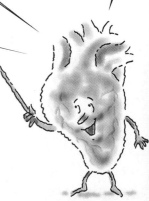

Prototype pro

Class IA antiarrhythmics: Quinidine gluconate

Actions
• Causes direct and indirect effects on cardiac tissue
• Decreases automaticity, conduction velocity, and membrane responsiveness
• Prolongs effective refractory period

Indications
• Atrial fibrillation, flutter, and tachycardia
• Premature atrial and ventricular contractions
• Paroxysmal supraventricular tachycardia

Nursing considerations
• Monitor for adverse effects, such as vertigo, headache, arrhythmias, electrocardiogram changes (specifically, a widening QRS complex and prolonged QT interval), hypotension, heart failure, tinnitus, diarrhea, nausea, vomiting, hematologic disorders, hepatotoxicity, respiratory arrest, angioedema, fever, and temporary hearing loss.
• Frequently monitor pulse and blood pressure.
• Keep in mind that anticoagulation may be performed before treatment.

A chain reaction

This increase in conduction rate can produce dangerous increases in ventricular heart rate if rapid atrial activity is present, as in a patient with atrial fibrillation. In turn, the increased ventricular heart rate can offset the ability of the antiarrhythmics to convert atrial arrhythmias to a regular rhythm.

Pharmacotherapeutics

Class IA antiarrhythmics are used to treat certain arrhythmias, such as premature ventricular contractions, ventricular tachycardia, atrial fibrillation, atrial flutter, and paroxysmal atrial tachycardia. (See *Class IA antiarrhythmics: Quinidine gluconate.*)

Drug interactions

Class IA antiarrhythmics can interact with other drugs in various ways:
• Disopyramide taken with macrolide antibiotics, such as clarithromycin and erythromycin, increases the risk of QT-interval prolongation, which may lead to an increased risk of arrhythmias, especially polymorphic ventricular tachycardia.
• Disopyramide plus verapamil may produce added myocardial depression and should be avoided in patients with heart failure.
• Class IA antiarrhythmics combined with other antiarrhythmics, such as beta-adrenergic blockers, increase the risk of arrhythmias.
• Quinidine plus neuromuscular blockers causes increased skeletal muscle relaxation.
• Quinidine increases the risk of digoxin toxicity.

• Rifampin, phenytoin, and phenobarbital can reduce the effects of quinidine and disopyramide.
• Sodium bicarbonate and cimetidine may increase the level of quinidine.
• Azole antifungals may increase the risk of cardiovascular events when used with quinidine; they shouldn't be used together.
• Grapefruit may delay the absorption of quinidine.

Adverse reactions

Class IA antiarrhythmics, especially quinidine, commonly produce GI signs and symptoms, such as diarrhea, cramping, nausea, vomiting, anorexia, and bitter taste.

Good news, bad news

Ironically, not only do class IA antiarrhythmics treat arrhythmias, but they can also induce arrhythmias, especially conduction delays that may worsen existing heart blocks.

Nursing process

These nursing process steps are appropriate for patients undergoing treatment with class IA antiarrhythmics.

Assessment
• Assess the patient's arrhythmia before therapy and regularly thereafter.
• Monitor the ECG continuously when therapy starts and when the dosage is adjusted. Specifically, monitor for ventricular arrhythmias and ECG changes (widening QRS complexes and a prolonged QT interval).
• Monitor the patient's vital signs frequently, and assess for signs of toxicity and adverse reactions.
• Measure apical pulse rate and blood pressure before giving the drug.
• Monitor serum drug levels as indicated.
• Monitor blood studies, such as liver function tests, as indicated.
• Be alert for adverse reactions and drug interactions.
• Evaluate the patient's and family's knowledge of drug therapy.
• Monitor the patient's intake and output.
• Evaluate the patient's serum electrolyte levels.

Key nursing diagnoses
• Decreased cardiac output related to arrhythmias or myocardial depression
• Risk for injury related to adverse reactions
• Deficient knowledge related to drug therapy

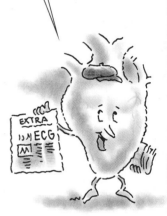

Have you heard the news? Class IA antiarrhythmics can induce arrhythmias as well as treat them.

Planning outcome goals

- Cardiac output will improve as evidenced by stable blood pressure, cardiac monitoring, and adequate urine output.
- Complications from adverse reactions will be diminished.
- The patient will verbalize an understanding of drug therapy.

Implementation

- Don't crush sustained-release tablets.
- Notify the prescriber about adverse reactions.
- Use I.V. forms of these drugs to treat acute arrhythmias.

Evaluation

- Patient maintains adequate cardiac output as evidenced by normal vital signs and adequate tissue perfusion.
- Patient has no serious adverse reactions.
- Patient and his family demonstrate an understanding of drug therapy. (See *Teaching about antiarrhythmics*.)

Education edge

Teaching about antiarrhythmics

If antiarrhythmics are prescribed, review these points with the patient and his caregivers:

- Antiarrhythmic drug therapy helps stop irregular beats in the heart and helps it to beat more effectively.
- It's important to take the drug exactly as prescribed. You may need to use an alarm clock or other reminders if the medication needs to be taken at odd hours around the clock.
- Take your pulse before each dose. Notify your prescriber if your pulse is irregular or less than 60 beats/minute.
- Avoid hazardous activities that require mental alertness if adverse central nervous system reactions occur.
- Limit fluid and salt intake if the prescribed drug causes fluid retention.
- Quinidine and disopyramide should be taken with food if GI upset occurs.
- Verapamil should be taken on an empty stomach or 1 to 2 hours after a meal.
- Some medications, such as quinidine, require you to limit intake of such foods as citrus juices, milk, and vegetables as well as avoid over-the-counter (OTC) drugs (such as antacids) that make urine alkaline.

- Report adverse effects, such as constipation or diarrhea, chest pain, difficulty breathing, ringing in the ears, swelling, unusually slow or fast pulse, sudden irregular pulse, or rash, to your prescriber.
- If tiredness occurs, space activities throughout the day and take periodic rest periods to help conserve energy.
- If nausea, vomiting, or loss of appetite occurs, eat small, frequent meals or take the drug with meals, if appropriate.
- Some medications, such as disopyramide, may make you more sensitive to light, so avoid prolonged exposure to sunlight.
- Avoid OTC medications as well as herbal products unless approved by your prescriber. Many of these drugs and preparations can interfere with the action of antiarrhythmics.
- It's important to follow up with the prescriber to help evaluate heart rhythm and response to the drug.
- Don't stop taking the medication on your own; talk to your prescriber regarding any concerns.

Class IB antiarrhythmics

Class IB antiarrhythmics include mexiletine and lidocaine; the latter is used to treat acute ventricular arrhythmias.

Pharmacokinetics

Mexiletine is absorbed well from the GI tract after oral administration.

It's (un)bound to happen

Lidocaine is distributed widely throughout the body, including the brain. Lidocaine and mexiletine are moderately bound to plasma proteins. (Remember, only the portion of a drug that's unbound can produce a response.)

Class IB antiarrhythmics are metabolized in the liver and excreted in the urine. Mexiletine also is excreted in breast milk.

Pharmacodynamics

Class IB drugs work by blocking the rapid influx of sodium ions during the depolarization phase of the heart's depolarization-repolarization cycle. This results in a decreased refractory period, which reduces the risk of arrhythmias.

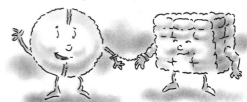

Don't worry! Plasma proteins like him can keep some antiarrhythmics occupied but my "unbound" portion will still get the job done.

Make an IB-line for the ventricle

Because class IB antiarrhythmics affect the Purkinje fibers (fibers in the conduction system of the heart) and myocardial cells in the ventricles, they're only used to treat ventricular arrhythmias. (See *Class IB antiarrhythmics: Lidocaine.*)

Prototype pro

Class IB antiarrhythmics: Lidocaine

Actions
- Decreases depolarization, automaticity, and excitability in the ventricles during diastole by direct action on the tissues, especially the Purkinje network

Indications
- Ventricular arrhythmias

Nursing considerations
- Monitor for adverse effects, such as confusion, tremor, restlessness, seizures, hypotension, new arrhythmias, cardiac arrest, tinnitus, blurred vision, respiratory depression, and anaphylaxis.
- Monitor serum lidocaine levels for toxicity.
- Monitor electrolytes, blood urea nitrogen, and creatinine levels.

Pharmacotherapeutics

Class IB antiarrhythmics are used to treat ventricular ectopic beats, ventricular tachycardia, and ventricular fibrillation.

Drug interactions

Class IB antiarrhythmics may exhibit additive or antagonistic effects when administered with other antiarrhythmics, such as phenytoin, propranolol, procainamide, and quinidine.

In addition:
• Rifampin may reduce the effects of mexiletine.
• Theophylline plasma levels are increased when theophylline is given with mexiletine.
• Use of a beta-adrenergic blocker or disopyramide with mexiletine may reduce the contractility of the heart.

Adverse reactions

Adverse reactions to class IB antiarrhythmics include:
• drowsiness
• light-headedness
• paresthesia
• sensory disturbances
• hypotension
• bradycardia.

Adverse reactions to mexiletine also include hypotension, atrioventricular block, bradycardia, confusion, ataxia, and double vision, nausea, vomiting, tremors, and dizziness.

In addition, lidocaine toxicity can cause seizures and respiratory and cardiac arrest.

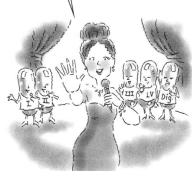

Stop! In the name of rhythm… Combining class IB antiarrhythmics with other antiarrhythmics can cause additive or antagonistic effects. And that would totally throw our rhythm off!

Nursing process

These nursing process steps are appropriate for patients undergoing treatment with class IB antiarrhythmics.

Assessment

• Assess the patient's arrhythmia before therapy and regularly thereafter.
• Monitor the ECG continuously when therapy starts and when the dosage is adjusted. A patient receiving the drug via infusion must be on a cardiac monitor and attended at all times.
• Monitor the patient's vital signs frequently, especially ECG and blood pressure.
• Assess for adverse reactions and signs of toxicity. As blood levels of lidocaine increase, nervousness, confusion, dizziness, tinnitus, somnolence, paresthesia, and circumoral numbness may oc-

cur. Acute toxicity may result in seizures, cardiovascular collapse, and respiratory arrest.
• Measure apical pulse rate and blood pressure before giving the drug.
• Monitor serum drug levels as indicated. Therapeutic levels for lidocaine are 2 to 5 mcg/ml.
• Monitor blood studies as indicated, such as liver function tests and blood urea nitrogen (BUN) and creatinine levels.
• Evaluate the patient's and family's knowledge of drug therapy.

Key nursing diagnoses
• Decreased cardiac output related to arrhythmias or myocardial depression
• Risk for injury related to adverse reactions
• Deficient knowledge related to drug therapy

Planning outcome goals
• Cardiac output will improve as evidenced by stable blood pressure, cardiac monitoring, and adequate urine output.
• Complications from adverse reactions will be diminished.
• The patient will verbalize an understanding of drug therapy.

Implementation
• Use an infusion-control device to administer the infusion. If giving lidocaine, don't exceed 4 mg/minute; a faster rate greatly increases the risk of toxicity.
• Dilute concentrated forms for I.V. infusion.
• If administering the drug via the I.M. route (alternative route for lidocaine), give it in the deltoid area.
• Remember that I. M. injections increase creatine kinase (CK) levels. The CK-MM isoenzyme (which originates in skeletal muscle, not cardiac muscle) level increases significantly in patients who receive an I.M. injection.
• Don't crush sustained-release tablets.
• Be aware that sustained-release and extended-release medications aren't interchangeable.
• Take safety precautions if adverse CNS reactions occur.
• Notify the prescriber about adverse reactions. If signs of lidocaine toxicity occur, stop the drug at once and notify the prescriber. Continued infusion could lead to seizures, cardiovascular collapse, coma, and respiratory arrest.
• Use I.V. forms of these drugs to treat acute arrhythmias. Discontinue the drug and notify the prescriber if arrhythmias worsen or if ECG changes, such as widening QRS complex or substantially prolonged PR interval, are evident.
• Provide patient teaching.

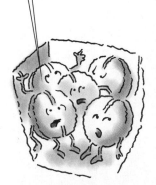

Keep in mind that you shouldn't crush sustained-release tablets—and we're all feeling a bit crushed in here!

Evaluation
- Patient maintains adequate cardiac output as evidenced by normal vital signs and adequate tissue perfusion.
- Patient has no serious adverse reactions.
- Patient and his family state an understanding of drug therapy.

Class IC antiarrhythmics

Class IC antiarrhythmics are used to treat certain severe, refractory (resistant) ventricular arrhythmias. Class IC antiarrhythmics include:
- flecainide acetate
- propafenone hydrochloride
- moricizine (a class I antiarrhythmic drug that shares class IA, IB, and IC properties).

Pharmacokinetics

After oral administration, class IC antiarrhythmics are absorbed well, distributed in varying degrees, and probably metabolized by the liver. They're excreted primarily by the kidneys, except for propafenone, which is excreted primarily in feces. (See *Class IC antiarrhythmics: Propafenone*.)

After oral administration, about 38% of moricizine is absorbed. It undergoes extensive metabolism, with less than 1% of a dose excreted unchanged in the urine. Moricizine is highly protein bound, leaving only a small portion of the drug free to produce its antiarrhythmic effect.

Pharmacodynamics

Class IC antiarrhythmics primarily slow conduction along the heart's conduction system. Moricizine decreases the fast inward current of sodium ions of the action potential, depressing the depolarization rate and effective refractory period.

Pharmacotherapeutics

Like class IB antiarrhythmics, class IC antiarrhythmic drugs are used to treat life-threatening ventricular arrhythmias. They're also used to treat supraventricular arrhythmias (abnormal heart rhythms that originate above the bundle branches of the heart's conduction system).

Treating troublesome tachycardia

Flecainide and propafenone may also be used to prevent paroxysmal supraventricular tachycardia (PSVT) in patients without

Prototype pro

Class IC antiarrhythmics: Propafenone

Actions
- Reduces inward sodium current in Purkinje and myocardial cells
- Decreases excitability, conduction velocity, and automaticity in atrioventricular (AV) nodal, His-Purkinje, and intraventricular tissue
- Prolongs refractory period in AV nodal tissue

Indications
- Ventricular arrhythmias

Nursing considerations
- Administer with food to minimize adverse GI reactions.
- Notify the prescriber if the QRS complex increases by more than 25%.
- During use with digoxin, monitor the electrocardiogram and digoxin levels frequently.

structural heart disease. Moricizine is used to manage life-threatening ventricular arrhythmias such as sustained ventricular tachycardia.

Drug interactions

Class IC antiarrhythmics may exhibit additive effects when administered with other antiarrhythmics. Here are some other interactions:
• When used with digoxin, flecainide and propafenone increase the risk of digoxin toxicity.
• Quinidine increases the effects of propafenone.
• Cimetidine may increase the plasma level and the risk of toxicity of moricizine.
• Propranolol or digoxin given with moricizine may increase the PR interval.
• Theophylline levels may be reduced in the patient receiving moricizine.
• Propafenone increases the serum concentration and effects of metoprolol and propranolol.
• Warfarin may increase the level of propafenone.

Adverse reactions

Class IC antiarrhythmics can produce serious adverse reactions, including the development of new arrhythmias and aggravation of existing arrhythmias (especially moricizine). These drugs aren't given to patients with structural heart defects because of a high incidence of resulting mortality. Other cardiovascular adverse reactions include palpitations, shortness of breath, chest pain, heart failure, and cardiac arrest.

Because propafenone has beta-adrenergic blocking properties, it may also cause bronchospasm.

Can't stomach it

GI adverse reactions include abdominal pain, heartburn, nausea, and vomiting.

Nursing process

These nursing process steps are appropriate for patients undergoing treatment with class IC antiarrhythmics.

Assessment
• Assess the patient's arrhythmia before therapy and regularly thereafter.
• Monitor the ECG continuously when therapy starts and when the dosage is adjusted.

- Monitor the patient's vital signs frequently, and assess for signs of toxicity and adverse reactions.
- Measure the apical pulse rate and blood pressure before giving the drug.
- Monitor serum drug levels as indicated.
- Monitor blood studies, such as liver function tests, as indicated.
- Be alert for adverse reactions and drug interactions.
- Evaluate the patient's and family's knowledge of drug therapy.

Key nursing diagnoses

- Decreased cardiac output related to arrhythmias or myocardial depression
- Risk for injury related to adverse reactions
- Deficient knowledge related to drug therapy

Planning outcome goals

- Cardiac output will improve as evidenced by stable blood pressure, cardiac monitoring, and adequate urine output.
- Complications from adverse reactions will be diminished.
- The patient will verbalize an understanding of drug therapy.

Implementation

- Don't crush sustained-release tablets.
- Take safety precautions if adverse CNS reactions occur.
- Notify the prescriber about adverse reactions.
- Use I.V. forms of these drugs to treat acute arrhythmias.
- Administer the drug with food to minimize adverse reactions as indicated.
- Notify the prescriber if the PR interval or QRS complex increases by more than 25%. A reduction in dosage may be necessary.
- Monitor the ECG and digoxin levels frequently if used with digoxin.
- Provide patient teaching.

Evaluation

- Patient maintains adequate cardiac output as evidenced by normal vital signs and adequate tissue perfusion.
- Patient has no serious adverse reactions.
- Patient and his family state an understanding of drug therapy.

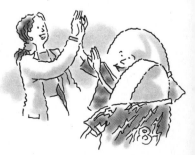

You may be Class II antiarrhythmics, but you're still first rate with me!

Class II antiarrhythmics

Class II antiarrhythmics are composed of beta-adrenergic antagonists, which are also known as *beta-adrenergic blockers* or *beta blockers*. Beta-adrenergic blockers used as antiarrhythmics include:

- acebutolol (not commonly used)
- esmolol
- propranolol.

Pharmacokinetics

Acebutolol and propranolol are absorbed almost entirely from the GI tract after an oral dose. Esmolol, which can only be given I.V., is immediately available throughout the body.

No breaking and entering

Acebutolol and esmolol have low lipid solubility. That means that they can't penetrate the blood-brain barrier (highly fatty cells that act as barriers between the blood and brain). Propranolol has high lipid solubility and readily crosses the blood-brain barrier.

Just a little gets the job done

Propranolol undergoes significant first-pass effect, leaving only a small portion of this drug available to be distributed to the body.

Esmolol is metabolized exclusively by red blood cells (RBCs), with only 1% excreted in the urine. Approximately 50% of acebutolol is excreted in feces. Propranolol's metabolites are excreted in urine as well.

Pharmacodynamics

Class II antiarrhythmics block beta-adrenergic receptor sites in the conduction system of the heart. As a result, the ability of the SA node to fire spontaneously (automaticity) is slowed. The ability of the AV node and other cells to receive and conduct an electrical impulse to nearby cells (conductivity) is also reduced.

Cutting back on contractions

Class II antiarrhythmics also reduce the strength of the heart's contractions. When the heart beats less forcefully, it doesn't require as much oxygen to do its work.

Pharmacotherapeutics

Class II antiarrhythmics slow ventricular rates in patients with atrial flutter, atrial fibrillation, and paroxysmal atrial tachycardia.

Drug interactions

Class II antiarrhythmics can cause a variety of drug interactions:
- Administering class II antiarrhythmics with phenothiazines and other antihypertensive drugs increases the antihypertensive effect.

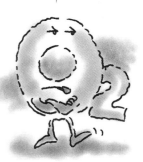

Hmph! I know when I'm not needed.

• Administration with nonsteroidal anti-inflammatory drugs (NSAIDs) can cause fluid and water retention, decreasing the anti-hypertensive effects of the drug.
• The effects of sympathomimetics may be reduced when taken with class II antiarrhythmics.

Depressing news

• Beta-adrenergic blockers given with verapamil can depress the heart, causing hypotension, bradycardia, AV block, and asystole.
• Beta-adrenergic blockers reduce the effects of sulfonylureas.
• The risk of digoxin toxicity increases when digoxin is taken with esmolol.

Adverse reactions

Common adverse reactions to class II antiarrhythmics include:
• arrhythmias
• bradycardia
• heart failure
• hypotension
• GI reactions, such as nausea, vomiting, and diarrhea
• bronchoconstriction
• fatigue.

Nursing process

These nursing process steps are appropriate for patients undergoing treatment with class II antiarrhythmics.

Assessment

• Assess the patient's arrhythmia before therapy and regularly thereafter.
• Monitor the ECG continuously when therapy starts, when the dosage is adjusted, and especially during I.V. therapy.
• Monitor the patient's vital signs frequently, and assess for signs of toxicity and adverse reactions.
• Measure the apical pulse rate and blood pressure before giving the drug.
• Monitor serum drug levels as indicated.
• Monitor blood studies, such as liver function tests, as indicated.
• Be alert for adverse reactions and drug interactions.
• Evaluate the patient's and family's knowledge of drug therapy.
• Monitor the patient's intake and output and daily weight.

Key nursing diagnoses

• Decreased cardiac output related to arrhythmias or myocardial depression

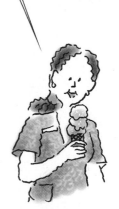

Monitor the patient's intake and output and daily weight. I may go a little overboard on the intake here if I'm not careful!

• Risk for injury related to adverse reactions
• Deficient knowledge related to drug therapy

Planning outcome goals

• Cardiac output will improve as evidenced by stable blood pressure, cardiac monitoring, and adequate urine output.
• Complications from adverse reactions will be diminished.
• The patient will demonstrate correct drug administration.

Implementation

• Don't crush sustained-release tablets.
• Take safety precautions if adverse CNS reactions occur.
• Notify the prescriber about adverse reactions.
• Use I.V. forms of these drugs for treating acute arrhythmias; they may be given as a loading dose I.V. or diluted with normal saline solution and given by intermittent infusion.
• Check the apical pulse before giving the drug. If you detect extremes in pulse rate, withhold the drug and call the prescriber immediately.
• Administer the drug with meals as indicated.
• Before any surgical procedure, notify the anesthesiologist that the patient is receiving this drug.
• Don't discontinue the I.V. form of the drug abruptly.
• Provide patient teaching.

Evaluation

• Patient maintains adequate cardiac output as evidenced by normal vital signs and adequate tissue perfusion.
• Patient has no serious adverse reactions.
• Patient and his family state an understanding of drug therapy.

Class III antiarrhythmics

Class III antiarrhythmics are used to treat ventricular arrhythmias. Drugs in this class include amiodarone, dofetilide, ibutilide, and sotalol.

Class distinctions

Sotalol is a nonselective (not having a specific affinity for a receptor) beta-adrenergic blocker (class II) that also has class III properties. The class III antiarrhythmic effects are more predominant, especially at higher doses, so sotalol is usually listed as a class III antiarrhythmic.

Pharmacokinetics

The absorption of class III antiarrhythmics varies widely.

Slow but sure

After oral administration, amiodarone is absorbed slowly at widely varying rates. This drug is distributed extensively and accumulates in many sites, especially in organs with a rich blood supply and fatty tissue. It's highly protein bound in plasma, mainly to albumin. Sotalol is also slowly absorbed, with the amount varying between 60% and 100% with minimal protein binding.

Absolute absorption

Dofetilide is very well absorbed from the GI tract, with almost 100% overall absorption and with approximately 70% being bound to plasma proteins. Ibutilide is administered I.V. only, with absorption of 100%.

Pharmacodynamics

Although the exact mechanism of action isn't known, class III antiarrhythmics are thought to suppress arrhythmias by converting a unidirectional block to a bidirectional block. They have little or no effect on depolarization. These drugs delay repolarization and lengthen the refractory period and duration of the action potential.

Pharmacotherapeutics

Class III antiarrhythmics are used for ventricular arrhythmias. Dofetilide and ibutilide are used for symptomatic atrial fibrillation and flutter. Amiodarone is the first-line drug of choice for ventricular tachycardia and ventricular fibrillation. (See *Class III antiarrhythmics: Amiodarone*, page 204.)

Drug interactions

These drug interactions can occur with class III antiarrhythmics:
• Amiodarone increases quinidine, procainamide, and phenytoin levels.
• Amiodarone increases the risk of digoxin toxicity.
• Cimetidine may increase the level of amiodarone.
• The effects of warfarin are enhanced when taken with amiodarone.
• Ibutilide shouldn't be administered within 4 hours of other class I or class III antiarrhythmics because of the potential for prolonged refractory state.

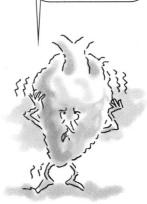

All this talk about "life-threatening arrhythmias" and other drug interactions is really stressing me out!

Prototype pro

Class III antiarrhythmics: Amiodarone

Actions
• Thought to prolong the refractory period and duration of action potential and to decrease repolarization

Indications
• Life-threatening ventricular tachycardia and ventricular fibrillation
• Suppression of supraventricular tachycardias

Nursing considerations
• Be aware that the drug poses major and potentially life-threatening management problems in patients at risk for sudden death and should be used only in patients with documented, life-threatening, recurrent ventricular arrhythmias who are nonresponsive to adequate doses of other antiarrhythmics or when alternative drugs can't be tolerated.
• Know that amiodarone can cause fatal toxicities, including hepatic and pulmonary toxicity.
• Be aware that the drug causes vision impairment; most adults taking amiodarone develop corneal microdeposits, and cases of optic neuritis have been reported.
• Administer an oral loading dose in three equal doses; give with meals to decrease GI intolerance.
• Only give the drug I.V. if the patient is closely monitored for cardiac function and resuscitation equipment is available.
• Oral forms of the drug shouldn't be taken with grapefruit juice because it interferes with drug metabolism.

• Dofetilide shouldn't be administered with cimetidine, ketoconazole, megestrol, prochlorperazine, trimethoprim, sulfamethoxazole, or verapamil because the combination may induce life-threatening arrhythmias.
• Sotalol shouldn't be administered with dolasetron or droperidol because of an increased risk of life-threatening arrhythmias.
• Severe hypotension may develop when I.V. amiodarone is administered too rapidly.

Adverse reactions

Adverse reactions to class III antiarrhythmics, especially amiodarone, vary widely and commonly lead to drug discontinuation. A common adverse effect is aggravation of arrhythmias.

Other adverse reactions vary by drug:
• Amiodarone may also produce hypotension, bradycardia, nausea, and anorexia. Severe pulmonary toxicity occurs in 15% of patients and can be fatal. Vision disturbances and corneal microdeposits may also occur.
• Ibutilide may cause sustained ventricular tachycardia, QT-interval prolongation, hypotension, nausea, and headache.
• Sotalol may cause AV block, bradycardia, ventricular arrhythmias, bronchospasm, and hypotension.

Nursing process

These nursing process steps are appropriate for patients undergoing treatment with class III antiarrhythmics.

Assessment

- Assess the patient's arrhythmia before therapy and regularly thereafter.
- Monitor the ECG continuously when therapy starts and when the dosage is adjusted.
- Monitor the patient's vital signs frequently, and assess for signs of toxicity and adverse reactions.
- Measure the patient's apical pulse rate and blood pressure before giving the drug.
- Monitor serum drug levels as indicated.
- Monitor blood studies, such as liver function tests, as indicated.
- Be alert for adverse reactions and drug interactions.
- Evaluate the patient's and family's knowledge of drug therapy.

Key nursing diagnoses

- Decreased cardiac output related to arrhythmias or myocardial depression
- Risk for injury related to adverse reactions
- Deficient knowledge related to drug therapy

Planning outcome goals

- Cardiac output will improve as evidenced by stable blood pressure, cardiac monitoring, and adequate urine output.
- Complications from adverse reactions will be diminished.
- The patient will verbalize an understanding of drug therapy.

Implementation

- During and after administration, make sure proper equipment and facilities, such as cardiac monitoring, intracardiac pacing, a cardioverter-defibrillator, and medication for treatment of sustained ventricular tachycardia, are available.
- Correct hypokalemia and hypomagnesemia before therapy to reduce the risk of arrhythmias.

A stable situation

- Remember that admixtures and approved diluents are chemically and physically stable for 24 hours at room temperature or 48 hours if refrigerated.
- Don't crush sustained-release tablets.
- Be aware that sustained-release and extended-release medications aren't interchangeable.
- Take safety precautions if adverse CNS reactions occur.

- Notify the prescriber about adverse reactions.
- Use I.V. forms of the drug to treat acute arrhythmias.
- Provide patient teaching.

Evaluation

- Patient maintains adequate cardiac output as evidenced by normal vital signs and adequate tissue perfusion.
- Patient has no serious adverse reactions.
- Patient states the importance of compliance with therapy.

Class IV antiarrhythmics

Class IV antiarrhythmics are composed of calcium channel blockers. Calcium channel blockers used to treat arrhythmias include verapamil and diltiazem.

One mission

Verapamil and diltiazem are used to treat supraventricular arrhythmias with rapid ventricular response rates (rapid heart rate in which the rhythm originates above the ventricles).

Pharmacokinetics

Class IV antiarrhythmics are rapidly and completely absorbed from the GI tract after P.O. administration; only about 20% to 35% reaches systemic circulation. About 90% of the circulating drug is bound to plasma proteins. Class IV antiarrhythmics are metabolized in the liver and excreted in the urine as unchanged drug and active metabolites.

Pharmacodynamics

Class IV antiarrhythmics inhibit calcium ion influx across cardiac and smooth muscle cells, thus decreasing myocardial contractility and oxygen demand. They also dilate coronary arteries and arterioles.

Pharmacotherapeutics

This class of drugs is used to relieve angina, lower blood pressure, and restore normal sinus rhythm.

Drug interactions

These drug interactions may occur with class IV antiarrhythmics:
- Furosemide forms a precipitate when mixed with diltiazem injection. Give through separate I.V. lines.

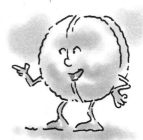

Class IV antiarrhythmics are used to relieve angina, lower blood pressure, and restore normal sinus rhythm.

- Anesthetics may potentiate the effects of class IV antiarrhythmics.
- Cyclosporine levels may be increased by diltiazem, resulting in toxicity; avoid using these drugs together.
- Diltiazem may increase levels of digoxin. Monitor the patient and drug levels.
- Cimetidine may inhibit diltiazem metabolism, resulting in toxicity.
- Propranolol and other beta-adrenergic blockers may precipitate heart failure or prolong cardiac conduction time with diltiazem and, therefore, should be used together cautiously.
- Antihypertensives and quinidine may cause hypotension when used with verapamil; monitor blood pressure.
- Disopyramide, flecainide, and propranolol and other beta-adrenergic blockers may cause heart failure when used with verapamil.
- Verapamil may decrease lithium levels.
- Rifampin may decrease the effects of verapamil.
- Black catechu may cause additive effects when used with verapamil.

Don't drink and...

- Grapefruit juice may increase verapamil levels.
- Verapamil enhances the effects of alcohol; discourage concurrent use.

Adverse reactions

The following adverse effects can occur when taking class IV antiarrhythmics.

Mild effects

- Dizziness
- Headache
- Hypotension
- Constipation
- Nausea
- Rash

Serious effects

- Heart failure
- Bradycardia
- AV block
- Ventricular asystole
- Ventricular fibrillation
- Pulmonary edema

Nursing process

These nursing process steps are appropriate for patients undergoing treatment with class IV antiarrhythmics.

Assessment

• Obtain a history of the patient's underlying condition before therapy, and reassess regularly thereafter.
• Assess the patient's arrhythmia before therapy and regularly thereafter.
• Monitor the ECG continuously when therapy starts and when the dosage is adjusted.
• Monitor the patient's vital signs frequently, and assess for signs of toxicity and adverse reactions.
• Measure the patient's apical pulse rate and blood pressure before giving the drug.
• Monitor the patient's intake and output.
• Monitor serum drug levels as indicated.
• Monitor blood studies, such as liver function tests, as indicated.
• Be alert for adverse reactions and drug interactions.
• Evaluate the patient's and family's knowledge of drug therapy.

Key nursing diagnoses

• Decreased cardiac output related to arrhythmias or myocardial depression
• Risk for injury related to adverse reactions
• Deficient knowledge related to drug therapy

Planning outcome goals

• Cardiac output will improve as evidenced by stable blood pressure, cardiac monitoring, and adequate urine output.
• Complications from adverse reactions will be diminished.
• The patient will verbalize an understanding of drug therapy.

Implementation

• Don't crush sustained-release tablets.
• Know that sustained-release and extended-release drug forms aren't interchangeable.

Forget the fluids

• Fluid and sodium intake may need to be restricted to minimize edema.
• Take safety precautions if adverse CNS reactions occur.
• Notify the prescriber about adverse reactions.
• Use I.V. forms of the drug for treating acute arrhythmias; cardiac monitoring is required during administrations.

• Withhold the dose and notify the prescriber if the patient's systolic pressure drops below 90 mm Hg or his heart rate drops to less than 60 beats/minute, or follow the prescriber's ordered parameters for withholding the medication.
• Help the patient walk because dizziness can occur.
• If the drugs are being used to terminate supraventricular tachycardia, the prescriber may have the patient perform vagal maneuvers after receiving the drug.
• Provide patient teaching.

Evaluation

• Patient maintains adequate cardiac output as evidenced by normal vital signs and adequate tissue perfusion.
• Patient has no serious adverse reactions.
• Patient states the importance of compliance with therapy.

Adenosine

Adenosine is an injectable antiarrhythmic drug indicated for acute treatment of PSVT.

Pharmacokinetics

After I.V. administration, adenosine probably is distributed rapidly throughout the body and metabolized inside RBCs as well as in vascular endothelial cells.

Pharmacodynamics

Adenosine depresses the pacemaker activity of the SA node, reducing heart rate and the ability of the AV node to conduct impulses from the atria to the ventricles.

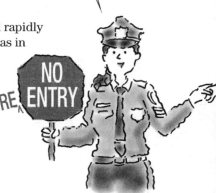

Adenosine is especially effective against reentry tachycardias that involve the AV node.

Pharmacotherapeutics

Adenosine is especially effective against reentry tachycardias (when an impulse depolarizes an area of heart muscle and returns and repolarizes it) that involve the AV node.

Packs a punch against PSVT

Adenosine is also effective in more than 90% of PSVT cases. It's predominantly used to treat arrhythmias associated with accessory bypass tracts (brief periods of rapid heart rate in which the rhythm's origin is above the ventricle), as in Wolff-Parkinson-White syndrome, a condition in which strands of heart tissue formed during fetal development abnormally connect structures such as the atria and ventricles, bypassing normal conduction. This condition is also known as a *preexcitation syndrome*.

Drug interactions

Adenosine has various drug interactions:
• Methylxanthines antagonize the effects of adenosine so that the patient may need larger doses of adenosine.
• Dipyridamole and carbamazepine potentiate the effects of adenosine, which may call for smaller doses of adenosine.
• When adenosine is administered with carbamazepine, the risk of heart block increases.
• Caffeine and theophylline may decrease adenosine's effects.

Adverse reactions

Adenosine many cause facial flushing, shortness of breath, dyspnea, and chest discomfort.

Nursing process

These nursing process steps are appropriate for patients undergoing treatment with adenosine.

Assessment
• Assess the patient's arrhythmia before therapy and regularly thereafter.
• Monitor the ECG continuously when therapy starts and when the dosage is adjusted.
• Monitor the patient's vital signs frequently, and assess for signs of toxicity and adverse reactions.
• Measure the apical pulse rate and blood pressure before giving the drug.
• Be alert for adverse reactions and drug interactions.
• Evaluate the patient's and family's knowledge of drug therapy.

Key nursing diagnoses
• Decreased cardiac output related to arrhythmias or myocardial depression
• Risk for injury related to adverse reactions
• Deficient knowledge related to drug therapy

Planning outcome goals
• Cardiac output will improve as evidenced by stable blood pressure, cardiac monitoring, and adequate urine output.
• Complications from adverse reactions will be diminished.
• The patient will verbalize an understanding of drug therapy.

Implementation

• If the solution is cold, check for crystals that may form. If crystals are visible, gently warm the solution to room temperature. Don't use unclear solutions.

Speed is key

• Give rapidly for effective drug action. Give directly into the vein if possible. If an I.V. line is used, inject the drug into the most proximal port and follow with a rapid saline flush to ensure that the drug reaches systemic circulation quickly.
• If ECG disturbances occur, withhold the drug, obtain a rhythm strip, and notify the prescriber immediately.
• Tell the patient that he may feel flushing or chest pain that lasts for 1 to 2 minutes after the drug is injected.
• Take safety precautions if adverse CNS reactions occur.
• Notify the prescriber about adverse reactions.

Evaluation

• Patient maintains adequate cardiac output as evidenced by normal vital signs and adequate tissue perfusion.
• Patient has no serious adverse reactions.
• Patient states the importance of compliance with therapy.

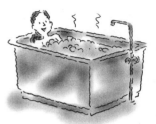

If crystals form in a cold solution, gently warm the solution to room temperature. This is my favorite way to warm up!

Antianginal drugs

Although angina's cardinal symptom is chest pain, the drugs used to treat angina aren't typically analgesics. Rather, antianginal drugs treat angina by reducing myocardial oxygen demand (reducing the amount of oxygen the heart needs to do its work), by increasing the supply of oxygen to the heart, or both. (See *How antianginal drugs work*, page 212.)

The three classes of antianginal drugs discussed in this section include:
• nitrates (for treating acute angina)
• beta-adrenergic blockers (for long-term prevention of angina)
• calcium channel blockers (used when other drugs fail to prevent angina).

Nitrates

Nitrates are the drugs of choice for relieving acute angina. Nitrates commonly prescribed to treat angina include:
• amyl nitrite
• isosorbide dinitrate

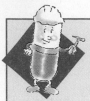

How antianginal drugs work

Angina occurs when the coronary arteries, the heart's primary source of oxygen, supply insufficient oxygen to the myocardium. This increases the heart's workload, increasing heart rate, preload (blood volume in the ventricles at end of diastole), afterload (pressure in the arteries leading from the ventricles), and force of myocardial contractility. The antianginal drugs relieve angina by decreasing one or more of these four factors. This diagram summarizes how antianginal drugs affect the cardiovascular system.

Afterload
Decreased by calcium channel blockers and nitrates

Heart rate
Decreased by beta-adrenergic blockers and some calcium channel blockers

Preload
Decreased by nitrates

Contractility
Decreased by beta-adrenergic blockers and calcium channel blockers

- isosorbide mononitrate
- nitroglycerin.

Pharmacokinetics

Nitrates can be administered in a variety of ways.

All absorbed...

Nitrates given sublingually (under the tongue), buccally (in the pocket of the cheek), as chewable tablets, as lingual aerosols (sprayed onto or under the tongue), or via inhalation (amyl nitrite) are absorbed almost completely because of the rich blood supply of the mucous membranes of the mouth.

...half-absorbed...

Swallowed nitrate capsules are absorbed through the mucous membranes of the GI tract, and only about half the dose enters circulation.

Transdermal nitrates (a patch or ointment placed on the skin) are absorbed slowly and in varying amounts, depending on the quantity of drug applied, the location where the patch is applied, the surface area of skin used, and the circulation to the skin.

...or not absorbed at all

I.V. nitroglycerin, which doesn't need to be absorbed, goes directly into circulation. (See *Nitrates: Nitroglycerin*.)

Pharmacodynamics

Nitrates cause the smooth muscle of the veins and, to a lesser extent, the arteries to relax and dilate. Nitrates work in the following way:
• When the veins dilate, less blood returns to the heart.
• This, in turn, reduces the amount of blood in the ventricles at the end of diastole, when the ventricles are full. (This blood volume in the ventricles just before contraction is called *preload*.)
• By reducing preload, nitrates reduce ventricular size and ventricular wall tension (the left ventricle doesn't have to stretch as much to pump blood). This, in turn, reduces the oxygen requirements of the heart.

Lighten the load

The arterioles provide the most resistance to the blood pumped by the left ventricle (called *peripheral vascular resistance*). Nitrates decrease afterload by dilating the arterioles, reducing resistance, easing the heart's workload, and easing the demand for oxygen.

Pharmacotherapeutics

Nitrates are used to relieve and prevent angina.

The short story...

Rapidly absorbed nitrates, such as nitroglycerin, are the drugs of choice for relief of acute angina because they have a rapid onset of action, are easy to take, and are inexpensive.

Prototype pro

Nitrates: Nitroglycerin

Actions
• Relaxes vascular smooth muscle
• Causes general vasodilation

Indications
• Acute or chronic anginal attacks

Nursing considerations
• Monitor for adverse effects, such as headache, dizziness, orthostatic hypotension, tachycardia, flushing, palpitations, and hypersensitivity reactions.
• Monitor vital signs closely.
• Treat headaches with acetaminophen or aspirin.

Nitrates are used to treat acute angina because of their rapid onset of action.

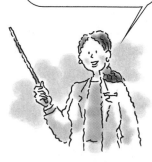

...or the long one

Longer-acting nitrates, such as the daily nitroglycerin transdermal patch, are convenient and can be used to prevent chronic angina. Oral nitrates are also used because they seldom produce serious adverse reactions.

Drug interactions

These drug interactions may occur with nitrates:
• Severe hypotension can result when nitrates interact with alcohol.
• Sildenafil shouldn't be taken within 24 hours of nitrates because of possible enhanced hypotensive effects.
• Absorption of sublingual nitrates may be delayed when taken with an anticholinergic drug.
• Marked orthostatic hypotension (a drop in blood pressure when a person stands up) with light-headedness, fainting, or blurred vision may occur when calcium channel blockers and nitrates are used together.

Adverse reactions

Most adverse reactions to nitrates are caused by changes in the cardiovascular system. The reactions usually disappear when the dosage is reduced.

My aching head...

Headache is the most common adverse reaction. Hypotension may occur, accompanied by dizziness and increased heart rate.

Nursing process

These nursing process steps are appropriate for patients undergoing treatment with nitrates.

Assessment
• Monitor vital signs. With I.V. nitroglycerin, monitor blood pressure and pulse rate every 5 to 15 minutes while adjusting the dosage and every hour thereafter.
• Monitor the effectiveness of the prescribed drug.
• Observe for adverse reactions.

Key nursing diagnoses
• Risk for injury related to adverse reactions
• Excess fluid volume related to adverse cardiovascular effects
• Deficient knowledge related to drug therapy

Planning outcome goals
• Risk of injury to the patient will be minimized.
• Fluid volume will remain within normal limits as evidenced by vital signs, cardiac monitoring, and urine output.
• The patient will demonstrate correct drug administration.

Implementation
• Tablets may be given on an empty stomach, either 30 minutes before or 1 to 2 hours after meals. Tell the patient to swallow tablets whole, not chew them.
• Have the patient sit or lie down when receiving the first nitrate dose. Take his pulse and blood pressure before giving the dose and when the drug action starts.
• Don't give a beta-adrenergic blocker or calcium channel blocker to relieve acute angina.
• Withhold the dose and notify the prescriber if the patient's heart rate is less than 60 beats/minute or his systolic blood pressure drops below 90 mm Hg, or follow the prescriber's ordered parameters for withholding the medication.
• Dilute I.V. nitroglycerin with D_5W or normal saline solution for injection, using a glass bottle. Avoid the use of I.V. filters because the drug binds to plastic. Special nonabsorbent polyvinyl chloride tubing is available from the manufacturer. Administer the drug with an infusion control device. Concentration shouldn't exceed 400 mcg/ml.
• Administer sublingual nitroglycerin tablets at the first sign of an attack, placing the medication under the tongue until it's completely absorbed. The dose can be repeated every 10 to 15 minutes up to three doses.
• Place topical ointments on paper as prescribed; then place the paper on a nonhairy area and cover it with plastic. Remove excess ointment from the previous site when applying the next dose. Remember to rotate application sites and make sure you don't get any ointment on your fingers.
• Remove a transdermal patch before defibrillation. Aluminum backing on the patch may explode with electric current.
• Be aware that the drug may initially cause headache until tolerance develops or the dosage is minimized.

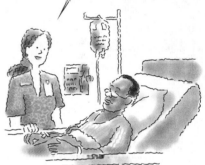

Have the patient sit or lie down when receiving the first nitrate dose.

Evaluation
• Patient sustains no injury from adverse reactions.
• Patient maintains normal fluid balance.
• Patient and his family demonstrate an understanding of drug therapy. (See *Teaching about antianginals*, page 216.)

Education edge

Teaching about antianginals

If antianginals are prescribed, review these points with the patient and his caregivers:
• It's essential to understand how to use the prescribed form of the drug.
• Take the drug regularly, as prescribed, and have it accessible at all times.
• Don't discontinue the drug abruptly without your prescriber's approval. Coronary vasospasm can occur.
• If taking nitrates, you may need an additional dose before anticipated stress or at bedtime if angina is nocturnal. Check with your prescriber.
• Use caution when wearing a transdermal patch near a microwave oven. Leaking radiation may heat the metallic backing of the patch and cause burns.
• Avoid alcohol during drug therapy.
• Change to an upright position slowly. Go up and down stairs carefully, and lie down at the first sign of dizziness.
• Store nitrates in a cool, dark place in a tightly closed container. To ensure freshness, replace sublingual tablets every 3 months and remove the cotton because it absorbs the drug.

• Store sublingual tablets in their original container or another container specifically approved for this use, and carry the container in a jacket pocket or purse, not in a pocket close to the body.
• As indicated, take your pulse before taking the medication, such as with beta-adrenergic blockers and calcium channel blockers. Withhold the dose and alert your prescriber if your pulse rate is below 60 beats/minute.
• If taking nitroglycerin sublingually, go to the emergency department if three tablets taken 5 minutes apart don't relieve anginal pain.
• Report serious or persistent adverse reactions to your prescriber.
• Avoid alcohol.
• Place the buccal tablet between your lip and gum above the incisors or between your cheek and gum. Don't swallow or chew the tablet.

Beta-adrenergic antagonists

Beta-adrenergic antagonists (also called *beta-adrenergic blockers*) are used for long-term prevention of angina and are one of the main types of drugs used to treat hypertension. Beta-adrenergic blockers include:
• atenolol
• carvedilol
• metoprolol tartrate
• nadolol
• propranolol hydrochloride.

Pharmacokinetics

Metoprolol and propranolol are absorbed almost entirely from the GI tract, whereas less than half the dose of atenolol or nadolol is absorbed. These beta-adrenergic blockers are distributed widely. Propranolol is highly protein bound; the other beta-adrenergic

Prototype pro

Beta$_1$- and beta$_2$-adrenergic blockers: Propranolol

Actions
• Reduces cardiac oxygen demand by blocking catecholamine-induced increases in heart rate, blood pressure, and force of myocardial contraction
• Depresses renin secretion and prevents vasodilation of cerebral arteries
• Relieves anginal and migraine pain, lowers blood pressure, restores normal sinus rhythm, and helps limit myocardial infarction (MI) damage

Indications
• Angina pectoris
• Mortality reduction after MI
• Supraventricular, ventricular, and atrial arrhythmias
• Tachyarrhythmias caused by excessive catecholamine action during anesthesia, hyperthyroidism, or pheochromocytoma
• Hypertension
• Prevention of frequent, severe, uncontrollable, or disabling migraine or vascular headache
• Essential tremor
• Hypertrophic cardiomyopathy

Nursing considerations
• Check the patient's apical pulse before giving the drug. If you detect extremes in pulse rate, withhold the drug and call the prescriber immediately.
• Give the drug with meals. Food may increase the drug's absorption.
• Before any surgical procedure, notify the anesthesiologist that the patient is receiving propranolol. The drug shouldn't be stopped before surgery, especially for patients with cardiovascular disorders or pheochromocytoma.
• Notify the prescriber if the patient develops severe hypotension; a vasopressor may be prescribed.
• Be aware that geriatric patients may have increased adverse reactions and may need dosage adjustment.
• Don't stop the drug abruptly.
• For overdose, give I.V. atropine, I.V. isoproterenol, or glucagon; refractory cases may require a pacemaker.

Prototype pro

Beta$_1$-adrenergic blockers: Metoprolol

Actions
• Competes with beta-adrenergic agonists for available beta-adrenergic receptor sites

Indications
• Hypertension
• Angina pectoris

Nursing considerations
• Monitor for adverse reactions, such as fatigue, dizziness, bradycardia, hypotension, heart failure, and atrioventricular block.
• Withhold the drug as ordered if the apical pulse is less than 60 beats/minute.
• Monitor blood pressure frequently.

blockers are poorly protein bound. (See *Beta$_1$- and beta$_2$-adrenergic blockers: Propranolol* and *Beta$_1$-adrenergic blockers: Metoprolol.*)

Propranolol and metoprolol are metabolized in the liver, and their metabolites are excreted in urine. Carvedilol is metabolized in the liver and excreted in the bile and feces. Atenolol and nadolol aren't metabolized and are excreted unchanged in urine and feces.

Pharmacodynamics

Beta-adrenergic blockers decrease blood pressure and block beta-adrenergic receptor sites in the heart muscle and conduction system. This decreases heart rate and reduces the force of the heart's contractions, resulting in a lower demand for oxygen.

Pharmacotherapeutics

Beta-adrenergic blockers are indicated for the long-term prevention of angina. Metoprolol may be given I.V. in acute coronary syndrome, followed by an oral dose. Carvedilol and metoprolol are indicated for heart failure. Beta-adrenergic blockers are also first-line therapy for treating hypertension.

Drug interactions

Several drugs interact with beta-adrenergic blockers:
• Antacids delay absorption of beta-adrenergic blockers.
• NSAIDs can decrease the hypotensive effects of beta-adrenergic blockers.
• Lidocaine toxicity may occur when the drug is taken with beta-adrenergic blockers.
• The requirements for insulin and oral antidiabetic drugs can be altered by beta-adrenergic blockers.
• The ability of theophylline to produce bronchodilation is impaired by nonselective beta-adrenergic blockers.

Adverse reactions

Adverse reactions to beta-adrenergic blockers include:
• bradycardia, angina, heart failure, and arrhythmias, especially AV block
• fainting
• fluid retention
• peripheral edema
• shock
• nausea and vomiting
• diarrhea
• significant constriction of the bronchioles.

Not so fast...

Suddenly stopping a beta-adrenergic blocker may trigger angina, hypertension, arrhythmias, and acute myocardial infarction (MI).

Nursing process

These nursing process steps are appropriate for patients undergoing treatment with beta-adrenergic blockers.

Assessment
- Assess the patient's arrhythmia before therapy and regularly thereafter.
- Monitor the ECG continuously when therapy starts, when the dosage is adjusted, and particularly during I.V. therapy.
- Monitor the patient's vital signs frequently; assess for signs of toxicity and adverse reactions.
- Measure the apical pulse rate and blood pressure before giving the drug.
- Monitor serum drug levels as indicated.
- Monitor blood studies, such as liver function tests, as indicated.
- Be alert for adverse reactions and drug interactions.
- Evaluate the patient's and family's knowledge of drug therapy.

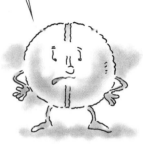

Watch your patient closely for drug interactions. You know, I don't always get along with just any old drug.

Key nursing diagnoses
- Decreased cardiac output related to arrhythmias or myocardial depression
- Risk for injury related to adverse reactions
- Deficient knowledge related to drug therapy

Planning outcome goals
- Cardiac output will improve as evidenced by stable blood pressure, cardiac monitoring, and adequate urine output.
- Complications from adverse reactions will be diminished.
- The patient will verbalize an understanding of drug therapy.

Implementation
- Don't crush sustained-release tablets.
- Be aware that sustained-released and extended-release medications aren't interchangeable.
- Take safety precautions if adverse CNS reactions occur.
- Notify the prescriber about adverse reactions.
- Use I.V. forms of the drug for treating acute arrhythmias. I.V. forms may be given as a loading dose I.V. or may be diluted with normal saline solution and given by intermittent infusion.
- Check the apical pulse before giving the drug. If you detect an extreme pulse rate, withhold the drug and call the prescriber immediately.
- Know that the drug may be given with meals as indicated.
- Before any surgical procedure, notify the anesthesiologist that the patient is receiving this drug.
- Don't discontinue the drug abruptly.
- Provide patient teaching.

Evaluation
- Patient maintains adequate cardiac output as evidenced by normal vital signs and adequate tissue perfusion.
- Patient has no serious adverse reactions.
- Patient states the importance of compliance with therapy.

Calcium channel blockers

Calcium channel blockers are commonly used to prevent angina that doesn't respond to drugs in either of the other antianginal classes. Several of the calcium channel blockers are also used as antiarrhythmics and in the treatment of hypertension.

Calcium channel blockers used to treat angina include:
- amlodipine besylate
- diltiazem
- nicardipine
- nifedipine
- verapamil.

Pharmacokinetics

When administered orally, calcium channel blockers are absorbed quickly and almost completely. Because of the first-pass effect, however, the bioavailability of these drugs is much lower. Calcium channel blockers are highly bound to plasma proteins.

Through the liver in a jiffy

All calcium channel blockers are metabolized rapidly and almost completely in the liver.

Pharmacodynamics

Calcium channel blockers prevent the passage of calcium ions across the myocardial cell membrane and vascular smooth muscle cells. This causes dilation of the coronary and peripheral arteries, which decreases the force of the heart's contractions and reduces the workload of the heart. (See *How calcium channel blockers work*.)

Putting on the brakes

By preventing arterioles from constricting, calcium channel blockers also reduce afterload, resulting in a decreased oxygen demand of the heart.

Some calcium channel blockers (diltiazem and verapamil) also reduce the heart rate by slowing conduction through the SA and AV nodes. A slower heart rate reduces the heart's need for additional oxygen.

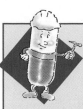

Pharm function

How calcium channel blockers work

Calcium channel blockers increase myocardial oxygen supply and slow cardiac impulse formation. Apparently, the drugs produce these effects by blocking the slow calcium channel. This action inhibits the influx of extra-cellular calcium ions across both myocardial and vascular smooth-muscle cell membranes. Calcium channel blockers achieve this blockade without changing serum calcium concentrations.

No calcium = dilation
This calcium blockade causes the coronary arteries (and, to a lesser extent, the peripheral arteries and arterioles) to dilate, decreasing afterload and increasing myocardial oxygen supply.

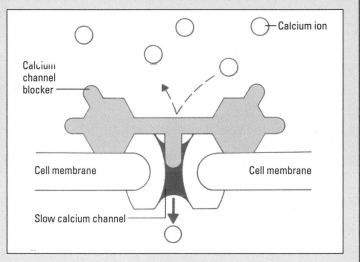

Pharmacotherapeutics

Calcium channel blockers are used only for long-term prevention of angina, not for short-term relief of chest pain. Calcium channel blockers are particularly effective for preventing Prinzmetal's angina. (See *Calcium channel blockers: Verapamil*, page 222.)

Drug interactions

These drug interactions can occur with calcium channel blockers:
• Calcium salts and vitamin D reduce the effectiveness of calcium channel blockers.
• Nondepolarizing blocking drugs may enhance the muscle-relaxant effect when taken with calcium channel blockers.
• Verapamil and diltiazem increase the risk of digoxin toxicity and enhance the action of carbamazepine.

Adverse reactions

As with other antianginal drugs, cardiovascular reactions are the most common and serious adverse reactions to calcium channel blockers. Possible adverse reactions include orthostatic hypotension, heart failure, hypotension, and arrhythmias, such as bradycardia and AV block. Other possible adverse reactions include

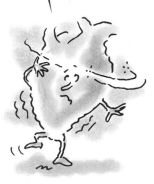

Such adverse reactions! Headache, flushing, weakness, dizziness... Ohhh...

Prototype pro

Calcium channel blockers: Verapamil

Actions
• Inhibits calcium ion influx across the cardiac and smooth-muscle cells
• Reduces myocardial contractility and oxygen demand
• Dilates coronary arteries and arterioles

Indications
• Angina relief
• Decreased blood pressure
• Abnormal sinus rhythm

Nursing considerations
• A patient with severely compromised cardiac function or one taking beta-adrenergic blockers should receive lower doses of verapamil.
• Monitor cardiac rhythm and blood pressure during the start of therapy and with dose adjustments.
• Notify the prescriber if signs and symptoms of heart failure occur, such as swelling of the hands and feet and shortness of breath.

dizziness, headache, flushing, weakness, and persistent peripheral edema.

Nursing process

These nursing process steps are appropriate for patients undergoing treatment with calcium channel blockers.

Assessment
• Obtain a history of the patient's underlying condition before therapy, and reassess regularly thereafter.
• Assess the patient's arrhythmia before therapy and regularly thereafter.
• Monitor the ECG continuously when therapy starts and when the dosage is adjusted.
• Monitor the patient's vital signs frequently, and assess for signs of toxicity and adverse reactions.
• Measure the apical pulse rate and blood pressure before giving the drug.
• Monitor serum drug levels as indicated.
• Monitor blood studies, such as liver function tests, as indicated.
• Be alert for adverse reactions and drug interactions.
• Evaluate the patient's and family's knowledge of drug therapy.

Key nursing diagnoses
• Decreased cardiac output related to arrhythmias or myocardial depression
• Risk for injury related to adverse reactions
• Deficient knowledge related to drug therapy

Planning outcome goals

- Cardiac output will improve as evidenced by stable blood pressure, cardiac monitoring, and adequate urine output.
- Complications from adverse reactions will be diminished.
- The patient will verbalize an understanding of drug therapy.

Implementation

- Don't crush sustained-release tablets.
- Be aware that sustained-released and extended-release medications aren't interchangeable.
- Take safety precautions if adverse CNS reactions occur.
- Notify the prescriber about adverse reactions.
- Know that I.V. forms are used for treating acute arrhythmias; cardiac monitoring is required during administration.
- If the patient's systolic pressure is below 90 mm Hg or his heart rate drops below 60 beats/minute, withhold the dose and notify the prescriber or follow the prescriber's ordered parameters for withholding the medication.

Help your patient walk the walk

- Assist the patient with ambulation during the start of therapy because dizziness can occur.
- If the drug is being used to terminate supraventricular tachycardia, the prescriber may have the patient perform vagal maneuvers after receiving the drug.
- Advise the patient that fluid and sodium intake may need to be restricted to minimize edema.
- Provide patient teaching.

Evaluation

- Patient maintains adequate cardiac output as evidenced by normal vital signs and adequate tissue perfusion.
- Patient has no serious adverse reactions.
- Patient states the importance of compliance with therapy.

Antihypertensive drugs

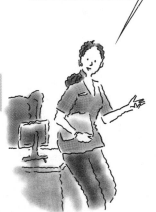

Antihypertensive drugs are used to treat hypertension. That makes sense!

Antihypertensive drugs are used to treat hypertension, a disorder characterized by elevation in systolic blood pressure, diastolic blood pressure, or both.

A word to the wise

According to the Seventh Report of the Joint National Committee on Prevention, Detection, Evaluation, and Treatment of High Blood Pressure, several classes of drugs have been shown in clini-

cal trials to be effective in treating hypertension. Diuretics, primarily thiazide diuretics, are used as initial therapy in treating most patients with hypertension. (These drugs will be discussed in chapter 8.) Other classes of drugs used to treat hypertension include:
- angiotensin-converting enzyme (ACE) inhibitors
- angiotensin-receptor blockers (ARBs)
- beta-adrenergic antagonists
- calcium channel blockers.

If these drugs are ineffective, treatment continues with sympatholytic drugs (other than beta-adrenergic blockers), direct vasodilators, selective aldosterone-receptor antagonists, or a combination of drugs.

Angiotensin-converting enzyme inhibitors

ACE inhibitors reduce blood pressure by interrupting the renin-angiotensin activating system (RAAS). Commonly prescribed ACE inhibitors include:
- benazepril
- captopril (see *ACE inhibitors: Captopril*)
- enalapril
- enalaprilat
- fosinopril sodium
- lisinopril
- moexipril

Prototype pro

ACE inhibitors: Captopril

Actions
- Thought to inhibit angiotensin-converting enzyme (ACE), preventing conversion of angiotensin I to angiotensin II (reduced formation of angiotensin II decreases peripheral arterial resistance, thus decreasing aldosterone secretion)

Indications
- Sodium and water retention
- High blood pressure
- Impaired renal function in patients with diabetes

Nursing considerations
- Monitor white blood cell and differential counts before therapy, every 2 weeks for the first 3 months of therapy, and periodically thereafter.
- Give the drug 1 hour before meals because food may reduce drug absorption.
- Withhold the dose and notify the prescriber if the patient develops fever, sore throat, leukopenia, hypotension, or tachycardia.
- Keep in mind that light-headedness and syncope can develop in hot weather, with inadequate fluid intake, vomiting, diarrhea, and excessive perspiration.

- quinapril hydrochloride
- ramipril
- trandolapril.

Pharmacokinetics

ACE inhibitors are absorbed from the GI tract, distributed to most body tissues, metabolized somewhat in the liver, and excreted by the kidneys. Ramipril also is excreted in feces. Enalaprilat is the only I.V. ACE inhibitor available.

Pharmacodynamics

ACE inhibitors work by preventing the conversion of angiotensin I to angiotensin II. Angiotensin II is a potent vasoconstrictor that increases peripheral resistance and promotes the excretion of aldosterone (which promotes sodium and water retention). As angiotensin II is reduced, arterioles dilate, reducing peripheral vascular resistance.

By reducing aldosterone secretion, ACE inhibitors promote the excretion of sodium and water, reducing the amount of blood the heart needs to pump and reducing blood pressure.

Pharmacotherapeutics

ACE inhibitors may be used alone or in combination with other agents, such as a thiazide diuretic, to treat hypertension. They're commonly used when beta-adrenergic blockers or diuretics are ineffective.

Captopril, enalapril, fosinopril, lisinopril, quinapril, ramipril, and trandolapril are also indicated for use in heart failure for the following situations:
- left ventricular systolic failure (unless contraindicated or intolerant)
- left ventricular systolic dysfunction without symptoms of heart failure
- after acute MI (especially in patients with prior myocardial injury) to reduce mortality
- left ventricular dysfunction (recent or remote) to prevent or delay the development of left ventricular dilation and overt heart failure
- combined use with beta-adrenergic blockers to produce complementary effects
- combined use with diuretics if fluid retention persists.

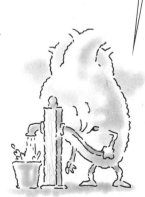

ACE inhibitors reduce the amount of blood I need to pump. Thank goodness! Pumping can be hard work!

Multiple MI uses

Lisinopril, ramipril, and trandolapril are also indicated for use in patients who have had an MI to improve survival and to reduce morbidity and mortality in patients with left ventricular dysfunction.

Historically speaking...

Ramipril is also indicated to prevent major cardiovascular events in patients with a history of vascular disease or diabetes. It's also used to reduce overall cardiovascular risk, including death, nonfatal MI, nonfatal stroke, and complications of diabetes.

Drug interactions

ACE inhibitors can cause several different types of interactions with other cardiovascular drugs:
• All ACE inhibitors enhance the hypotensive effects of diuretics and other antihypertensives such as beta-adrenergic blockers. They can also increase serum lithium levels, possibly resulting in lithium toxicity.
• When ACE inhibitors are used with potassium-sparing diuretics, potassium supplements, or potassium-containing salt substitutes, hyperkalemia may occur.
• ACE inhibitors may interact with other medications, both prescribed and over the counter. For example, patients taking ACE inhibitors should avoid taking NSAIDs. In addition to decreasing the antihypertensive effects of ACE inhibitors, NSAIDs may also alter renal function.
• Food decreases the absorption of ACE inhibitors.

On their own

Captopril, enalapril, and lisinopril may become less effective when administered with NSAIDs. Antacids may impair the absorption of fosinopril, and quinapril may reduce the absorption of tetracycline.

Adverse reactions

ACE inhibitors can cause these adverse reactions:
• headache
• fatigue
• dry, nonproductive, persistent cough
• angioedema
• GI reactions
• increased serum potassium concentrations
• tickling in the throat
• transient elevations of BUN and serum creatinine levels (indicators of kidney function).

They can cause problems with fetal circulation and shouldn't be administered during the second or third trimester of pregnancy.

Captopril cautions

Captopril may cause protein in the urine, reduced neutrophils and granulocytes (types of white blood cells [WBCs]), rash, loss of taste, hypotension, or a severe allergic reaction.

Nursing process

These nursing process steps are appropriate for patients undergoing treatment with ACE inhibitors.

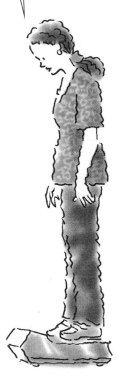

Be sure to monitor the weight of a patient taking ACE inhibitors.

Assessment
• Obtain a baseline blood pressure and pulse rate and rhythm, and recheck regularly.
• Monitor the patient for adverse reactions and drug interactions.
• Monitor the patient's weight and fluid and electrolyte status.
• Assess the patient's underlying condition before therapy and regularly thereafter.
• Monitor laboratory results, including WBC and differential, potassium level, and renal function (BUN and creatinine clearance levels and urinalysis).
• Monitor the patient's compliance with treatment.
• Observe the patient's tolerance of the drug's therapeutic effects. The dosage may need to be increased.

Potential patch problems

• Monitor a transdermal patch for dermatitis, and ask the patient about pruritus. Keep in mind that the patch can require several days to take effect and that interim oral therapy may be needed.

Key nursing diagnoses
• Risk for injury related to orthostatic hypotension
• Risk for injury related to presence of hypertension
• Deficient knowledge related to drug therapy

Planning outcome goals
• Blood pressure will be maintained within acceptable limits.
• Risk for injury will be minimized.
• The patient will verbalize an understanding of drug therapy.

Implementation
• If giving orally, administer the drug before meals as indicated.
• Follow the manufacturer's guidelines when mixing and administering parenteral drugs.
• Prevent or minimize orthostatic hypotension by helping the patient to get up slowly and by telling the patient not to make sudden movements.

- Maintain the patient's nonpharmacologic therapies, such as sodium restriction, calorie reduction, stress management, and exercise program.
- Keep in mind that drug therapy may be given to lower blood pressure rapidly in some hypertensive emergency situations.
- Know that the dosage is usually adjusted to the patient's blood pressure and tolerance.
- To improve adherence of a transdermal patch, apply an adhesive overlay. Place the patch at a different site each week.

Avoiding an electrifying experience

- Remove a transdermal patch before defibrillation to prevent arcing.
- Periodic eye examinations are recommended.

Evaluation

- Patient sustains no trauma from orthostatic hypotension.
- Patient sustains no injury.
- Patient and his family demonstrate an understanding of drug therapy.

Angiotensin II receptor blocking agents

ARBs lower blood pressure by blocking the vasoconstrictive effects of angiotensin II. Available ARBs include:

- losartan
- valsartan
- irbesartan
- candesartan cilexetil
- telmisartan
- eprosartan
- olmesartan.

Pharmacokinetics

ARBs have varying pharmacokinetic properties, and all are highly bound to plasma proteins.

Pharmacodynamics

ARBs act by interfering with the RAAS. They selectively block the binding of angiotensin II to the angiotensin II receptor. This prevents the vasoconstricting and aldosterone-secreting effects of angiotensin II (a potent vasoconstrictor), resulting in a blood pressure decrease.

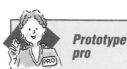

Prototype pro

Angiotensin II receptor blockers: Losartan

Actions
- Inhibits vasoconstricting and aldosterone-secreting effects of angiotensin II by selectively blocking binding of angiotensin II to receptor sites in many tissues, including vascular smooth muscle and adrenal glands

Indications
- High blood pressure

Nursing considerations
- Monitor blood pressure before therapy and regularly thereafter.
- Regularly assess kidney function (creatinine and blood urea nitrogen levels).

No inhibitions

ARBs don't inhibit the production of ACE that's responsible for the conversion of angiotensin I to angiotensin II, nor do they cause a breakdown in bradykinin (a vasodilator). (See *Angiotensin II receptor blockers: Losartan.*)

Pharmacotherapeutics

ARBs may be used alone or in combination with other agents, such as a diuretic, for the treatment of hypertension. Valsartan may also be used as an alternative to ACE inhibitors or for the management of heart failure. Irbesartan and losartan are indicated for patients with type 2 diabetes because of their inherent renal protective effect.

Drug interactions

These drug interactions may occur with ARBs:
• Losartan taken with fluconazole may increase levels of losartan, leading to increased hypotensive effects.
• NSAIDs reduce the antihypertensive effects of ARBs.
• Rifampin may increase metabolism of losartan, leading to decreased antihypertensive effect.
• Potassium supplements can increase the risk of hyperkalemia when used with ARBs.
• Losartan taken with lithium may increase lithium levels.

Adverse reactions

Adverse effects of ARBs include:
• headache
• fatigue
• cough and tickling in the throat
• angioedema
• GI reactions
• increased serum potassium
• transient elevations of BUN and serum creatinine levels.
    ARBs shouldn't be used during the second and third trimester of pregnancy; this can result in injury to and death of the fetus.

Nursing process

These nursing process steps are appropriate for patients undergoing treatment with ARBs.

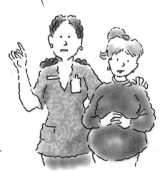

ARBs shouldn't be used during the second and third trimesters because of the risk of injury or death of the fetus.

Assessment

- Obtain a baseline blood pressure and pulse rate and rhythm; recheck regularly.
- Monitor the patient for adverse reactions.
- Monitor the patient's weight and fluid and electrolyte status.
- Observe the patient's compliance with treatment.
- Observe the patient's tolerance of the drug, and monitor the drug's therapeutic effects. The dosage may need to be adjusted.
- Monitor a transdermal patch for dermatitis; ask the patient about pruritus. Keep in mind that the patch can require several days to take effect and that the patient may need interim oral therapy.

Key nursing diagnoses

- Risk for injury related to orthostatic hypotension
- Risk for injury related to the presence of hypertension
- Deficient knowledge related to drug therapy

Planning outcome goals

- Blood pressure will be maintained within acceptable limits.
- Risk for injury will be minimized.
- The patient will verbalize correct drug administration.

Implementation

- If giving orally, administer the drug with food or at bedtime as indicated.
- Follow the manufacturer's guidelines when mixing and administering parenteral drugs.
- Prevent or minimize orthostatic hypotension by helping the patient to get up slowly and by telling the patient not to make sudden movements.
- Maintain the patient's nonpharmacologic therapies, such as sodium restriction, calorie reduction, stress management, and exercise program.
- Keep in mind that drug therapy may be given to lower blood pressure rapidly in some hypertensive emergency situations.
- Know that the dosage is usually adjusted to the patient's blood pressure and tolerance.
- To improve adherence of a transdermal patch, apply an adhesive overlay. Place the patch at a different site each week.
- Remove a transdermal patch before defibrillation to prevent arcing.
- Periodic eye examinations are recommended.

The patient on ARBs should maintain nonpharmacologic therapies, including an exercise program. Let's keep up the pace!

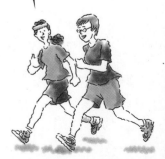

Evaluation

- Patient sustains no trauma from orthostatic hypotension.

• Patient sustains no injury.
• Patient and his family demonstrate an understanding of drug therapy.

Beta-adrenergic antagonists

Beta-adrenergic antagonists, or beta-adrenergic blockers, are one of the main types of drugs used to treat hypertension, including ocular hypertension. They're also used for long-term prevention of angina. Beta-adrenergic blockers used for hypertension include:
• acebutolol
• atenolol
• betaxolol
• bisoprolol
• carteolol
• metoprolol tartrate
• nadolol
• pindolol
• propranolol hydrochloride
• timolol.

Pharmacokinetics

The pharmacokinetics of beta-adrenergic blockers varies by drug. Acebutolol, betaxolol, carteolol, metoprolol, pindolol, propranolol, and timolol are absorbed almost entirely from the GI tract, whereas less than half of atenolol or nadolol is absorbed. GI tract absorption of bisoprolol is approximately 80%.

Acebutolol, carteolol, propranolol, metoprolol, and timolol are metabolized in the liver, and their metabolites are excreted in urine. Atenolol and nadolol aren't metabolized and are excreted unchanged in urine and feces. Betaxolol is metabolized in the liver and is primarily excreted in urine. Bisoprolol is partially eliminated by renal pathways. Approximately 50% of the drug is excreted in the urine and about 2% in feces. Pindolol is metabolized in the liver (about 65% of the dose), and 35% to 50% of the dose is excreted unchanged in urine.

Pharmacodynamics

Beta-adrenergic blockers decrease blood pressure and block beta-adrenergic receptor sites in the heart muscle and conduction system. This decreases heart rate and reduces the force of the heart's contractions, resulting in a lower demand for oxygen.

Pharmacotherapeutics

Beta-adrenergic blockers are used as first-line therapy for treating hypertension and are also indicated for the long-term prevention of angina.

The "eyes" have it

Betaxolol, carteolol, and timolol are also used for ocular hypertension.

Drug interactions

Several drugs interact with beta-adrenergic blockers:
• Antacids delay absorption of beta-adrenergic blockers.
• NSAIDs can decrease the hypotensive effects of beta-adrenergic blockers.
• Lidocaine toxicity may occur when the drug is taken with beta-adrenergic blockers.
• The requirements for insulin and oral antidiabetic drugs can be altered by beta-adrenergic blockers.
• The ability of theophylline to produce bronchodilation is impaired by nonselective beta-adrenergic blockers.
• Hypotensive effects may be increased when beta-adrenergic blockers are administered with diuretics.

Adverse reactions

Adverse reactions to beta-adrenergic blockers include:
• bradycardia, angina, heart failure, and arrhythmias, especially AV block
• fainting
• fluid retention
• peripheral edema
• dizziness
• shock
• nausea and vomiting
• diarrhea
• significant constriction of the bronchioles.

Slow to a halt

Suddenly stopping a beta-adrenergic blocker may trigger angina, hypertension, arrhythmias, and acute MI.

Nursing process

These nursing process steps are appropriate for patients undergoing treatment with beta-adrenergic blockers.

Assessment

- Obtain a baseline blood pressure and pulse rate and rhythm; recheck regularly.
- Monitor the ECG when therapy starts, when the dosage is adjusted, and particularly during I.V. therapy.
- Monitor the patient's vital signs frequently; assess for signs of toxicity and adverse reactions.
- Measure the apical pulse rate and blood pressure before giving the drug.
- Monitor blood studies, such as liver function tests, as indicated.
- Be alert for adverse reactions and drug interactions.
- Evaluate the patient's and family's knowledge of drug therapy.

Key nursing diagnoses

- Risk for injury related to orthostatic hypotension
- Risk for injury related to presence of hypertension
- Deficient knowledge related to drug therapy

Planning outcome goals

- Blood pressure will be maintained within acceptable limits.
- Risk for injury will be minimized.
- The patient will verbalize an understanding of drug therapy.

Implementation

- Don't crush sustained-release tablets.
- Be aware that sustained-released and extended-release medications aren't interchangeable.
- Take safety precautions if adverse CNS reactions occur.
- Notify the prescriber about adverse reactions.
- Know that the dosage is usually adjusted to the patient's blood pressure and tolerance.
- Prevent or minimize orthostatic hypotension by helping the patient to get up slowly and by telling the patient not to make sudden movements.
- Use I.V. forms of the drug for treating severe hypertension. I.V. forms may be given as a loading dose I.V. or may be diluted with normal saline solution and given by intermittent infusion.
- If systolic blood pressure is below 90 mm Hg or heart rate is below 60 beats/minute, withhold the dose and notify the prescriber or follow the prescriber's ordered parameters for withholding the medication.
- Know that the drug may be given with meals as indicated.
- Before any surgical procedure, notify the anesthesiologist that the patient is receiving this drug.
- Don't discontinue I.V. administration abruptly.
- Provide patient teaching.

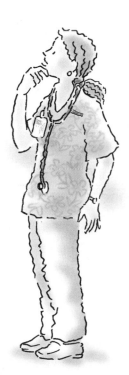

Evaluation

- Blood pressure is maintained within acceptable limits.
- Patient sustains no injury from orthostatic hypotension.
- Patient and his family demonstrate an understanding of drug therapy.

Calcium channel blockers

Calcium channel blockers are commonly used to treat hypertension. Several are also used to treat arrhythmias and to prevent angina that doesn't respond to other antianginal drugs.

Calcium channel blockers used to treat hypertension include:

- amlodipine besylate
- diltiazem
- felodipine
- isradipine
- nicardipine
- nifedipine
- nisoldipine
- verapamil.

Pharmacokinetics

When administered orally, calcium channel blockers are absorbed quickly and almost completely. Because of the first-pass effect, however, the bioavailability of these drugs is much lower. Food decreases amlodipine absorption by 30%, and high-fat foods increase the peak concentration of nisoldipine. Calcium channel blockers are highly bound to plasma proteins.

All calcium channel blockers are metabolized rapidly and almost completely in the liver and are primarily excreted in urine.

Pharmacodynamics

Calcium channel blockers prevent the passage of calcium ions across the myocardial cell membrane and vascular smooth-muscle cells. This causes dilation of the coronary and peripheral arteries, which decreases the force of the heart's contractions and reduces the workload of the heart and decreases blood pressure. By preventing arterioles from constricting, calcium channel blockers also reduce afterload, resulting in a decreased oxygen demand of the heart.

No need for extra O_2

Some calcium channel blockers (diltiazem and verapamil) also reduce the heart rate by slowing conduction through the SA and AV nodes. A slower heart rate reduces the heart's need for additional oxygen.

Pharmacotherapeutics

Calcium channel blockers are used to treat hypertension and for long-term prevention of angina. They shouldn't be used for short-term relief of chest pain. Calcium channel blockers are particularly effective for preventing Prinzmetal's angina.

Drug interactions

These drug interactions can occur with calcium channel blockers:
• Calcium salts and vitamin D reduce the effectiveness of calcium channel blockers.
• Nondepolarizing blocking drugs may enhance the muscle-relaxant effect when taken with calcium channel blockers.
• Verapamil and diltiazem increase the risk of digoxin toxicity, enhance the action of carbamazepine, and can produce myocardial depression.

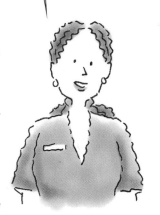

Calcium channel blockers are particularly effective for preventing Prinzmetal's angina.

Adverse reactions

Possible adverse reactions include headache, dizziness, weakness, orthostatic hypotension, heart failure, hypotension, peripheral edema, palpitations, and arrhythmias such as tachycardia. Bradycardia and AV block also occur with diltiazem and verapamil.

Nursing process

These nursing process steps are appropriate for patients undergoing treatment with calcium channel blockers.

Assessment
• Obtain a history of the patient's underlying condition before therapy, and reassess regularly thereafter.
• Obtain a baseline blood pressure and pulse rate and rhythm; recheck regularly.
• Monitor the ECG when therapy starts and when the dosage is adjusted.
• Monitor the patient's vital signs frequently, and assess for signs of toxicity and adverse reactions.
• Measure the apical pulse rate and blood pressure before giving the drug.
• Monitor serum drug levels as indicated.
• Monitor blood studies, such as liver function tests, as indicated.
• Be alert for adverse reactions and drug interactions.
• Evaluate the patient's and family's knowledge of drug therapy.

Key nursing diagnoses

- Risk for injury related to orthostatic hypotension
- Risk for injury related to adverse reactions
- Deficient knowledge related to drug therapy

Planning outcome goals

- Risk for injury will be minimized.
- Complications from adverse reactions will be diminished.
- The patient will verbalize an understanding of drug therapy.

Implementation

- Don't crush sustained-release tablets.
- Be aware that sustained-released and extended-release medications aren't interchangeable.
- Take safety precautions if adverse CNS reactions occur.
- Notify the prescriber about adverse reactions.
- If the patient's systolic pressure is below 90 mm Hg or his heart rate drops below 60 beats/minute, withhold the dose and notify the prescriber or follow the prescriber's ordered parameters for withholding the medication.
- Assist the patient with ambulation during the start of therapy because dizziness can occur.
- Advise the patient that fluid and sodium intake may need to be restricted to minimize edema.

Evaluation

- Patient sustains no injury from orthostatic hypotension.
- Patient has no serious adverse reactions.
- Patient and his family demonstrate an understanding of drug therapy.

Diuretic drugs

Diuretic drugs include several classes of diuretics that reduce blood pressure by increasing urine output and decreasing edema, circulating blood volume, and cardiac output. See Chapter 8 for specific information on the various types of diuretics.

Sympatholytic drugs

Sympatholytic drugs include several different types of drugs that reduce blood pressure by inhibiting or blocking the sympathetic nervous system. They're classified by their site or mechanism of action and include:

Prototype pro

Centrally acting sympatholytics: Clonidine

Actions
• Inhibits central vasomotor centers, decreasing sympathetic outflow to the heart, kidneys, and peripheral vasculature
• Decreases peripheral vascular resistance
• Decreases systolic and diastolic blood pressure
• Decreases heart rate

Indications
• High blood pressure

Nursing considerations
• The drug is adjusted to the patient's blood pressure and tolerance.
• When stopping therapy in a patient receiving both clonidine and a beta-adrenergic blocker, gradually withdraw the beta-adrenergic blocker first to minimize adverse reactions.
• Discontinuing clonidine for surgery isn't recommended.

Prototype pro

Alpha-adrenergic blockers: Doxazosin

Actions
• Acts on peripheral vasculature to produce vasodilation

Indications
• High blood pressure

Nursing considerations
• The dosage must be increased gradually, with adjustments every 2 weeks for hypertension.
• Monitor blood pressure.
• Monitor the electrocardiogram for arrhythmias.

• central-acting sympathetic nervous system inhibitors (clonidine hydrochloride and methyldopa) (see *Centrally acting sympatholytics: Clonidine*)
• alpha-adrenergic blockers (doxazosin, phentolamine, prazosin, and terazosin) (see *Alpha-adrenergic blockers: Doxazosin*)
• mixed alpha- and beta-adrenergic blockers (carvedilol and labetalol)
• norepinephrine depletors (guanadrel sulfate, guanethidine monosulfate, and reserpine). However, these drugs are rarely used.

Pharmacokinetics

Most sympatholytic drugs are absorbed well from the GI tract, distributed widely, metabolized in the liver, and excreted primarily in urine.

Pharmacodynamics

All sympatholytic drugs inhibit stimulation of the sympathetic nervous system. This causes dilation of the peripheral blood vessels or decreased cardiac output, thereby reducing blood pressure.

Pharmacotherapeutics

If blood pressure can't be controlled by beta-adrenergic blockers and diuretics, an alpha-adrenergic blocker (such as prazosin) or an alpha-beta blocker (such as labetalol) may be used.

Try and try again

If the patient still fails to achieve the desired blood pressure, the prescriber may add a drug from a different class, substitute a drug in the same class, or increase the drug dosage.

Drug interactions

Sympatholytic drugs can create the following drug interactions:
• Clonidine plus tricyclic antidepressants may increase blood pressure.
• Clonidine taken with CNS depressants may worsen CNS depression.
• Carvedilol taken with antidiabetic agents may result in an increased hypoglycemic effect.
• Carvedilol taken with calcium channel blockers and digoxin may result in increased digoxin levels.
• Carvedilol taken with rifampin decreases levels of carvedilol.

Adverse reactions

Sympatholytic drugs can also produce significant adverse reactions. Possible adverse reactions to sympatholytic drugs vary by type. For example, alpha-adrenergic blockers may cause hypotension.

Central problems

Adverse reactions to central-acting drugs include:
• depression
• drowsiness
• edema
• liver dysfunction
• numbness and tingling
• vertigo.

"G" whiz

Adverse reactions to guanadrel include:
• difficulty breathing
• excessive urination
• fainting or dizziness
• orthostatic hypotension
• drowsiness
• diarrhea
• headache.
   Adverse reactions to guanethidine include:
• decreased heart contractility
• diarrhea
• fluid retention
• orthostatic hypotension.

Reserpine results

Adverse reactions to reserpine include:
- abdominal cramps
- diarrhea
- angina
- blurred vision
- bradycardia
- bronchoconstriction
- decreased libido
- depression
- drowsiness
- edema
- nasal congestion
- weight gain.

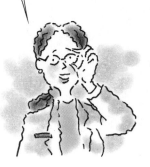

Look sharp! Adverse reactions to reserpine include abdominal cramps, diarrhea, angina, and blurred vision.

Nursing process

These nursing process steps are appropriate for patients undergoing treatment with sympatholytics.

Assessment
- Obtain a baseline blood pressure and pulse rate and rhythm; recheck regularly.
- Monitor the patient for adverse reactions.
- Monitor the patient's weight and fluid and electrolyte status.
- Monitor the patient's compliance with treatment.
- Observe the patient's tolerance of the drug, and monitor for the drug's therapeutic effects. The patient may require a dosage adjustment.
- Monitor a transdermal patch for dermatitis and ask about pruritus. Keep in mind that the patch can require several days to take effect and that interim oral therapy may be needed.

Key nursing diagnoses
- Risk for injury related to orthostatic hypotension
- Risk for injury related to presence of hypertension
- Deficient knowledge related to drug therapy

Planning outcome goals
- Blood pressure will be maintained within acceptable limits.
- Risk for injury to the patient will be minimized.
- The patient will verbalize an understanding of drug therapy.

Implementation
- If giving orally, administer the drug with food or at bedtime as indicated.

- Follow the manufacturer's guidelines when mixing and administering parenteral drugs.
- Prevent or minimize orthostatic hypotension by helping the patient to get up slowly and by telling the patient not to make sudden movements.
- Maintain the patient's nonpharmacologic therapies, such as sodium restriction, calorie reduction, stress management, and exercise program.
- Keep in mind that drug therapy may be given to lower blood pressure rapidly in some hypertensive emergency situations.
- Keep in mind that the dosage is usually adjusted to the patient's blood pressure and tolerance.
- To improve adherence of a transdermal patch, apply an adhesive overlay. Place the patch at a different site each week.
- Remove a transdermal patch before defibrillation to prevent arcing.
- Periodic eye examinations are recommended.

Evaluation

- Patient sustains no trauma from orthostatic hypotension.
- Patient sustains no injury.
- Patient and his family demonstrate an understanding of drug therapy. (See *Teaching about antihypertensives.*)

Education edge

Teaching about antihypertensives

If antihypertensives are prescribed, review these points with the patient and his caregivers:
- Take the drug exactly as prescribed. Don't stop the drug abruptly. Abrupt discontinuation may cause severe rebound hypertension.
- The last oral dose is usually administered at bedtime.
- The transdermal patch usually adheres despite showering and other routine daily activities. Use an adhesive overlay to improve skin adherence if necessary. Place the patch at a different site each week.
- The drug can cause drowsiness, but tolerance to this adverse effect will develop.

- Be aware of the adverse reactions caused by this drug, and notify your prescriber of serious or persistent reactions (dizziness, coughing, lightheadedness, hypotension).
- Avoid sudden changes in position to prevent dizziness, lightheadedness, or fainting, which are signs of orthostatic hypotension.
- Avoid hazardous activities until the full effects of the drug are known. Also avoid physical exertion, especially in hot weather.
- Consult with your prescriber before taking any over-the-counter medications or herbal remedies; serious drug interactions can occur.
- Comply with therapy.

Direct vasodilators

Direct vasodilators decrease systolic and diastolic blood pressure. They act on arteries, veins, or both. Examples of these drugs include:
- diazoxide
- hydralazine
- minoxidil
- nitroprusside.

Hypertension that hangs on tight

Hydralazine and minoxidil are usually used to treat resistant or refractory hypertension. Diazoxide and nitroprusside are reserved for use in hypertensive crisis. (See *Vasodilators: Nitroprusside,* page 242.)

Pharmacokinetics

Most vasodilating drugs are absorbed rapidly and distributed well. They're all metabolized in the liver, and most are excreted by the kidneys.

Pharmacodynamics

The direct vasodilators relax peripheral vascular smooth muscles, causing the blood vessels to dilate. This lowers blood pressure by increasing the diameter of the blood vessels, reducing total peripheral resistance.

Pharmacotherapeutics

Vasodilating drugs are rarely used alone to treat hypertension. Rather, they're usually used in combination with other drugs to treat the patient with moderate to severe hypertension (hypertensive crisis).

Drug interactions

Few drug interactions occur with vasodilating drugs. Some that may occur, however, include the following:
- The antihypertensive effects of hydralazine and minoxidil are increased when they're given with other antihypertensive drugs, such as methyldopa or reserpine.
- Vasodilating drugs may produce additive effects when given with nitrates, such as isosorbide dinitrate or nitroglycerin.

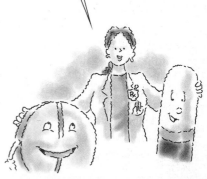

Successful treatment of hypertension usually requires a team approach.

Adverse reactions

Direct vasodilators commonly produce adverse reactions related to reflex activation of the sympathetic nervous system. As blood pressure falls, the sympathetic nervous system is stimulated, producing such compensatory measures as vasoconstriction and tachycardia.

Other reactions to sympathetic stimulation include:
- palpitations
- angina
- edema
- breast tenderness
- fatigue
- headache
- rash
- severe pericardial effusion.

Nursing process

These nursing process steps are appropriate for patients undergoing treatment with direct vasodilating drugs.

Assessment
- Obtain a baseline blood pressure and pulse rate and rhythm; recheck regularly.
- Because excessive doses or rapid infusion of more than 15 mcg/kg/minute of nitroprusside can cause cyanide toxicity, check thiocyanate levels every 72 hours. Levels above 100 mcg/ml may cause toxicity. Watch for profound hypotension, metabolic acidosis, dyspnea, headache, loss of consciousness, ataxia, and vomiting.
- Monitor the patient for adverse reactions and drug interactions.
- Monitor the patient's weight and fluid and electrolyte status.
- Observe the patient's compliance with the treatment.
- Observe the patient's tolerance of the drug, and monitor the drug's therapeutic effects. The dosage may need to be adjusted.
- Monitor a transdermal patch for dermatitis and ask the patient about pruritus. Keep in mind that the patch can require several days to take effect and that interim oral therapy may be needed.

Key nursing diagnoses
- Risk for injury related to orthostatic hypotension
- Risk for injury related to presence of hypertension
- Deficient knowledge related to drug therapy

Planning outcome goals
- Blood pressure will be maintained within acceptable limits.

Prototype pro

Vasodilators: Nitroprusside

Actions
- Relaxes arteriolar and venous smooth muscle

Indications
- High blood pressure
- Increased preload and afterload

Nursing considerations
- Monitor thiocyanate levels every 72 hours; excessive doses or rapid infusion (more than 15 mcg/kg/minute) can cause cyanide toxicity.
- Monitor for adverse effects and signs of cyanide toxicity, including profound hypotension, metabolic acidosis, dyspnea, headache, loss of consciousness, ataxia, and vomiting.
- Monitor blood pressure every 5 minutes at the start of infusion and every 15 minutes thereafter.
- An I.V. infusion must be wrapped in foil because it's sensitive to light.

- Risk for injury will be minimized.
- The patient will demonstrate an understanding of drug therapy.

Implementation

- If giving orally, administer the drug with food or at bedtime as indicated.
- Follow the manufacturer's guidelines when mixing and administering parenteral drugs.
- Prevent or minimize orthostatic hypotension by helping the patient to get up slowly and by telling the patient not to make sudden movements.

Curses! Foiled again

- Keep in mind that nitroprusside is sensitive to light; wrap I.V. solutions of this drug in foil. A fresh solution should have a faint brownish tint. Discard the drug after 24 hours.
- Infuse I.V. forms with an infusion pump, usually piggybacked through a peripheral line with no other medications.
- If administering I.V., check blood pressure every 5 minutes at the start of the infusion and every 15 minutes thereafter with nitroprusside and titrate the dosage according to blood pressure parameters ordered by the doctor. If severe hypotension occurs, stop the infusion and notify the prescriber. Effects of the drug quickly reverse.
- If cyanide toxicity occurs, stop the drug immediately and notify the prescriber.
- Maintain the patient's nonpharmacologic therapies, such as sodium restriction, calorie reduction, stress management, and exercise program.
- Keep in mind that drug therapy may be given to lower blood pressure rapidly in some hypertensive emergency situations.
- Know that the dosage is usually adjusted to the patient's blood pressure and tolerance.
- To improve adherence of a transdermal patch, apply an adhesive overlay. Place the patch at a different site each week.
- Remove a transdermal patch before defibrillation to prevent arcing.
- Periodic eye examinations are recommended.

Evaluation

- Patient sustains no injury from orthostatic hypotension.
- Patient sustains no injury.
- Patient and his family demonstrate an understanding of drug therapy.

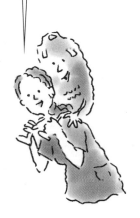

I.V. infusions of the drug are usually piggybacked through a peripheral line with no other medications.

Selective aldosterone-receptor antagonist

Eplerenone, the only selective aldosterone-receptor antagonist, produces sustained increases in plasma renin and serum aldosterone. This inhibits the negative feedback mechanism of aldosterone on renin secretion. It selectively binds to mineralocorticoids receptors. The result is an antihypertensive effect.

Pharmacokinetics

Eplerenone has a plasma protein binding of 50% and is primarily bound to alpha-1-acid glycoproteins after oral administration. Its metabolism is controlled by the cytochrome P450 isoform 3A4 (CYP3A4), and less than 5% of the dose is excreted unchanged in urine and feces.

Pharmacodynamics

Eplerenone blocks the binding of aldosterone, an important part of the RAAS. Aldosterone causes increases in blood pressure through sodium reabsorption.

Pharmacotherapeutics

Eplerenone is used to lower blood pressure.

Drug interactions

Eplerenone levels may be increased when the drug is taken with inhibitors of CYP3A4 (erythromycin, saquinavir, verapamil, and fluconazole).

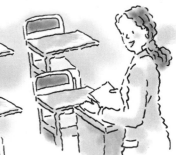

Eplerenone is in a class by itself!

Adverse reactions

Eplerenone may cause hyperkalemia, which may result in arrhythmias.

Nursing process

These nursing process steps are appropriate for patients undergoing treatment with a selective aldosterone-receptor antagonist.

Assessment

• Obtain a baseline blood pressure and pulse rate and rhythm; recheck regularly.
• Monitor the patient for adverse reactions.
• Monitor the patient's weight and fluid and electrolyte status, including his potassium levels.
• Monitor the patient's compliance with treatment.

Key nursing diagnoses

- Risk for injury related to orthostatic hypotension
- Risk for injury related to presence of hypertension
- Deficient knowledge related to drug therapy

Planning outcome goals

- Blood pressure will be maintained within acceptable limits.
- Risk for injury will be minimized.
- The patient will verbalize an understanding of drug therapy.

Implementation

- If giving orally, administer the drug with food or at bedtime as indicated.
- Prevent or minimize orthostatic hypotension by helping the patient to get up slowly and by telling the patient not to make sudden movements.
- Don't give the patient potassium supplements or salt substitutes that contain potassium.
- Maintain the patient's nonpharmacologic therapies, such as sodium restriction, calorie reduction, stress management, and exercise program.
- Know that the dosage is usually adjusted to the patient's blood pressure and tolerance.
- Periodic eye examinations are recommended.

Evaluation

- Patient sustains no trauma from orthostatic hypotension.
- Patient sustains no injury.
- Patient and his family demonstrate an understanding of drug therapy.

Antilipemic drugs

Antilipemic drugs are used to lower abnormally high blood levels of lipids, such as cholesterol, triglycerides, and phospholipids. The risk of developing coronary artery disease increases when serum lipid levels are elevated. These drugs are used in combination with lifestyle changes, such as proper diet, weight loss, and exercise, and treatment of any underlying disorder.

Antilipemic drug classes include:

- bile-sequestering drugs
- fibric acid derivatives
- HMG-CoA reductase inhibitors
- nicotinic acid
- cholesterol absorption inhibitors.

Bile-sequestering drugs

The bile-sequestering drugs are cholestyramine, colesevelam, and colestipol hydrochloride. These drugs are resins that remove excess bile acids from the fat deposits under the skin.

Pharmacokinetics

Bile-sequestering drugs aren't absorbed from the GI tract. Instead, they remain in the intestine, where they combine with bile acids for about 5 hours and are eventually excreted in feces.

Pharmacodynamics

The bile-sequestering drugs lower blood levels of low-density lipoproteins (LDLs). These drugs combine with bile acids in the intestines to form an insoluble compound that's then excreted in feces. The decreasing level of bile acid in the gallbladder triggers the liver to synthesize more bile acids from their precursor, cholesterol.

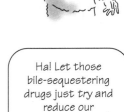

Would you care for a side of bile-sequestering drugs with your low-fat meal?

Calling all cholesterol!

As cholesterol leaves the bloodstream and other storage areas to replace the lost bile acids, blood cholesterol levels decrease. Because the small intestine needs bile acids to emulsify lipids and form chylomicrons, absorption of all lipids and lipid-soluble drugs decreases until the bile acids are replaced.

Pharmacotherapeutics

Bile-sequestering drugs are the drugs of choice for treating type IIa hyperlipoproteinemia (familial hypercholesterolemia) in a patient who isn't able to lower LDL levels through dietary changes. A patient whose blood cholesterol levels indicate a severe risk of coronary artery disease is most likely to require one of these drugs as a supplement to his diet.

Drug interactions

Bile-sequestering drugs produce the following drug interactions:
• Bile acid–binding resins of bile-sequestering drugs may interfere with the absorption of digoxin, oral phosphate supplements, and hydrocortisone.
• Bile-sequestering drugs may decrease absorption of propranolol, tetracycline, furosemide, penicillin G, hydrochlorothiazide, and gemfibrozil.

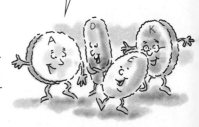

Ha! Let those bile-sequestering drugs just try and reduce our absorption!

• Bile-sequestering drugs may reduce absorption of lipid-soluble vitamins, such as A, D, E, and K. Poor absorption of vitamin K can affect prothrombin time significantly, increasing the risk of bleeding.

Adverse reactions

Short-term adverse reactions to bile-sequestering drugs are relatively mild. More severe reactions can result from long-term use. Adverse GI effects with long-term therapy include severe fecal impaction, vomiting, diarrhea, and hemorrhoid irritation.

Less likely

Rarely, peptic ulcers and bleeding, gallstones, and inflammation of the gallbladder may occur.

Nursing process

These nursing process steps are appropriate for patients undergoing treatment with bile-sequestering drugs.

Assessment
• Assess the patient's cholesterol level and pruritus before therapy as appropriate.
• Monitor blood cholesterol and lipid levels before and periodically during therapy. Monitor the drug's effectiveness by checking cholesterol and triglyceride levels every 4 weeks or by asking the patient whether pruritus has diminished or abated as appropriate.
• Monitor creatine kinase (CK) levels when therapy begins and every 6 months thereafter. Also check CK levels if a patient who takes a cholesterol synthesis inhibitor complains of muscle pain.
• Monitor the patient for adverse reactions and drug interactions.
• Monitor the patient for fat-soluble vitamin deficiency because long-term use may be linked to deficiency of vitamins A, D, E, and K and folic acid.
• Evaluate the patient's and family's knowledge of drug therapy.

Key nursing diagnoses
• Risk for injury related to adverse drug effects
• Health-seeking behaviors related to elevated serum cholesterol
• Deficient knowledge related to drug therapy

Planning outcome goals
• Adverse drug effects will be minimized.
• Cholesterol levels will be lowered to acceptable levels.
• The patient will verbalize an understanding of drug therapy.

Education edge

Teaching about antilipemics

If antilipemics are prescribed, review these points with the patient and his caregivers:
• Take the drug exactly as prescribed. If you take a bile-sequestering drug, never take the dry form. Esophageal irritation or severe constipation may result.
• Use a large glass and sprinkle the powder on the surface of a preferred beverage. Let the mixture stand a few minutes; then stir thoroughly. The best diluents are water, milk, and juice (especially pulpy fruit juice). Mixing with carbonated beverages may result in excess foaming. After drinking this preparation, swirl a small additional amount of liquid in the same glass and then drink it to ensure ingestion of the entire dose.
• Diet is very important in controlling serum lipid levels. Maintain proper dietary management of serum lipids (restricting to-

tal fat and cholesterol intake) as well as control of other cardiac disease risk factors.
• Drink 2 to 3 qt (2 to 3 L) of fluid daily, and report persistent or severe constipation.
• Weight control, exercise, and smoking cessation programs may be appropriate.
• If you also take bile acid resin, take fenofibrate 1 hour before or 4 to 6 hours after bile acid resin.
• When taking fenofibrate, promptly report symptoms of unexplained muscle weakness, pain, or tenderness, especially if accompanied by malaise or fever.
• Have periodic eye examinations.
• Don't crush or chew extended-release tablets.

Implementation
• If severe constipation develops, decrease the dosage, add a stool softener, or discontinue the drug.
• Give all other drugs at least 1 hour before or 4 to 6 hours after cholestyramine to avoid blocking their absorption.

Mixing it up

• Mix powder forms of bile-sequestering drugs with 120 to 180 ml of liquid. Never administer dry powder alone because the patient may accidentally inhale it.
• To mix the powder, sprinkle it on the surface of a preferred beverage or wet food (soup, applesauce, crushed pineapple). Let it stand for a few minutes, and then stir it to obtain uniform suspension. Know that mixing with carbonated beverages may result in excess foaming. Use a large glass and mix slowly.

Evaluation
• Patient doesn't exhibit injury from adverse drug effects.
• Patient maintains adequate cholesterol levels.
• Patient and his family demonstrate an understanding of drug therapy. (See *Teaching about antilipemics*.)

Fibric acid derivatives

Fibric acid is produced by several fungi. Two derivatives of this acid are fenofibrate and gemfibrozil. These drugs are used to reduce high triglyceride levels and, to a lesser extent, high LDL levels.

Pharmacokinetics

Fenofibrate and gemfibrozil are absorbed readily from the GI tract and are highly protein bound. Fenofibrate undergoes rapid hydrolysis, and gemfibrozil undergoes extensive metabolism in the liver. Both drugs are excreted in urine.

Pharmacodynamics

Although the exact mechanism of action for these drugs isn't known, researchers believe that fibric acid derivatives may:
• reduce cholesterol production early in its formation
• mobilize cholesterol from the tissues
• increase cholesterol excretion
• decrease synthesis and secretion of lipoproteins
• decrease synthesis of triglycerides.

A silver lining

Gemfibrozil produces two other effects:
• It increases high-density lipoprotein (HDL) levels in the blood (remember, this is "good" cholesterol).
• It increases the serum's capacity to dissolve additional cholesterol.

Pharmacotherapeutics

Fibric acid drugs are used primarily to reduce triglyceride levels, especially very-low-density triglycerides, and secondarily to reduce blood cholesterol levels.

Because of their ability to reduce triglyceride levels, fibric acid derivatives are useful in treating patients with types II, III, IV, and mild type V hyperlipoproteinemia.

Drug interactions

These drug interactions may occur:
• Fibric acid drugs may displace acidic drugs, such as barbiturates, phenytoin, thyroid derivatives, and cardiac glycosides.
• The risk of bleeding increases when fibric acid derivatives are taken with oral anticoagulants.
• Fibric acid derivatives can lead to adverse GI effects.

Adverse reactions

Adverse reactions to fibric acid drugs include headache, dizziness, blurred vision, arrhythmias, thrombocytopenia, and rash. GI effects include epigastric pain, dyspepsia, nausea, vomiting, and diarrhea or constipation.

Nursing process

These nursing process steps are appropriate for patients undergoing treatment with fibric acid derivatives.

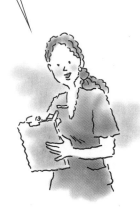

Here's a checklist for you: Fibric acid drugs can cause headache, dizziness, blurred vision, arrhythmias, thrombocytopenia, rash, and GI effects.

Assessment
- Assess the patient's cholesterol level and pruritus before therapy as appropriate.
- Monitor blood cholesterol and lipid levels before and periodically during therapy. Monitor the drug's effectiveness by checking cholesterol and triglyceride levels every 4 weeks or by asking the patient whether pruritus has diminished or abated as appropriate.
- Assess liver function tests before starting therapy and periodically thereafter.
- Monitor CK levels when therapy begins and every 6 months thereafter. Also check CK levels if a patient who takes a cholesterol synthesis inhibitor complains of muscle pain.
- Monitor the patient for adverse reactions and drug interactions.
- Monitor the patient for fat-soluble vitamin deficiency because long-term use may be linked to deficiency of vitamins A, D, E, and K and folic acid.
- If the patient is taking fenofibrate, monitor him for muscle pain, tenderness, or weakness, especially if he develops malaise or fever.
- Evaluate the patient's and family's knowledge of drug therapy.

Key nursing diagnoses
- Risk for injury related to adverse drug effects
- Health-seeking behaviors related to elevated serum cholesterol
- Deficient knowledge related to drug therapy

Planning outcome goals
- Adverse drug effects will be minimized.
- Cholesterol levels will be lowered to acceptable levels.
- The patient will verbalize an understanding of drug therapy.

Implementation
- If severe constipation develops, decrease the dosage, add a stool softener, or discontinue the drug.
- Administer a daily fibric acid derivative at prescribed times.

• Withdraw therapy in a patient who doesn't have an adequate response after 2 months of treatment with the maximum dosage.
• Give fenofibrate with meals to increase bioavailability.
• Give gemfibrozil 30 minutes before breakfast and dinner.
• Evaluate renal function and triglyceride levels of a patient with severe renal impairment before dosage increases.
• Reinforce the importance of adhering to a triglyceride-lowering diet.
• Instruct the patient who also takes bile acid resin to take fenofibrate 1 hour before or 4 to 6 hours after bile acid resin.

Evaluation

• Patient doesn't exhibit injury from adverse drug effects.
• Patient maintains adequate cholesterol levels.
• Patient and his family demonstrate an understanding of drug therapy.

HMG-CoA reductase inhibitors

As their name implies, 3-hydroxy-3-methylglutaryl coenzyme A (HMG-CoA) reductase inhibitors (also known as the *statins*) lower lipid levels by interfering with cholesterol synthesis. These drugs include atorvastatin calcium, fluvastatin sodium, lovastatin, pravastatin sodium, and simvastatin. (See *Antilipemics: Atorvastatin.*)

Pharmacokinetics

With the exception of pravastatin, HMG-CoA reductase inhibitors are highly bound to plasma proteins. All undergo extensive first-pass metabolism. Their specific pharmacokinetic properties vary slightly.

Pharmacodynamics

HMG-CoA reductase inhibitors inhibit the enzyme that's responsible for the conversion of HMG-CoA to mevalonate, an early rate-limiting step in the biosynthesis of cholesterol.

Pharmacotherapeutics

Statin drugs are used primarily to reduce LDLs and also to reduce total blood cholesterol levels. These agents also produce a mild increase in HDLs.

Because of their ability to lower cholesterol levels, statins are indicated for the treatment of primary hypercholesterolemia (types IIa and IIb).

Prototype pro

Antilipemics: Atorvastatin

Actions
• Inhibits HMG-CoA. reductase

Indications
• High plasma cholesterol and lipoprotein levels

Nursing considerations
• Use the drug only after diet and other nonpharmacologic treatments prove ineffective.
• Restrict the patient to a standard low-cholesterol diet before and during therapy.
• Before starting treatment, perform a baseline lipid profile to exclude secondary causes of hypercholesterolemia. Liver function test results and lipid levels should be obtained before therapy, after 6 and 12 weeks, or following a dosage increase and periodically thereafter.
• Before starting treatment, a baseline creatine kinase may be performed and the patient should be routinely monitored for myopathy, which may be an indication of rhabdomyolysis.

Event preventer

As a result of their effect on LDL and total cholesterol, these drugs are indicated for primary and secondary prevention of cardiovascular events.

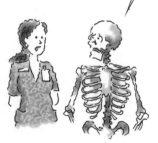

I know statins help produce LDL levels, but I'm not too crazy about the joint pain they can cause.

Drug interactions

These drug interactions may occur:
• Atorvastatin, simvastatin, or lovastatin when combined with niacin, erythromycin, clarithromycin, immunosuppressant drugs (especially cyclosporine), gemfibrozil, itraconazole, ketoconazole, or fluconazole may increase the risk of myopathy (muscle wasting and weakness) or rhabdomyolysis (potentially fatal breakdown of skeletal muscle, causing renal failure).
• All HMG-CoA reductase inhibitors should be administered 1 hour before or 4 hours after bile-sequestering (cholestyramine, colestipol, colesevelam).
• Lovastatin and simvastatin may increase the risk of bleeding when administered with warfarin.

Adverse reactions

HMG-CoA reductase inhibitors may alter liver function studies, increasing aspartate aminotransferase, alanine aminotransferase, alkaline phosphatase, and bilirubin levels. Other hepatic effects may include pancreatitis, hepatitis, and cirrhosis.

Oh, the pain of it all...

Myalgia is the most common musculoskeletal effect, although arthralgia and muscle cramps may also occur. Myopathy and rhabdomyolysis are rare but potentially severe reactions that may occur with these drugs.

Possible adverse GI reactions include nausea, vomiting, diarrhea, abdominal pain, flatulence, and constipation.

Nursing process

These nursing process steps are appropriate for patients undergoing treatment with HMG-CoA reductase inhibitors.

Assessment

• Assess the patient's cholesterol level and pruritus before therapy as appropriate.
• Monitor blood cholesterol and lipid levels before and periodically during therapy. Monitor the drug's effectiveness by checking cholesterol and triglyceride levels every 4 weeks or by asking the patient whether pruritus has diminished or abated as appropriate.

• Monitor CK levels when therapy begins and every 6 months thereafter. Also check CK levels if a patient who takes a cholesterol synthesis inhibitor complains of muscle pain.
• Liver function tests should be performed at the start of therapy and periodically thereafter. A liver biopsy may be performed if enzyme level elevations persist.
• Monitor the patient for adverse reactions and drug interactions.
• Monitor the patient for fat-soluble vitamin deficiency because long-term use may be linked to deficiency of vitamins A, D, E, and K and folic acid.
• Evaluate the patient's and family's knowledge of drug therapy.

Key nursing diagnoses
• Risk for injury related to adverse drug effects
• Health-seeking behaviors related to elevated serum cholesterol
• Deficient knowledge related to drug therapy

Planning outcome goals
• Risk for adverse GI effects will be minimized.
• Cholesterol levels will be lowered to acceptable levels.
• The patient will verbalize correct drug administration.

Implementation
• If severe constipation develops, decrease the dosage, add a stool softener, or discontinue the drug.
• Give the drug before meals and at bedtime as applicable. Give lovastatin with an evening meal, simvastatin in the evening, and fluvastatin and pravastatin at bedtime.

Evaluation
• Patient doesn't exhibit injury from adverse drug effects.
• Patient maintains adequate cholesterol levels.
• Patient and his family demonstrate an understanding of drug therapy.

Nicotinic acid

Also known as *niacin*, nicotinic acid is a water-soluble vitamin that decreases triglyceride and apolipoprotein B-100 levels and increases HDL levels. The drug is available in immediate-release and extended-release tablets.

Pharmacokinetics

Nicotinic acid is moderately bound to plasma proteins; its overall binding ranges from 60% to 70%. The drug undergoes rapid metabolism by the liver to active and inactive metabolites. About 75% of the drug is excreted in urine.

Pharmacodynamics

The way that nicotinic acid lowers triglyceride and apolipoprotein levels is unknown. However, it may work by inhibiting hepatic synthesis of lipoproteins that contain apolipoprotein B-100, promoting lipoprotein lipase activity, reducing free fatty acid mobilization from adipose tissue, and increasing fecal elimination of sterols.

Pharmacotherapeutics

Nicotinic acid is used primarily as an adjunct to lower triglyceride levels in patients with type IV or V hyperlipidemia who are at high risk for pancreatitis. The drug also may be used to lower cholesterol and LDL levels in patients with hypercholesterolemia. It's commonly used with other antilipemics to meet LDL goals and to increase the HDL level for patients who have a lower-than-desired HDL level.

Just say no

This antilipemic is contraindicated in patients who are hypersensitive to nicotinic acid and in those with hepatic dysfunction, active peptic ulcer disease, or arterial bleeding. Also, because nicotinic acid can cause hyperglycemia, it's not prescribed for patients with diabetes.

Drug interactions

These drug interactions can occur with nicotinic acid:
• Together, nicotinic acid and an HMG-CoA reductase inhibitor may increase the risk of muscle wasting and weakness, myopathy, or life-threatening breakdown of skeletal muscle, causing renal failure or rhabdomyolysis.
• A bile-sequestering drug, such as cholestyramine or colestipol, can bind with nicotinic acid and decrease its effectiveness.
• When given with nicotinic acid, kava may increase the risk of hepatotoxicity.

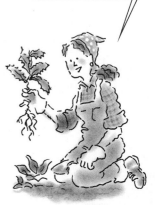

Giving kava with nicotinic acid may increase the risk of hepatotoxicity.

Adverse reactions

High doses of nicotinic acid may produce vasodilation and cause flushing. Extended-release forms tend to produce less severe vasodilation than immediate-release forms. To help minimize flushing, aspirin may be given 30 minutes before nicotinic acid, or the extended-release form may be given at night.

Nicotinic acid can cause hepatotoxicity; the risk of this adverse reaction is greater with extended-release forms. Other adverse effects include nausea, vomiting, diarrhea, and epigastric or substernal pain.

Nursing process

These nursing process steps are appropriate for patients undergoing treatment with nicotinic acid.

Assessment

• Assess the patient's cholesterol level and pruritus before therapy, as appropriate.
• Monitor blood cholesterol and lipid levels before and periodically during therapy. Monitor the drug's effectiveness by checking cholesterol and triglyceride levels every 4 weeks or by asking the patient whether pruritus has diminished or abated as appropriate.
• Monitor CK levels when therapy begins and every 6 months thereafter. Also check CK levels if a patient who takes a cholesterol synthesis inhibitor complains of muscle pain.
• Monitor the patient for adverse reactions and drug interactions.
• Monitor the patient for fat-soluble vitamin deficiency because long-term use may be linked to deficiency of vitamins A, D, E, and K and folic acid.
• Evaluate the patient's and family's knowledge of drug therapy.

Key nursing diagnoses

• Risk for injury related to adverse drug effects
• Health-seeking behaviors related to elevated serum cholesterol
• Deficient knowledge related to drug therapy

Planning outcome goals

• Adverse drug effects will be minimized.
• Cholesterol levels will be lowered to acceptable levels.
• The patient will verbalize an understanding of drug therapy.

Implementation

• If severe constipation develops, decrease the dosage, add a stool softener, or discontinue the drug.
• Administer aspirin as appropriate to help reduce flushing.
• Know that timed-released niacin or niacinamide may prevent excessive flushing that occurs with large dosages. However, timed-release niacin has been linked to hepatic dysfunction, even at dosages as low as 1 g daily.
• Give the drug with meals to minimize GI adverse effects.

• To decrease flushing, advise the patient to take the drug with a low-fat snack and to avoid taking it after alcohol, hot beverages, hot or spicy foods, a hot shower, or exercise.

Evaluation
• Patient doesn't exhibit injury from adverse drug effects.
• Patient maintains adequate cholesterol levels.
• Patient and his family demonstrate an understanding of drug therapy.

Cholesterol absorption inhibitors

As their name implies, cholesterol absorption inhibitors inhibit the absorption of cholesterol and related phytosterols from the intestine. Ezetimibe is the drug that falls under this class.

Pharmacokinetics

Ezetimibe is absorbed and extensively conjugated to an active form and is highly bound to plasma proteins. The drug is primarily metabolized in the small intestine and is excreted by the biliary and renal routes.

Pharmacodynamics

Ezetimibe reduces blood cholesterol levels by inhibiting the absorption of cholesterol by the small intestine.

On the edge

The drug works at the brush border of the small intestine to inhibit cholesterol absorption. This leads to a decrease in delivery of intestinal cholesterol to the liver, causing a reduction in hepatic cholesterol stores and an increase in clearance from the blood.

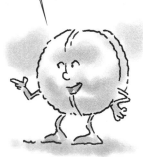

Ezetimibe reduces blood cholesterol levels by inhibiting the absorption of cholesterol by the small intestine.

Pharmacotherapeutics

Ezetimibe may be administered alone as adjunctive therapy to diet for treatment of primary hypercholesterolemia and homozygous sitosterolemia. The drug is also indicated as adjunctive therapy, administered in addition to HMG-CoA reductase inhibitors, for the treatment of primary hypercholesterolemia and homozygous familial hypercholesterolemia.

Helping things along

Ezetimibe helps to further lower total cholesterol and LDL and further increase HDL cholesterol in patients who can't achieve their desired goals following maximum-dose HMG-CoA reductase inhibitor therapy.

Drug interactions

Cholestyramine may decrease the effectiveness of ezetimibe. Fenofibrate, gemfibrozil, and cyclosporine lead to an increased level of ezetimibe.

Adverse reactions

The most common adverse reactions to ezetimibe include:
• fatigue
• abdominal pain
• diarrhea
• pharyngitis
• sinusitis
• arthralgia and back pain
• cough.
    When ezetimibe is given with an HMG-CoA reductase inhibitor, the most common adverse reactions are:
• chest or abdominal pain
• dizziness
• headache
• diarrhea
• pharyngitis
• sinusitis
• upper respiratory infection
• arthralgia, myalgia, and back pain.

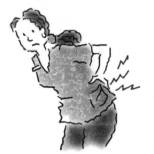

Whether you take ezetimibe alone or with HMG-CoA, it can sometimes cause back pain. Ouch!

Nursing process

These nursing process steps are appropriate for patients undergoing treatment with cholesterol absorption inhibitors.

Assessment

• Assess the patient's cholesterol level and pruritus before therapy as appropriate.
• Monitor blood cholesterol and lipid levels before and periodically during therapy. Monitor the drug's effectiveness by checking cholesterol and triglyceride levels every 4 weeks or by asking the patient whether pruritus has diminished or abated as appropriate.
• Monitor CK levels when therapy begins and every 6 months thereafter. Also check CK levels if a patient who takes a cholesterol synthesis inhibitor complains of muscle pain.
• Be alert for adverse reactions and drug interactions.

- Monitor the patient for fat-soluble vitamin deficiency because long-term use may be linked to deficiency of vitamins A, D, E, and K and folic acid.
- Evaluate the patient's and family's knowledge of drug therapy.

Key nursing diagnoses
- Risk for injury related to adverse drug effects
- Health-seeking behaviors related to elevated serum cholesterol
- Deficient knowledge related to drug therapy

Planning outcome goals
- Adverse drug effects will be minimized.
- Cholesterol levels will be lowered to acceptable levels.
- The patient will verbalize correct drug administration.

Implementation
- If severe constipation develops, decrease the dosage, add a stool softener, or discontinue the drug.
- Teach the patient how to follow a cholesterol-lowering diet as appropriate.

Evaluation
- Patient doesn't exhibit injury from adverse drug effects.
- Patient maintains adequate cholesterol levels.
- Patient and his family demonstrate an understanding of drug therapy.

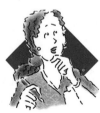

Quick quiz

1.   A patient is receiving digoxin for treatment of atrial fibrillation. When you enter the room to give the medication, you find the patient irritable and complaining of nausea and blurred vision. She's also disoriented to place and time. The most appropriate action at this time is to:

- A.   attempt to reorient the patient while helping her take the digoxin.
- B.   return to the room later and see whether the patient will take the medication.
- C.   withhold the digoxin and notify the prescriber about your assessment findings.
- D.   check the medication profile for possible drug interactions after giving the digoxin to the patient.

Answer: C. Irritability, nausea, blurred vision, and confusion are signs and symptoms of digoxin toxicity. The digoxin dose should be withheld, the prescriber notified, and the digoxin level checked. You should try to reorient the patient and prepare for possible emergency treatment pending the laboratory results.

2. A patient comes to the emergency department complaining of chest pains, which started 1 hour ago while he was mowing the lawn. Nitroglycerin was given sublingually as prescribed. Which of the following adverse reactions would be most likely to occur?

    A.   Hypotension
    B.   Dizziness
    C.   GI distress
    D.   Headache

Answer: D. The most common adverse reaction to nitrates is headache. Nitrates dilate the blood vessels in the meningeal layers between the brain and cranium. Hypotension, dizziness, and GI distress may occur, but the likelihood varies with each patient.

3. Which adverse reaction associated with ACE inhibitors is common and can lead to disruption of therapy?

    A.   Constipation
    B.   Cough
    C.   Sexual dysfunction
    D.   Tachycardia

Answer: B. A common adverse reaction, cough causes discontinuation of ACE inhibitor therapy because it disrupts the patient's sleep patterns.

4. A patient is taking an HMG-CoA reductase inhibitor. Which of the following tests should be performed at the start of therapy and periodically thereafter?

    A.   Liver function
    B.   Electrolyte levels
    C.   Complete blood count
    D.   ECG

Answer: A. Because increased liver enzyme levels may occur in patients receiving long-term HMG-CoA therapy, liver function test results should be monitored.

Scoring

☆☆☆   If you answered all four questions correctly, A+! You're aces with ACE inhibitors and all of the other cardiovascular drugs.

☆☆   If you answered three questions correctly, cool! Cardiovascular drugs aren't causing you any complications.

☆   If you answered fewer than three questions correctly, stay mellow! This is a complex chapter, and it might just require another dose.

Respiratory drugs

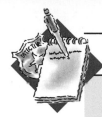

Just the facts

In this chapter, you'll learn:

♦ classes of drugs used to treat respiratory disorders

♦ uses and varying actions of these drugs

♦ absorption, distribution, metabolization, and excretion of these drugs

♦ drug interactions and adverse reactions to these drugs.

Drugs and the respiratory system

The respiratory system, which extends from the nose to the pulmonary capillaries, performs the essential function of gas exchange between the body and its environment. In other words, it takes in oxygen and expels carbon dioxide.

Drugs used to improve respiratory symptoms are available in inhalation and systemic formulations. These include:

• beta$_2$-adrenergic agonists
• anticholinergics
• corticosteroids
• leukotriene modifiers
• mast cell stabilizers
• methylxanthines
• expectorants
• antitussives
• decongestants.

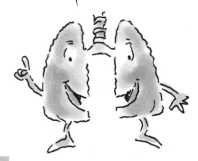

Are you ready to learn about respiratory system drugs? Then take a deep breath and let's get started.

Beta$_2$-adrenergic agonists

Beta$_2$-adrenergic agonists are used for the treatment of symptoms associated with asthma and chronic obstructive pulmonary dis-

ease (COPD). Agents in this class can be divided into two categories:
- short-acting
- long-acting.

The short...

Short-acting beta$_2$-adrenergic agonists include:
- albuterol (systemic, inhalation)
- levalbuterol (inhalation)
- metaproterenol (inhalation)
- pirbuterol (inhalation)
- terbutaline (systemic).

...and long of it

Long-acting beta$_2$-adrenergic agonists include:
- salmeterol (inhalation)
- formoterol (inhalation).

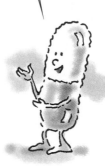

Beta-adrenergic agonists can be short- or long-acting.

Pharmacokinetics (how drugs circulate)

Beta$_2$-adrenergic agonists are minimally absorbed from the GI tract. Inhaled formulations generally exert their effects locally. After inhalation, beta$_2$-adrenergic agonists appear to be absorbed over several hours from the respiratory tract. These drugs don't cross the blood-brain barrier. They're extensively metabolized in the liver to inactive compounds and are rapidly excreted in urine and feces.

Pharmacodynamics (how drugs act)

Beta$_2$-adrenergic agonists increase levels of cyclic adenosine monophosphate through the stimulation of beta$_2$-adrenergic receptors in the smooth muscle, resulting in bronchodilation. Beta$_2$-adrenergic agonists may lose their selectivity at higher doses, which can increase the risk of toxicity. Inhaled agents are preferred because they act locally in the lungs, resulting in fewer adverse effects than systemically absorbed formulations.

Pharmacotherapeutics (how drugs are used)

Short-acting inhaled beta$_2$-adrenergic agonists are the drugs of choice for fast relief of symptoms in asthmatic patients. They're primarily used on an as-needed basis for asthma and COPD and are also effective for exercise-induced asthma.

From morning till night

Some patients with COPD use short-acting inhaled beta$_2$-adrenergic agonists around the clock on a specified schedule. However, excessive use of these agents may indicate poor asthma control, requiring reassessment of the therapeutic regimen.

Strictly regimented

Long-acting agents are more appropriately used with anti-inflammatory agents, specifically inhaled corticosteroids, to help control asthma. They must be administered on schedule in order to be most effective. They're especially useful when a patient exhibits nocturnal asthmatic symptoms. Because of their delayed onset, long-acting beta$_2$-adrenergic agonists aren't used for acute symptoms. They're also ineffective against the chronic inflammation associated with asthma.

Drug interactions

Interactions with beta$_2$-adrenergic agonists aren't as common when using inhaled formulations. Beta-adrenergic blockers decrease the bronchodilating effects of the beta$_2$-adrenergic agonists and, therefore, these drugs should be used together cautiously.

Adverse reactions

Adverse reactions to short-acting beta$_2$-adrenergic agonists include paradoxical bronchospasm, tachycardia, palpitations, tremors, and dry mouth.

Adverse reactions to long-acting beta$_2$-adrenergic agonists include bronchospasm, tachycardia, palpitations, hypertension, and tremors.

Nursing process

These nursing process steps are appropriate for patients undergoing treatment with beta$_2$-adrenergic agonists.

Assessment
- Assess the patient's respiratory condition before therapy and regularly thereafter.
- Assess peak flow readings before starting treatment and periodically thereafter.
- Be alert for adverse reactions and drug interactions.
- Evaluate the patient's and family's knowledge of drug therapy.

Key nursing diagnoses
- Ineffective breathing pattern related to respiratory condition
- Impaired gas exchange related to underlying condition
- Deficient knowledge related to drug therapy

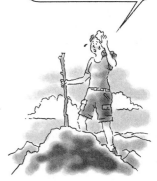

Assess...whew! ...peak flow readings before starting treatment and then periodically.

Education edge

Teaching about bronchodilators

If bronchodilators are prescribed, review these points with the patient and his caregivers:

• Take the drug as directed. Note that some medications should be taken every 12 hours, even if you're feeling better, and other drugs, such as albuterol, should only be used in an acute attack.

• Take the drug 30 to 60 minutes before exercise as directed to prevent exercise-induced bronchospasm.

• Contact your prescriber if the medication no longer provides sufficient relief or if you need more than four inhalations per day. This may be a sign that asthma symptoms are worsening. Don't increase the dosage of the drug.

• If you're taking an inhaled corticosteroid, continue to use it as directed by the prescriber.

• Don't take bronchodilators with other drugs, over-the-counter preparations, or herbal remedies without your prescriber's consent.

• Follow these instructions for using a metered-dose inhaler as appropriate:

– Clear your nasal passages and throat.

– Breathe out, expelling as much air from lungs as possible.

– Place the mouthpiece well into mouth, and inhale deeply as you release the dose from the inhaler.

– Hold your breath for several seconds, remove the mouthpiece, and exhale slowly.

• Avoid accidentally spraying the medication into your eyes. Temporary blurring of vision may result.

• If more than one inhalation is ordered, wait at least 2 minutes between each subsequent inhalation.

• If you use a corticosteroid inhaler, use the bronchodilator first, and then wait about 5 minutes before using the corticosteroid. This process allows the bronchodilator to open air passages for maximum effectiveness of the corticosteroid.

• Take a missed dose as soon as you remember, unless it's almost time for the next dose; in that case, skip the missed dose. Don't double the dose.

Planning outcome goals

• Breathing pattern will improve as evidenced by regular and even respiratory rate and rhythm.

• Gas exchange will be adequate as evidenced by improved peak flow rates, oxygen saturation, and arterial blood gas (ABG) levels.

• The patient will demonstrate correct drug administration.

Implementation

• Report insufficient relief or worsening condition.

• Obtain an order for a mild analgesic if a drug-induced headache occurs.

• Don't use long-acting beta$_2$-adrenergic agonists for reversing bronchospasm during an acute asthma attack.

• For the inhalation formulation, teach the patient to hold his breath for several seconds after inhalation and wait at least 2 minutes before taking another inhalation of the drug.

Evaluation
- Patient exhibits normal breathing pattern.
- Patient exhibits improved gas exchange.
- Patient and family understand drug therapy. (See *Teaching about bronchodilators.*)

Anticholinergics

Anticholinergics competitively antagonize the actions of acetylcholine and other cholinergic agonists at receptors. Although oral anticholinergics generally aren't used to treat asthma and other COPDs because of their tendency to thicken secretions and form mucus plugs in the airways one anticholinergic—ipratropium—is used for COPD.

Ipratropium

Inhaled ipratropium bromide is a bronchodilator used primarily in patients suffering from COPD. It may also be used as an adjunct to beta$_2$-adrenergic agonists.

Pharmacokinetics

Ipratropium is minimally absorbed from the GI tract. It exerts its effects locally.

Pharmacodynamics

Ipratropium blocks the parasympathetic nervous system rather than stimulating the sympathetic nervous system. To exert its anticholinergic effects, this drug inhibits muscarinic receptors, which results in bronchodilation.

Pharmacotherapeutics

Ipratropium is used in patients with COPD. It may also be used as an adjunctive therapy for the treatment of asthma; however, it's less effective as a form of long-term management. It's commonly used in combination with a short-acting beta$_2$-adrenergic agonist on a scheduled basis. It's also used to treat rhinorrhea and is available a a nasal spray.

Drug interactions

Drug interactions aren't as likely when using an inhaled formulation of ipratropium. Use antimuscarinic and anticholinergic agents cautiously with ipratropium.

Adverse reactions

The most common adverse reactions to anticholinergics include:
- nervousness
- tachycardia
- nausea and vomiting
- dizziness
- headache
- paradoxical bronchospasm with excessive use.

Nursing process

These nursing process steps are appropriate for patients undergoing treatment with anticholinergics.

Assessment

- Assess the patient's respiratory condition before therapy and regularly thereafter.
- Assess peak flow readings before starting treatment and periodically thereafter.
- Be alert for adverse reactions and drug interactions.
- Evaluate the patient's and family's knowledge of drug therapy.

Key nursing diagnoses

- Ineffective breathing pattern related to respiratory condition
- Impaired gas exchange related to underlying condition
- Deficient knowledge related to drug therapy

Planning outcome goals

- Breathing pattern will improve as evidenced by regular and even respiratory rate and rhythm.
- Gas exchange will be adequate as evidenced by improved peak flow rates, oxygen saturation, and ABG levels.
- The patient will demonstrate correct drug administration.

Implementation

- Report insufficient relief or a worsening condition.
- Obtain an order for a mild analgesic if a drug-induced headache occurs.

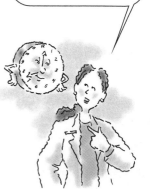

Watch that clock! Keep in mind that total inhalations shouldn't exceed 12 in 24 hours, and total nasal sprays shouldn't exceed 8 in each nostril in 24 hours.

Acutely ineffective

- Be aware that the drug isn't effective for treating acute episodes of bronchospasm when rapid response is needed.
- Monitor the medication regimen. Total inhalations shouldn't exceed 12 in 24 hours, and total nasal sprays shouldn't exceed 8 in each nostril in 24 hours.
- If more than one inhalation is ordered, 2 minutes should elapse between inhalations. If more than one type of inhalant is ordered, always give the bronchodilator first and wait 5 minutes before administering the other inhalant.
- Give the drug on time to ensure maximal effect.
- Notify the prescriber if the drug fails to relieve bronchospasms.
- Provide patient teaching.

Evaluation
- Patient exhibits normal breathing pattern.
- Patient exhibits improved gas exchange.
- Patient and family understand drug therapy.

Corticosteroids

Corticosteroids are anti-inflammatory agents available in both inhaled and systemic formulations for the short- and long-term control of asthma symptoms. This class consists of many drugs with differing potencies.

The nose knows

Inhaled corticosteroids include:
- beclomethasone dipropionate
- budesonide
- flunisolide
- fluticasone propionate
- triamcinolone acetonide.

Over the lips, past the gums

Oral corticosteroids include:
- prednisolone
- prednisone.

A vein attempt

I.V. corticosteroids include:
- methylprednisolone sodium succinate
- hydrocortisone sodium succinate.

Before you give that drug

Corticosteroid warning

Consider these points about special populations before administering corticosteroids:

• Growth should be monitored in children, especially when taking systemic agents or higher doses of inhaled agents.

• Older patients may benefit from specific medications, diet, and exercise intended to prevent osteoporosis while on these agents, especially when receiving higher doses of inhaled steroids or systemic agents.

• Patients with diabetes may require closer monitoring of blood glucose while on steroids.

• Corticosteroid levels are negligible in the breast milk of mothers who are receiving less than 20 mg/day of oral prednisone. The amount found in breast milk can be minimized if the mother waits at least 4 hours after taking prednisone to breast-feed the infant.

• To reduce the risk of adverse effects occurring with the inhaled agents, use the lowest possible doses to maintain control. Spacers should be used to administer doses, and patients should rinse their mouths out following administration.

Pharmacokinetics

Inhaled corticosteroids are minimally absorbed, although absorption increases as the dose is increased. Oral prednisone is readily absorbed and extensively metabolized in the liver to the active metabolite, prednisolone. I.V. forms have a rapid onset.

Pharmacodynamics

Corticosteroids inhibit the production of cytokines, leukotrienes, and prostaglandins; the recruitment of eosinophils; and the release of other inflammatory mediators. They also have various effects elsewhere in the body that cause many of the long-term adverse effects associated with these agents. (See *Corticosteroid warning.*)

Pharmacotherapeutics

Corticosteroids are the most effective agents available for the long-term treatment and prevention of asthma exacerbations. Systemic formulations are commonly reserved for moderate to severe acute exacerbations but are also used in those with severe asthma that's refractory to other measures. Systemic corticosteroids should be used at the lowest effective dosage and for the shortest possible period to avoid adverse effects.

Inhaled corticosteroids remain the mainstay of therapy to prevent future exacerbations for most asthmatics with mild to severe disease. Use of inhaled corticosteroids reduces the need for systemic steroids in many patients, thus reducing the risk of serious

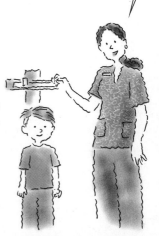

Growth should be monitored in children taking corticosteroids, especially when they take systemic agents or higher doses of inhaled agents.

long-term adverse effects. Inhaled corticosteroids shouldn't be used for acute symptoms; rather, short-acting inhaled beta$_2$-adrenergic agonists should be used.

Drug interactions

Interactions aren't likely when using inhaled formulations. Hormonal contraceptives, ketoconazole, and macrolide antibiotics can increase the activity of corticosteroids in general and may require a dosage decrease of the steroid. Barbiturates, cholestyramine, and phenytoin can decrease the effectiveness of corticosteroids and may require a dosage increase of the steroid.

Adverse reactions

Possible adverse reactions to inhaled corticosteroids include:
* mouth irritation
* oral candidiasis
* upper respiratory tract infection
* cough and hoarseness.
    Possible adverse reactions to oral corticosteroids include:
* hyperglycemia
* nausea and vomiting
* headache
* insomnia
* growth suppression in children.

Nursing process

These nursing process steps are appropriate for patients undergoing treatment with corticosteroids.

Assessment

* Assess the patient's respiratory condition before therapy and regularly thereafter.
* Assess peak flow readings before starting treatment and periodically thereafter.
* Be alert for adverse reactions and drug interactions.
* Evaluate the patient's and family's knowledge of drug therapy.

Key nursing diagnoses

* Ineffective breathing pattern related to respiratory condition
* Impaired gas exchange related to underlying condition
* Deficient knowledge related to drug therapy

Planning outcome goals

• Breathing pattern will improve as evidenced by regular and even respiratory rate and rhythm.
• Gas exchange will be adequate as evidenced by improved peak flow rates, oxygen saturation, and ABG levels.
• The patient will demonstrate correct drug administration.

Implementation

• Report insufficient relief or worsening of condition.
• Give oral doses with food to prevent GI irritation.
• Take precautions to avoid exposing the patient to infection.
• Don't stop the drug abruptly.
• Notify the prescriber of severe or persistent adverse reactions.
• Avoid prolonged use of corticosteroids, especially in children.

Evaluation

• Patient exhibits normal breathing pattern.
• Patient exhibits improved gas exchange.
• Patient and family understand drug therapy.

Leukotriene modifiers

Leukotriene modifiers are used for the prevention and long-term control of mild asthma. There are two types:
• *Leukotriene receptor antagonists* include zafirlukast and montelukast.
• *Leukotriene formation inhibitors* include zileuton. (See *Leukotriene modifiers: Zafirlukast.*)

Pharmacokinetics

All leukotriene modifiers are extensively metabolized, have a rapid absorption, and are highly protein bound (more than 90%).

Factoring in food

Zafirlukast's absorption is decreased by food. Montelukast has a rapid absorption from the GI tract and may be given with food. Administration of zileuton with food doesn't affect the rate of absorption. Patients with hepatic impairment may require a dosage adjustment.

Pharmacodynamics

Leukotrienes are substances that are released from mast cells, eosinophils, and basophils. They can result in smooth-muscle con-

Prototype pro

Leukotriene modifiers: Zafirlukast

Actions
• Selectively competes for leukotriene receptor sites, blocking inflammatory action

Indications
• Prophylaxis and long-term management of asthma

Nursing considerations
• This drug isn't indicated for reversing bronchospasm in acute asthma attacks.
• Give cautiously to elderly patients and those with hepatic impairment.
• Drug absorption is decreased by food; give the drug 1 hour before or 2 hours after meals.
• Monitor liver function studies in patients with suspected hepatic dysfunction. The drug may need to be discontinued if hepatic dysfunction is confirmed.

traction of the airways, increased permeability of the vasculature, increased secretions, and activation of other inflammatory mediators.

Leukotrienes are inhibited by two different mechanisms:

☝ The leukotriene receptor antagonists (zafirlukast and montelukast) are competitive inhibitors of the leukotriene D4 and E4 receptors that inhibit leukotriene from interacting with its receptor and blocking its action.

✌ The leukotriene formation inhibitor (zileuton) inhibits the production of 5-lipoxygenase, an enzyme that inhibits the formation of leukotrienes, which are known to contribute to swelling, bronchoconstriction, and mucus secretion seen in patients with asthma.

Pharmacotherapeutics

Leukotriene modifiers are primarily used to prevent and control asthma exacerbations in patients with mild to moderate disease. They aren't effective in terminating an acute asthma attack. They may also be used as steroid-sparing agents in some patients.

Drug interactions

The following drug interactions occur with leukotriene modifiers:
• Because zafirlukast inhibits cytochrome P450 2C9 (CYP2C9), increased toxicity can result when the drug is used with phenytoin or warfarin.
• Zafirlukast and zileuton inhibit CYP3A4 and could result in increased toxicity if used with amlodipine, atorvastatin, carbamazepine, clarithromycin, cyclosporine, erythromycin, hormonal contraceptives, itraconazole, ketoconazole, lovastatin, nelfinavir, nifedipine, ritonavir, sertraline, simvastatin, or warfarin.
• Because zileuton inhibits CYP1A2, increased toxicity can result if it's administered with amitriptyline, clozapine, desipramine, fluvoxamine, imipramine, theophylline, or warfarin.
• Zafirlukast, zileuton, and montelukast are metabolized by CYP2C9. Increased toxicity can result if these drugs are administered with amiodarone, cimetidine, fluconazole, fluoxetine, fluvoxamine, isoniazid, metronidazole, or voriconazole.
• Leukotrienes have a decreased effectiveness when given with carbamazepine, phenobarbital, phenytoin, primidone, or rifampin.
• Zileuton and montelukast are metabolized by CYP3A4. Increased toxicity can result if these drugs are given with amiodarone, cimetidine, clarithromycin, cyclosporine, erythromycin, fluoxetine, fluvoxamine, itraconazole, ketoconazole, metronidazole, or voriconazole.

• Zileuton and montelukast are metabolized by CYP3A4. Decreased effectiveness can result if administered with carbamazepine, efavirenz, garlic supplements, modafinil, nevirapine, oxcarbazepine, phenobarbital, phenytoin, primidone, rifabutin, rifampin, or St. John's wort.
• Zileuton is metabolized by CYP1A2. Increased toxicity can result if administered with cimetidine, clarithromycin, erythromycin, fluvoxamine, or isoniazid. Decreased effectiveness can result if administered with carbamazepine, phenobarbital, phenytoin, primidone, rifampin, ritonavir, or St. John's wort. If the patient is a smoker, nicotine can result in decreased effectiveness of zileuton.

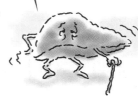

Zileuton is contraindicated in patients with active liver disease—which actually makes me feel more inactive.

Adverse reactions

Adverse reactions to leukotriene modifiers include:
• headache
• dizziness
• nausea and vomiting
• myalgia
• cough.
    Zileuton is contraindicated in patients with active liver disease.

Nursing process

These nursing process steps are appropriate for patients undergoing treatment with leukotriene modifiers.

Assessment

• Assess the patient's respiratory condition before therapy and regularly thereafter.
• Assess peak flow readings before starting treatment and periodically thereafter.
• Use cautiously in patients with hepatic impairment.
• Be alert for adverse reactions and drug interactions.
• Evaluate the patient's and family's knowledge of drug therapy.

Key nursing diagnoses

• Ineffective breathing pattern related to respiratory condition
• Impaired gas exchange related to underlying condition
• Deficient knowledge related to drug therapy

Planning outcome goals

• Breathing pattern will improve as evidenced by regular and even respiratory rate and rhythm.
• Gas exchange will be adequate as evidenced by improved peak flow rates, oxygen saturation, and ABG levels.
• The patient will demonstrate correct drug administration.

Implementation
- Report insufficient relief or worsening of condition.
- Don't use these drugs for reversing bronchospasm during an acute asthma attack.
- Administer zafirlukast 1 hour before or 2 hours after meals.

Evaluation
- Patient exhibits normal breathing pattern.
- Patient exhibits improved gas exchange.
- Patient and family understand drug therapy.

Mast cell stabilizers

Mast cell stabilizers are used for the prevention and long-term control of asthma, especially in pediatric patients and patients with mild disease. These drugs aren't effective in the management of an acute asthma attack.

Medications in this class include nedocromil and cromolyn sodium.

Pharmacokinetics

Mast cell stabilizers are minimally absorbed from the GI tract. Inhaled formulations exert effects locally.

Pharmacodynamics

The mechanism of action of mast cell stabilizers is poorly understood, but these agents seem to inhibit the release of inflammatory mediators by stabilizing the mast cell membrane, possibly through the inhibition of chloride channels.

Pharmacotherapeutics

Mast cell stabilizers control the inflammatory process and are used for the prevention and long-term control of asthma symptoms. They're the agents of choice for children and patients with exercise-induced asthma.

Handling hay fever

The intranasal form of cromolyn is used to treat seasonal allergies.

Drug interactions

There are no known drug interactions for nedocromil or cromolyn sodium.

Adverse reactions

Adverse reactions to inhaled mast cell stabilizers may include:
• pharyngeal and tracheal irritation
• cough
• wheezing
• bronchospasm
• headache.

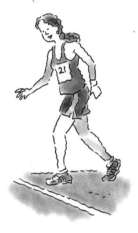

With the proper medication, exercise-induced asthma doesn't have to stop you in your tracks.

Nursing process

These nursing process steps are appropriate for patients undergoing treatment with mast cell stabilizers.

Assessment

• Assess the patient's respiratory condition before therapy and regularly thereafter.
• Assess peak flow readings before starting treatment and periodically thereafter.
• Be alert for adverse reactions and drug interactions.
• Evaluate the patient's and family's knowledge of drug therapy.

Key nursing diagnoses

• Ineffective breathing pattern related to respiratory condition
• Impaired gas exchange related to underlying condition
• Deficient knowledge related to drug therapy

Planning outcome goals

• Breathing pattern will improve as evidenced by regular and even respiratory rate and rhythm.
• Gas exchange will be adequate as evidenced by improved peak flow rates, oxygen saturation, and ABG levels.
• The patient will demonstrate correct drug administration.

Implementation

• Report insufficient relief or worsening of condition.
• Don't use these drugs for reversing bronchospasm during an acute asthma attack.
• Obtain an order for a mild analgesic if a drug-induced headache occurs.
• Monitor for adverse effects of therapy.

Evaluation

- Patient exhibits normal breathing pattern.
- Patient exhibits improved gas exchange.
- Patient and family understand drug therapy.

Methylxanthines

Methylxanthines, also called *xanthines*, are used to treat breathing disorders. Examples of methylxanthines include:

- anhydrous theophylline
- aminophylline
- oxtriphylline.

Aminophylline and oxtriphylline are theophylline derivatives. Theophylline is the most commonly used oral methylxanthine. Aminophylline is preferred when I.V. methylxanthine treatment is required.

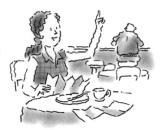

High-fat meals can increase theophylline concentrations and increase the risk of toxicity. Waiter! I'll have a salad with low-fat dressing, please.

Pharmacokinetics

When methylxanthines are given as an oral solution or a rapid-release tablet, they're absorbed rapidly and completely. They're converted in the body to an active form, which is principally theophylline. High-fat meals can increase theophylline concentrations and increase the risk of toxicity.

pH scale weighs in

Absorption of slow-release forms of theophylline depends on the patient's gastric pH. Food can also alter absorption. When converting patient dosages from I.V. aminophylline to theophylline by mouth (P.O.), the dosage is decreased by 20%.

Theophylline is approximately 56% protein bound in adults and 36% protein bound in neonates. It readily crosses the placental barrier and is secreted in breast milk. Smokers and patients on dialysis may need higher doses.

Theophylline is metabolized primarily in the liver by the CYP1A2 enzyme and, in adults and children, about 10% of a dose is excreted unchanged in urine. Therefore, no dosage adjustment is required in a patient with renal insufficiency. Elderly patients and patients with liver dysfunction may require lower doses. Because infants have immature livers with reduced metabolic functioning, as much as one-half of a dose may be excreted unchanged in their urine. Theophylline levels need to be collected to evaluate efficacy and avoid toxicity. The therapeutic serum concentration is 10 to 20 mcg/ml (SI, 44 to 111 µmol/L). Levels need to be assessed when a dose is initiated or changed, and when drugs are added or removed from a patient's medication regimen.

Pharmacodynamics

Methylxanthines work in several ways.

Taking it easy

Methylxanthines decrease airway reactivity and relieve bronchospasm by relaxing bronchial smooth muscle. It's thought that theophylline inhibits phosphodiesterase (PDE), resulting in smooth-muscle relaxation as well as bronchodilation and a decrease in inflammatory mediators (namely mast cells, T cells, and eosinophils). Much of theophylline's toxicity may be due to increased catecholamine release.

Driven to breathe

In nonreversible obstructive airway disease (chronic bronchitis, emphysema, and apnea), methylxanthines appear to increase the sensitivity of the brain's respiratory center to carbon dioxide and stimulate the respiratory drive.

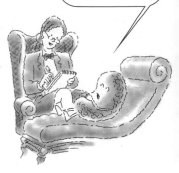

So you're telling me methylxanthines increase your sensitivity to carbon dioxide?

Yes, and it always ends up stimulating my respiratory drive!

Pumped up

In chronic bronchitis and emphysema, these drugs reduce fatigue of the diaphragm, the respiratory muscle that separates the abdomen from the thoracic cavity. They also improve ventricular function and, therefore, the heart's pumping action.

Pharmacotherapeutics

Methylxanthines are used as second- or third-line agents for the long-term control of and presentation of symptoms related to:
- asthma
- chronic bronchitis
- emphysema.

Oh baby

Theophylline has been used to treat neonatal apnea (periods of not breathing in a neonate) and has been effective in reducing severe bronchospasm in infants with cystic fibrosis.

Drug interactions

Theophylline drug interactions occur with those substances that inhibit or induce the CYP1A2 enzyme system:
- Inhibitors of CYP1A2 decrease the metabolism of theophylline, thus increasing the serum concentration. This results in increased

adverse reactions or toxicity. The dose of theophylline may need to be reduced. Examples of CYP1A2 inhibitors include ketoconazole, erythromycin, clarithromycin, cimetidine, isoniazid, fluvoxamine, hormonal contraceptives, ciprofloxacin, ticlopidine, and zileuton.

• Inducers of CYP1A2 increase the metabolism of theophylline, decreasing the serum concentration. This results in possible therapeutic failure. The dose of theophylline may need to be increased. Examples of CYP1A2 inducers include rifampin, carbamazepine, phenobarbital, phenytoin, and St. John's wort.

• Smoking cigarettes or marijuana increases theophylline elimination, decreasing its serum concentration and effectiveness.

• Taking adrenergic stimulants or drinking beverages that contain caffeine or caffeinelike substances may result in additive adverse reactions to theophylline or signs and symptoms of methylxanthine toxicity.

• Activated charcoal may decrease theophylline levels.

• Receiving halothane, enflurane, isoflurane, and methoxyflurane with theophylline and theophylline derivatives increases the risk of cardiac toxicity.

• Theophylline and its derivatives may reduce the effects of lithium by increasing its rate of excretion.

• Thyroid hormones may reduce theophylline levels; antithyroid drugs may increase theophylline levels.

Adverse reactions

Adverse reactions to methylxanthines may be transient or symptomatic of toxicity.

Gut reactions

Adverse GI system reactions include:
• nausea and vomiting
• abdominal cramping
• epigastric pain
• anorexia
• diarrhea.

Nerve racking

Adverse central nervous system (CNS) reactions include:
• headache
• irritability, restlessness, and anxiety
• insomnia
• dizziness.

Sleep tight, little one. Theophylline is used to treat neonatal apnea.

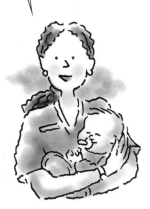

Heart of the matter

Adverse cardiovascular reactions include:
- tachycardia
- palpitations
- arrhythmias.

Nursing process

These nursing process steps are appropriate for patients undergoing treatment with methylxanthines.

Assessment

- Assess the patient's respiratory condition before therapy and regularly thereafter.
- Assess peak flow readings before starting treatment and periodically thereafter.
- Be alert for adverse reactions and drug interactions.
- Monitor vital signs and measure fluid intake and output. Expected clinical effects include improvement in the quality of pulse and respirations.
- The xanthine metabolism rate varies among individuals; the dosage is determined by monitoring the patient's response, tolerance, pulmonary function, and serum theophylline level.
- Evaluate the patient's and family's knowledge of drug therapy.

Key nursing diagnoses

- Ineffective breathing pattern related to respiratory condition
- Impaired gas exchange related to underlying condition
- Deficient knowledge related to drug therapy

Planning outcome goals

- Breathing pattern will improve as evidenced by regular and even respiratory rate and rhythm.
- Gas exchange will be adequate as evidenced by improved peak flow rates, oxygen saturation, and ABG levels.
- The patient will verbalize an understanding of drug therapy.

Implementation

- Report insufficient relief or worsening of condition.
- Give P.O. doses around the clock, using a sustained-release product at bedtime.
- Use a commercially available infusion solution for I.V. use, or mix the drug in dextrose 5% in water (D_5W). Use an infusion pump for a continuous infusion.

Education edge

Teaching about methylxanthines

If methylxanthines are prescribed, review these points with the patient and his caregivers:
• Don't dissolve, crush, or chew sustained-release products.
• For a child who can't swallow capsules, sprinkle the contents of capsules over soft food and instruct the child to swallow without chewing.
• Follow instructions for drug administration and dosage schedule.
• Relieve GI symptoms by taking the oral form of the drug with a full glass of water after meals.
• Take the drug regularly as directed. Don't take extra medication.

• Dizziness may occur at the start of therapy, especially in an elderly patient.
• Change position slowly and avoid hazardous activities during drug therapy.
• Check with your prescriber before using other drugs.
• If you're a smoker while on drug therapy and then you quit, notify your prescriber; your dosage may need to be reduced.
• Report signs and symptoms of toxicity to your prescriber, including tachycardia, anorexia, nausea, vomiting, diarrhea, restlessness, irritability, and headache.
• Have blood levels monitored periodically.
• Avoid foods with caffeine.

Smoked out

• Know that the dosage may need to be increased in cigarette smokers and in habitual marijuana smokers because smoking causes the drug to be metabolized faster.
• Know that the daily dose may need to be decreased in patients with heart failure or hepatic disease and in elderly patients because metabolism and excretion may be decreased.
• Monitor the patient's vital signs.
• Measure and record the patient's intake and output.
• Tell the patient to avoid caffeine.

Evaluation

• Patient exhibits normal breathing pattern.
• Patient exhibits improved gas exchange.
• Patient and family understand drug therapy. (See *Teaching about methylxanthines*.)

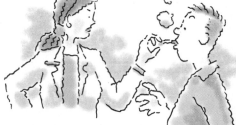

Expectorants

Expectorants increase bronchial secretions, which, in turn, thin mucus so that it's cleared more easily out of airways.

Guaifenesin

The most commonly used expectorant is guaifenesin, a common component of over-the-counter (OTC) cold and flu medications.

Pharmacokinetics

Guaifenesin is absorbed through the GI tract, metabolized by the liver, and excreted primarily by the kidneys.

Pharmacodynamics

By increasing the production of respiratory tract fluids, guaifenesin reduces the thickness, adhesiveness, and surface tension of mucus, making it easier to clear from the airways. It also provides a soothing effect on mucous membranes of the respiratory tract. The result is a more productive cough.

Pharmacotherapeutics

Guaifenesin helps make mucus easier to cough up and is used for the relief of symptoms caused by productive coughs from many disorders, such as:
- colds
- minor bronchial irritation
- bronchitis
- influenza
- sinusitis
- bronchial asthma
- emphysema.

Drug interactions

Guaifenesin isn't known to have specific drug interactions.

Adverse reactions

Adverse reactions to guaifenesin include:
- vomiting (if taken in large doses)
- diarrhea
- drowsiness
- nausea
- abdominal pain
- headache
- hives or skin rash.

Nursing process

These nursing process steps are appropriate for patients undergoing treatment with an expectorant.

Assessment

• Assess the patient's sputum production before and after giving the drug.
• Be alert for adverse reactions and drug interactions.
• Monitor the patient's hydration level if adverse GI reactions occur.
• Evaluate the patient's and family's knowledge of drug therapy.

Key nursing diagnoses

• Ineffective airway clearance related to underlying condition
• Risk for deficient fluid volume related to adverse GI reactions
• Deficient knowledge related to drug therapy

Planning outcome goals

• The patient will have a patent airway.
• Fluid volume will be adequate as exhibited by blood pressure, pulse, and urine output.
• The patient will verbalize an understanding of drug therapy.

Implementation

• Administer the medication as directed; give with a full glass of water as appropriate.

The acid test

• Be aware that the drug may interfere with laboratory tests for 5-hydroxyindoleacetic acid and vanillylmandelic acid.
• Report ineffectiveness of the drug to the prescriber; also report if the patient's cough persists or if signs and symptoms worsen.
• Encourage the patient to perform deep-breathing exercises.
• Advise the patient not to take other medications, OTC products, or herbal remedies unless approved by the prescriber or a pharmacist.

Evaluation

• Patient's lungs are clear, and respiratory secretions are normal.
• Patient maintains adequate hydration.
• Patient and family understand drug therapy.

Antitussives

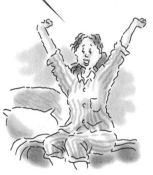

Antitussives are used to relieve a dry, nonproductive cough, allowing for a good night's sleep.

Antitussive drugs suppress or inhibit coughing. They're typically used to treat dry, nonproductive coughs. The major antitussives include:

• benzonatate
• codeine
• dextromethorphan hydrobromide
• hydrocodone bitartrate.

Pharmacokinetics

Antitussives are absorbed well through the GI tract, metabolized in the liver, and excreted in urine. Opioid antitussives are excreted in breast milk and should be used during pregnancy only if the benefits outweigh the risks.

Pharmacodynamics

Antitussives act in slightly different ways:
• Benzonatate acts by anesthetizing stretch receptors throughout the bronchi, alveoli, and pleura.
• Codeine, dextromethorphan, and hydrocodone suppress the cough reflex by direct action on the cough center in the medulla of the brain, thus lowering the cough threshold.

Pharmacotherapeutics

The uses of these drugs vary slightly, but each treats a serious, nonproductive cough that interferes with a patient's ability to rest or carry out activities of daily living.

Testing 1, 2, 3

Benzonatate relieves cough caused by pneumonia, bronchitis, the common cold, and chronic pulmonary diseases such as emphysema. It can also be used during bronchial diagnostic tests, such as bronchoscopy, when the patient must avoid coughing.

And the winner is...

Dextromethorphan is the most widely used cough suppressant in the United States and may provide better antitussive activity than codeine. Its popularity may stem from the fact that it isn't associated with sedation, respiratory depression, or addiction at usual dosages.

When the going gets tough

The opioid antitussives (typically codeine and hydrocodone) are usually reserved for treating intractable cough, but can be used for less serious coughs.

Drug interactions

Antitussives may interact with other drugs in the following ways:
• Codeine and hydrocodone may cause excitation, an extremely elevated temperature, hypertension or hypotension, and coma when taken with monoamine oxidase (MAO) inhibitors.
• Dextromethorphan use with MAO inhibitors may produce excitation, an elevated body temperature, hypotension, and coma.

Dangerous depression

• Codeine may cause increased CNS depression—including drowsiness, lethargy, stupor, respiratory depression, coma, and death—when taken with other CNS depressants, including alcohol, barbiturates, sedative-hypnotics, and phenothiazines.

Adverse reactions

Benzonatate can cause different kinds of adverse reactions than the opioid antitussives, codeine, dextromethorphan, and hydrocodone.

Benzonatate

Benzonatate needs to be swallowed whole; chewing or crushing can produce a local anesthetic effect on the mouth and throat, which can compromise the airway. The following reactions can also occur when taking benzonatate:
• dizziness
• sedation
• headache
• nasal congestion
• burning in the eyes
• GI upset or nausea
• constipation
• skin rash, eruptions, or itching
• chills
• chest numbness.

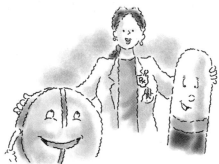

Different types of antitussives can cause different kinds of adverse reactions.

Opioid antitussives

Common adverse reactions include nausea, vomiting, sedation, dizziness, and constipation. Other reactions include:

- pupil constriction
- bradycardia or tachycardia
- hypotension
- stupor
- seizures
- circulatory collapse
- respiratory arrest.

Nursing process

These nursing process steps are appropriate for patients undergoing treatment with antitussives.

Assessment

- Obtain a history of the patient's cough.
- Be alert for adverse reactions and drug interactions.
- Monitor the patient's hydration level if adverse GI reactions occur.
- Evaluate the patient's and family's knowledge of drug therapy.

Key nursing diagnoses

- Ineffective airway clearance related to underlying condition
- Fatigue related to presence of nonproductive cough
- Deficient knowledge related to drug therapy

Planning outcome goals

- The patient will have a patent airway.
- The patient will state that fatigue is lessened.
- The patient will verbalize an understanding of drug therapy.

Implementation

- Report ineffectiveness of the drug to the prescriber; also report if the patient's cough persists or if signs and symptoms worsen.
- Encourage the patient to perform deep-breathing exercises.
- Advise the patient not to take other medications, OTC products, or herbal remedies until talking with the prescriber or a pharmacist.
- Tell the patient taking an opioid antitussive to avoid driving and drinking alcohol.

Evaluation

- Patient's lungs are clear, and respiratory secretions are normal.
- Patient's cough is relieved.
- Patient and family understand drug therapy.

Decongestants

Decongestants may be classified as systemic or topical, depending on how they're administered.

How swell!

As sympathomimetic drugs, systemic decongestants stimulate the sympathetic nervous system to reduce swelling of the respiratory tract's vascular network. Systemic decongestants include:
- ephedrine
- phenylephrine
- pseudoephedrine.

In the clear

Topical decongestants are also powerful vasoconstrictors. When applied directly to swollen mucous membranes of the nose, they provide immediate relief from nasal congestion. Topical decongestants include:
- ephedrine, epinephrine, and phenylephrine (sympathomimetic amines)
- naphazoline, oxymetazoline, tetrahydrozoline, and xylometazoline (imidazoline derivatives of sympathomimetic amines)
- desoxyephedrine and propylhexedrine.

Pharmacokinetics

The pharmacokinetic properties of decongestants vary. When taken orally, the systemic decongestants are absorbed readily from the GI tract and widely distributed throughout the body into various tissues and fluids, including cerebrospinal fluid, the placenta, and breast milk.

All in a day's work

Systemic decongestants are slowly and incompletely metabolized by the liver and excreted largely unchanged in the urine within 24 hours of oral administration.

In the neighborhood

Topical decongestants act locally on the alpha-adrenergic receptors of the vascular smooth muscle in the nose, causing the arterioles to constrict. As a result of this local action, absorption of the drug becomes negligible.

Pharmacodynamics

The properties of systemic and topical decongestants vary slightly.

Direct and to the point

The systemic decongestants cause vasoconstriction by directly stimulating alpha-adrenergic receptors in the blood vessels of the body. They also cause contraction of urinary and GI sphincters, dilation of the pupils of the eyes, and decreased secretion of insulin.

Indirect hit

These drugs may also act indirectly, resulting in the release of norepinephrine from storage sites in the body, which leads to peripheral vasoconstriction.

On a clear day...

Like systemic decongestants, topical decongestants stimulate alpha-adrenergic receptors in the smooth muscle of the blood vessels in the nose, resulting in vasoconstriction. The combination of reduced blood flow to the nasal mucous membranes and decreased capillary permeability reduces swelling. This action improves respiration by helping to drain sinuses, clear nasal passages, and open eustachian tubes.

> When it comes to beating decongestion, we're a winning team!

Pharmacotherapeutics

Systemic and topical decongestants are used to relieve the symptoms of swollen nasal membranes resulting from:
- allergic rhinitis (hay fever)
- vasomotor rhinitis
- acute coryza (profuse discharge from the nose)
- sinusitis
- the common cold.

It's a group effort

Systemic decongestants are usually given with other drugs, such as antihistamines, antimuscarinics, antipyretic-analgesics, and antitussives.

Advantage, topical

Topical decongestants provide two major advantages over systemics: minimal adverse reactions and rapid symptom relief.

Drug interactions

Because they produce vasoconstriction, which reduces drug absorption, drug interactions involving topical decongestants seldom occur. However, systemic decongestants may interact with other drugs:

• Increased CNS stimulation may occur when systemic decongestants are taken with other sympathomimetic drugs, including epinephrine, norepinephrine, dopamine, dobutamine, isoproterenol, metaproterenol, and terbutaline.

• When taken with MAO inhibitors, systemic decongestants may cause severe hypertension or a hypertensive crisis, which can be life-threatening. These drugs shouldn't be used together.

• Alkalinizing drugs may increase the effects of pseudoephedrine by reducing its urinary excretion.

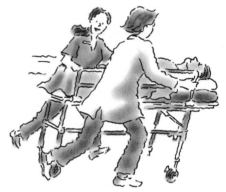

Taking MAO inhibitors with systemic decongestants may cause severe hypertension, even a hypertensive crisis.

Adverse reactions

Most adverse reactions to decongestants result from CNS stimulation and include:

• nervousness
• restlessness and insomnia
• nausea
• palpitations and tachycardia
• difficulty urinating
• elevated blood pressure.

Systemic decongestants

Systemic decongestants also exacerbate hypertension, hyperthyroidism, diabetes, benign prostatic hyperplasia, glaucoma, and heart disease.

Topical decongestants

The most common adverse reaction associated with prolonged use (more than 5 days) of topical decongestants is rebound nasal congestion. Other reactions include burning and stinging of the nasal mucosa, sneezing, and mucosal dryness or ulceration.

Nursing process

These nursing process steps are appropriate for patients undergoing treatment with decongestants.

Assessment

• Assess the patient's condition before and after giving the drug.
• Assess the patient's nares for signs of bleeding.
• Be alert for adverse reactions and drug interactions.
• Monitor the patient's hydration level if adverse GI reactions occur.
• Evaluate the patient's and family's knowledge of drug therapy.

Key nursing diagnoses

• Ineffective airway clearance related to underlying condition
• Risk for deficient fluid volume related to adverse GI reactions
• Deficient knowledge related to drug therapy

Planning outcome goals

• The patient will have a patent airway.
• Fluid volume will be adequate as exhibited by blood pressure, pulse, and urine output.
• The patient will demonstrate correct drug administration.

Implementation

• Report ineffectiveness of the drug to the prescriber; also report if the patient's cough persists or if signs and symptoms worsen.
• Encourage the patient to perform deep-breathing exercises.
• Advise the patient not to take other medications, OTC products, or herbal remedies until talking with the prescriber or a pharmacist.
• Identify and correct hypoxia, hypercapnia, and acidosis, which may reduce drug effectiveness or increase adverse reactions, before or during ephedrine administration.
• Don't crush or break extended-release forms of the drug.
• Give the last dose at least 2 hours before bedtime to minimize insomnia.
• Instruct the patient to limit his use of intranasal forms to 3 to 5 days to prevent rebound congestion.

Evaluation

• Patient's lungs are clear, and respiratory secretions are normal.
• Patient maintains adequate hydration.
• Patient and family understand drug therapy.

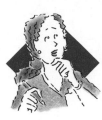

Quick quiz

1. You're instructing a patient with asthma about the use of bronchodilators. You should teach the patient:

    A.   to take the medication 4 hours before exercise to prevent exercise-induced bronchospasm.

    B.   to take only the specific drugs prescribed for acute bronchospasm, usually a short-acting $beta_2$-adrenergic agonist such as albuterol.

    C.   to double the dose of the medication in the event of a missed dose.

    D.   that long-acting $beta_2$ agonists, such as salmeterol, are effective in the treatment of acute asthma attacks.

Answer: B. Short-acting $beta_2$-adrenergic agonists are used in the treatment of acute bronchospasm. Long-acting agents aren't effective in acute attacks. To prevent exercise-induced asthma, medication should be taken 30 to 60 minutes before exercise.

2. Which anticholinergic agent is used to treat patients with COPD?

    A.   Atropine

    B.   Guaifenesin

    C.   Budesonide

    D.   Ipratropium bromide

Answer: D. Inhaled ipratropium bromide is an anticholinergic agent used as a bronchodilator in patients with COPD.

3. Which leukotriene modifier's absorption is decreased by food and should be given 1 hour before or 2 hours after meals?

    A.   Zileuton

    B.   Montelukast

    C.   Zafirlukast

    D.   Nedocromil

Answer: C. Absorption of zafirlukast is decreased by food, and it must be given 1 hour before meals or 2 hours after meals.

Scoring

☆☆☆   If you answered all three questions correctly, good job! You can take a deep breath and move on to the next chapter.

☆☆   If you answered two questions correctly, you're as relaxed as bronchial smooth muscle on xanthines.

☆   If you answered fewer than two questions correctly, you may need another dose of the chapter to clear your head about respiratory drugs.

Gastrointestinal drugs

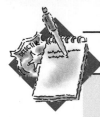

Just the facts

In this chapter, you'll learn:

♦ classes of drugs used to improve GI function

♦ uses and varying actions of these drugs

♦ absorption, distribution, metabolization, and excretion of these drugs

♦ drug interactions and adverse reactions to these drugs.

Drugs and the gastrointestinal system

The GI tract is basically a hollow, muscular tube that begins at the mouth and ends at the anus; it encompasses the pharynx, esophagus, stomach, and the small and large intestines. Its primary functions are to digest and absorb foods and fluids and excrete metabolic waste.

Roll call

Classes of drugs used to improve GI function include:
• antiulcer drugs
• adsorbent, antiflatulent, and digestive drugs
• antidiarrheal and laxative drugs
• obesity drugs
• antiemetic drugs.

Antiulcer drugs

A peptic ulcer is a circumscribed lesion in the mucosal membrane, developing in the lower esophagus, stomach, duodenum, or jejunum.

Common culprits

The major causes of peptic ulcers include:
- bacterial infection with *Helicobacter pylori*
- the use of nonsteroidal anti-inflammatory drugs (NSAIDs)
- hypersecretory states such as Zollinger-Ellison syndrome (a condition in which excessive gastric acid secretion causes peptic ulcers)
- cigarette smoking, which causes hypersecretion and impairs ulcer healing
- a genetic predisposition, which accounts for 20% to 50% of patients with peptic ulcers.

Busting bacteria or bolstering balance

Antiulcer drugs are formulated to eradicate *H. pylori* or restore the balance between acid and pepsin secretions and the GI mucosal defense. (See *Where drugs affect GI secretions.*) These drugs include:
- systemic antibiotics
- antacids
- histamine-2 (H_2) receptor antagonists
- proton pump inhibitors
- other antiulcer drugs, such as misoprostol and sucralfate.

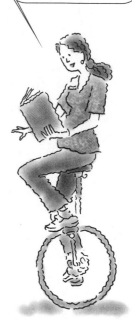

It says here that antiulcer drugs can restore the balance between acid and pepsin secretions and the GI mucosal defense.

Systemic antibiotics

H. pylori is a gram-negative bacteria that's thought to be a major causative factor in peptic ulcer formation and gastritis (inflammation of the stomach lining). Eradicating the bacteria promotes ulcer healing and decreases recurrence.

It takes two

Successful treatment involves the use of two or more antibiotics in combination with other drugs. Systemic antibiotics used to treat *H. pylori* include:
- amoxicillin
- clarithromycin
- metronidazole
- tetracycline.

Pharmacokinetics (how drugs circulate)

Systemic antibiotics are variably absorbed from the GI tract.

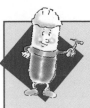

Pharm function

Where drugs affect GI secretions

Antiulcer drugs and digestive drugs that affect GI secretions can decrease secretory activity, block the action of secretions, form a protective coating on the lining, or replace missing enzymes. The illustration below depicts where these types of GI drugs act.

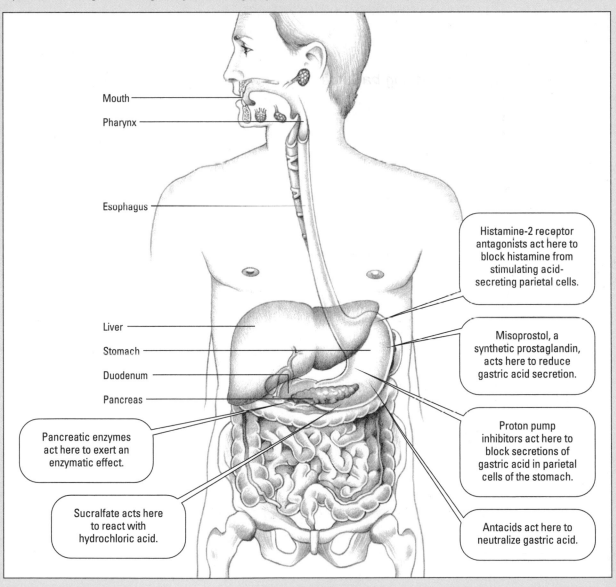

Mouth

Pharynx

Esophagus

Liver

Stomach

Duodenum

Pancreas

Histamine-2 receptor antagonists act here to block histamine from stimulating acid-secreting parietal cells.

Misoprostol, a synthetic prostaglandin, acts here to reduce gastric acid secretion.

Pancreatic enzymes act here to exert an enzymatic effect.

Proton pump inhibitors act here to block secretions of gastric acid in parietal cells of the stomach.

Sucralfate acts here to react with hydrochloric acid.

Antacids act here to neutralize gastric acid.

Got milk?

Food, especially dairy products, decreases the absorption of tetracycline but doesn't significantly delay the absorption of the other antibiotics.

All of these antibiotics are distributed widely and are excreted primarily in urine.

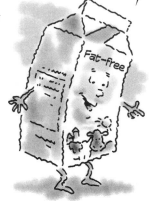

Dairy products and other foods decrease the absorption of the antibiotic tetracycline.

Pharmacodynamics (how drugs act)

Antibiotics act by treating the *H. pylori* infection. They're usually combined with an H_2-receptor antagonist or a proton pump inhibitor to decrease stomach acid and further promote healing.

Pharmacotherapeutics (how drugs are used)

Systemic antibiotics are indicated for *H. pylori* eradication to reduce the risk of a duodenal ulcer.

Sounds like a plan

Treatment plans that use at least two antimicrobial drugs and a proton pump inhibitor for 14 days and then continue the proton pump inhibitor for 6 more weeks help to reduce acid in patients with peptic ulcers.

Drug interactions

Tetracycline and metronidazole can interact with many other drugs. For example, tetracycline increases digoxin levels and, when combined with methoxyflurane, increases the risk of nephrotoxicity. Metronidazole and tetracycline increase the risk of bleeding when taken with oral anticoagulants.

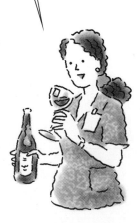

Don't combine metronidazole with alcohol. A severe reaction may occur.

Adverse reactions

Antibiotics used to improve GI tract function may lead to adverse reactions, such as those listed here:
• Metronidazole, clarithromycin, and tetracycline commonly cause mild GI disturbances.
• Clarithromycin and metronidazole may produce abnormal tastes.
• Metronidazole may cause a disulfiram-like reaction (nausea, vomiting, headache, cramps, flushing) when combined with alcohol. Discourage concomitant use.
• Amoxicillin may cause diarrhea.

Nursing process

These nursing process steps are appropriate for patients undergoing treatment with systemic antibiotics.

Assessment

• Assess the patient's infection before therapy and regularly thereafter.
• Assess signs and symptoms of the patient's ulcer.
• Watch for edema, especially in the patient who's also receiving corticosteroids; antibiotics, such as metronidazole, may cause sodium retention.
• Assess for adverse reactions and drug interactions.
• Identify risk factors for peptic ulcer disease, such as cigarette smoking, stress, and drug therapy with irritating medications (aspirin, other NSAIDs, corticosteroids, or antineoplastics).
• Assess the patient's and family's understanding of drug therapy.

Key nursing diagnoses

• Ineffective health maintenance related to presence of susceptible organisms
• Risk for deficient fluid volume related to drug-induced adverse GI reactions
• Deficient knowledge related to drug therapy

Planning outcome goals

• The patient's overall health status will improve.
• Stable vital signs and the patient's urine output will indicate improved fluid volume status.
• The patient and his family will demonstrate an understanding of drug therapy.

Implementation

• Administer drugs as appropriate for the patient's condition and diagnosis.
• Use measures to prevent or minimize peptic ulcer disease and gastric acid–induced esophageal disorders.
• Observe the patient for improvement in signs and symptoms.
• Instruct the patient to take the full course of antibiotics.

Evaluation

• Patient is free from infection.
• Patient maintains adequate hydration throughout therapy.
• Patient and his family demonstrate an understanding of drug therapy. (See *Teaching about antiulcer drugs*, page 296.)

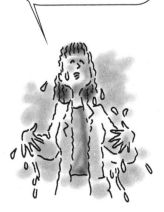

Make sure to evaluate for adequate hydration in the patient taking systemic antibiotics. I think I might be adequately hydrated!

Teaching about antiulcer drugs

If antiulcer drugs are prescribed, review these points with the patient and his caregivers:
• Elevate the head of the bed.
• Avoid abdominal distention by eating small meals.
• Don't lie down for 1 to 2 hours after eating.
• Decrease intake of fats, chocolate, citric juices, coffee, and alcohol.
• Avoid smoking.
• As possible, take steps to avoid obesity, constipation, and other conditions that increase intra-abdominal pressure.
• Take medications with enough water to avoid irritating the esophagus.
• Take antiulcer drugs as directed; underuse decreases their effectiveness and overuse increases adverse effects.

• Swallow capsules whole unless otherwise instructed; some medications can be sprinkled on applesauce if they're difficult to swallow.
• Take medications with or without food as prescribed, when applicable.
• Eat a well-balanced diet.
• Get adequate rest.
• Exercise regularly.
• Avoid gastric irritants as well as nonsteroidal anti-inflammatory drugs.
• Reduce psychological stress; employ stress management techniques as needed.
• Don't take other medications, over-the-counter preparations, or herbal remedies without first consulting with the prescriber.

Antacids

Antacids are over-the-counter (OTC) medications used in combination with other drugs to treat peptic ulcers. Types of antacids include:
• aluminum carbonate gel
• calcium carbonate
• magaldrate (aluminum-magnesium complex)
• magnesium hydroxide and aluminum hydroxide
• simethicone.

Pharmacokinetics

Antacids work locally in the stomach by neutralizing gastric acid. They don't need to be absorbed to treat peptic ulcers. Antacids are distributed throughout the GI tract and are eliminated primarily in feces.

Pharmacodynamics

The acid-neutralizing action of antacids reduces the total amount of acid in the GI tract, allowing peptic ulcers time to heal.

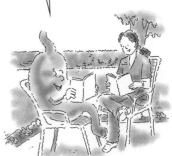

By reducing the amount of acid in the GI tract, antacids allow peptic ulcers time to heal. Which gives me some time to relax...

Pepsin, a digestive enzyme, acts more effectively when the stomach is highly acidic; therefore, as acidity drops, pepsin action is also reduced.

Myth buster

Contrary to popular belief, antacids don't work by coating peptic ulcers or the lining of the GI tract.

Pharmacotherapeutics

Antacids are primarily prescribed to relieve pain and are used adjunctively in peptic ulcer disease.

Churn, churn, churn

Antacids also relieve symptoms of acid indigestion, heartburn, dyspepsia (burning or indigestion), and gastroesophageal reflux disease (GERD), where the contents of the stomach and duodenum flow back into the esophagus.

Foiling phosphate absorption

Antacids may be used to control hyperphosphatemia (elevated blood phosphate levels) in kidney failure. Because calcium binds with phosphate in the GI tract, calcium carbonate antacids prevent phosphate absorption. (See *Antacids: Aluminum hydroxide.*)

Drug interactions

All antacids can interfere with the absorption of oral drugs if given at the same time. Absorption of digoxin, phenytoin, ketoconazole, iron salts, isoniazid, quinolones, and tetracycline may be reduced if taken within 2 hours of antacids. If a patient is taking an antacid in addition to other drugs, separate the drugs' administration times.

Adverse reactions

All adverse reactions to antacids are dose related and include:
- diarrhea
- constipation
- electrolyte imbalances
- aluminum accumulation in serum.

Nursing process

These nursing process steps are appropriate for patients undergoing treatment with antacids.

Prototype pro

Antacids: Aluminum hydroxide

Actions
- Reduces total acid load in the GI tract
- Elevates gastric pH to reduce pepsin activity
- Strengthens the gastric mucosal barrier
- Increases esophageal sphincter tone

Indications
- GI discomfort

Nursing considerations
- Shake suspensions well.
- When administering through a nasogastric tube, make sure that the tube is patent and placed correctly; after instilling, flush the tube with water to ensure passage to the stomach and to clear the tube.
- Don't give other oral drugs within 2 hours of antacid administration. This may cause premature release of enteric-coated drugs in the stomach.

Assessment
- Assess the patient's condition before therapy and regularly thereafter.
- Record the number and consistency of stools.
- Assess the patient for adverse reactions.
- Monitor the patient receiving long-term, high-dose aluminum carbonate and aluminum hydroxide for fluid and electrolyte imbalance, especially if he's on a sodium-restricted diet.
- Monitor phosphate levels in the patient receiving aluminum carbonate or aluminum hydroxide.
- Watch for signs of hypercalcemia in the patient receiving calcium carbonate.
- Monitor magnesium levels in the patient with mild renal impairment who takes magaldrate.

Key nursing diagnoses
- Constipation or diarrhea related to adverse effects of antacids
- Ineffective protection related to drug-induced electrolyte imbalance
- Deficient knowledge related to drug therapy

Planning outcome goals
- The patient's underlying symptoms will improve.
- Laboratory studies will show normal electrolyte balance.
- The patient and his family will demonstrate an understanding of antacid therapy.

Implementation
- Manage constipation with laxatives or stool softeners, or ask the prescriber about switching the patient to a magnesium preparation.
- If the patient suffers from diarrhea, obtain an order for an antidiarrheal as needed, and ask the prescriber about switching the patient to an antacid containing aluminum.
- Shake the container of a liquid form well.
- When giving the drug through a nasogastric (NG) tube, make sure that the tube is patent and placed correctly. After instilling the drug, flush the tube with water to ensure passage to the stomach and to clear the tube.

Evaluation
- Patient regains a normal bowel elimination pattern.
- Patient maintains a normal electrolyte balance.
- Patient and his family demonstrate an understanding of drug therapy. (See *Teaching about antacids*.)

> Laxatives, stool softeners, or antidiarrheals may be ordered to counteract the effects of antacids.

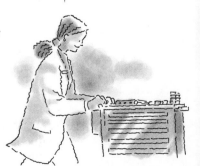

Education edge

Teaching about antacids

If antacids are prescribed, review these points with the patient and his caregivers:
• Don't take antacids indiscriminately or switch antacids without the prescriber's consent.
• Don't take calcium carbonate with milk or other foods high in vitamin D.

• Shake the suspension form well before taking it.
• Some antacids, such as aluminum hydroxide, may color stools white or cause white streaks.
• To prevent constipation, increase fluid and roughage intake and increase activity level.

H$_2$-receptor antagonists

H$_2$-receptor antagonists are commonly prescribed antiulcer drugs in the United States. Drugs in this category include:
• cimetidine
• famotidine
• nizatidine
• ranitidine.

Pharmacokinetics

Cimetidine, nizatidine, and ranitidine are absorbed rapidly and completely from the GI tract. Famotidine isn't completely absorbed. Food and antacids may reduce the absorption of H$_2$-receptor antagonists.

H$_2$-receptor antagonists are distributed widely throughout the body, metabolized by the liver, and excreted primarily in urine.

> Food and antacids may reduce my absorption, making it more difficult for me to achieve my peak performance.

Pharmacodynamics

H$_2$-receptor antagonists block histamine from stimulating the acid-secreting parietal cells of the stomach.

Really in a bind

Acid secretion in the stomach depends on the binding of gastrin, acetylcholine, and histamine to receptors on the parietal cells. If the binding of any one of these substances is blocked, acid secretion is reduced. By binding with H$_2$ receptors, H$_2$-receptor antagonists block the action of histamine in the stomach and reduce acid secretion. (See *H$_2$-receptor antagonists: Famotidine*, page 300.)

Pharmacotherapeutics

H_2-receptor antagonists are used therapeutically to:
- promote healing of duodenal and gastric ulcers
- provide long-term treatment of pathologic GI hypersecretory conditions such as Zollinger-Ellison syndrome
- reduce gastric acid production and prevent stress ulcers in severely ill patients and in those with reflux esophagitis or upper GI bleeding.

Drug interactions

H_2-receptor antagonists may interact with antacids and other drugs:
- Antacids reduce the absorption of cimetidine, nizatidine, ranitidine, and famotidine.
- Cimetidine may increase the blood levels of oral anticoagulants, propranolol (and possibly other beta-adrenergic blockers), benzodiazepines, tricyclic antidepressants, theophylline, procainamide, quinidine, lidocaine, phenytoin, calcium channel blockers, cyclosporine, carbamazepine, and opioid analgesics by reducing their metabolism in the liver and their subsequent excretion.
- Cimetidine taken with carmustine increases the risk of bone marrow toxicity.
- Cimetidine inhibits ethyl alcohol metabolism in the stomach, resulting in higher blood alcohol levels.

Adverse reactions

Using H_2-receptor antagonists may lead to adverse reactions, especially in elderly patients or in patients with altered hepatic or renal function:

A rash of reactions

- Cimetidine and ranitidine may produce headache, dizziness, malaise, muscle pain, nausea, diarrhea or constipation, rashes, itching, loss of sexual desire, gynecomastia (cimetidine), and impotence.
- Famotidine and nizatidine produce few adverse reactions, with headache being the most common, followed by constipation or diarrhea and rash.

Nursing process

These nursing process steps are appropriate for patients undergoing treatment with H_2-receptor antagonists.

Prototype pro

H_2-receptor antagonists: Famotidine

Actions
- Inhibits histamine's action at H_2 receptors in gastric parietal cells
- Reduces gastric acid output and concentration regardless of the stimulating agent (histamine, food, insulin, caffeine, betazole, or pentagastrin) or basal conditions

Indications
- Gastroesophageal reflux disease
- Zollinger-Ellison syndrome
- Duodenal ulcer
- Gastric ulcer
- Heartburn

Nursing considerations
- Monitor for adverse effects such as headache.
- Monitor for signs of GI bleeding such as blood in the patient's feces.

Assessment
- Assess for adverse reactions, especially hypotension and arrhythmias.
- Periodically monitor laboratory tests, such as complete blood count and renal and hepatic studies.

Key nursing diagnoses
- Impaired tissue integrity related to the patient's underlying condition
- Decreased cardiac output related to adverse cardiovascular effects (cimetidine)
- Deficient knowledge related to drug therapy

Planning outcome goals
- The patient's tissue integrity will improve as evidenced by a reduction in underlying symptoms.
- The patient will maintain adequate cardiac output as evidenced by stable vital signs and adequate urine output.
- The patient and his family will demonstrate an understanding of drug therapy.

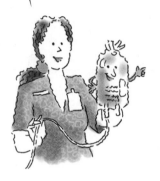

Be aware! Exceeding the recommended infusion rates when administering H_2-receptor antagonists I.V. increases the risk of adverse cardiovascular effects.

Implementation
- Administer a once-daily dose at bedtime to promote compliance. Twice-daily doses should be administered in the morning and evening; multiple doses, with meals and at bedtime.
- Don't exceed the recommended infusion rates when administering H_2-receptor antagonists I.V.; doing so increases the risk of adverse cardiovascular effects. Continuous I.V. infusion may suppress acid secretion more effectively.
- Administer antacids at least 1 hour before or after H_2-receptor antagonists. Antacids can decrease drug absorption.
- Anticipate dosage adjustments for the patient with renal disease.
- Avoid stopping the drug abruptly.

Evaluation
- Patient experiences decrease in or relief from upper GI symptoms with drug therapy.
- Patient maintains a normal heart rhythm.
- Patient and his family demonstrate an understanding of drug therapy. (See *Teaching about H_2-receptor antagonists*, page 302.)

Education edge

Teaching about H₂-receptor antagonists

If histamine-2 (H₂) receptor antagonists are prescribed, review these points with the patient and his caregivers:
• Take the drug with a snack if desired.
• Take the drug as prescribed; don't stop taking the drug suddenly.
• If taking the drug once daily, take it at bedtime for best results.
• Continue to take the drug even after pain subsides to allow for adequate healing.
• If the prescriber approves, you may also take antacids, especially at the beginning of therapy when pain is severe.
• Don't take antacids within 1 hour of taking an H₂-receptor antagonist.

• Don't take the drug for more than 8 weeks unless specifically ordered to do so by the prescriber.
• Don't self-medicate for heartburn longer than 2 weeks without consulting the prescriber.
• Be aware of possible adverse reactions, and report unusual effects.
• Avoid smoking during therapy; smoking stimulates gastric acid secretion and worsens the disease.
• Immediately report black tarry stools, diarrhea, confusion, or rash.
• Don't take other drugs, over-the-counter products, or herbal remedies without first consulting with the prescriber or a pharmacist.

Proton pump inhibitors

Proton pump inhibitors disrupt chemical binding in stomach cells to reduce acid production, lessening irritation and allowing peptic ulcers to better heal. They include:
• esomeprazole
• lansoprazole
• omeprazole
• pantoprazole
• rabeprazole.

Pharmacokinetics

Proton pump inhibitors are given orally in enteric-coated formulas to bypass the stomach because they're highly unstable in acid. They dissolve in the small intestine and are rapidly absorbed. Esomeprazole, lansoprazole, and pantoprazole can also be given I.V.

Bound and determined

These drugs are highly protein bound and extensively metabolized by the liver to inactive compounds and then eliminated in urine.

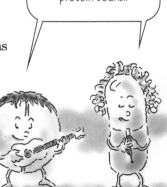

We just want to be-eee-eee-ee-eeee protein bound!

Pharmacodynamics

Proton pump inhibitors block the last step in gastric acid secretion by combining with hydrogen, potassium, and adenosine triphosphate in the parietal cells of the stomach. (See *Proton pump inhibitors: Omeprazole.*)

Pharmacotherapeutics

Proton pump inhibitors are indicated for:
- short-term treatment of active gastric ulcers
- active duodenal ulcers
- erosive esophagitis
- symptomatic GERD that isn't responsive to other therapies
- active peptic ulcers associated with *H. pylori* infection (in combination with antibiotics)
- long-term treatment of hypersecretory states such as Zollinger-Ellison syndrome.

Drug interactions

Proton pump inhibitors may interfere with the metabolism of diazepam, phenytoin, and warfarin, causing increased half-lives and elevated plasma concentrations of these drugs.

Proton pump interpHerence

Proton pump inhibitors may also interfere with the absorption of drugs that depend on gastric pH for absorption, such as ketoconazole, digoxin, ampicillin, and iron salts.

Adverse reactions

Adverse reactions to proton pump inhibitors include:
- abdominal pain
- diarrhea
- nausea and vomiting.

Nursing process

These nursing process steps are appropriate for patients undergoing treatment with proton pump inhibitors.

Assessment

- Assess the patient's condition before therapy and regularly thereafter.
- Assess the patient for adverse reactions and drug interactions.
- Monitor the patient's hydration status if adverse GI reactions occur.

Prototype pro

Proton pump inhibitors: Omeprazole

Actions
- Inhibits activity of acid (proton) pump and binds to hydrogen, potassium, and adenosine triphosphate, located at the secretory surface of the gastric parietal cells, to block gastric acid formation

Indications
- Gastroesophageal reflux disease
- Zollinger-Ellison syndrome
- Duodenal ulcer
- Gastric ulcer
- *Helicobacter pylori* infection

Nursing considerations
- Monitor the patient for adverse effects, such as headache, dizziness, and nausea.
- Administer the drug 30 minutes before meals.

• Assess the patient's and family's knowledge of drug therapy.

Key nursing diagnoses
• Impaired tissue integrity related to upper gastric disorder
• Risk for deficient fluid volume related to drug-induced adverse GI reactions
• Deficient knowledge related to drug therapy

Planning outcome goals
• The patient's tissue integrity will improve as evidenced by a reduction in presenting symptoms.
• The patient will maintain adequate fluid volume as evidenced by stable vital signs and urine output.
• The patient and his family will demonstrate an understanding of drug therapy.

Implementation
• Administer the drug 30 minutes before meals.
• Dosage adjustments aren't needed for patients with renal or hepatic impairment.
• Tell the patient to swallow capsules whole and not to open or crush them.
• When giving I.V. esomeprazole, lansoprazole, or pantoprazole, check the package insert and your facility's policy for reconstitution, compatibility, and infusion time information.

Evaluation
• Patient responds well to therapy.

> Remember: Give proton pump inhibitors 30 minutes before meals.

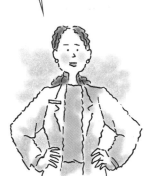

Education edge

Teaching about proton pump inhibitors

If proton pump inhibitors are prescribed, review these points with the patient and his caregivers:
• Take the drug before eating; however, oral pantoprazole may be taken with or without food.
• Swallow the tablets or capsules whole; don't crush or chew them. These formulations are delayed-release and long-acting; opening, crushing, or chewing them destroys the drug's effects.
• If swallowing capsules is difficult, lansoprazole capsules can be opened and mixed with 60 ml of apple, orange, vegetable, or tomato juice. Capsule contents can also be sprinkled on 1 table-spoon of applesauce, pudding, cottage cheese, or yogurt. Swallow the mixture immediately without chewing the granules.
• Observe for the drug's effects; if symptoms persist or adverse reactions (such as headache, diarrhea, abdominal pain, and nausea or vomiting) occur, notify the prescriber.
• Don't take over-the-counter preparations, other prescription drugs, or herbal remedies without first consulting with the prescriber.

• Patient maintains adequate hydration throughout therapy.
• Patient and his family demonstrate an understanding of drug therapy. (See *Teaching about proton pump inhibitors.*)

Other antiulcer drugs

Research on the usefulness of other drugs in treating peptic ulcer disease continues. Two other antiulcer drugs currently in use are:
• misoprostol (a synthetic prostaglandin E_1)
• sucralfate.

Pharmacokinetics

Each of these drugs has slightly different pharmacokinetic properties.

An active acid

After an oral dose, misoprostol is absorbed extensively and rapidly. It's metabolized to misoprostol acid, which is clinically active, meaning it can produce a pharmacologic effect. Misoprostol acid is highly protein bound and is excreted primarily in urine.

Goes on by the GI

Sucralfate is minimally absorbed from the GI tract. It's excreted in feces.

Pharmacodynamics

The actions of these drugs vary.

Reduce and boost

Misoprostol protects against peptic ulcers caused by NSAIDs by reducing the secretion of gastric acid and by boosting the production of gastric mucus, a natural defense against peptic ulcers.

A sticky situation

Sucralfate works locally in the stomach, rapidly reacting with hydrochloric acid to form a thick, pastelike substance that adheres to the gastric mucosa and especially to ulcers. By binding to the ulcer site, sucralfate actually protects the ulcer from the damaging effects of acid and pepsin to promote healing. This binding usually lasts for 6 hours.

Pharmacotherapeutics

Each of these drugs has its own therapeutic uses.

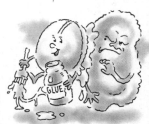

Once I get into the stomach, I stick like glue to ulcers like you!

Attention to prevention

Misoprostol prevents peptic ulcers caused by NSAIDs in patients at high risk for complications resulting from gastric ulcers.

To treat and prevent

Sucralfate is used for short-term treatment (up to 8 weeks) of duodenal or gastric ulcers and prevention of recurrent ulcers or stress ulcers.

Drug interactions

Misoprostol and sucralfate may interact with other drugs:
• Antacids may bind with misoprostol or decrease its absorption. However, this effect doesn't appear to be clinically significant.
• Cimetidine, digoxin, norfloxacin, phenytoin, fluoroquinolones, ranitidine, tetracycline, and theophylline decrease the absorption of sucralfate.
• Antacids may reduce the binding of sucralfate to the gastric and duodenal mucosa, reducing its effectiveness.

Adverse reactions

Adverse reactions to misoprostol include:
• diarrhea (common and usually dose-related)
• abdominal pain
• gas
• indigestion
• nausea and vomiting
• spontaneous abortion (women of childbearing age shouldn't become pregnant while taking misoprostol).
    Adverse reactions to sucralfate include:
• constipation
• nausea and vomiting
• metallic taste.

Nursing process

These nursing process steps are appropriate for patients undergoing treatment with the antiulcer drugs misoprostol and sucralfate.

Assessment

• Assess the patient's condition before therapy and regularly thereafter.
• Assess for adverse reactions and drug interactions.

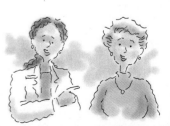

Make sure you discuss contraceptive methods or alternative treatment with women who are taking misoprostol. This drug can harm the fetus if pregnancy occurs.

Pregnancy precaution

- If a female patient is taking misoprostol, the drug can cause danger to the fetus if pregnancy occurs; discuss contraceptive methods or alternative treatment.
- Monitor the patient's hydration status if adverse GI reactions occur.
- Assess the patient's and family's understanding of drug therapy.

Key nursing diagnoses

- Impaired tissue integrity related to upper gastric disorder
- Risk for deficient fluid volume related to drug-induced adverse GI reactions
- Deficient knowledge related to drug therapy

Planning outcome goals

- The patient's tissue integrity will improve as evidenced by a reduction in presenting symptoms.
- The patient will maintain adequate fluid volume as evidenced by stable vital signs and urine output.
- The patient and his family will demonstrate an understanding of drug therapy.

Implementation

- Administer sucralfate 1 hour before meals and at bedtime.
- Administer misoprostol with food.
- Tell the patient to continue the prescribed regimen at home to ensure complete healing. Explain that pain and ulcerative symptoms may subside within the first few weeks of therapy.
- Urge the patient to avoid cigarette smoking because it may increase gastric acid secretion and worsen disease.

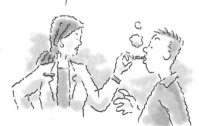

No butts about it! Cigarette smoking may increase gastric acid secretions and worsen ulcers.

The spice of life

- Tell the patient to avoid alcohol, chocolate, spicy foods, or anything that irritates his stomach.
- Elevate the head of the bed for comfort.
- Tell the patient to avoid large meals within 2 hours before bedtime.
- In women, start misoprostol therapy on the second or third day of the next normal menses to ensure that the patient isn't pregnant.

Evaluation

- Patient responds well to therapy.
- Patient maintains adequate hydration throughout therapy.
- Patient and his family demonstrate an understanding of drug therapy.

Adsorbent, antiflatulent, and digestive drugs

Adsorbent, antiflatulent, and digestive drugs aid healthy GI function. They're used to fight undesirable toxins, acids, and gases in the GI tract.

Adsorbent drugs

Natural and synthetic adsorbent drugs, or adsorbents, are prescribed as antidotes for the ingestion of toxins, substances that can lead to poisoning or overdose.

It's no picnic

The most commonly used clinical adsorbent is activated charcoal, a black powder residue obtained from the distillation of various organic materials.

Pharmacokinetics

Quick action required

Activated charcoal must be administered soon after toxic ingestion because activated charcoal can only bind with drugs or poisons that haven't yet been absorbed from the GI tract. Activated charcoal, which isn't absorbed or metabolized by the body, is excreted unchanged in feces.

A vicious cycle

After initial absorption, some poisons move back into the intestines, where they're reabsorbed. Activated charcoal may be administered repeatedly to break this cycle.

Pharmacodynamics

Because adsorbent drugs attract and bind toxins in the intestine, they inhibit toxins from being absorbed from the GI tract. However, this binding doesn't change toxic effects caused by earlier absorption of the poison.

Pharmacotherapeutics

Activated charcoal is a general-purpose antidote used for many types of acute oral poisoning. It isn't indicated in acute poisoning from mineral acids, alkalines, cyanide, ethanol, methanol, iron,

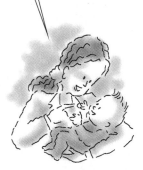

> Adsorbent drugs are used as antidotes to toxins.

> Children younger than age 1 shouldn't be given activated charcoal.

sodium chloride alkali, inorganic acids, or organic solvents. It also shouldn't be used in children younger than age 1. It shouldn't be used if the patient has a risk of GI obstruction, perforation, or hemorrhage; decreased or absent bowel sounds; or a history of recent GI surgery.

Drug interactions

Activated charcoal can decrease the absorption of oral medications; therefore, these medications (other than those used to treat the ingested toxin) shouldn't be taken orally within 2 hours of taking activated charcoal. Drugs used to induce vomiting, such as ipecac syrup, may decrease the effectiveness of activated charcoal. If these drugs are used together to treat oral poisoning, activated charcoal should be used only after vomiting has stopped.

Adverse reactions

Activated charcoal turns stool black and may cause constipation. A laxative such as sorbitol is usually given with activated charcoal to prevent constipation and improve taste.

Nursing process

These nursing process steps are appropriate for patients undergoing treatment with adsorbent drugs.

Assessment

• Obtain a history of the substance reportedly ingested, including time of ingestion, if possible. Activated charcoal isn't effective for all drugs and toxic substances.
• Assess for adverse reactions and drug interactions.
• Assess the patient's and family's knowledge of drug therapy.

Key nursing diagnoses

• Risk for injury related to ingestion of toxic substance or overdose
• Risk for deficient fluid volume related to drug-induced vomiting
• Deficient knowledge related to drug therapy

Planning outcome goals

• The patient's risk of injury will be minimized.
• The patient will maintain adequate fluid volume status as evidenced by stable vital signs and urine output.
• The patient and his family will demonstrate an understanding of drug therapy.

Implementation

• Don't give the drug to a semiconscious or unconscious patient unless the airway is protected and an NG tube is in place for instillation.
• Mix the powdered form with tap water to form the consistency of thick syrup. Add a small amount of fruit juice or flavoring to make it more palatable.
• Give by NG tube after lavage if needed.

Down with dairy

• Don't give the drug in ice cream, milk, or sherbet; these may reduce absorption.
• Repeat the dose if the patient vomits shortly after administration.
• Keep airway, oxygen, and suction equipment nearby.
• Follow treatment with a stool softener or laxative to prevent constipation.
• Tell the patient that his stools will be black.

Evaluation

• Patient doesn't experience injury from ingesting toxic substance or from overdose.
• Patient exhibits no signs of deficient fluid volume.
• Patient and his family demonstrate an understanding of drug therapy.

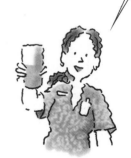

Here's a tip: Once you've mixed the powdered form of the adsorbent with tap water, add a small amount of fruit juice to make it more palatable.

Antiflatulent drugs

Antiflatulent drugs, or antiflatulents, disperse gas pockets in the GI tract. They're available alone or in combination with antacids. The major antiflatulent drug currently in use is simethicone.

Pharmacokinetics

Simethicone isn't absorbed from the GI tract. It's distributed only in the intestinal lumen and is eliminated intact in feces.

Pharmacodynamics

Simethicone creates foaming action in the GI tract. It produces a film in the intestines that disperses mucus-enclosed gas pockets and helps prevent their formation.

Pharmacotherapeutics

Simethicone is prescribed to treat conditions in which excess gas is a problem, such as:

- functional gastric bloating
- postoperative gaseous bloating
- diverticular disease
- spastic or irritable colon
- the swallowing of air.

Drug interactions

Simethicone doesn't interact significantly with other drugs.

Adverse reactions

Simethicone doesn't cause any known adverse reactions. It has, however, been associated with excessive belching or flatus.

Nursing process

These nursing process steps are appropriate for patients undergoing treatment with antiflatulent drugs.

Assessment
- Assess the patient's condition before therapy and regularly thereafter.
- Assess for adverse GI reactions.
- Assess the patient's and family's knowledge of drug therapy.

Key nursing diagnoses
- Acute pain related to gas in the GI tract
- Deficient knowledge related to drug therapy

Planning outcome goals
- The patient's pain will decrease.
- The patient and his family will demonstrate an understanding of drug therapy.

Implementation
- Make sure that the patient chews the tablet form before swallowing.

A shaky situation
- If giving the suspension form, make sure to shake the bottle or container thoroughly to distribute the solution.
- Inform the patient that the drug doesn't prevent gas formation.
- Encourage the patient to change his position frequently and to ambulate to help pass flatus.

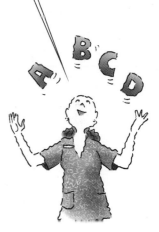

Antiflatulent drugs treat excess air or gas in the stomach or intestine. And that's how you spell relief!

Evaluation

- Patient's gas pain is relieved.
- Patient and his family demonstrate an understanding of drug therapy.

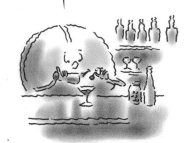

Here's your suspension—shaken, not stirred.

Digestive drugs

Digestive drugs (also called *digestants*) aid digestion in patients who are missing enzymes or other substances needed to digest food. Digestive drugs that function in the GI tract, liver, and pancreas include:

- dehydrocholic acid
- pancreatic enzymes (pancreatin, pancrelipase, lipase, protease, and amylase).

Pharmacokinetics

Digestive drugs aren't absorbed; they act locally in the GI tract and are excreted in feces.

Pharmacodynamics

The action of digestive drugs resembles the action of the body substances they replace. Dehydrocholic acid, a bile acid, increases the output of bile in the liver.

The enzyme effect

The pancreatic enzymes replace missing or deficient normal pancreatic enzymes. They exert their effect in the duodenum and upper jejunum of the upper GI tract. These drugs contain trypsin to digest proteins, amylase to digest carbohydrates, and lipase to digest fats.

Pharmacotherapeutics

Because their action resembles the action of the body substances they replace, each digestive drug has its own indication.

Go with the flow

Dehydrocholic acid, a bile acid, provides temporary relief from constipation and promotes bile flow.

For the enzyme impaired

Pancreatic enzymes are administered to patients with insufficient levels of pancreatic enzymes, such as those with pancreatitis or cystic fibrosis. They may also be used to treat steatorrhea (a disorder of fat metabolism characterized by fatty, foul-smelling stools). (See *Pancreatic enzymes warning*.)

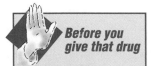

Before you give that drug

Pancreatic enzymes warning

Pancreatic enzymes should be given before meals. This ensures that the drug is available in the small intestine to help digestion. Giving pancreatic enzymes at another time, such as 1 hour or more after eating or during a meal, decreases the drug's effectiveness.

Drug interactions

Antacids reduce the effects of pancreatic enzymes and shouldn't be given at the same time. Pancreatic enzymes may also decrease the absorption of folic acid and iron.

Adverse reactions

Adverse reactions to dehydrocholic acid include:
* abdominal cramping
* biliary colic (with gallstone obstruction of the biliary duct)
* diarrhea.
  Adverse reactions to pancreatic enzymes include:
* diarrhea
* nausea
* abdominal cramping.

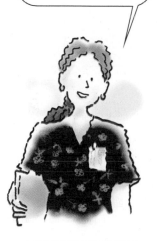

Patients with pancreatitis or cystic fibrosis may require pancreatic enzyme administration because their bodies may not produce enough on their own.

Nursing process

These nursing process steps are appropriate for patients undergoing treatment with digestive drugs.

Assessment

* Assess the patient's condition before therapy and regularly thereafter. A decrease in the number of bowel movements and improved stool consistency indicate effective therapy.
* Monitor the patient's diet to ensure a proper balance of fat, protein, and starch intake. This helps avoid indigestion. The dosage varies according to the degree of maldigestion and malabsorption, the amount of fat in the diet, and the enzyme activity of the drug.
* Assess the patient's and family's knowledge of drug therapy.
* Assess the patient's and family's knowledge and attitudes about nutrition.

Key nursing diagnoses

* Imbalanced nutrition: Less than body requirements related to the condition
* Noncompliance related to long-term therapy
* Deficient knowledge related to drug therapy

Planning outcome goals

* The patient's nutritional status will improve as evidenced by laboratory tests and weight.
* The patient will comply with the prescribed drug regimen.
* The patient and his family will demonstrate an understanding of drug therapy.

A balanced diet, including adequate fat, protein, and starch intake, will prevent indigestion.

Implementation
- Administer the drug before or with each meal as applicable.
- For older infants, the powdered form may be mixed with applesauce and given before meals.
- Avoid contact with or inhalation of the powder form; it may be irritating.
- Older children may take capsules with food.
- Tell the patient not to crush or chew enteric-coated dosage forms. Capsules containing enteric-coated microspheres may be opened and their contents sprinkled on a small amount of soft food, such as applesauce. Follow administration with a glass of water or juice.
- Review food preferences and diet orders with the patient and his family.
- Provide food and fluids that the patient enjoys at times he prefers, if possible.
- Treat signs and symptoms or disorders that may interfere with nutrition, such as pain, nausea, vomiting, or diarrhea.
- Consult with a dietitian if special diets are ordered. Provide foods the patient likes, selecting nutritionally better choices that fall within the prescribed diet.

Evaluation
- Patient maintains normal digestion of fats, carbohydrates, and proteins.
- Patient complies with the prescribed drug regimen.
- Patient and his family demonstrate an understanding of drug therapy. (See *Teaching about digestive drugs.*)

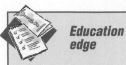

Education edge

Teaching about digestive drugs

If digestive drugs are prescribed, review these points with the patient and his caregivers:
- Exercise and stay active to aid the digestion and improve appetite.
- Minimize the use of strong pain medications and sedatives because these drugs may cause drowsiness and deter eating and drinking.
- Have routine check-ups to monitor weight, fluid intake, urine output, and laboratory studies and to assess nutritional outcome.

Antidiarrheal and laxative drugs

Diarrhea and constipation represent the two major symptoms related to disturbances of the large intestine.

Antidiarrheals act systemically or locally and include:
- opioid-related drugs
- kaolin and pectin (a combination drug and the only one that acts locally).

Laxatives stimulate defecation and include:
- hyperosmolar drugs
- dietary fiber and related bulk-forming substances
- emollients
- stimulants
- lubricants.

5-HT$_3$-receptor antagonists are used to treat irritable bowel syndrome (IBS), a disorder of the colon that's characterized by constipation or diarrhea.

Opioid-related drugs

> Opioid-related drugs decrease the wavelike movement of peristalsis. Cowabunga!

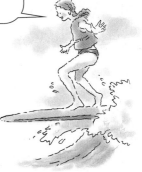

Opioid-related drugs decrease peristalsis (involuntary, progressive wavelike intestinal movement that pushes fecal matter along) in the intestines and include:
- diphenoxylate with atropine
- loperamide.

Pharmacokinetics

Diphenoxylate with atropine is readily absorbed from the GI tract. However, loperamide isn't absorbed well after oral administration.

Both drugs are distributed in serum, metabolized in the liver, and excreted primarily in feces. Diphenoxylate with atropine is metabolized to difenoxin, its biologically active major metabolite.

Pharmacodynamics

Diphenoxylate with atropine and loperamide slow GI motility by depressing the circular and longitudinal muscle action (peristalsis) in the large and small intestines. These drugs also decrease expulsive contractions throughout the colon.

Pharmacotherapeutics

Diphenoxylate with atropine and loperamide are used to treat acute, nonspecific diarrhea. Loperamide is also used to treat chronic diarrhea. (See *Antidiarrheals: Loperamide*.)

Drug interactions

Diphenoxylate with atropine, and loperamide may enhance the depressant effects of barbiturates, alcohol, opioids, tranquilizers, and sedatives.

Adverse reactions

Adverse reactions to diphenoxylate with atropine and loperamide include:
- nausea
- vomiting
- abdominal discomfort or distention
- drowsiness
- fatigue
- central nervous system (CNS) depression
- tachycardia
- paralytic ileus (reduced or absent peristalsis in the intestines).

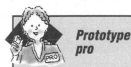

Prototype pro

Antidiarrheals: Loperamide

Actions
- Inhibits peristaltic activity, prolonging transit of intestinal contents

Indications
- Diarrhea

Nursing considerations
- Monitor the drug's effect on bowel movements.
- If giving by nasogastric tube, flush the tube to clear it and to ensure the drug's passage to the stomach.
- Oral liquids are available in different concentrations. Check the dosage carefully.
- For children, consider an oral liquid that doesn't contain alcohol.

Nursing process

These nursing process steps are appropriate for patients undergoing treatment with opioid-related drugs.

Assessment

• Assess the patient's condition before therapy and regularly thereafter.
• Assess the patient's diarrhea before therapy and regularly thereafter.
• Monitor the patient's fluid and electrolyte balance.
• Monitor the patient's hydration status if adverse GI reactions occur.
• Evaluate the patient for adverse reactions.
• Assess the patient's and family's knowledge of drug therapy.

Key nursing diagnoses

• Diarrhea related to the underlying condition
• Risk for deficient fluid volume related to GI upset
• Deficient knowledge related to drug therapy

Planning outcome goals

• The patient will have normal bowel movements.
• The patient will maintain adequate fluid balance as evidenced by intake and output.
• The patient and his family will demonstrate an understanding of drug therapy.

Implementation

• Administer the drug exactly as prescribed.
• Correct fluid and electrolyte disturbances before starting the drug; dehydration may increase the risk of delayed toxicity in some cases.
• Use naloxone to treat respiratory depression caused by overdose.
• Take safety precautions if the patient experiences adverse CNS reactions.
• Notify the prescriber about serious or persistent adverse reactions.

Evaluation

• Patient's diarrhea is relieved.
• Patient maintains adequate hydration.
• Patient and his family demonstrate an understanding of drug therapy. (See *Teaching about antidiarrheals*.)

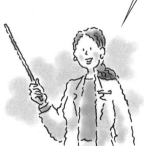

Before giving antidiarrheals, make sure you correct fluid and electrolyte disturbances, which may cause dehydration.

Education edge

Teaching about antidiarrheals

If antidiarrheals are prescribed, review these points with the patient and his caregivers:
• Take the drug exactly as prescribed; be aware that excessive use of opium preparations can lead to dependence.
• Notify your prescriber if diarrhea lasts for more than 2 days, if acute abdominal signs and symptoms occur, or if the drug is ineffective.

• Avoid hazardous activities that require alertness if central nervous system depression occurs.
• Maintain intake of fluids and electrolytes, up to 2 to 3 qt (2 to 3 L) per day.
• Avoid food and fluids that can irritate the GI tract while diarrhea is present.
• Schedule rest periods and decrease activity while diarrhea persists to reduce peristalsis.

Kaolin and pectin

Kaolin and pectin mixtures are locally acting OTC antidiarrheals. They work by adsorbing irritants and soothing the intestinal mucosa.

Pharmacokinetics

Kaolin and pectin aren't absorbed and, therefore, aren't distributed throughout the body. They're excreted in feces.

Pharmacodynamics

Kaolin and pectin act as adsorbents, binding with bacteria, toxins, and other irritants on the intestinal mucosa.

A kinder, gentler pH

Pectin decreases the pH in the intestinal lumen and provides a soothing effect on irritated mucosa.

Pharmacotherapeutics

Kaolin and pectin are used to relieve mild to moderate acute diarrhea.

Just a stopgap

They also may be used to temporarily relieve chronic diarrhea until the cause is determined and definitive treatment starts.

Drug interactions

These antidiarrheals can interfere with the absorption of digoxin or other drugs from the intestinal mucosa if administered at the same time.

Adverse reactions

Kaolin and pectin mixtures cause few adverse reactions. However, constipation may occur, especially in elderly or debilitated patients or in cases of overdose or prolonged use.

Nursing process

These nursing process steps are appropriate for patients undergoing treatment with kaolin and pectin.

Assessment
• Assess the patient's condition before therapy and regularly thereafter.
• Assess the patient's diarrhea before therapy and regularly thereafter.
• Monitor fluid and electrolyte balance.
• Assess the patient for adverse reactions.
• Assess the patient's and family's knowledge of drug therapy.

Key nursing diagnoses
• Diarrhea related to the underlying condition
• Risk for deficient fluid volume related to GI upset
• Deficient knowledge related to drug therapy

Planning outcome goals
• The patient will have normal bowel movements.
• The patient will maintain adequate fluid balance as evidenced by intake and output.
• The patient and his family will demonstrate an understanding of drug therapy.

Implementation
• Administer the drug exactly as prescribed.
• Correct fluid and electrolyte disturbances before starting the drug; dehydration may increase the risk of delayed toxicity in some cases.
• Take safety precautions if the patient experiences adverse CNS reactions.
• Notify the prescriber about serious or persistent adverse reactions.

Kaolin and pectin may cause constipation, especially in elderly or debilitated patients.

Evaluation
- Patient's diarrhea is relieved.
- Patient maintains adequate hydration.
- Patient and his family demonstrate an understanding of drug therapy.

Hyperosmolar laxatives

Hyperosmolar laxatives work by drawing water into the intestine, thereby promoting bowel distention and peristalsis. They include:
- glycerin
- lactulose
- saline compounds, such as magnesium salts, sodium biphosphate, sodium phosphate, polyethylene glycol (PEG), and electrolytes.

Pharmacokinetics

The pharmacokinetic properties of hyperosmolar laxatives vary. Glycerin is placed directly into the colon by enema or suppository and isn't absorbed systemically.

Intestine marks the spot

Lactulose enters the GI tract orally and is minimally absorbed. As a result, the drug is distributed only in the intestine. It's metabolized by bacteria in the colon and excreted in feces.

Saline away

After saline compounds are introduced into the GI tract orally or as an enema, some of their ions are absorbed. Absorbed ions are excreted in urine, the unabsorbed drug in feces.

And then there's PEG

PEG is a nonabsorbable solution that acts as an osmotic drug but doesn't alter electrolyte balance.

Pharmacodynamics

Hyperosmolar laxatives produce a bowel movement by drawing water into the intestine. Fluid accumulation distends the bowel and promotes peristalsis and a bowel movement. (See *Hyperosmolar laxatives: Magnesium hydroxide*, page 320.)

Pharmacotherapeutics

The uses of hyperosmolar laxatives vary:
- Glycerin is helpful in bowel retraining.

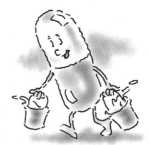

I come bearing water to help promote peristalsis!

Prototype pro

Hyperosmolar laxatives: Magnesium hydroxide

Actions
- Reduces total acid in the GI tract
- Elevates gastric pH to reduce pepsin activity
- Strengthens the gastric mucosal barrier
- Increases esophageal sphincter tone

Indications
- Upset stomach
- Constipation
- Inadequate magnesium level

Nursing considerations
- Monitor the drug's effect on bowel movements.
- Shake the suspension well. Give the drug with a large amount of water when used as a laxative.
- When used with a nasogastric tube, make sure the tube is placed properly and is patent. After instilling the drug, flush the tube with water to ensure passage to the stomach and to maintain tube patency.

- Lactulose is used to treat constipation and help reduce ammonia production and absorption from the intestines in liver disease.
- Saline compounds are used when prompt and complete bowel evacuation is required.

Drug interactions

Hyperosmolar laxatives don't interact significantly with other drugs. However, the absoprtion of oral drugs administered 1 hour before PEG is significantly decreased.

Adverse reactions

Adverse reactions to hyperosmolar laxatives involve fluid and electrolyte imbalances.
Adverse reactions to glycerin include:
- weakness
- fatigue.
Lactulose may cause these adverse reactions:
- abdominal distention, gas, and abdominal cramps
- nausea and vomiting
- diarrhea
- hypokalemia
- hypovolemia
- increased blood glucose level.
Adverse reactions to saline compounds include:
- weakness
- lethargy

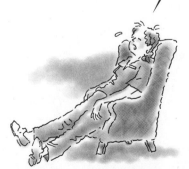

Adverse reactions to glycerin includes weakness and fatigue.

- dehydration
- hypernatremia
- hypermagnesemia
- hyperphosphatemia
- hypocalcemia
- cardiac arrhythmias
- shock.
    These adverse reactions may occur with PEG:
- nausea
- abdominal fullness
- explosive diarrhea
- bloating.

Nursing process

These nursing process steps are appropriate for patients undergoing treatment with hyperosmolar laxatives.

Assessment
- Obtain a baseline assessment of the patient's bowel patterns and GI history before giving a laxative.
- Determine whether the patient maintains adequate fluid intake and diet and whether he exercises.
- Assess the patient's bowel pattern throughout therapy. Assess bowel sounds and color and consistency of stools.
- Monitor the patient's fluid and electrolyte status during administration.
- Assess for adverse reactions and drug interactions.
- Assess the patient's and family's knowledge of drug therapy.

Key nursing diagnoses
- Diarrhea related to adverse GI effects
- Acute pain related to abdominal discomfort
- Deficient knowledge related to drug therapy

Planning outcome goals
- The patient will maintain regular bowel movements.
- The patient's pain will decrease.
- The patient and his family will demonstrate an understanding of drug therapy.

Implementation
- Time drug administration so that bowel evacuation doesn't interfere with scheduled activities or sleep.
- Shake suspensions well; give with a large amount of water as applicable.

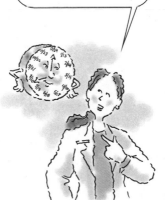

Schedule laxative administration so that the drug's effects don't interfere with the patient's activities or sleep.

• If administering the drug through an NG tube, make sure that the tube is placed properly and is patent. After instilling the drug, flush the tube with water to ensure passage to the stomach and to maintain tube patency.

• Don't crush enteric-coated tablets.

• Make sure that the patient has easy access to a bedpan or bathroom.

• Institute measures to prevent constipation.

Evaluation

• Patient regains normal bowel elimination pattern.

• Patient states that pain is relieved with stool evacuation.

• Patient and his family demonstrate an understanding of drug therapy.

Dietary fiber and related bulk-forming laxatives

A high-fiber diet is the most natural way to prevent or treat constipation. Dietary fiber is the part of plants not digested in the small intestine.

Close resemblance

Bulk-forming laxatives, which resemble dietary fiber, contain natural and semisynthetic polysaccharides and cellulose. These laxatives include:

• methylcellulose

• polycarbophil

• psyllium hydrophilic mucilloid.

Pharmacokinetics

Dietary fiber and bulk-forming laxatives aren't absorbed systemically. The polysaccharides in these drugs are converted by intestinal bacterial flora into osmotically active metabolites that draw water into the intestine. Dietary fiber and bulk-forming laxatives are excreted in feces.

Pharmacodynamics

Dietary fiber and bulk-forming laxatives increase stool mass and water content, promoting peristalsis. (See *Bulk-forming laxatives: Psyllium.*)

Pharmacotherapeutics

Bulk-forming laxatives are used to:

• treat simple cases of constipation, especially constipation resulting from a low-fiber or low-fluid diet

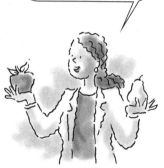

A high-fiber diet is the most natural way to prevent or treat constipation, but bulk-forming laxatives can offer a little help if nature isn't cooperating!

Prototype pro

Bulk-forming laxatives: Psyllium

Actions
• Absorbs water and expands to increase bulk and moisture content of stool, thus encouraging peristalsis and bowel movements

Indications
• Constipation

Nursing considerations
• Mix the drug with at least 8 oz (240 ml) of cold, pleasant-tasting liquid such as orange juice to mask grittiness. Stir only a few seconds. Have the patient drink the mixture immediately, before it congeals. Follow administration with another glass of liquid.
• Psyllium may reduce the patient's appetite if taken before meals.
• This drug isn't absorbed systemically and is nontoxic.
• Psyllium is useful in debilitated patients and in patients with postpartum constipation, irritable bowel syndrome, or diverticular disease. It's also used to treat chronic laxative abuse and combined with other laxatives to empty the colon before barium enema examination.
• Advise patients with diabetes to check the drug's label and to use a brand that doesn't contain sugar.

• aid patients recovering from acute myocardial infarction (MI) or cerebral aneurysms who need to avoid Valsalva's maneuver (forced expiration against a closed airway) and maintain soft stool
• manage patients with IBS and diverticulosis.

Drug interactions

Decreased absorption of digoxin, warfarin, and salicylates occurs if these drugs are taken within 2 hours of fiber or bulk-forming laxatives.

Adverse reactions

Adverse reactions to dietary fiber and related bulk-forming laxatives include:
• flatulence
• a sensation of abdominal fullness
• intestinal obstruction
• fecal impaction (hard feces that can't be removed from the rectum)
• esophageal obstruction (if sufficient liquid hasn't been administered with the drug)
• severe diarrhea.

Nursing process

These nursing process steps are appropriate for patients undergoing treatment with dietary fiber and bulk-forming laxatives.

Assessment

- Obtain a baseline assessment of the patient's bowel patterns and GI history before giving a laxative.
- Assess the patient for adverse reactions and drug interactions.
- Monitor the patient's bowel pattern throughout therapy. Assess bowel sounds and color and consistency of stools.
- Assess the patient's fluid and electrolyte status during administration.
- Determine whether the patient maintains adequate fluid intake and diet and whether he exercises regularly.
- Assess the patient's and family's knowledge of drug therapy.

Key nursing diagnoses

- Diarrhea related to adverse GI effects
- Acute pain related to abdominal discomfort
- Deficient knowledge related to drug therapy

Planning outcome goals

- The patient will maintain regular bowel movements.
- The patient's pain will decrease.
- The patient and his family will demonstrate an understanding of drug therapy.

Implementation

- Time drug administration so that the drug's effects don't interfere with scheduled activities or sleep.
- Mix drugs as directed and give with a large amount of water, as applicable.
- Don't crush enteric-coated tablets.
- Keep in mind that the laxative effect usually occurs in 12 to 24 hours but may be delayed for up to 3 days.
- Make sure that the patient has easy access to a bedpan or bathroom.
- Institute measures to prevent constipation.

Evaluation

- Patient regains normal bowel elimination pattern.
- Patient states that pain is relieved with stool evacuation.
- Patient and his family demonstrate an understanding of drug therapy.

Emollient laxatives

Emollient laxatives—also known as *stool softeners*—include the calcium, potassium, and sodium salts of docusate.

Pharmacokinetics

Administered orally, emollient laxatives are absorbed and excreted through bile in feces.

Pharmacodynamics

Emollient laxatives emulsify the fat and water components of feces in the small and large intestines. This detergent action allows water and fats to penetrate the stool, making it softer and easier to eliminate. Emollients also stimulate electrolyte and fluid secretion from intestinal mucosal cells. (See *Emollient laxatives: Docusate.*)

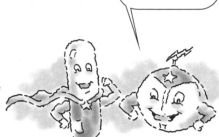

Prepare to emulsify!

Pharmacotherapeutics

Emollient laxatives are the drugs of choice for softening stools in patients who should avoid straining during a bowel movement, including those with:
- recent MI or surgery
- disease of the anus or rectum
- increased intracranial pressure (ICP)
- hernias.

Drug interactions

Taking oral doses of mineral oil with oral emollient laxatives increases the systemic absorption of mineral oil. This increased absorption may result in tissue deposits of the oil.

Prototype pro

Emollient laxatives: Docusate

Actions
- Reduces surface tension of interfacing liquid contents of the bowel, promoting incorporation of additional liquid into stool, thus forming a softer mass

Indications
- Stool softener for patients who should avoid straining during a bowel movement

Nursing considerations
- Monitor the drug's effect on bowel movements.

- Be alert for adverse reactions and drug interactions.
- This drug is the laxative of choice for patients who shouldn't strain during defecation (including those recovering from myocardial infarction or rectal surgery), for patients with rectal or anal disease that makes passage of firm stool difficult, and for patients with postpartum constipation.
- Discontinue the drug if abdominal cramping occurs and notify the prescriber.
- Docusate doesn't stimulate intestinal peristaltic movements.

Proceed with caution

Because emollient laxatives may enhance the absorption of many oral drugs, drugs with low margins of safety (narrow therapeutic index) should be administered cautiously.

Adverse reactions

Although adverse reactions to emollient laxatives seldom occur, they may include:
• a bitter taste
• diarrhea
• throat irritation
• mild, transient abdominal cramping.

Nursing process

These nursing process steps are appropriate for patients undergoing treatment with emollient laxatives.

Assessment

• Obtain a baseline assessment of the patient's bowel patterns and GI history before giving a laxative.
• Assess the patient for adverse reactions and drug interactions.
• Monitor the patient's bowel pattern throughout therapy. Assess bowel sounds and color and consistency of stools.
• Assess the patient's fluid and electrolyte status during administration.
• Determine whether the patient maintains adequate fluid intake and diet and whether he exercises.
• Assess the patient's and family's knowledge of drug therapy.

Key nursing diagnoses

• Diarrhea related to adverse GI effects
• Acute pain related to abdominal discomfort
• Deficient knowledge related to drug therapy

Planning outcome goals

• The patient will maintain regular bowel movements.
• The patient's pain will decrease.
• The patient and his family will demonstrate an understanding of drug therapy.

Implementation

• Time drug administration so that bowel evacuation doesn't interfere with scheduled activities or sleep.
• Shake suspensions well; give with a large amount of water as applicable.

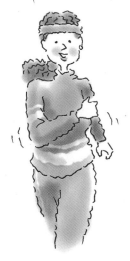

Determine whether the patient maintains adequate fluid intake and diet and whether he exercises.

Don't forget to flush

- If administering the drug through an NG tube, make sure that the tube is placed properly and is patent. After instilling the drug, flush the tube with water to ensure passage to the stomach and to maintain tube patency.
- Don't crush enteric-coated tablets.
- Make sure that the patient has easy access to a bedpan or bathroom.
- Institute measures to prevent constipation.

Evaluation

- Patient regains normal bowel elimination pattern.
- Patient states that pain is relieved with stool evacuation.
- Patient and his family demonstrate an understanding of drug therapy.

Stimulant laxatives

Stimulant laxatives, also known as *irritant cathartics*, include:
- bisacodyl
- cascara sagrada
- castor oil
- senna.

Pharmacokinetics

Stimulant laxatives are minimally absorbed and are metabolized in the liver. The metabolites are excreted in urine and feces.

Pharmacodynamics

Stimulant laxatives stimulate peristalsis and produce a bowel movement by irritating the intestinal mucosa or stimulating nerve endings of the intestinal smooth muscle.

Powering up peristalsis

Castor oil also increases peristalsis in the small intestine.

Pharmacotherapeutics

Stimulant laxatives are the preferred drugs for emptying the bowel before general surgery, sigmoidoscopic or proctoscopic procedures, and radiologic procedures such as barium studies of the GI tract.

> Stimulant laxatives are used to empty the bowel before general surgery, sigmoidoscopic or proctoscopic procedures, and radiologic procedures.

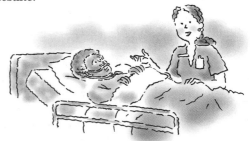

Conquering constipation

Besides their use before surgery and procedures, stimulant laxatives are used to treat constipation caused by prolonged bed rest, neurologic dysfunction of the colon, and constipating drugs such as opioids.

Drug interactions

No significant drug interactions occur with stimulant laxatives. However, because stimulant laxatives produce increased intestinal motility, they reduce the absorption of other oral drugs administered at the same time, especially sustained-release forms.

Adverse reactions

Adverse reactions to stimulant laxatives include:
• weakness
• nausea
• abdominal cramps
• mild inflammation of the rectum and anus
• urine discoloration (with cascara sagrada or senna use).

Nursing process

These nursing process steps are appropriate for patients undergoing treatment with stimulant laxatives.

Assessment
• Obtain a baseline assessment of the patient's bowel patterns and GI history before giving a laxative.
• Assess the patient for adverse reactions and drug interactions.
• Monitor the patient's bowel pattern throughout therapy. Assess bowel sounds and color and consistency of stools.
• Assess the patient's fluid and electrolyte status during administration.
• Determine whether the patient maintains adequate fluid intake and diet and whether he exercises.
• Assess the patient's and family's knowledge of drug therapy.

Key nursing diagnoses
• Diarrhea related to adverse GI effects
• Acute pain related to abdominal discomfort
• Deficient knowledge related to drug therapy

Planning outcome goals
• The patient will maintain regular bowel movements.

• The patient's pain will decrease.
• The patient and his family will demonstrate an understanding of drug therapy.

Implementation

• Time drug administration so that bowel evacuation doesn't interfere with scheduled activities or sleep.
• Shake suspensions well; give with a large amount of water as indicated.
• If administering the drug through an NG tube, make sure that the tube is placed properly and is patent. After instilling the drug, flush the tube with water to ensure passage to the stomach and to maintain tube patency.
• Don't crush enteric-coated tablets.
• Make sure that the patient has easy access to a bedpan or bathroom.
• Institute measures to prevent constipation.

Evaluation

• Patient regains normal bowel elimination pattern.
• Patient states that pain is relieved with stool evacuation.
• Patient and his family demonstrate an understanding of drug therapy.

Lubricant laxatives

Mineral oil is the main lubricant laxative in current clinical use.

Pharmacokinetics

In its nonemulsified form, mineral oil is minimally absorbed; the emulsified form is about half absorbed.

Mineral oil on the move

Absorbed mineral oil is distributed to the mesenteric lymph nodes, intestinal mucosa, liver, and spleen. Mineral oil is metabolized by the liver and excreted in feces. (See *Lubricant laxatives: Mineral oil.*)

Pharmacodynamics

Mineral oil lubricates the stool and the intestinal mucosa and prevents water reabsorption from the bowel lumen. The increased fluid content of feces increases peristalsis. Rectal administration by enema also produces distention.

Prototype pro

Lubricant laxatives: Mineral oil

Actions
• Increases water retention in stool by creating a barrier between the colon wall and feces that prevents colonic reabsorption of fecal water

Indications
• Constipation

Nursing considerations
• Monitor the drug's effect on bowel movements.
• Be alert for adverse reactions and drug interactions.
• Give the drug on an empty stomach.
• Give the drug with fruit juice or a carbonated drink to disguise its taste.

Pharmacotherapeutics

Mineral oil is used to treat constipation and maintain soft stools when straining is contraindicated, such as after a recent MI (to avoid Valsalva's maneuver), eye surgery (to prevent increased pressure in the eye), or cerebral aneurysm repair (to avoid increased ICP). Administered orally or by enema, mineral oil is also used to treat patients with fecal impaction.

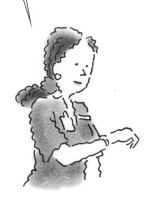

You can minimize drug interactions by giving mineral oil at least 2 hours before other drugs.

Drug interactions

To minimize drug interactions, administer mineral oil at least 2 hours before other drugs. These drug interactions may occur:
• Mineral oil may impair the absorption of many oral drugs, including fat-soluble vitamins, hormonal contraceptives, and anticoagulants.
• Mineral oil may interfere with the antibacterial activity of nonabsorbable sulfonamides.

Adverse reactions

Adverse reactions to mineral oil include:
• nausea
• vomiting
• diarrhea
• abdominal cramping.

Nursing process

These nursing process steps are appropriate for patients undergoing treatment with lubricant laxatives.

Assessment

• Obtain a baseline assessment of the patient's bowel patterns and GI history before giving a laxative.
• Assess the patient for adverse reactions and drug interactions.
• Monitor the patient's bowel pattern throughout therapy. Assess bowel sounds and color and consistency of stools.
• Assess the patient's fluid and electrolyte status during administration.
• Determine whether the patient maintains adequate fluid intake and diet and whether he exercises.
• Assess the patient's and family's knowledge of drug therapy.

Key nursing diagnoses

• Diarrhea related to adverse GI effects
• Acute pain related to abdominal discomfort
• Deficient knowledge related to drug therapy

Education edge

Teaching about laxatives

If laxatives are prescribed, review these points with the patient and his caregivers:
• Therapy should be short term. Abuse or prolonged use can result in nutritional imbalances.
• Diet, exercise, and fluid intake are important in maintaining normal bowel function and preventing or treating constipation.
• Drink at least 6 to 10 glasses (8 oz each) of fluid daily, unless contraindicated.
• Exercise regularly to help with bowel elimination.
• Stool softeners and bulk-forming laxatives may take several days to achieve results.

• If using a bulk-forming laxative, remain active and drink plenty of fluids.
• Stimulant laxatives may cause harmless urine discoloration.
• Include foods high in fiber, such as bran and other cereals, fresh fruit, and vegetables, in your diet.
• Frequent or prolonged use of some laxatives can result in dependence.
• Never take laxatives when experiencing acute abdominal pain, nausea, or vomiting. A ruptured appendix or other serious complication may result.
• Notify the prescriber if signs and symptoms persist or if the laxative doesn't work.

Planning outcome goals
• The patient will maintain regular bowel movements.
• The patient's pain will decrease.
• The patient and his family will demonstrate an understanding of drug therapy.

Implementation
• Time drug administration so that bowel evacuation doesn't interfere with scheduled activities or sleep.
• When giving mineral oil by mouth, give it on an empty stomach.
• Perform rectal administration according to facility protocol.
• Make sure that the patient has easy access to a bedpan or bathroom.
• Institute measures to prevent constipation.

Evaluation
• Patient regains normal bowel elimination pattern.
• Patient states that pain is relieved with stool evacuation.
• Patient and his family demonstrate an understanding of drug therapy. (See *Teaching about laxatives*.)

Selective 5-HT$_3$-receptor antagonists

Alosetron, a selective antagonist of serotonin 5-HT$_3$ receptors, is used for short-term treatment of severe diarrhea-predominant IBS in women. Blocking 5-HT$_3$ receptors helps decrease the pain associated with IBS. Access to alosetron, however, is limited.

Restricted use only

The drug is available through a restricted marketing program because serious adverse bowel effects have been reported. Only doctors enrolled in the prescribing program for alosetron can write a prescription for it.

Pharmacokinetics

Alosetron is rapidly absorbed after oral administration. It's metabolized by the cytochrome P450 pathway.

Pharmacodynamics

Alosetron selectively inhibits 5-HT$_3$ receptors on enteric neurons in the GI tract. By inhibiting activation of these cation channels, neuronal depolarization is blocked, resulting in decreased visceral pain, colonic transit, and GI secretions—factors that usually contribute to the symptoms of IBS.

The fine print

Alosetron hasn't been studied in pregnant women or nursing mothers. The risks and benefits should be evaluated before giving alosetron to these patients. Older adults may be sensitive to the effects of alosetron, which may increase the risk of serious constipation.

Pharmacotherapeutics

Alosetron is used for the short-term treatment of women with IBS whose primary symptom is diarrhea that has lasted longer than 6 months and has not responded to conventional treatment. Don't give this drug if the patient is constipated. Stop the drug if constipation develops. This drug is not indicated for men.

Drug interactions

Studies have shown that alosetron inhibits cytochrome P450 1A2 (CYP1A2) and *N*-acetyltransferase by 30%. Although clinical trials haven't been conducted, the inhibition of *N*-acetyltransferase may have clinical significance when alosetron is given with such drugs as isoniazid, procainamide, and hydralazine. Avoid using alosetron with other drugs that decrease GI motility to prevent the risk of constipation.

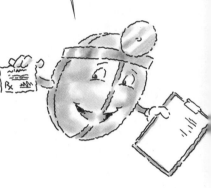

Because of the potential for serious adverse effects, alosetron is prescribed only by doctors enrolled in the drug's prescribing program.

Adverse reactions

Alosetron has produced serious, and sometimes fatal, adverse reactions, including:
- ischemic colitis
- serious complications of constipation including obstruction, perforation, and toxic megacolon.

Nursing process

These nursing process steps are appropriate for patients undergoing treatment with a selective 5-HT$_3$-receptor antagonist.

Assessment
- Obtain a baseline assessment of the patient's bowel patterns and GI history before starting therapy.
- Assess the patient for adverse reactions and drug interactions.

A collection of contraindications
- Assess the patient for contraindications to alosetron, such as constipation, intestinal obstruction, stricture, toxic megacolon, GI perforation, GI adhesions, ischemic colitis, impaired intestinal circulation, thrombophlebitis, hypercoagulable state, Crohn's disease, ulcerative colitis, or diverticulitis.
- Monitor the patient's bowel pattern throughout therapy. Assess bowel sounds and color and consistency of stools.
- Assess the patient's fluid and electrolyte status during administration.
- Determine whether the patient maintains adequate fluid intake and diet and whether she exercises.
- Assess the patient's and family's knowledge of drug therapy.

Key nursing diagnoses
- Diarrhea related to adverse GI effects
- Acute pain related to abdominal discomfort
- Deficient knowledge related to drug therapy

Planning outcome goals
- The patient will maintain regular bowel movements.
- The patient's pain will decrease.
- The patient and her family will demonstrate an understanding of drug therapy.

Implementation
- Time drug administration so that bowel evacuation doesn't interfere with scheduled activities or sleep.

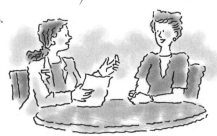

Because you're a woman, alosetron may be indicated for your IBS.

• Make sure that the patient has easy access to a bedpan or bathroom.
• Institute measures to prevent constipation.
• Inform the patient of the risks and benefits of the drug.
• Explain to the patient that she must enroll in the drug's prescribing program and sign a patient-physician agreement to participate in therapy.

Evaluation

• Patient regains normal bowel elimination pattern.
• Patient states that pain is relieved with stool evacuation.
• Patient and her family demonstrate an understanding of drug therapy.

Obesity drugs

Obesity drugs can help morbidly obese patients who have health problems that will likely improve with weight loss. These drugs are used in combination with a weight management program that includes diet, physical activity, and behavioral modification. They should be used only for improving health, not for cosmetic weight loss.

Obesity drugs include:
• appetite suppressants (phentermine hydrochloride and sibutramine)
• fat blockers (orlistat)

Pharmacokinetics

Phentermine is rapidly absorbed from the intestine and distributed throughout the body. It's excreted in urine. Sibutramine is rapidly absorbed from the intestine and rapidly distributed to most body tissues. It's metabolized in the liver and excreted in the urine and feces. Orlistat isn't absorbed systemically; its action occurs in the GI tract, and it's excreted in the feces.

Pharmacodynamics

The appetite suppressants phentermine and sibutramine increase the amount of norepinephrine and dopamine in the brain, which suppresses appetite.

Caught in a bind

The fat-blocking drug orlistat works differently. It binds to gastric and pancreatic lipases in the GI tract, making them unavailable to break down fats. This prevents absorption of 30% of the fat ingested in a meal.

Pharmacotherapeutics

Appetite suppressants and fat blockers are used primarily in morbidly obese patients for whom weight loss will improve health and prevent death.

Drug interactions

Obesity drugs have the following interactions:
• Appetite suppressants taken with cardiovascular stimulants may increase risk of hypertension and arrhythmias.
• When taken with CNS stimulants, appetite suppressants can result in anxiety and insomnia.
• Appetite suppressants taken with serotonergic drugs (including selective serotonin reuptake inhibitors such as fluoxetine, triptan antimigraine drugs such as sumatriptan, lithium, and dextromethorphan, which is commonly found in cough syrup) can cause agitation, confusion, hypomania, impaired coordination, loss of consciousness, nausea, and tachycardia.
• Taking orlistat with fat-soluble vitamins blocks vitamin absorption.

Adverse reactions

Phentermine hydrochloride can cause nervousness, dry mouth, constipation, and hypertension. Adverse effects of sibutramine include dry mouth, headache, insomnia, nervousness, constipation, hypertension, tachycardia, and palpitations.

In the short run

Orlistat causes abdominal pain, oily spotting, fecal urgency, flatulence with discharge, fatty stools, fecal incontinence, and increased defecation although these effects usually subside after a few weeks.

Nursing process

These nursing process steps are appropriate for patients undergoing treatment with obesity drugs.

Assessment

• Assess patient for factors and health risks related to excess weight, such as cardiovascular disease, diabetes, and sleep apnea.
• Determine the patient's blood pressure and pulse rate before starting therapy with phentermine or sibutramine.

• Assess the patient for adverse reactions.
• Assess such laboratory values as cholesterol levels and blood sugar.
• Assess the patient's caloric intake before starting therapy.
• Measure the patient's weight, waist circumference, and body mass index.
• Assess the patient's motivation to adhere to a weight-management program.

Key nursing diagnoses
• Imbalanced nutrition: More than body requirements related to excessive caloric intake
• Disturbed body image related to excessive weight
• Deficient knowledge related to drug therapy

Planning outcome goals
• The patient will decrease his caloric intake.
• The patient will experience a positive body image with weight loss.
• The patient will verbalize an understanding of drug therapy.

Implementation
• Explain to the patient that phentermine is for short-term use only. Don't give this drug to a patient with hypertension, cardiovascular disease, or a history of drug abuse.
• Assess the patient taking phentermine for agitation and anxiety.
• Don't give sibutramine to patients with cardiovascular disorders or severe renal or hepatic dysfunction. Use the drug cautiously in patients taking mediation to increase blood pressure and pulse rate as well as in patients with impaired hepatic function, narrow-angle glaucoma, or a history of drug abuse.
• Because orlistat prevents absorption of fat-soluble vitamins—including A, D, E, and K—make sure the patient takes a multivitamin daily 2 hours before or after taking orlistat.
• Monitor the blood pressure of the patient taking phentermine or sibutramine at regular intervals throughout therapy.
• Promote exercise and healthy eating as part of an overall strategy to lose weight.

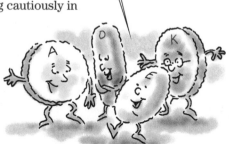

Orlistat prevents the absorption of fat-soluble vitamins, so make sure you administer us daily 2 hours before or after orlistat.

Evaluation
• Patient decreases caloric intake and loses weight.
• Patient regains a positive body image.

Education edge

Teaching about obesity drugs

If obesity drugs are prescribed, review these points with the patient and his caregivers:

• Take an appetite suppressant in the morning to decrease your appetite during the day and to prevent the drug from interfering with sleep at night.

• If you're taking sibutramine, take it once daily in the morning, with or without food. Have your blood pressure and heart rate checked at regular intervals, and notify your health care provider if you develop rash, hives, or another allergic reaction.

• If you're taking phentermine, take it 30 minutes before meals or as a single dose in the morning. Avoid caffeine. Keep in mind that the drug may lose its effectiveness over time; you should not use it for more than 3 months.

• If you're taking orlistat, take one capsule with each main meal (or up to 1 hour after a meal) three times a day. If you miss a meal, skip that dose. Take a multivitamin that contains fat-soluble vitamins A, D, E, and K daily, at least 2 hours before or after taking orlistat.

• Patient verbalizes an understanding of drug therapy. (See *Teaching about obesity drugs*.)

Antiemetic drugs

Antiemetic drugs decrease nausea, reducing the urge to vomit.

Antiemetics

The major antiemetics include:

• antihistamines, including dimenhydrinate, diphenhydramine hydrochloride, buclizine hydrochloride, cyclizine hydrochloride, hydroxyzine hydrochloride, hydroxyzine pamoate, meclizine hydrochloride, and trimethobenzamide hydrochloride

• phenothiazines, including chlorpromazine hydrochloride, perphenazine, prochlorperazine maleate, promethazine hydrochloride, and thiethylperazine maleate

• serotonin receptor ($5\text{-}HT_3$) antagonists, including ondansetron, dolasetron, granisetron, and palonosetron.

#1 nausea fighter

Ondansetron is currently the antiemetic of choice in the United States.

Pharmacokinetics

The pharmacokinetic properties of antiemetics may vary slightly. Oral antihistamine antiemetics are absorbed well from the GI tract and are metabolized primarily by the liver. Their inactive metabolites are excreted in urine.

Phenothiazines and serotonin receptor antagonists are absorbed well and extensively metabolized by the liver. They are excreted in urine and feces.

Pharmacodynamics

The action of antiemetics may vary.

Mechanism unknown

The mechanism of action that produces the antiemetic effect of antihistamines is unclear.

The trigger zone

Phenothiazines produce their antiemetic effect by blocking the dopaminergic receptors in the chemoreceptor trigger zone in the brain. (This area of the brain, near the medulla, stimulates the vomiting center in the medulla, causing vomiting.) These drugs may also directly depress the vomiting center.

Two spots to block

The serotonin receptor antagonists block serotonin stimulation centrally in the chemoreceptor trigger zone and peripherally in the vagal nerve terminals, both of which stimulate vomiting.

Pharmacotherapeutics

The uses of antiemetics may vary.

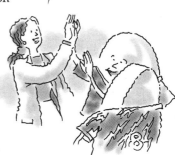

Way to block those vomit-inducing receptors, antiemetics!

Motion potion

With the exception of trimethobenzamide, the antihistamines are specifically used for nausea and vomiting caused by inner ear stimulation. As a consequence, these drugs prevent or treat motion sickness. They usually prove most effective when given before activities that produce motion sickness and are much less effective when nausea or vomiting has already begun.

Much more severe

Phenothiazines and serotonin receptor antagonists control severe nausea and vomiting from various causes. They're used when vomiting becomes severe and potentially hazardous, such as postsurgical or viral nausea and vomiting. Both types of drugs are also

Other antiemetics

Here are other antiemetics currently in use.

Scopolamine

Scopolamine prevents motion sickness, but its use is limited because of its sedative and anticholinergic effects. One scopolamine transdermal preparation, Transderm-Scop, is highly effective without producing the usual adverse effects.

Metoclopramide

Metoclopramide hydrochloride is principally used to treat GI motility disorders, including gastroparesis in diabetic patients. It's also used to prevent chemotherapy-induced nausea and vomiting.

Dronabinol

Dronabinol, a purified derivative of cannabis, is a schedule II drug (meaning it has a high potential for abuse) used to treat the nausea and vomiting resulting from cancer chemotherapy in patients who don't respond adequately to conventional antiemetics. It's also been used to stimulate the appetite in patients with acquired immunodeficiency syndrome. However, dronabinol can accumulate in the body, and the patient can develop tolerance or physical and psychological dependence.

Aprepitant

Aprepitant is used to prevent chemotherapy-induced nausea and vomiting. It works by blocking neurokinin receptors in the brain. It's given 1 hour before chemotherapy for the first 3 days of treatment.

prescribed to control the nausea and vomiting resulting from cancer chemotherapy and radiotherapy. (See *Other antiemetics*)

Drug interactions

Antiemetics may have many significant interactions:
• Antihistamines and phenothiazines can produce additive CNS depression and sedation when taken with CNS depressants, such as barbiturates, tranquilizers, antidepressants, alcohol, and opioids.
• Antihistamines can cause additive anticholinergic effects, such as constipation, dry mouth, vision problems, and urine retention, when taken with anticholinergic drugs, including tricyclic antidepressants, phenothiazines, and antiparkinsonian drugs.
• Phenothiazine antiemetics taken with anticholinergic drugs increase the anticholinergic effect and decrease antiemetic effects.
• Droperidol plus phenothiazine antiemetics increase the risk of extrapyramidal effects (abnormal involuntary movements).

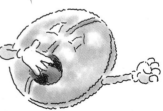

Antihistamines and phenothiazines can produce additive CNS depression and sedation when taken with CNS depressants.

Adverse reactions

The use of these antiemetic drugs may lead to adverse reactions:
• Antihistamine and phenothiazine antiemetics produce drowsiness; paradoxical CNS stimulation may also occur.

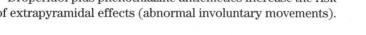

• CNS effects associated with phenothiazine and serotonin receptor antagonist antiemetics include confusion, anxiety, euphoria, agitation, depression, headache, insomnia, restlessness, and weakness.
• The anticholinergic effect of antiemetics may cause constipation, dry mouth and throat, painful or difficult urination, urine retention, impotence, and visual and auditory disturbances.
• Hypotension and orthostatic hypotension with an increased heart rate, fainting, and dizziness are common adverse reactions to phenothiazines.

Nursing process

These nursing process steps are appropriate for patients undergoing treatment with antiemetics.

Assessment

• Assess the patient's condition before therapy and regularly thereafter.
• Assess for adverse reactions and drug interactions.
• Assess the patient's and family's knowledge of drug therapy.

Key nursing diagnoses

• Ineffective health maintenance related to the underlying condition
• Risk for deficient fluid volume related to the underlying condition
• Deficient knowledge related to drug therapy

Planning outcome goals

• The patient will exhibit improved health as evidenced by decreased vomiting.
• The patient will maintain adequate fluid volume balance as evidenced by intake and output, vital signs, and electrolyte evaluations.
• The patient and his family will demonstrate an understanding of drug therapy.

Implementation

• Monitor the patient for the drug's effect.
• Administer the drug as directed to promote GI effectiveness and relieve distress.
• Give I.M. injections deeply into large muscle mass. Rotate injection sites.
• Don't give antiemetics subcutaneously.

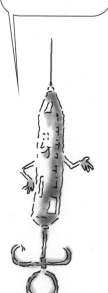

It isn't my job! Don't give antiemetics subcutaneously.

• For prevention of motion sickness, tell the patient to take the drug 30 to 60 minutes before travel.
• Warn the patient to avoid alcohol and hazardous activities until the drug's CNS effects are known.
• Stop the drug 4 days before allergy skin tests.

Evaluation
• Patient responds well to therapy.
• Patient maintains fluid volume.
• Patient and his family demonstrate an understanding of drug therapy.

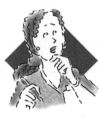

Quick quiz

1. A patient is taking calcium carbonate for peptic ulcer disease. You should monitor the patient for:
    A.   hypercalcemia.
    B.   hypocalcemia.
    C.   hyperkalemia.
    D.   hypokalemia.

Answer: A. Watch for signs of hypercalcemia in the patient receiving calcium carbonate.

2. Which adverse reaction is common and usually dose related in patients taking misoprostol?
    A.   Diarrhea
    B.   Nausea
    C.   Vomiting
    D.   Bloating

Answer: A. Misoprostol commonly causes diarrhea. This reaction is usually dose related.

3. Which drug or drug type may interact with the H_2-receptor antagonist cimetidine?
    A.   Hormonal contraceptives
    B.   Antilipemic agents
    C.   Digoxin
    D.   Oral anticoagulants

Answer: D. Cimetidine may increase the blood levels of oral anticoagulants by reducing their metabolism in the liver and excretion.

4. A patient is admitted to the emergency department with salicylate poisoning. Which drug should the nurse anticipate giving the patient?

    A.   Chlorpromazine
    B.   Activated charcoal
    C.   Magnesium citrate
    D.   Docusate

Answer: B. Activated charcoal is a general-purpose antidote that's used for various types of acute oral poisoning.

5. Which drug is used to treat IBS in women whose primary bowel symptom is diarrhea?

    A.   Alosetron
    B.   Bisacodyl
    C.   Famotidine
    D.   Docusate

Answer: A. Alosetron is a selective 5-HT$_3$-receptor antagonist that's used for the short-term treatment of IBS in women whose primary bowel symptom is severe diarrhea.

Scoring

★★★ If you answered all five questions correctly, thumbs up! Your knowledge of GI drugs is gastronomical.

★★ If you answered four questions correctly, nice work! You certainly aren't lacking learning in the laxative department.

★ If you answered fewer than four questions correctly, don't panic. You may need some more time to digest the material.

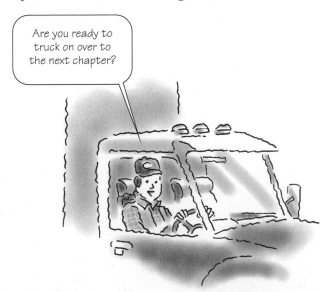

Genitourinary drugs

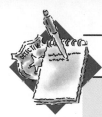

Just the facts

In this chapter, you'll learn:

♦ classes of drugs used to treat genitourinary (GU) disorders

♦ uses and varying actions of these drugs

♦ absorption, distribution, metabolization, and excretion of these drugs

♦ drug interactions and adverse reactions to these drugs.

Drugs and the genitourinary system

The GU system consists of the reproductive system (the sex organs) and the urinary system, which includes the kidneys, ureters, bladder, and urethra. The kidneys perform most of the work of the urinary system.

Multitalented

The kidneys perform several vital tasks, including:
• disposing of wastes and excess ions in the form of urine
• filtering blood, which regulates its volume and chemical makeup
• helping to maintain fluid, electrolyte, and acid-base balances
• producing several hormones and enzymes
• converting vitamin D to a more active form
• helping to regulate blood pressure and volume by secreting renin.

Helping hands

Types of drugs used to treat GU disorders include:
• diuretics
• urinary tract antispasmodics
• erectile dysfunction therapy drugs
• hormonal contraceptives.

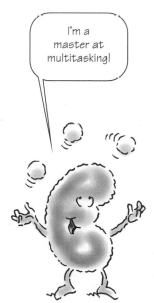

I'm a master at multitasking!

Diuretics

Diuretics trigger the excretion of water and electrolytes from the kidneys, making these drugs a primary choice in the treatment of renal disease, edema, hypertension, and heart failure.

Thiazide and thiazide-like diuretics

Derived from sulfonamides, thiazide and thiazide-like diuretics are used to treat edema and to prevent the development and recurrence of renal calculi. They're also used for such cardiovascular diseases as hypertension and heart failure.

Thiazide diuretics include:
- bendroflumethiazide
- chlorothiazide
- hydrochlorothiazide
- hydroflumethiazide
- methyclothiazide
- polythiazide.

Thiazide-like diuretics include:
- chlorthalidone
- indapamide
- metolazone.

Pharmacokinetics (how drugs circulate)

Thiazide diuretics are absorbed rapidly but incompletely from the GI tract after oral administration. They cross the placenta and are secreted in breast milk. These drugs differ in how well they're metabolized, but all are excreted primarily in urine. (See *Thiazide diuretics: Hydrochlorothiazide.*)

Thiazide-like diuretics are absorbed from the GI tract. Chlorthalidone is 90% bound to erythrocytes; little is known about its metabolism. Indapamide is distributed widely into body tissues and metabolized in the liver. Little is also known about the metabolism of metolazone. All of these drugs are primarily excreted in urine. (See *Thiazide-like diuretics: Indapamide*, page 346.)

Pharmacodynamics (how drugs act)

Thiazide and thiazide-like diuretics promote the excretion of water by preventing the reabsorption of sodium in the kidneys. As the kidneys excrete the excess sodium, they excrete water along with it. These drugs also increase the excretion of chloride, potassium, and bicarbonate, which can result in electrolyte imbalances.

Prototype pro

Thiazide diuretics: Hydrochlorothiazide

Actions
- Interferes with sodium transport across tubules of the cortical diluting segment of the nephron
- Increases renal excretion of sodium, chloride, water, potassium, and calcium
- Increases bicarbonate, magnesium, phosphate, bromide, and iodide excretion
- Decreases excretion of ammonia, causing increased serum ammonia levels

Indications
- Edema
- Hypertension

Nursing considerations
- Monitor for adverse effects, such as pancreatitis, hematologic disorders, and electrolyte imbalances, especially hypokalemla (symptoms of hypokalemia include leg cramps and muscle aches).
- Frequently monitor weight and blood pressure.

With long-term use, thiazide diuretics also lower blood pressure by causing arteriolar vasodilation.

Turning down the volume

Initially, diuretic drugs decrease circulating blood volume, leading to reduced cardiac output. However, if therapy is maintained, cardiac output stabilizes but plasma fluid volume decreases.

Pharmacotherapeutics (how drugs are used)

Thiazides are used for the long-term treatment of hypertension; they're also used to treat edema caused by kidney or liver disease, mild or moderate heart failure, and corticosteroid and estrogen therapy. Because these drugs decrease the level of calcium in urine, they may be used alone or with other drugs to prevent the development and recurrence of renal calculi.

Pointing out a paradox

In patients with diabetes insipidus (a disorder characterized by excessive urine production and excessive thirst resulting from reduced secretion of antidiuretic hormone), thiazides paradoxically decrease urine volume, possibly through sodium depletion and plasma volume reduction.

Drug interactions

Drug interactions related to thiazide and thiazide-like diuretics result in altered fluid volume, blood pressure, and serum electrolyte levels:

Prototype pro

Thiazide-like diuretics: Indapamide

Actions
• Interferes with sodium transport across the tubules of the cortical diluting segment in the nephron, thereby increasing renal excretion of sodium, chloride, water, potassium, and calcium

Indications
• Nephrotic syndrome
• Edema and ascites caused by hepatic cirrhosis

• Hypertension
• Diabetes insipidus, especially nephrogenic diabetes insipidus
• Edema from right-sided heart failure
• Mild to moderate left-sided heart failure

Nursing considerations
• Give the drug in the morning to prevent nocturia.
• Indapamide may be used with a potassium-sparing diuretic to prevent potassium loss.

• These drugs may decrease excretion of lithium, causing lithium toxicity.
• Nonsteroidal anti-inflammatory drugs, including cyclooxygenase 2 (COX-2) inhibitors, may reduce the antihypertensive effect of these diuretics.
• Use of these drugs with other potassium-depleting drugs and digoxin may cause an additive effect, increasing the risk of digoxin toxicity.
• These diuretics may increase the response to skeletal muscle relaxants.
• Use of these drugs may increase blood glucose levels, requiring higher doses of insulin or oral antidiabetic drugs.
• These drugs may produce additive hypotension when used with antihypertensives.

Adverse reactions

The most common adverse reactions to thiazide and thiazide-like diuretics are reduced blood volume, orthostatic hypotension, hypokalemia, hyperglycemia, and hyponatremia.

Nursing process

These nursing process steps are appropriate for patients undergoing treatment with thiazide and thiazide-like diuretics.

Administering thiazide diuretics along with antihypertensives can result in additive hypotension. I don't like the way this is adding up!

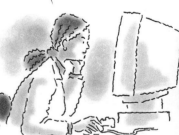

Assessment
- Monitor digoxin levels if the patient is receiving digoxin concurrently with a thiazide or thiazide-like diuretic.
- Monitor the patient's intake, output, and serum electrolyte levels regularly.
- Carefully monitor the patient for signs and symptoms of hypokalemia, such as drowsiness, paresthesia, muscle cramps, and hyporeflexia.

Weighing in

- Weigh the patient each morning immediately after he voids and before breakfast, using the same scale and making sure he's wearing the same type of clothing. Weight provides a reliable indicator of the patient's response to diuretic therapy.
- If the patient has diabetes, monitor his blood glucose levels because diuretics may cause hyperglycemia.
- Because these drugs aren't as effective when serum creatinine and blood urea nitrogen (BUN) levels rise to more than twice their normal levels, monitor these levels regularly. Also monitor blood uric acid levels.

Key nursing diagnoses
- Risk for deficient fluid volume related to excessive diuresis
- Deficient knowledge related to diuretic therapy

Planning outcome goals
- The patient will maintain a normal fluid volume as evidenced by having a blood pressure and heart rate within the normal range.
- Adverse effects of the diuretic will be minimized.
- The patient will demonstrate correct drug administration.

Implementation
- Give the drug in the morning to prevent nocturia from disrupting the patient's sleep.
- Consult a dietitian about providing the patient with a high-potassium diet.
- Administer potassium supplements as prescribed to maintain the patient's serum potassium level within an acceptable range.
- Keep a urinal or bedpan within reach of the patient or ensure that a bathroom is easily accessible.

Evaluation
- Patient maintains adequate hydration.
- Patient states the importance of taking the diuretic early in the day to prevent nocturia.

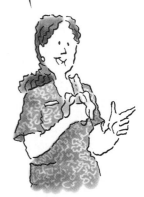

Pardon me for talking with my mouth full, but make sure patients taking thiazide and thiazide-like diuretics consume plenty of potassium-rich foods.

Education edge

Teaching about diuretics

If diuretics are prescribed, review these points with the patient and his caregivers:
• Make sure you understand the rationale for therapy and the importance of following the prescribed regimen.
• Take the drug at the same time each day to prevent nocturia. You may take the drug with food to minimize GI irritation.
• Seek your practitioner's approval before taking any other drug, including over-the-counter medications and herbal remedies.
• Record your weight each morning after voiding and before breakfast, in the same type of clothing, and using the same scale.
• Be aware of adverse effects, and report signs and symptoms promptly, especially chest, back, or leg pain; shortness of

breath; increased fluid accumulation or weight gain (more than 2 lb [0.9 kg]) daily; or excess water loss (as evidenced by a weight loss of more than 2 lb daily). Also watch for photosensitivity reactions, which usually occur 10 to 14 days after initial sun exposure.
• Avoid high-sodium foods (such as lunch meat, smoked meats, and processed cheeses) and don't add table salt to foods.
• If you're taking a potassium-depleting diuretic, include potassium-rich foods (such as bananas, oranges, and potatoes) in your diet. If you're taking a potassium-sparing diuretic, you don't need to add extra potassium-rich foods.
• Keep follow-up appointments to monitor the effectiveness of therapy.

• Patient and his family demonstrate an understanding of diuretic therapy. (See *Teaching about diuretics*.)

Loop diuretics

Loop (high ceiling) diuretics are highly potent drugs. They include bumetanide, ethacrynic acid, and furosemide.

Pharmacokinetics

Loop diuretics are absorbed well in the GI tract and are rapidly distributed. These diuretics are highly protein bound. They undergo partial or complete metabolism in the liver, except for furosemide, which is excreted primarily unchanged. Loop diuretics are excreted primarily by the kidneys.

Pharmacodynamics

Loop diuretics are the most potent diuretics available, producing the greatest volume of diuresis (urine production). Bumetanide—which is 40 times more potent than furosemide—is the shortest-acting diuretic. Loop diuretics also have a high potential for causing severe adverse reactions. (See *Loop diuretics warning*.)

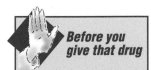

Before you give that drug

Loop diuretics warning

Loop diuretics, with the exception of ethacrynic acid, contain sulfa. A patient who has an allergy to sulfa may experience an allergic reaction to loop diuretics. Use with caution, and alert the patient to this possibility.

Prototype pro

Loop diuretics: Furosemide

Actions
• Inhibits sodium and chloride reabsorption in the ascending loop of Henle, thus increasing renal excretion of sodium, chloride, and water
• Increases excretion of potassium (like thiazide diuretics)
• Produces greater maximum diuresis and electrolyte loss than a thiazide diuretic

Indications
• Acute pulmonary edema
• Edema
• Hypertension

Nursing considerations
• Monitor for adverse effects, such as pancreatitis, hematologic disorders, and electrolyte imbalances (especially hypokalemia).
• Monitor weight and blood pressure frequently.
• Signs of hypokalemia may include leg cramps and muscle aches.

The scoop on the loop

Loop diuretics received their name because they act primarily on the thick, ascending loop of Henle (the part of the nephron responsible for concentrating urine) to increase the secretion of sodium, chloride, and water. These drugs also inhibit sodium, chloride, and water reabsorption in the proximal tubule.

Pharmacotherapeutics

Loop diuretics are used to treat edema associated with renal disease, hepatic cirrhosis, and heart failure, as well as to treat hypertension (usually with a potassium-sparing diuretic or potassium supplement to prevent hypokalemia). (See *Loop diuretics: Furosemide.*)

Ethacrynic acid may also be used for the short-term management of ascites due to malignancy, idiopathic edema, or lymphedema. Furosemide may be used with mannitol to treat cerebral edema.

Drug interactions

Loop diuretics produce a variety of drug interactions:
• The risk of ototoxicity (damage to the organs of hearing) increases when aminoglycosides and cisplatin are taken with loop diuretics (especially with high doses of furosemide).

• Loop diuretics reduce the hypoglycemic effects of oral antidiabetic drugs, possibly resulting in hyperglycemia.
• These drugs may increase the risk of lithium toxicity.
• The risk of electrolyte imbalances that can trigger arrhythmias increases when cardiac glycosides and loop diuretics are taken together.
• Use with digoxin may cause additive toxicity, increasing the risk of digoxin toxicity and arrhythmias.

Adverse reactions

The most common adverse reactions involve fluid and electrolyte imbalances, including metabolic alkalosis, hypovolemia, hypochloremia, hypochloremic alkalosis, hyperglycemia, hyperuricemia, dehydration, hyponatremia, hypokalemia, and hypomagnesemia.

The list goes on...

Loop diuretics may also cause transient deafness, tinnitus, diarrhea, nausea, vomiting, abdominal pain, impaired glucose tolerance, dermatitis, paresthesia, hepatic dysfunction, photosensitivity, and orthostatic hypotension.

I said, loop diuretics may cause transient deafness!

Nursing process

These nursing process steps are appropriate for patients undergoing treatment with loop diuretics.

Assessment
• Monitor the patient's blood pressure and pulse rate (especially during rapid diuresis) to detect signs of hypovolemia. Establish baseline values before therapy begins, and watch for significant changes.

Baseline basics

• Establish a baseline complete blood count (CBC) (including a white blood cell [WBC] count), liver function test results, and levels of serum electrolytes, carbon dioxide, magnesium, BUN, and creatinine. Review periodically.
• Assess the patient for evidence of excessive diuresis, including hypotension, tachycardia, poor skin turgor, excessive thirst, and dry or cracked mucous membranes.
• Monitor the patient for edema and ascites. Observe the legs of ambulatory patients and the sacral area of patients on bed rest.
• Monitor and record the patient's weight and intake and output carefully every 24 hours.

• If the patient is receiving digoxin and loop diuretics concurrently, monitor serum digoxin levels.

Key nursing diagnoses
• Risk for deficient fluid volume related to excessive diuresis
• Risk for injury related to electrolyte imbalance
• Deficient knowledge related to diuretic therapy

Planning outcome goals
• The patient will maintain a normal fluid volume as evidenced by having a blood pressure and heart rate within the normal range.
• The patient won't exhibit adverse effects of electrolyte imbalance.
• The patient will demonstrate correct diuretic therapy administration.

Implementation
• Give the diuretic in the morning to ensure that major diuresis occurs before bedtime. To prevent nocturia, don't administer later than 6 p.m.
• Administer I.V. doses slowly over 1 to 2 minutes to prevent hypotension.
• Watch closely for changes in the patient's sodium and potassium levels.

Dosage details

• If ordered, reduce the dosage for a patient with hepatic dysfunction and increase the dosage for a patient with renal impairment, oliguria, or decreased diuresis. (Inadequate urine output may result in circulatory overload, causing water intoxication, pulmonary edema, and heart failure). If ordered, increase the dosage of insulin or oral hypoglycemic in a diabetic patient and reduce the dosage of other antihypertensive drugs.
• Weigh the patient each morning immediately after he voids and before breakfast, using the same scale and making sure he's wearing the same type of clothing. Weight provides a reliable indicator of the patient's response to diuretic therapy.
• Keep a urinal or bedpan within reach of the patient or ensure that the bathroom is easily accessible.
• Give the diuretic with food or milk to prevent GI upset.
• Instruct the patient to use sunscreen and wear protective clothing to prevent photosensitivity reactions.

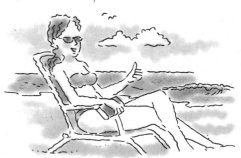

Tell the patient to use sunscreen and wear protective clothing to avoid a photosensitivity reaction.

Evaluation

- Patient maintains adequate hydration.
- Patient's electrolyte levels remain within normal limits.
- Patient and his family demonstrate an understanding of diuretic therapy.

Potassium-sparing diuretics

Potassium-sparing diuretics have weaker diuretic and antihypertensive effects than other diuretics but provide the advantage of conserving potassium. These drugs include amiloride, spironolactone, and triamterene.

Pharmacokinetics

Potassium-sparing diuretics are only available orally and are absorbed in the GI tract. They're metabolized by the liver (except for amiloride, which isn't metabolized) and excreted primarily in urine.

Pharmacodynamics

The direct action of potassium-sparing diuretics on the distal tubule of the kidneys results in urinary excretion of sodium, water, bicarbonate, and calcium. The drug also decreases the excretion of potassium and hydrogen ions. These effects lead to reduced blood pressure and increased serum potassium levels.

Compare and contrast

Structurally similar to aldosterone, spironolactone acts as an aldosterone antagonist. Aldosterone promotes the retention of sodium and water and the loss of potassium, whereas spironolactone counteracts these effects by competing with aldosterone for receptor sites. As a result, sodium, chloride, and water are excreted and potassium is retained.

Pharmacotherapeutics

Potassium-sparing diuretics are used to treat:
- edema
- diuretic-induced hypokalemia in patients with heart failure
- cirrhosis
- nephrotic syndrome (abnormal condition of the kidneys)
- heart failure
- hypertension.

A hairy situation

Spironolactone also is used to treat hyperaldosteronism (excessive secretion of aldosterone) and hirsutism (excessive hair growth), including hirsutism associated with Stein-Leventhal (polycystic ovary) syndrome. Potassium-sparing diuretics are commonly used with other diuretics to potentiate their action or counteract their potassium-wasting effects.

Drug interactions

Giving potassium-sparing diuretics with potassium supplements or angiotensin-converting enzyme inhibitors increases the risk of hyperkalemia. Concurrent use of spironolactone and digoxin increases the risk of digoxin toxicity.

Adverse reactions

Few adverse drug reactions occur with potassium-sparing diuretics. However, their potassium-sparing effects can lead to hyperkalemia, especially if given with a potassium supplement or high-potassium diet.

Nursing process

These nursing process steps are appropriate for patients undergoing treatment with potassium-sparing diuretics.

Assessment

• Monitor the patient's blood pressure and heart rate, especially during rapid diuresis. Establish baseline values before therapy begins, and watch for significant changes.
• Establish a baseline CBC (including WBC count), liver function test results, and levels of serum electrolytes, carbon dioxide, magnesium, BUN, and creatinine. Review periodically.
• Assess the patient for evidence of excessive diuresis: hypotension, tachycardia, poor skin turgor, excessive thirst, or dry and cracked mucous membranes.
• Monitor the patient for signs and symptoms of hyperkalemia, such as confusion, hyperexcitability, muscle weakness, flaccid paralysis, arrhythmias, abdominal distention, and diarrhea.
• Monitor the patient for edema and ascites. Observe the legs of ambulatory patients and the sacral area of patients on bed rest.
• Weigh the patient each morning immediately after he voids and before breakfast, using the same scale and making sure he's wearing the same type of clothing. Weight provides a reliable indicator of the patient's response to diuretic therapy.

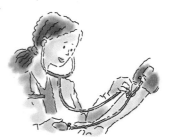

Establish a baseline blood pressure value before therapy begins.

• Monitor and record the patient's intake and output carefully every 24 hours.

Key nursing diagnoses
• Risk for deficient fluid volume related to excessive diuresis
• Risk for injury related to electrolyte imbalance
• Deficient knowledge related to diuretic therapy

Planning outcome goals
• The patient will maintain a normal fluid volume as evidenced by having a blood pressure and heart rate within the normal range.
• The patient won't demonstrate adverse effects of electrolyte imbalance.
• The patient will demonstrate correct diuretic therapy administration.

Implementation
• Give the diuretic in the morning or early afternoon to prevent nocturia from disrupting the patient's sleep.
• Keep a urinal or bedpan within reach of the patient or ensure that a bathroom is easily accessible.
• If ordered, reduce the dosage for a patient with hepatic dysfunction and increase the dosage for a patient with renal impairment, oliguria, or decreased diuresis. (Inadequate urine output may result in circulatory overload, causing water intoxication, pulmonary edema, and heart failure). If ordered, increase the dosage of insulin or oral hypoglycemic in a diabetic patient and reduce the dosage of other antihypertensive drugs.

Drop that banana!

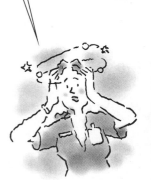

Potassium-sparing diuretics may cause dizziness and headache. I'm not feeling very well…

• Instruct the patient to avoid salt substitutes and potassium-rich foods, except with practitioner approval. Consult a dietitian.
• For maximum effectiveness, administer amiloride with food; administer triamterene after meals.
• Because potassium-sparing diuretics may cause dizziness, headache, or vision disturbances, advise the patient to avoid driving or performing activities requiring mental alertness or physical dexterity until his response to the diuretic is known.

Evaluation
• Patient maintains adequate hydration.
• Patient's electrolyte levels remain within normal limits.
• Patient and his family demonstrate an understanding of diuretic therapy.

Osmotic diuretics

Osmotic diuretics cause diuresis through osmosis, moving fluid into the extracellular spaces. They include mannitol and urea.

Pharmacokinetics

Administered I.V. for rapid distribution, osmotic diuretics are freely filtered by the glomeruli of the kidney—except for mannitol, which is only slightly metabolized. Osmotic diuretics are excreted primarily in urine.

Pharmacodynamics

Osmotic diuretics receive their name because they increase the osmotic pressure of the glomerular filtrate, which inhibits the reabsorption of sodium and water. They create an osmotic gradient in the glomerular filtrate and the blood. In the glomerular filtrate, the gradient prevents sodium and water reabsorption. In the blood, the gradient allows fluid to be drawn from the intracellular into the intravascular spaces.

Pharmacotherapeutics

Osmotic diuretics are used to treat acute renal failure and cerebral edema and to reduce intracranial and intraocular pressure. Mannitol is used to promote diuresis in acute renal failure and to promote urinary excretion of toxic substances.

Drug interactions

Taking osmotic diuretics with lithium may increase renal excretion of lithium, which in turn decreases the effectiveness of lithium. Patients taking both drugs require lithium level monitoring.

Adverse reactions

Osmotic diuretics may cause hyponatremia, dehydration, circulatory overload (from osmotic effects), and thrombophlebitis or local irritation at the infusion site.

The pressure's building...

Mannitol may cause rebound increased intracranial pressure (ICP) 8 to 12 hours after diuresis. It also may cause chest pain, blurred vision, rhinitis, thirst, and urine retention.

Nursing process

These nursing process steps are appropriate for patients undergoing treatment with osmotic diuretics.

Assessment

• Monitor the patient's blood pressure and heart rate, especially during rapid diuresis. Establish baseline values before therapy begins, and watch for significant changes.
• Monitor the patient's vital signs, urine output, and central venous pressure for signs of circulatory overload and fluid volume depletion.
• Assess the patient for circulatory overload when urine output is less than 30 ml/hour.
• Assess the patient's neurologic status and ICP for signs of increased ICP.

Key nursing diagnoses

• Risk for deficient fluid volume related to excessive diuresis
• Risk for injury related to electrolyte imbalance or circulatory overload
• Deficient knowledge related to diuretic therapy

Planning outcome goals

• The patient will maintain a normal fluid volume as evidenced by having a blood pressure and heart rate within a normal range.
• The patient won't exhibit adverse effects of electrolyte imbalance or circulatory overload.
• The patient will demonstrate correct diuretic therapy administration.

Implementation

• Administer osmotic diuretics in an I.V. solution slowly over 3 minutes to several hours, depending on the reason for giving the drug and the concentration of the solution.

An irritating problem

• Take steps to avoid infiltration because osmotic diuretics may cause mild irritation or even necrosis.
• Be especially alert for changes in the patient's sodium and potassium levels.
• Give the diuretic in the morning to ensure that major diuresis occurs before bedtime. To prevent nocturia, don't administer later than 6 p.m.
• Monitor intake and output carefully. Use an indwelling catheter for accurate evaluation of diuresis if necessary.

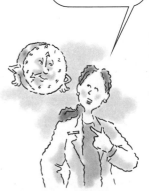

To prevent nocturia, don't administer diuretics after 6 p.m.

• Weigh the patient each morning immediately after he voids and before breakfast, using the same scale and making sure he's wearing the same type of clothing. Weight provides a reliable indicator of the patient's response to diuretic therapy.

Evaluation
• Patient maintains adequate hydration.
• Patient's electrolyte levels remain within normal limits.
• Patient and his family demonstrate an understanding of diuretic therapy.

Carbonic anhydrase inhibitors

Carbonic anhydrase inhibitors are diuretics that block the action of carbonic anhydrase. They include acetazolamide and methazolamide.

Pharmacokinetics

Carbonic anhydrase inhibitors are absorbed through the GI tract. Some systemic absorption also occurs after ophthalmic administration. They're distributed in tissues with high carbonic anhydrase content, such as erythrocytes, plasma, kidneys, eyes, liver, and muscle. Carbonic anhydrase inhibitors are excreted by the kidneys in urine.

Pharmacodynamics

In the kidneys, carbonic anhydrase inhibitors decrease the availability of hydrogen ions, which blocks the sodium-hydrogen exchange mechanisms. As a result, urinary excretion of sodium, potassium, bicarbonate, and water increases.

Don't lose your sense of humor

In the eyes, carbonic anhydrase inhibition reduces aqueous humor production, which reduces intraocular pressure.

Pharmacotherapeutics

Carbonic anhydrase inhibitors are used for diuresis and to treat glaucoma. Acetazolamide may also be used to treat epilepsy and acute mountain sickness.

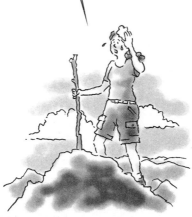

Acetazolamide... (huff)...may be used... (puff)...to treat acute mountain sickness...

Drug interactions

Carbonic anhydrase inhibitors produce a variety of drug interactions:

• Salicylates may cause carbonic anhydrase inhibitor toxicity, including central nervous system depression and metabolic acidosis.

• Diflunisal may increase intraocular pressure when given with a carbonic anhydrase inhibitor.

• Acetazolamide used concurrently with cyclosporine may increase cyclosporine levels and the risk of neurotoxicity.

• Acetazolamide used concurrently with primidone may decrease serum and urine levels of primidone.

Adverse reactions

Carbonic anhydrase inhibitors may cause hypokalemia, metabolic acidosis, and other electrolyte imbalances.

Nursing process

These nursing process steps are appropriate for patients undergoing treatment with carbonic anhydrase inhibitors.

Assessment

• Monitor the patient's blood pressure and heart rate, especially during rapid diuresis. Establish baseline values before therapy begins, and watch for significant changes.

• Establish a baseline CBC (including WBC count), liver function test results, and levels of serum electrolytes (especially potassium, bicarbonate, chloride, and magnesium), carbon dioxide, magnesium, BUN, and creatinine. Review periodically.

• Assess the patient for evidence of excessive diuresis: hypotension, tachycardia, poor skin turgor, excessive thirst, or dry and cracked mucous membranes.

• Monitor and record the patient's intake and output carefully.

Key nursing diagnoses

• Risk for deficient fluid volume related to excessive diuresis

• Risk for injury related to electrolyte imbalance

• Deficient knowledge related to diuretic therapy

Planning outcome goals

• The patient will maintain a normal fluid volume as evidenced by having a blood pressure and heart rate within a normal range.

Look on the positive side: Establishing baseline serum electrolyte levels will help to highlight any imbalances that may crop up!

• The patient won't exhibit adverse effects of electrolyte imbalance.
• The patient will demonstrate correct diuretic therapy administration.

Implementation
• Use cautiously in patients who are allergic to sulfonamides because a cross-sensitivity reaction may occur.

You're feeling very sleepy...
• Give the diuretic in the morning or early afternoon, if possible, to prevent nocturia from disrupting the patient's sleep.
• Weigh the patient each morning immediately after he voids and before breakfast, using the same scale and making sure he's wearing the same type of clothing. Weight provides a reliable indicator of the patient's response to diuretic therapy.
• Keep a urinal or bedpan within reach of the patient or ensure that a bathroom is easily accessible.
• Tell the patient to take the medication with food to prevent GI upset.

Evaluation
• Patient maintains adequate hydration.
• Patient's electrolyte levels remain within normal limits.
• Patient and his family demonstrate an understanding of diuretic therapy.

Urinary tract antispasmodics

Urinary tract antispasmodics help decrease urinary tract muscle spasms. They include darifenacin, flavoxate, oxybutynin, solifenacin, tolterodine, and trospium.

Pharmacokinetics
Flavoxate, oxybutynin, tolterodine, darifenacin, and solifenacin are most often administered orally and are rapidly absorbed. Trospium is administered orally but is poorly absorbed. Oxybutynin is also available as a dermal patch. These drugs are all widely distributed, metabolized in the liver, and excreted in urine. Urinary tract antispasmodics also cross the placenta and are excreted in breast milk.

Pharmacodynamics

Urinary tract antispasmodics relieve smooth muscle spasms by inhibiting parasympathetic activity, which causes the detrusor and urinary muscles to relax. Flavoxate and oxybutynin also exhibit many anticholinergic effects.

Pharmacotherapeutics

Urinary tract antispasmodics are used for patients with overactive bladders who have symptoms of urinary frequency, urgency, or incontinence.

Urgent symptoms

Trospium is also indicated for patients with overactive bladders who have symptoms of urge urinary incontinence, and oxybutynin acts as an antispasmodic for uninhibited or reflex neurogenic bladder. (See *How oxybutynin works*.)

Drug interactions

Urinary tract antispasmodics have few drug interactions:
• Use with anticholinergic agents may increase dry mouth, constipation, and other anticholinergic effects.
• Urinary tract antispasmodics may decrease the effectiveness of phenothiazines and haloperidol.
• Trospium may interfere with the elimination of certain drugs excreted through the kidneys (such as digoxin, metformin, and vancomycin), resulting in increased blood levels of these drugs.

Adverse reactions

Possible adverse reactions to urinary tract antispasmodics include:
• blurred vision
• headache
• somnolence
• urinary retention
• dry mouth
• dyspepsia
• constipation
• nausea
• vomiting
• weight gain
• pain
• acute and secondary angle closure glaucoma.

Pharm function

How oxybutynin works

When acetylcholine is released within the bladder, it attaches to receptors on the surface of smooth muscle in the bladder, stimulating bladder contractions. Oxybutynin suppresses these involuntary contractions by blocking the release of acetylcholine. This anticholinergic effect is what makes oxybutynin useful in the treatment of overactive bladder.

Antispasmodics can cause several adverse reactions, including headache and somnolence. I think I'll just try to sleep until my headache goes away...

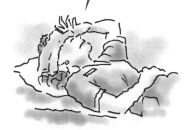

Nursing process

These nursing process steps are appropriate for patients undergoing treatment with urinary tract antispasmodics.

Assessment

• Assess the patient's signs and symptoms before beginning therapy.
• Make sure the patient undergoes periodic cystometry to evaluate his response to therapy.
• Monitor the patient's intake and output.

Key nursing diagnoses

• Risk for urge urinary incontinence related to overactive bladder
• Deficient knowledge related to drug therapy
• Situational low self-esteem related to incontinence

Planning outcome goals

• The patient will demonstrate increased comfort and fewer episodes of incontinence.
• The patient will demonstrate correct drug administration.
• The patient will voice feelings related to incontinence and its effect on self-esteem.

Implementation

• Administer the drug as prescribed.
• Offer small, frequent meals to help prevent nausea.
• Administer trospium at least 1 hour before meals or on an empty stomach.

Drink up!

• Unless contraindicated, encourage the patient to increase his fluid intake to 2 to 3 L per day.

Evaluation

• Patient has relief from incontinence.
• Patient and his family demonstrate an understanding of urinary tract antispasmodic therapy. (See *Teaching about urinary tract antispasmodics*, page 362.)
• Patient has improved self-esteem.

Education edge

Teaching about urinary tract antispasmodics

If urinary tract antispasmodics are prescribed, review these points with the patient and his caregivers:

• Take the drug with meals to help decrease GI upset.

• This drug may decrease your ability to sweat; use caution in a situation that could cause you to overheat.

• Take the drug whole; don't chew, crush, or cut the tablet.

• Suck on hard candy or ice chips to relieve dry mouth while taking this drug.

• Drink adequate fluids to help prevent constipation.

• Notify the practitioner if you can't urinate, develop a fever or severe constipation, or experience blurring of your vision.

Erectile dysfunction therapy drugs

Erectile dysfunction therapy drugs treat penile erectile dysfunction that results from a lack of blood flowing through the corpus cavernosum. This type of erectile dysfunction usually stems from vascular and neurologic conditions. Drugs used for erectile dysfunction include alprostadil, sildenafil, tadalafil, and vardenafil.

Pharmacokinetics

Erectile dysfunction drugs are well absorbed in the GI tract. Distribution of these drugs isn't known. The majority of these drugs—including sildenafil, tadalafil, and vardenafil—are given orally, metabolized in the liver, and excreted in feces.

An exceptional drug

Alprostadil is the exception: it's administered directly into the corpus cavernosum, metabolized in the lungs, and excreted in urine.

Pharmacodynamics

Sildenafil, tadalafil, and vardenafil selectively inhibit the phosphodiesterase type 5 receptors, which causes an increase in blood levels of nitric oxide. This increase in nitric oxide levels activates the cGMP enzyme, which relaxes smooth muscles and allows blood to flow into the corpus cavernosum, causing an erection.

Alprostadil acts locally, promoting smooth muscle relaxation, which causes an increase in blood flow to the corpus cavernosum and produces an erection.

Pharmacotherapeutics

Alprostadil, sildenafil, tadalafil, and vardenafil are all used in the treatment of erectile dysfunction. Sildenafil is also indicated for the treatment of pulmonary arterial hypertension.

Drug interactions

Erectile dysfunction drugs may interact with other drugs in the following ways:
• Nitrates and alpha-adrenergic blockers used in combination with erectile dysfunction drugs may cause severe hypotension and potentially serious cardiac events.
• Ketoconazole, itraconazole, and erythromycin may result in increased levels of vardenafil or tadalafil.
• Protease inhibitors, such as indinavir or ritonavir, may cause increased tadalafil or vardenafil levels.

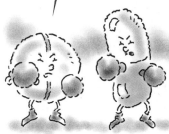

Sometimes we just can't get along: Nitrates and alpha-adrenergic blockers used with erectile dysfunction drugs can cause severe hypotension and potentially serious cardiac events.

Adverse reactions

Sildenafil increases the risk of cardiovascular events by decreasing supine blood pressure and cardiac output. Patients with known cardiovascular disease have an increased risk of cardiovascular events, including myocardial infarction (MI), sudden cardiac death, ventricular arrhythmias, cerebrovascular hemorrhage, transient ischemic attack, and hypertension.

Other reactions to these drugs include headache, dizziness, flushing, dyspepsia, and vision changes. Prolonged erections (more than 4 hours) can result in irreversible damage to erectile tissue. Alprostadil can cause penile pain.

Nursing process

These nursing process steps are appropriate for patients undergoing treatment with erectile dysfunction drugs.

Assessment
• Assess the patient's cardiovascular risk.
• Monitor the patient's blood pressure, heart rate, and electrocardiogram.

Tweaking the dosage
• Assess the effects of the particular dosage the patient is receiving; the dosage for these drugs is highly individualized and should be adjusted based on the patient's response.

Key nursing diagnoses

- Risk for decreased cardiac output related to erectile dysfunction therapy
- Risk for injury related to prolonged erection
- Deficient knowledge related to drug therapy

Planning outcome goals

- The patient won't exhibit signs of decreased cardiac output as evidenced by a stable blood pressure and heart rate.
- Complications from prolonged erection will be diminished.
- The patient will demonstrate correct drug administration.

Implementation

- Explain to the patient that the drug won't protect against pregnancy or the transmission of sexually transmitted diseases.
- If the patient is also taking human immunodeficiency virus medications, warn him about the risk of adverse reactions, including hypotension and priapism.
- If the patient is taking alprostadil, teach him how to prepare and administer the drug. Review aseptic technique, warn him that bleeding at the injection site can increase the risk of transmitting blood-borne diseases to his partner, and explain that he should take the drug as directed.

Evaluation

- Patient maintains adequate cardiac output as evidenced by normal vital signs and adequate tissue perfusion.

Education edge

Teaching about erectile dysfunction drugs

If an erectile dysfunction drug is prescribed, review these points with the patient and his caregivers:

- This drug won't work without the presence of sexual stimulation.
- Take this drug 30 minutes to 4 hours before anticipated sexual activity.
- If you have an erection that lasts longer than 4 hours, seek medical attention; this can become a medical emergency.

- Tell all healthcare providers that you're taking this drug.
- Don't take this drug if you're also taking nitrates or alpha-adrenergic blockers for high blood pressure or angina.
- If you notice persistent or bothersome adverse reactions, notify your practitioner.
- Don't take this drug with alcohol.

- Patient has no serious injury from prolonged erection, if it occurs.
- Patient and his family demonstrate an understanding of erectile dysfunction drugs. (See *Teaching about erectile dysfunction drugs.*)

Hormonal contraceptives

Hormonal contraceptives inhibit ovulation. Contraceptives typically contain a combination of hormones. For example, ethinyl estradiol may be combined with desogestrel, drospirenone, levonorgestrel, norethindrone, norgestimate, or norgestrel. Also, mestranol may be combined with norethindrone. Ethinyl estradiol or ethynodiol diacetate may also be used alone as a contraceptive.

Pharmacokinetics

Hormonal contraceptives are absorbed from the GI tract and are widely distributed. They're metabolized in the kidneys and excreted in urine and feces.

Patch power

Some forms of hormonal contraceptives are available in a transdermal patch form. These contraceptives are absorbed through the skin but have the same distribution, metabolism, and excretion as orally administered contraceptives.

Pharmacodynamics

The primary mechanism of action of combination hormonal contraceptives (estrogen and progestin) is the suppression of gonadotropins, which inhibits ovulation. Estrogen suppresses secretion of follicle-stimulating hormone, which blocks follicular development and ovulation. Progestin suppresses the secretion of luteinizing hormone, which prevents ovulation, even if the follicle develops. Progestin also thickens the cervical mucus; this interferes with sperm migration and causes endometrial changes that prevent implantation of a fertilized ovum.

Pharmacotherapeutics

The primary purpose for taking hormonal contraceptives is the prevention of pregnancy in women. The combination of ethinyl estradiol and norgestimate is also used to treat moderate acne in females under age 15.

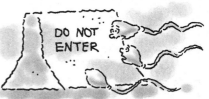

It looks like we're not welcome here, guys!

DO NOT ENTER

Drug interactions

Hormonal contraceptives can interact with other medications in various ways:

• Antibiotics, oxcarbazepine, phenobarbital, phenytoin, topiramate, and modafinil may decrease the effectiveness of oral contraceptives. A patient taking these drugs with a hormonal contraceptive needs to use a barrier contraceptive.
• Atorvastatin may increase serum estrogen levels.
• Cyclosporin and theophylline have an increased risk of toxicity when taken with hormonal contraceptives.
• Prednisone increases the therapeutic and possibly toxic effects of hormonal contraceptives.
• Several herbal medications can affect serum levels of hormonal contraceptives.

Adverse reactions

Potentially serious adverse reactions to hormonal contraceptives include arterial thrombosis, thrombophlebitis, pulmonary embolism, MI, cerebral hemorrhage or thrombosis, hypertension, gallbladder disease, and hepatic adenomas.

Other adverse reactions include:
• acne
• bleeding or spotting between menstrual periods
• bloating
• breast tenderness or enlargement
• changes in libido
• diarrhea
• difficulty wearing contact lenses
• unusual hair growth
• weight fluctuations
• upset stomach
• vomiting.

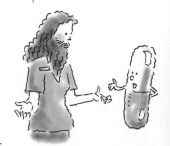

I know hormonal contraceptives can cause unusual hair growth, but this is ridiculous!

Nursing process

These nursing process steps are appropriate for patients undergoing treatment with hormonal contraceptives.

Assessment

• Monitor the patient's vital signs, especially blood pressure.
• Obtain a patient history. Hormonal contraceptive are contraindicated in patients with a history of thrombophlebitis or thromboembolic disorders, deep vein thrombosis, cerebrovascular accidents, coronary artery disease, known carcinoma of the breast, any estrogen-dependent neoplasm, abnormal genital bleeding, or cholestatic jaundice with pregnancy.

Proceed with caution

- Also assess for a history of smoking, fibrocystic breast disease or abnormal mammogram, migraines, high blood pressure, and diabetes. Hormonal contraceptives should be used with caution in patients with these conditions.
- Evaluate the patient's knowledge of hormonal contraceptives.

Key nursing diagnoses

- Risk for ineffective protection related to contraceptive therapy
- Risk for injury related to adverse reactions
- Deficient knowledge related to hormonal contraceptive therapy

Planning outcome goals

- The patient won't become pregnant.
- The patient won't experience adverse reactions.
- The patient will demonstrate an understanding of hormonal contraceptive therapy.

Implementation

- Teach the patient how to take her pills (21-, 28-, or 91-day packets) or how to apply the patch.
- Teach the patient about possible drug interactions and when she'll need to use an additional form of contraception.

Evaluation

- Patient shows no evidence of pregnancy while on hormonal contraceptives.
- Patient is free from adverse reactions.
- Patient and her family demonstrate an understanding of hormonal contraceptive therapy. (See *Teaching about hormonal contraceptives.*)

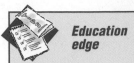

Education edge

Teaching about hormonal contraceptives

If a hormonal contraceptive is prescribed, review these points with the patient or her caregivers:
- Take this medication at the same time each day and as directed by your practitioner.
- If you miss two periods in a row, contact your practitioner; you may be pregnant.
- Notify your practitioner immediately if you have chest pain, difficulty breathing, leg pain, or severe abdominal pain or headache. These symptoms could indicate a serious adverse reaction.
- Notify your practitioner if you have persistent or bothersome adverse reactions.
- Don't take this drug if you think you're pregnant.

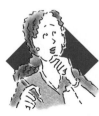

Quick quiz

1. When caring for a patient taking a hydrochlorothiazide, you should monitor the patient for:
    A. hypertension.
    B. hypernatremia.
    C. hypokalemia.
    D. hypoglycemia.

Answer: C. Watch for signs of hypokalemia in a patient receiving hydrochlorothiazide.

2. When teaching a patient about diuretics, you should tell him to:
- A. take the drug in the evening.
- B. call his practitioner if he loses more that 2 lb (0.9 kg) per day.
- C. eat a high-sodium diet.
- D. avoid sun exposure for several hours after taking the medication to prevent a photosensitivity reaction.

Answer: B. A weight loss of more that 2 lb per day indicates excessive diuresis.

3. Urinary tract antispasmodics are used to treat:
- A. overactive bladder.
- B. erectile dysfunction.
- C. hypertension.
- D. seizures.

Answer: A. Urinary tract antispasmodics are used to treat an overactive bladder.

4. When teaching a patient how to take hormonal contraceptives, which of the following instructions should you give?
- A. Take the drug in the morning.
- B. If you miss a dose, skip it and take it the next day.
- C. If you miss one menstrual period, stop taking the drug and take a pregnancy test.
- D. Use an additional form of birth control if you're taking certain antibiotics.

Answer: D. Advise the patient taking hormonal contraceptives to use an additional form of birth control if she's also taking certain antibiotics because antibiotics may decrease the effectiveness of hormonal contraceptives.

Scoring

☆☆☆ If you answered all four questions correctly, terrific! Everything's flowing smoothly for you when it comes to GU drugs.

☆☆ If you answered three questions correctly, super! Your stream of knowledge about GU drugs is impressive.

☆ If you answered fewer than three questions correctly, don't spaz out! Relax, review the chapter, and try again.

Hematologic drugs

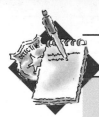

Just the facts

In this chapter, you'll learn:

♦ classes of drugs used to treat hematologic disorders

♦ uses and varying actions of these drugs

♦ absorption, distribution, metabolization, and excretion of these drugs

♦ drug interactions and adverse reactions to these drugs.

Drugs and the hematologic system

The hematologic system includes plasma (the liquid component of blood) and blood cells, such as red blood cells (RBCs), white blood cells, and platelets. Types of drugs used to treat disorders of the hematologic system include:
• hematinic drugs
• anticoagulant drugs
• thrombolytic drugs.

Hematinic drugs

Hematinic drugs provide essential building blocks for RBC production. They do so by increasing hemoglobin, the necessary element for oxygen transportation.

Taking aim at anemia

This section discusses hematinic drugs—iron, vitamin B_{12}, and folic acid—used to treat microcytic and macrocytic anemia as well as epoetin alfa and darbepoetin alfa, which are used to treat normocytic anemia.

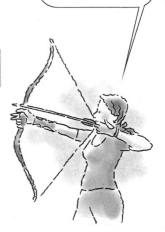

Hematinic drugs give me the tools I need to take aim at anemia.

Iron

Iron preparations are used to treat the most common form of anemia—iron deficiency anemia. Iron preparations discussed in this section include ferrous fumarate, ferrous gluconate, ferrous sulfate, iron dextran, iron sucrose, and sodium ferric gluconate complex.

Pharmacokinetics (how drugs circulate)

Iron is absorbed primarily from the duodenum and upper jejunum of the intestine. The formulations don't vary in their rate of absorption, but they do vary in the amount of elemental iron supplied.

What's in store?

The amount of iron absorbed depends partially on the body's stores of iron. When body stores are low or RBC production is accelerated, iron absorption may increase by 20% to 30%. On the other hand, when total iron stores are large, only about 5% to 10% of iron is absorbed.

Form and function

Enteric-coated preparations decrease iron absorption because, in that form, iron isn't released until after it leaves the duodenum. The lymphatic system absorbs the parenteral form after I.M. injections.

Iron is transported by the blood and bound to transferrin, its carrier plasma protein. About 30% of the iron is stored primarily as hemosiderin or ferritin in the reticuloendothelial cells of the liver, spleen, and bone marrow. About 66% of the total body iron is contained in hemoglobin. Excess iron is excreted in urine, stool, and sweat and through intestinal cell sloughing. Excess iron is also secreted in breast milk.

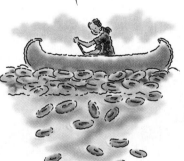

Iron is transported by the blood. It's an interesting way to travel!

Pharmacodynamics (how drugs act)

Although iron has other roles, its most important role is the production of hemoglobin. About 80% of the iron in the plasma goes to the bone marrow, where it's used for erythropoiesis (production of RBCs).

Pharmacotherapeutics (how drugs are used)

Oral iron therapy is used to prevent or treat iron deficiency anemia. It's also used to prevent anemia in children ages 6 months to 2 years because this is a period of rapid growth and development.

Baby makes two

A pregnant woman may need iron supplements to replace the iron used by the developing fetus. She should take oral iron therapy in the form of prenatal vitamins unless she's unable to take iron.

An alternate route

Parenteral iron therapy is used for patients who can't absorb oral preparations, aren't compliant with oral therapy, or have bowel disorders (such as ulcerative colitis or Crohn's disease). Patients with end-stage renal disease who receive hemodialysis may also receive parenteral iron therapy at the end of their dialysis session. Parenteral iron therapy corrects the iron store deficiency quickly; however, the anemia isn't corrected any faster than it would be with oral preparations.

Two of a kind

There are two parenteral iron products available. Iron dextran is given by either I.M. injection or slow continuous I.V. infusion. Iron sucrose is indicated for use in the hemodialysis patient and is administered by I.V. infusion.

Drug interactions

Iron absorption is reduced by antacids as well as by such foods as spinach, whole-grain breads, and cereals, coffee, tea, eggs, and milk products. Other drug interactions involving iron include the following:
• Tetracycline, demeclocycline, minocycline, oxytetracycline, doxycycline, methyldopa, quinolones, levofloxacin, norfloxacin, ofloxacin, gatifloxacin, lomefloxacin, moxifloxacin, sparfloxacin, ciprofloxacin, levothyroxine, and penicillamine absorption may be reduced when taken with oral iron preparations.
• Cholestyramine, cimetidine, magnesium trisilicate, and colestipol may reduce iron absorption in the GI tract.
• Cimetidine and other histamine-2 receptor antagonists may decrease GI absorption of iron.

Adverse reactions

The most common adverse reaction to iron therapy is gastric irritation and constipation. Iron preparations also darken the stool. The liquid form can stain the teeth. Parenteral iron has been associated with an anaphylactoid reaction. (See *Parenteral iron.*)

Nursing process

These nursing process steps are appropriate for patients undergoing treatment with iron.

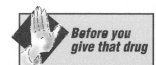

Before you give that drug

Parenteral iron

Before administering parenteral iron, be aware that it has been associated with an anaphylactoid reaction. Administer initial test doses before a full dose infusion to evaluate for potential reactions. Continue to monitor the patient closely because delayed reactions can occur up to 1 to 2 days later.

Signs and symptoms of an anaphylactoid reaction to parenteral iron include:
• arthralgia
• backache
• chest pain
• chills
• dizziness
• headache
• malaise
• fever
• myalgia
• nausea
• vomiting
• hypotension
• respiratory distress.

Assessment

- Assess the patient's iron deficiency before starting therapy.
- Monitor the iron's effectiveness by evaluating the patient's hemoglobin level, hematocrit, and reticulocyte count.
- Monitor the patient's health status.
- Assess for adverse reactions and drug interactions.
- Observe the patient for delayed reactions from therapy.
- Assess the patient's and family's knowledge of drug therapy.

Key nursing diagnoses

- Ineffective health maintenance related to iron deficiency
- Risk for injury related to the underlying condition
- Deficient knowledge related to drug therapy

Planning outcome goals

- The patient's iron deficiency will improve as evidenced by laboratory studies.
- The risk of injury to the patient will be minimized.
- The patient and his family will demonstrate an understanding of drug therapy.

Implementation

- Don't give iron dextran with oral iron preparations.

Testing, testing

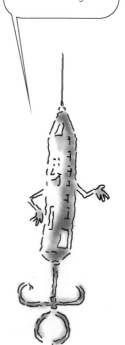

To give iron I.M., use a 19G or 20G needle that's 2″ to 3″ long.

- If I.M. or I.V. injections of iron are recommended, a test dose may be required in the facility.
- If administering iron I.M., use a 19G or 20G needle that's 2″ to 3″ long. Inject into the upper outer quadrant of the buttock. Use the Z-track method to avoid leakage into subcutaneous tissue and staining of the skin.
- Minimize skin staining with I.M. injections of iron by using a separate needle to withdraw the drug from its container.
- I.V. iron is given if the patient has insufficient muscle mass for deep I.M. injection, impaired absorption from muscle as a result of stasis or edema, the potential for uncontrolled I.M. bleeding from trauma (as in patients with hemophilia), or the need for massive and prolonged parenteral therapy (as in patients with chronic substantial blood loss).
- Promote a varied diet that's adequate in protein, calories, minerals, and electrolytes.
- Encourage foods high in iron as applicable to help delay the onset of iron deficiency anemia.
- Administer I.V. fluids and electrolytes as necessary to provide nutrients. Oral food intake or tube feedings are preferable to I.V. therapy.

Education edge

Teaching about hematinic drugs

If hematinic drugs are prescribed, review these points with the patient and his caregivers:
• The best source of minerals and electrolytes is a well-balanced diet that includes a variety of foods.
• Don't take over-the-counter preparations, other drugs, or herbal remedies without first talking to the prescriber or a pharmacist. Adverse interactions can occur with hematinic drugs. For example, herbal preparations of chamomile, feverfew, and St. John's wort may inhibit iron absorption.
• Keep all mineral and electrolyte substances out of the reach of children; accidental overdose can occur.

• Keep follow-up appointments for periodic blood tests and procedures to make sure treatment is appropriate.
• Take the drug as prescribed. Iron supplements should be taken with or after meals with 8 oz (237 ml) of fluid.
• Don't crush or chew slow-release tablets or capsules. Liquid preparations can be diluted with water and sipped through a straw.
• Rinse the mouth after taking liquid preparations to prevent staining of the teeth.
• Iron preparations may cause dark green or black stools.
• Get plenty of rest and rise slowly to avoid dizziness. Take rest periods during the day to conserve energy.

• Correct underlying disorders that contribute to mineral and electrolyte deficiency or excess.
• Promote measures to relieve anorexia, nausea, vomiting, diarrhea, pain, and other signs and symptoms.
• Arrange for a nutritional consult as needed.

Evaluation
• Patient's hemoglobin level, hematocrit, and reticulocyte counts are normal.
• Patient doesn't experience anaphylaxis.
• Patient and his family demonstrate an understanding of drug therapy. (See *Teaching about hematinic drugs*.)

Vitamin B$_{12}$

Vitamin B$_{12}$ preparations are used to treat pernicious anemia. Common vitamin B$_{12}$ preparations include cyanocobalamin and hydroxocobalamin.

Pharmacokinetics

Vitamin B$_{12}$ is available in parenteral, oral, and intranasal forms.

A pernicious problem

A substance called *intrinsic factor*, secreted by the gastric mucosa, is needed for vitamin B$_{12}$ absorption. People who have a deficiency of intrinsic factor develop a special type of anemia known as *vitamin B₁₂-deficiency pernicious anemia*. Because people with this disorder can't absorb vitamin B_{12}, an injectable or intranasal form of the drug is used to treat it.

Final destination: Liver

When cyanocobalamin is injected by the I.M. or subcutaneous (subQ) route, it's absorbed and binds to transcobalamin II for transport to the tissues. It's then transported in the bloodstream to the liver, where 90% of the body's vitamin B_{12} supply is stored. Although hydroxocobalamin is absorbed more slowly from the injection site, its uptake in the liver may be greater than that of cyanocobalamin.

Slow release

With either drug, the liver slowly releases vitamin B_{12} as needed. It's secreted in breast milk during lactation. About 3 to 8 mcg of vitamin B_{12} are excreted in bile each day and then reabsorbed in the ileum. Within 48 hours after a vitamin B_{12} injection, 50% to 95% of the dose is excreted unchanged in urine.

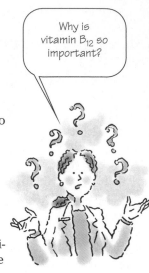

Why is vitamin B_{12} so important?

Pharmacodynamics

When vitamin B_{12} is administered, it replaces vitamin B_{12} that the body normally would absorb from the diet.

A must for myelin maintenance

This vitamin is essential for cell growth and replication and for the maintenance of myelin (nerve coverings) throughout the nervous system. Vitamin B_{12} also may be involved in lipid and carbohydrate metabolism.

Pharmacotherapeutics

Cyanocobalamin and hydroxocobalamin are used to treat pernicious anemia, a megaloblastic anemia characterized by decreased gastric production of hydrochloric acid and the deficiency of intrinsic factor, a substance normally secreted by the parietal cells of the gastric mucosa that's essential for vitamin B_{12} absorption.

Common ground

Intrinsic factor deficiencies are common in patients who have undergone total or partial gastrectomies or total ileal resection. Oral vitamin B_{12} preparations are used to supplement nutritional deficiencies of the vitamin.

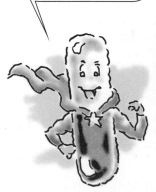

Because I'm essential for cell growth and replication and for maintaining myelin throughout the nervous system.

Drug interactions

Alcohol, aspirin, aminosalicylic acid, neomycin, chloramphenicol, and colchicine may decrease the absorption of oral cyanocobalamin.

Adverse reactions

No dose-related adverse reactions occur with vitamin B_{12} therapy. However, some rare reactions may occur when vitamin B_{12} is administered parenterally.

Don't be so (hyper)sensitive

Adverse reactions to parenteral administration can include hypersensitivity reactions that could result in mild diarrhea, itching, transient rash, hives, hypokalemia, polycythemia vera, peripheral vascular thrombosis, heart failure, pulmonary edema, anaphylaxis, or even death.

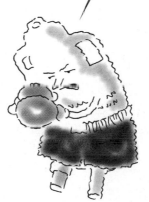

Adverse reactions to parenteral vitamin B_{12} can be a real knockout.

Nursing process

These nursing process steps are appropriate for patients undergoing treatment with vitamin B_{12}.

Assessment
- Assess the patient's vitamin B_{12} deficiency before therapy.
- Monitor the drug's effectiveness by evaluating the patient's hemoglobin level, hematocrit, and reticulocyte count.
- Monitor the patient's health status.
- Assess for adverse reactions and drug interactions.
- Observe the patient for delayed reactions to therapy.
- Assess the patient's and family's knowledge of drug therapy.

Key nursing diagnoses
- Ineffective health maintenance related to vitamin B_{12} deficiency
- Risk for injury related to the underlying condition
- Deficient knowledge related to drug therapy

Planning outcome goals
- The patient's vitamin B_{12} deficiency will improve as evidenced by laboratory studies.
- The risk of injury to the patient will be minimized.
- The patient and his family will demonstrate an understanding of drug therapy.

Implementation

• Promote a varied diet that's adequate in protein, calories, minerals, and electrolytes.

• Encourage foods high in iron as applicable to help delay the onset of iron deficiency anemia.

• Administer I.V. fluids and electrolytes as necessary to provide nutrients. Oral food intake or tube feedings are preferable to I.V. therapy.

• Correct underlying disorders that contribute to mineral and electrolyte deficiency or excess.

• Promote measures to relieve anorexia, nausea, vomiting, diarrhea, pain, and other signs and symptoms.

Evaluation

• Patient's hemoglobin level, hematocrit, and reticulocyte counts are normal.

• Patient's underlying condition and neurologic signs and symptoms improve.

• Patient and his family demonstrate an understanding of drug therapy.

Folic acid

Folic acid is given to treat megaloblastic anemia caused by folic acid deficiency. This type of anemia usually occurs in infants, adolescents, pregnant and lactating women, elderly persons, alcoholics, and those with intestinal or malignant diseases. Folic acid is also used as a nutritional supplement.

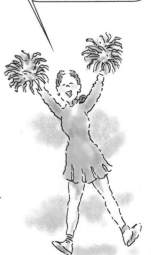

Three cheers for synthetic folic acid! It's readily absorbed even in patients with malabsorption syndromes.

Pharmacokinetics

Folic acid is absorbed rapidly in the first third of the small intestine and distributed into all body tissues. Synthetic folic acid is readily absorbed even in malabsorption syndromes.

Folic acid is metabolized in the liver. Excess folate is excreted unchanged in urine, and small amounts of folic acid are excreted in feces. Folic acid is also secreted in breast milk.

Pharmacodynamics

Folic acid is an essential component for normal RBC production and growth. A deficiency in folic acid results in megaloblastic anemia and low serum and RBC folate levels.

Pharmacotherapeutics

Folic acid is used to treat folic acid deficiency. Patients who are pregnant or undergoing treatment for liver disease, hemolytic anemia, alcohol abuse, skin disorders, or renal disorders typically need folic acid supplementation. Folic acid supplementation also reduces the risk of neural tube defects and colon cancer. Serum folic acid levels less than 5 mg indicate folic acid deficiency.

Drug interactions

These drug interactions may occur with folic acid:
• Methotrexate, sulfasalazine, hormonal contraceptives, aspirin, triamterene, pentamidine, and trimethoprim reduce the effectiveness of folic acid.

The anti anti-convulsant

• In large doses, folic acid may counteract the effects of anticonvulsants, such as phenytoin, potentially leading to seizures.

Adverse reactions

Adverse reactions to folic acid include:
• erythema
• itching
• rash
• anorexia
• nausea
• altered sleep patterns
• difficulty concentrating
• irritability
• overactivity.

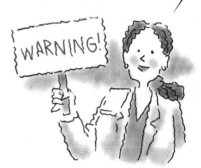

Seize this warning! Large doses of folic acid may counteract the effects of anticonvulsants.

Nursing process

These nursing process steps are appropriate for patients undergoing treatment with folic acid.

Assessment

• Assess the patient's folic acid deficiency before therapy.
• Monitor the therapy's effectiveness by evaluating the patient's hemoglobin level, hematocrit, and reticulocyte count.
• Monitor the patient's health status.
• Assess for adverse reactions and drug interactions.
• Observe the patient for delayed reactions to therapy.
• Assess the patient's and family's knowledge of drug therapy.

Key nursing diagnoses

• Ineffective health maintenance related to folic acid deficiency
• Risk for injury related to the underlying condition
• Deficient knowledge related to drug therapy

Planning outcome goals

• The patient's folic acid deficiency will improve as evidenced by laboratory studies.
• The risk of injury to the patient will be minimized.
• The patient and his family will demonstrate an understanding of drug therapy.

Implementation

• Promote a varied diet that's adequate in protein, calories, minerals, and electrolytes.
• Administer I.V. fluids and electrolytes as necessary to provide nutrients. Oral food intake or tube feedings are preferable to I.V. therapy.
• Correct underlying disorders that contribute to mineral and electrolyte deficiency or excess.
• Promote measures to relieve anorexia, nausea, vomiting, diarrhea, pain, and other signs and symptoms.
• If using the I.M. route, don't mix folic acid and other drugs in the same syringe.

Evaluation

• Patient's hemoglobin level, hematocrit, and reticulocyte counts are normal.
• Patient's underlying condition improves.
• Patient and his family demonstrate an understanding of drug therapy.

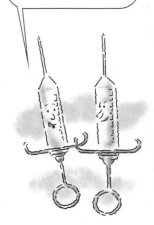

If you're using the I.M. route, don't mix folic acid and other drugs in the same syringe. You'll need both of us for proper administration.

Epoetin alfa and darbepoetin alfa

Erythropoietin is a substance that forms in the kidneys in response to hypoxia (reduced oxygen) and anemia. It stimulates RBC production (erythropoiesis) in the bone marrow. For the patient experiencing decreased erythropoietin production, epoetin alfa and darbepoetin alfa are glycoproteins that are used to stimulate RBC production.

Pharmacokinetics

Epoetin alfa and darbepoetin alfa may be given subQ or I.V.

Reaching the peak

After subQ administration, peak serum levels of epoetin alfa occur in 5 to 24 hours. The peak level of darbepoetin alfa occurs within 24 to 72 hours. The circulating half-life is 4 to 13 hours for epoetin alfa and 49 hours for darbepoetin alfa. The therapeutic effect of these drugs lasts for several days after administration. They're eliminated through the kidneys.

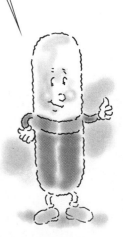

I'm SO stimulating! Epoetin alfa and darbepoetin alfa are used to stimulate RBC production.

Pharmacodynamics

Patients with conditions that decrease erythropoietin production (such as chronic renal failure) typically develop normocytic anemia. Epoetin alfa and darbepoetin alfa are structurally similar to erythropoietin. Therapy with these drugs corrects normocytic anemia within 5 to 6 weeks.

Pharmacotherapeutics

Epoetin alfa is used to:
• treat patients with anemia associated with chronic renal failure
• treat anemia associated with zidovudine therapy in patients with human immunodeficiency virus infection
• treat anemia in cancer patients receiving chemotherapy
• reduce the need for allogenic blood transfusions in patients undergoing surgery.

Darbepoetin alfa is indicated for anemia associated with chronic renal failure.

Drug interactions

No known drug interactions exist.

Adverse reactions

Hypertension is the most common adverse reaction to epoetin alfa and darbepoetin alfa. Other adverse reactions may include:
• headache
• joint pain
• nausea
• edema
• fatigue
• diarrhea
• vomiting
• chest pain
• skin reactions at the injection site
• weakness
• dizziness.

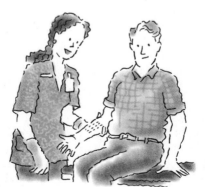

Epoetin alfa and darbepoetin alfa may cause skin reactions at the injection site.

Nursing process

These nursing process steps are appropriate for patients undergoing treatment with epoetin alfa or darbepoetin alfa.

Assessment

• Assess the patient's iron deficiency before starting therapy.

- Monitor the drug's effectiveness by evaluating the patient's hemoglobin level, hematocrit, and reticulocyte count.
- Monitor the patient's health status.
- Assess vital signs, especially blood pressure.
- Assess for adverse reactions and drug interactions.
- Observe the patient for delayed reactions to therapy.
- Assess the patient's and family's knowledge of drug therapy.

Key nursing diagnoses
- Ineffective health maintenance related to iron deficiency
- Risk for injury related to the underlying condition
- Deficient knowledge related to drug therapy

Planning outcome goals
- The patient's iron deficiency will improve as evidenced by laboratory studies.
- The risk of injury to the patient will be minimized.
- The patient and his family will demonstrate an understanding of drug therapy.

Implementation
- Give the I.V. form of the drug by direct injection.
- Additional heparin may be needed to prevent blood clotting if the patient is on dialysis.
- Promote a varied diet that's adequate in protein, calories, minerals, and electrolytes.

Delaying tactics
- Encourage foods high in iron as applicable to help delay the onset of iron deficiency anemia.
- Administer I.V. fluids and electrolytes as necessary to provide nutrients. Oral food intake or tube feedings are preferable to I.V. therapy.
- Correct underlying disorders that contribute to mineral and electrolyte deficiency or excess.
- Promote measures to relieve anorexia, nausea, vomiting, diarrhea, pain, and other signs and symptoms.
- Administer supplementation as necessary.

Evaluation
- Patient's hemoglobin level, hematocrit, and reticulocyte counts are normal.
- Patient's underlying condition improves.
- Patient and his family demonstrate an understanding of drug therapy.

Anticoagulant drugs

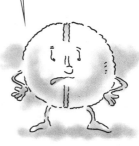

Blood trying to clot? I think not! Anticoagulant drugs reduce the blood's ability to clot.

Anticoagulant drugs are used to reduce the ability of the blood to clot. Major categories of anticoagulant drugs include:
- heparin
- oral anticoagulants
- antiplatelet drugs
- direct thrombin inhibitors
- factor Xa inhibitors.

Heparin and heparin derivatives

Heparin, prepared commercially from animal tissue, is an anti-thrombolytic agent used to prevent clot formation. Because it doesn't affect the synthesis of clotting factors, heparin can't dissolve already formed clots.

The lightweights

Low-molecular-weight heparins, such as dalteparin sodium and enoxaparin sodium, are derived by decomposing unfractionated heparin into simpler compounds. They were developed to prevent deep vein thrombosis (DVT), a blood clot in the deep veins (usually of the legs), in surgical patients. Their use is preferred because they can be given subQ and don't require as much monitoring as unfractionated heparin.

Pharmacokinetics

Because heparin and its derivatives aren't absorbed well from the GI tract, they must be administered parenterally. Unfractionated heparin is administered by continuous I.V. infusion. Low-molecular-weight heparins have the advantage of a prolonged circulating half-life. They can be administered subQ once or twice daily. Distribution is immediate after I.V. administration, but it isn't as predictable with subQ injection.

Low-molecular-weight heparins can be given subQ and don't require as much monitoring as unfractionated heparin. So bring on those fractions!

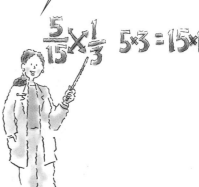

I.M. is out

Heparin and its derivatives aren't given I.M. because of the risk of local bleeding. These drugs metabolize in the liver. Their metabolites are excreted in urine. (See *Anticoagulant drugs: Heparin and heparin derivatives*, page 382.)

Pharmacodynamics

Heparin and heparin derivatives prevent the formation of new thrombi. Here's how heparin works:

Prototype pro

Anticoagulant drugs: Heparin and heparin derivatives

Actions
• Accelerates formation of an antithrombin III-thrombin complex
• Inactivates thrombin and prevents the conversion of fibrinogen to fibrin

Indications
• Deep vein thrombosis
• Pulmonary embolism
• Open-heart surgery
• Disseminated intravascular coagulation
• Unstable angina
• Post–myocardial infarction
• Cerebral thrombosis in evolving stroke
• Left ventricular thrombi
• Heart failure
• History of embolism and atrial fibrillation

Nursing considerations
• Monitor the patient for adverse effects, such as hemorrhage, prolonged clotting time, thrombocytopenia, and hypersensitivity reactions.
• Regularly inspect the patient for bleeding gums, bruises, petechiae, epistaxis, tarry stools, hematuria, and hematemesis.
• Effects can be neutralized by protamine sulfate.
• Monitor partial thromboplastin time regularly.

• Heparin inhibits the formation of thrombin and fibrin by activating antithrombin III.
• Antithrombin III then inactivates factors IXa, Xa, XIa, and XIIa in the intrinsic and common pathways. The end result is the prevention of a stable fibrin clot.
• In low doses, heparin increases the activity of antithrombin III against factor Xa and thrombin and inhibits clot formation.
• Much larger doses are necessary to inhibit fibrin formation after a clot has been formed. This relationship between dose and effect is the rationale for using low-dose heparin to prevent clotting.
• Whole blood clotting time, thrombin time, and partial thromboplastin time (PTT) are prolonged during heparin therapy. However, these times may be only slightly prolonged with low or ultra-low preventive dosages.

Pharmacotherapeutics

Heparin may be used in many clinical situations to prevent the formation of new clots or the extension of existing clots. These situations include:

• preventing or treating venous thromboemboli, characterized by inappropriate or excessive intravascular activation of blood clotting as well as extending embolisms
• treating disseminated intravascular coagulation, a complication of other diseases that results in accelerated clotting
• treating arterial clotting and preventing embolus formation in patients with atrial fibrillation, an arrhythmia in which ineffective atrial contractions cause blood to pool in the atria, increasing the risk of clot formation
• preventing thrombus formation and promoting cardiac circulation in an acute myocardial infarction (MI) by preventing further clot formation at the site of the already formed clot.

An out-of-body experience

Heparin can be used to prevent clotting whenever the patient's blood must circulate outside the body through a machine, such as the cardiopulmonary bypass machine and hemodialysis machine, as well as during extracorporeal circulation and blood transfusions.

No bones About it

Heparin is also useful for preventing clotting during intra-abdominal or orthopedic surgery. (These types of surgery, in many cases, activate the coagulation mechanisms excessively.) In fact, heparin is the drug of choice for orthopedic surgery. (See *Monitoring heparin therapy*.)

Pulling the plug on DVT

Low-molecular-weight heparins are used to prevent DVT.

Drug interactions

Watch for these drug interactions in patients taking heparin or heparin derivatives:
• Because heparin and heparin derivatives act synergistically with all the oral anticoagulants, the risk of bleeding increases when the patient takes both drugs together. The prothrombin time (PT) and International Normalized Ratio (INR), used to monitor the effects of oral anticoagulants, may also be prolonged.
• The risk of bleeding increases when the patient takes nonsteroidal anti-inflammatory drugs (NSAIDs), iron dextran, clopidogrel, cilostazol, or an antiplatelet drug, such as aspirin, ticlopidine, or dipyridamole, while also receiving heparin or its derivatives.
• Drugs that antagonize or inactivate heparin and heparin derivatives include antihistamines, digoxin, penicillins, cephalosporins, nitroglycerin, nicotine, phenothiazines, tetracycline hydrochloride, quinidine, neomycin sulfate, and I.V. penicillin.

Monitoring heparin therapy

Therapy with unfractionated heparin requires close monitoring. Dosage adjustments may be needed to ensure therapeutic effectiveness without increasing the risk of bleeding. Monitor partial thromboplastin time to measure the effectiveness of unfractionated heparin therapy. Also monitor platelet count to watch for heparin-induced thrombocytopenia.

When to switch

Heparin therapy is associated with thrombocytopenia. If heparin-induced thrombocytopenia develops, use thrombin inhibitors, such as lepirudin, argatroban, or bivalirudin, instead of heparin.

• Nicotine may inactivate heparin and heparin derivatives.
• Nitroglycerin may inhibit the effects of heparin and heparin derivatives.
• Protamine sulfate and administration of fresh frozen plasma counteract the effects of heparin and heparin derivatives.

Adverse reactions

One advantage of heparin and its derivatives is that they produce relatively few adverse reactions. These reactions can usually be prevented if the patient's PTT is maintained within the therapeutic range (1½ to 2½ times the control).

Reversal of fortune

Bleeding, the most common adverse effect, can be reversed easily by administering protamine sulfate, which binds to heparin and forms a stable salt with it. Other adverse effects include bruising, hematoma formation, necrosis of the skin or other tissue, and thrombocytopenia.

Put out that cigarette right now! Not only is smoking bad for you, but the nicotine may inactivate heparin!

Nursing process

These nursing process steps are appropriate for patients undergoing treatment with heparin or heparin derivatives.

Assessment
• Assess the patient for bleeding and other adverse reactions.
• Assess the patient's underlying condition before therapy.
• Monitor the patient's vital signs, hemoglobin level, hematocrit, platelet count, PT, INR, and PTT.
• Assess the patient's urine, stool, and emesis for blood.

Key nursing diagnoses
• Ineffective protection related to the drug's effects on the body's normal clotting and bleeding mechanisms
• Risk for deficient fluid volume related to bleeding
• Deficient knowledge related to drug therapy

Planning outcome goals
• The patient will have clotting times appropriate for drug therapy.
• The patient will maintain adequate fluid volume as evidenced by vital signs and laboratory studies.
• The patient and his family will demonstrate an understanding of drug therapy.

Implementation

- Carefully and regularly monitor PTT. Anticoagulation is present when PTT values are 1½ to 2 times the control values.
- Don't administer heparin I.M.; avoid I.M. injections of any anticoagulant, if possible.
- Keep protamine sulfate available to treat severe bleeding caused by the drug.
- Notify the prescriber about serious or persistent adverse reactions.
- Maintain bleeding precautions throughout therapy.
- Administer I.V. solutions using an infusion pump, as appropriate.
- Avoid excessive I.M. injection of other drugs, to minimize the risk of hematoma.

Evaluation

- Patient's health status improves.
- Patient has no evidence of bleeding or hemorrhaging.
- Patient and his family demonstrate an understanding of drug therapy.

Oral anticoagulants

The major oral anticoagulant used in the United States is the coumarin compound warfarin sodium.

Pharmacokinetics

Warfarin is absorbed rapidly and almost completely when it's taken orally.

Why the delay?

Despite its rapid absorption, warfarin's effects aren't seen for about 36 to 48 hours and it may take 3 to 4 days for the full effect to occur. This is because warfarin antagonizes the production of vitamin K–dependent clotting factors. Before warfarin can exhibit its full effect, the circulating vitamin K clotting factors must be exhausted.

Warfarin is bound extensively to plasma albumin, metabolized in the liver, and excreted in urine. Because warfarin is highly protein bound and metabolized in the liver, using other drugs at the same time may alter the amount of warfarin in the body. This may increase the risk of bleeding and clotting, depending on which drugs are used.

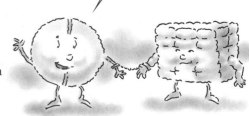

I'm extensively bound to plasma albumin. Stick with me, buddy, and you'll go places!

Pharmacodynamics

Oral anticoagulants alter the ability of the liver to synthesize vitamin K–dependent clotting factors, including prothrombin and factors VII, IX, and X. However, clotting factors already in the bloodstream continue to coagulate blood until they become depleted, so anticoagulation doesn't begin immediately.

Pharmacotherapeutics

Oral anticoagulants are prescribed to treat thromboembolism and, in this situation, are started while the patient is still receiving heparin. Warfarin, however, may be started without heparin in outpatients at high risk for thromboembolism. (See *Anticoagulant drugs: Warfarin.*)

The chosen one

Oral anticoagulants also are the drugs of choice to prevent DVT and treat patients with prosthetic heart valves or diseased mitral valves. They sometimes are combined with an antiplatelet drug, such as aspirin, clopidogrel, or dipyridamole, to decrease the risk of arterial clotting.

Drug interactions

Many patients who take oral anticoagulants also receive other drugs, placing them at risk for serious drug interactions:
• Many drugs, such as highly protein-bound medications, increase the effects of warfarin, resulting in an increased risk of bleeding. Examples include acetaminophen, allopurinol, amiodarone, cephalosporins, cimetidine, ciprofloxacin, clofibrate, danazol, diazoxide, disulfiram, erythromycin, fluoroquinolones, glucagon, heparin, ibuprofen, isoniazid, ketoprofen, metronidazole, miconazole, neomycin, propafenone, propylthiouracil, quinidine, streptokinase, sulfonamides, tamoxifen, tetracyclines, thiazides, thyroid drugs, tricyclic antidepressants, urokinase, and vitamin E.
• Drugs metabolized by the liver may increase or decrease the effectiveness of warfarin. Examples include barbiturates, carbamazepine, corticosteroids, corticotropin, mercaptopurine, nafcillin, hormonal contraceptives containing estrogen, rifampin, spironolactone, sucralfate, and trazodone.
• A diet high in vitamin K reduces the effectiveness of oral anticoagulants.
• The risk of phenytoin toxicity increases when phenytoin is taken with warfarin. Phenytoin may increase or decrease the effects of warfarin.

Prototype pro

Anticoagulant drugs: Warfarin

Actions
• Inhibits vitamin K–dependent activation of clotting factors II, VII, IX, and X formed in the liver

Indications
• Prevention of pulmonary embolism caused by deep vein thrombosis, myocardial infarction, rheumatic fever, prosthetic heart valves, or chronic atrial fibrillation

Nursing considerations
• Monitor the patient for adverse reactions, such as hemorrhage, prolonged clotting time, rash, fever, diarrhea, and hepatitis.
• Regularly inspect the patient for bleeding gums, bruises, petechiae, epistaxis, tarry stools, hematuria, and hematemesis.
• The drug's effects can be neutralized by vitamin K.
• Monitor prothrombin time regularly.

• Chronic alcohol abuse increases the risk of clotting in patients taking warfarin. Patients with acute alcohol intoxication have an increased risk of bleeding.
• Vitamin K and fresh frozen plasma reduce the effects of warfarin.

Adverse reactions

The primary adverse reaction to oral anticoagulant therapy is minor bleeding. Severe bleeding can occur, however, with the most common site being the GI tract. Bleeding into the brain may be fatal. Bruises and hematomas may form at arterial puncture sites (for example, after a blood gas sample is drawn). Neurosis or gangrene of the skin and other tissue can occur. Warfarin is contraindicated during pregnancy.

In reverse

The effects of oral anticoagulants can be reversed with phytonadione (vitamin K_1).

Nursing process

These nursing process steps are appropriate for patients undergoing treatment with oral anticoagulants.

Assessment
• Assess the patient's underlying condition before starting therapy.
• Monitor the patient closely for bleeding and other adverse reactions.
• Monitor the patient's vital signs, hemoglobin level, hematocrit, platelet count, PT, INR, and PTT.
• Assess the patient's urine, stool, and emesis for blood.

Key nursing diagnoses
• Ineffective protection related to the drug's effects on the body's normal clotting and bleeding mechanisms
• Risk for deficient fluid volume related to bleeding
• Deficient knowledge related to drug therapy

Planning outcome goals
• The patient's clotting times will respond appropriately to drug therapy.
• The patient will maintain adequate fluid volume as evidenced by vital signs and laboratory studies.
• The patient and his family will demonstrate an understanding of drug therapy.

Keep an eye on your patient's diet if he's taking oral anticoagulants. A diet high in vitamin K reduces the effectiveness of these drugs.

Education edge

Teaching about anticoagulant drugs

If anticoagulant drugs are prescribed, review these points with the patient and his caregivers:
• Take the drug exactly as prescribed. If taking warfarin, take it at night.
• If taking warfarin, have blood drawn for prothrombin time or International Normalized Ratio tests in the morning to ensure accurate results.
• Consult the prescriber before taking other drugs, including over-the-counter medications and herbal remedies.

• Institute ways to prevent bleeding during daily activities. For example, remove safety hazards from the home to reduce the risk of injury.
• Don't increase intake of green, leafy vegetables or other foods or multivitamins with vitamin K because vitamin K may antagonize the anticoagulant effects of the drug.
• Report bleeding or other adverse reactions promptly.
• Keep appointments for blood tests and follow-up examinations.
• Report planned or known pregnancy.

Implementation
• Carefully and regularly monitor PT and INR values.

Vital vitamin

• Keep vitamin K available to treat frank bleeding caused by warfarin.
• Notify the prescriber about serious or persistent adverse reactions.
• Maintain bleeding precautions throughout therapy.
• Administer the drug at the same time each day.

Evaluation
• Patient has no adverse change in health status.
• Patient has no evidence of bleeding or hemorrhaging.
• Patient and his family demonstrate an understanding of drug therapy. (See *Teaching about anticoagulant drugs.*)

Antiplatelet drugs

Antiplatelet drugs are used to prevent arterial thromboembolism, particularly in patients at risk for MI, stroke, and arteriosclerosis (hardening of the arteries). Antiplatelet drugs include:
• aspirin
• clopidogrel
• dipyridamole
• ticlopidine.

I.V. instances

I.V. antiplatelet drugs are used in the treatment of acute coronary syndromes and include the medications eptifibatide, tirofiban, and abciximab.

Pharmacokinetics

Oral antiplatelet drugs are absorbed very quickly and reach peak concentration between 1 and 2 hours after administration. Aspirin maintains its antiplatelet effect for approximately 10 days, or as long as platelets normally survive. The effects of clopidogrel last about 5 days.

Within minutes

Antiplatelet drugs administered I.V. are quickly distributed throughout the body. They're minimally metabolized and excreted unchanged in urine. The effects of the drugs are seen within 15 to 20 minutes of administration and last about 6 to 8 hours. Elderly patients and patients with renal failure may have decreased clearance of these drugs, prolonging their antiplatelet effect.

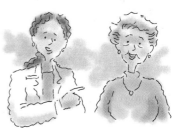

Elderly patients and patients with renal failure may have decreased clearance of antiplatelet drugs, which can prolong their antiplatelet effects.

Pharmacodynamics

Antiplatelet drugs interfere with platelet activity in different drug-specific and dosage-related ways.

Block that clot

Low dosages of aspirin appear to inhibit clot formation by blocking the synthesis of prostaglandin, which in turn prevents formation of the platelet-aggregating substance thromboxane A_2. Clopidogrel inhibits platelet aggregation by inhibiting platelet-fibrinogen binding.

Prevent that platelet

I.V. antiplatelet drugs block platelet function by inhibiting the glycoprotein IIa-IIIb receptor, which is the major receptor involved in platelet aggregation.

Dipyridamole may inhibit platelet aggregation through its ability to increase adenosine, which is a coronary vasodilator and platelet aggregation inhibitor.

In the early stages

Ticlopidine inhibits the binding of fibrinogen to platelets during the first stage of the clotting cascade.

Pharmacotherapeutics

Antiplatelet drugs have many different uses.

A familiar face

Aspirin is used in patients with a previous MI or unstable angina to reduce the risk of death, and in men to reduce the risk of transient ischemic attacks (TIAs) (temporary reduction in circulation to the brain).

Risky business

Clopidogrel is used to reduce the risk of an ischemic stroke or vascular death in patients with a history of a recent MI, stroke, or established peripheral artery disease. This drug is also used to treat acute coronary syndromes, especially in patients who undergo percutaneous transluminal coronary angioplasty (PTCA) or coronary artery bypass grafting.

Dynamic duos

Dipyridamole is used with a coumarin compound to prevent thrombus formation after cardiac valve replacement. Dipyridamole with aspirin has been used to prevent thromboembolic disorders in patients with aortocoronary bypass grafts (bypass surgery) or prosthetic (artificial) heart valves.

Ticlopidine is used to reduce the risk of thrombotic stroke in high-risk patients (including those with a history of frequent TIAs) and in patients who have already had a thrombotic stroke.

The list goes on

Eptifibatide is indicated in the treatment of acute coronary syndrome and in those patients undergoing percutaneous coronary intervention (PCI). Tirofiban is indicated in the treatment of acute coronary syndrome. Abciximab is indicated as an adjunct to PCI.

Drug interactions

Several drug interactions can occur in patients taking antiplatelet drugs:
• Antiplatelet drugs taken in combination with NSAIDs, heparin, or oral anticoagulants increase the risk of bleeding.
• Aspirin increases the risk of toxicity of methotrexate and valproic acid.
• Aspirin and ticlopidine may reduce the effectiveness of sulfinpyrazone to relieve signs and symptoms of gout.
• Antacids may reduce the plasma levels of ticlopidine.
• Cimetidine increases the risk of ticlopidine toxicity and bleeding.

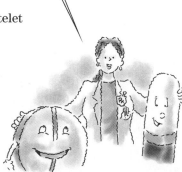

Drugs that interact with antiplatelet drugs include NSAIDs, heparin, oral anticoagulants, methotrexate, valproic acid, antacids, cimetidine, and salicylates in over-the-counter cold medicine compounds.

Don't mix and match

Because guidelines haven't been established for administering ticlopidine with heparin, oral anticoagulants, aspirin, or fibrinolytic drugs, discontinue these drugs before starting ticlopidine therapy.

Adverse reactions

Hypersensitivity reactions, particularly anaphylaxis, can occur. Bleeding is the most common adverse effect of I.V. antiplatelet drugs.

Adverse reactions to aspirin include:
- stomach pain
- heartburn
- nausea
- constipation
- blood in the stool
- slight gastric blood loss.

Clopidogrel may cause these adverse reactions:
- headache
- skin ulceration
- joint pain
- flulike symptoms
- upper respiratory tract infection.

These adverse reactions may occur with ticlopidine:
- diarrhea
- nausea
- dyspepsia
- rash
- elevated liver function test results
- neutropenia.

Dipyridamole may cause:
- headache
- dizziness
- nausea
- flushing
- weakness and fainting
- mild GI distress.

Nursing process

These nursing process steps are appropriate for patients undergoing treatment with antiplatelet drugs.

Assessment

- Assess the patient's underlying condition before starting therapy.

• Monitor the patient closely for bleeding and other adverse reactions.
• During long-term therapy with aspirin, monitor the patient's serum salicylate level and perform hearing assessments.
• Monitor the patient's vital signs, hemoglobin level, hematocrit, and platelet count.
• Assess the patient's urine, stool, and emesis for blood.

Key nursing diagnoses

• Ineffective protection related to the drug's effects on the body's normal clotting and bleeding mechanisms
• Risk for deficient fluid volume related to bleeding
• Deficient knowledge related to drug therapy

Planning outcome goals

• The patient's clotting times will respond appropriately to drug therapy.
• The patient will maintain adequate fluid volume as evidenced by vital signs and laboratory studies.
• The patient and his family will demonstrate an understanding of drug therapy.

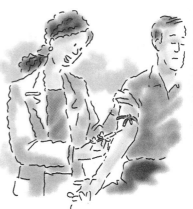

Patients receiving long-term aspirin therapy need to have their serum salicylate level monitored and their hearing checked.

Implementation

• Notify the prescriber about serious or persistent adverse reactions.
• Maintain bleeding precautions throughout therapy.
• Avoid excessive I.V., I.M., or subQ injection of other drugs to minimize the risk of hematoma.
• Give aspirin with food, milk, an antacid, or a large glass of water to reduce adverse GI reactions.
• Don't crush enteric-coated products.
• Withhold the dose and notify the prescriber if bleeding, salicylism (tinnitus, hearing loss), or adverse GI reactions develop.
• Stop antiplatelet drugs 5 to 7 days before elective surgery as appropriate.

Evaluation

• Patient has no adverse change in health status.
• Patient has no evidence of bleeding or hemorrhaging.
• Patient and his family demonstrate an understanding of drug therapy.

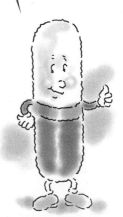

Don't crush enteric-coated drugs!

Direct thrombin inhibitors

Direct thrombin inhibitors are anticoagulant drugs used to prevent the formation of harmful blood clots in the body. Argatroban, bivalirudin, and lepirudin are examples of direct thrombin inhibitors.

Pharmacokinetics

Direct thrombin inhibitors are usually administered I.V., typically by continuous infusion. They're metabolized by the liver. Reduced dosages may be necessary in individuals with hepatic impairment. Effects on PTT become apparent within 4 to 5 hours of administration. Platelet count recovery becomes apparent within 3 days.

When you'll reach the peak

Direct thrombin inhibitors have a rapid onset after I.V. bolus administration. Bivalirudin reaches its peak response in 15 minutes and has a duration of 2 hours. Argatroban reaches peak levels in 1 to 3 hours; its duration lasts until the infusion stops. Peak levels of lepirudin occur in 10 minutes, and its duration also lasts until the infusion stops. Argatroban is excreted primarily in feces through biliary secretion. Bivalirudin and lepirudin are excreted renally.

Pharmacodynamics

Direct thrombin inhibitors interfere with the blood clotting mechanism by blocking the direct activity of soluble and clot-bound thrombin. When these drugs bind to thrombin, they inhibit:
• platelet activation, granule release, and aggregation
• fibrinogen cleavage
• fibrin formation and further activation of the clotting cascade.

Creating a complex

Lepirudin binds rapidly with thrombin to form tight complexes, but it doesn't inhibit other proteases.

No chance to react

Argatroban reversibly binds to the thrombin-active site and inhibits thrombin-induced reactions, including fibrin formation; coagulation factors V, VIII, and XIII activation; protein C activation; and platelet aggregation.

Hipper than heparin

Compared with heparin, direct thrombin inhibitors have three advantages:

 They have activity against clot-bound thrombin.

They have more predictable anticoagulant effects.

 They aren't inhibited by the platelet release reaction.

Pharmacotherapeutics

Argatroban and lepirudin are used to treat heparin-induced thrombocytopenia (HIT). Argatroban is administered in combination with aspirin to patients with HIT undergoing coronary interventions, such as PTCA, coronary stent placement, and atherectomy. However, the safety and effectiveness of argatroban for cardiac indications haven't been established for patients without HIT.

Bivalirudin bio

Bivalirudin has been approved for use in patients with unstable angina who are undergoing PTCA. It should be used in conjunction with aspirin therapy.

Keep track of contraindications

Bivalirudin is contraindicated in patients with cerebral aneurysm, intracranial hemorrhage, or general uncontrolled hemorrhage. In addition, the dosage may need to be reduced in those with impaired renal function because 20% of the drug is excreted unchanged in urine. Bivalirudin also increases the risk of hemorrhage in those with GI ulceration or hepatic disease. Hypertension may increase the risk of cerebral hemorrhage. Use bivalirudin with caution after recent surgery or trauma and during lactation.

Drug interactions

In addition, keep these points in mind:
• Parenteral anticoagulants should be discontinued before administering argatroban.
• Using argatroban and warfarin together has a combined effect on INR.
• If the patient previously received heparin, allow sufficient time for heparin's effect on the PTT to decrease before starting argatroban therapy.
• The safety and effectiveness of using argatroban and thrombolytic drugs together haven't been established.

Adverse reactions

Don't give direct thrombin inhibitors with drugs that may enhance the risk of bleeding. Patients at greatest risk for hemorrhage include those with severe hypertension, lumbar puncture, or spinal anesthesia; those undergoing major surgery, especially involving the brain, spinal cord, or eye; those with hematologic conditions associated with increased bleeding tendencies; and those with GI lesions. Use direct thrombin inhibitors cautiously in these patients.

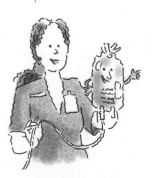

Don't give direct thrombin inhibitors with drugs that may enhance the risk of bleeding. Hemorrhage may occur.

The major adverse effect of direct thrombin inhibitors is bleeding with the possibility of major hemorrhage, although this rarely occurs.

Other adverse reactions include:
- intracranial hemorrhage
- retroperitoneal hemorrhage
- nausea, vomiting, abdominal cramps, and diarrhea
- headache
- hematoma at the I.V. infusion site.

Nursing process

These nursing process steps are appropriate for patients undergoing treatment with direct thrombin inhibitors.

Assessment
- Assess the patient's underlying condition before starting therapy.
- Monitor the patient closely for bleeding and other adverse reactions.
- Check PT, INR, and PTT.
- Monitor the patient's vital signs, hemoglobin level, hematocrit, and platelet count.
- Assess the patient's urine, stool, and emesis for blood.

Key nursing diagnoses
- Ineffective protection related to the drug's effects on the body's normal clotting and bleeding mechanisms
- Risk for deficient fluid volume related to bleeding
- Deficient knowledge related to drug therapy

Planning outcome goals
- The patient's clotting times will respond appropriately to drug therapy.
- The patient will maintain adequate fluid volume as evidenced by vital signs and laboratory studies.
- The patient and his family will demonstrate an understanding of drug therapy.

Implementation
- Notify the prescriber about serious or persistent adverse reactions.
- Maintain bleeding precautions throughout therapy.
- Administer I.V. solutions using an infusion pump as appropriate; dilute solutions according to the manufacturer's recommendations.

• Avoid excessive I.M., I.V., or subQ administration of other drugs to minimize the risk of hematoma.

Evaluation

• Patient has no adverse change in health status.
• Patient has no evidence of bleeding or hemorrhaging.
• Patient and his family demonstrate an understanding of drug therapy.

Factor Xa inhibitor drugs

Factor Xa inhibitor drugs are used to prevent DVT in patients undergoing total hip and knee replacement surgery or hip fracture surgery. The only factor Xa inhibitor drug available in the United States is fondaparinux.

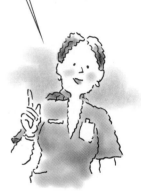

There's only one factor Xa inhibitor drug available in the United States: fondaparinux.

Pharmacokinetics

Fondaparinux is administered subQ and absorbed rapidly and completely. It's excreted primarily unchanged in urine. The peak effect is seen within 2 hours of administration and lasts for approximately 17 to 24 hours.

Pharmacodynamics

Fondaparinux binds to antithrombin III and potentiates by about 300 times the natural neutralization of factor Xa by antithrombin III.

Pardon me for interrupting

Factor Xa neutralization interrupts the coagulation cascade, which inhibits thrombin and thrombus formation.

Pharmacotherapeutics

Currently, fondaparinux is indicated for preventing DVT in patients undergoing total hip and knee replacement surgery and fractured hip surgery, and for the prevention or treatment of pulmonary embolism.

Drug interactions

Avoid giving factor Xa inhibitors with drugs that may enhance the risk of bleeding.

Adverse effects

Adverse effects that can occur with factor Xa inhibitor therapy include:

- bleeding
- nausea
- anemia
- fever
- rash
- constipation
- edema.

Nursing process

These nursing process steps are appropriate for patients undergoing treatment with factor Xa inhibitor drugs.

Assessment

- Assess the patient's underlying condition before starting therapy.
- Monitor the patient closely for bleeding and other adverse reactions.
- Check PT, INR, and PTT.
- Monitor the patient's vital signs, hemoglobin level, hematocrit, and platelet count.
- Assess the patient's urine, stool, and emesis for blood.

Key nursing diagnoses

- Ineffective protection related to the drug's effects on the body's normal clotting and bleeding mechanisms
- Risk for deficient fluid volume related to bleeding
- Deficient knowledge related to drug therapy

Planning outcome goals

- The patient's clotting times will respond appropriately to drug therapy.
- The patient will maintain adequate fluid volume as evidenced by vital signs and laboratory studies.
- The patient and his family will demonstrate an understanding of drug therapy.

Implementation

- Administer the drug by subQ injection into fatty tissue only; rotate injection sites.
- Don't mix the drug with other injections or infusions.
- Notify the prescriber about serious or persistent adverse reactions.
- Maintain bleeding precautions throughout therapy.
- Avoid excessive I.V., I.M., or subQ administration of other drugs to minimize the risk of hematoma.

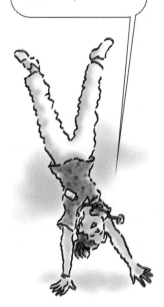

I don't think this is quite what they mean when they say to "rotate" injection sites for subQ administration of fondaparinux!

Evaluation
- Patient has no adverse change in health status.
- Patient has no evidence of bleeding or hemorrhaging.
- Patient and his family demonstrate an understanding of drug therapy.

Thrombolytic drugs

Thrombolytic drugs are used to dissolve a preexisting clot or thrombus, commonly in an acute or emergency situation. Some of the thrombolytic drugs currently used include alteplase, reteplase, tenecteplase, urokinase, and streptokinase.

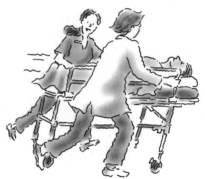

> Thrombolytic drugs are commonly used in acute or emergency situations.

Pharmacokinetics

After I.V. or intracoronary administration, thrombolytic drugs are distributed immediately throughout the circulation, quickly activating plasminogen (a precursor to plasmin, which dissolves fibrin clots).

In the blink of an eye

Alteplase, tenecteplase, reteplase, and urokinase are cleared rapidly from circulating plasma, primarily by the liver. Streptokinase is removed rapidly from the circulation by antibodies and the reticuloendothelial system (a body system involved in defending against infection and disposing products of cell breakdown). These drugs don't appear to cross the placental barrier.

Pharmacodynamics

Thrombolytic drugs convert plasminogen to plasmin, which lyses (dissolves) thrombi, fibrinogen, and other plasma proteins. (See *How alteplase helps restore circulation.*)

Pharmacotherapeutics

Thrombolytic drugs have several uses. They're used to treat certain thromboembolic disorders (such as acute MI, acute ischemic stroke, and peripheral artery occlusion) and have also been used to dissolve thrombi in arteriovenous cannulas (used in dialysis) and I.V. catheters to reestablish blood flow. (See *Thrombolytic drugs: Streptokinase*, page 400.)

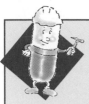

Pharm function

How alteplase helps restore circulation

When a thrombus forms in an artery, it obstructs the blood supply, causing ischemia and necrosis. Alteplase can dissolve a thrombus in either the coronary or pulmonary artery, restoring the blood supply to the area beyond the blockage.

Obstructed artery
A thrombus blocks blood flow through the artery, causing distal ischemia.

Inside the thrombus
Alteplase enters the thrombus, which consists of plasminogen bound to fibrin. Alteplase binds to the fibrin-plasminogen complex, converting the inactive plasminogen into active plasmin. This active plasmin digests the fibrin, dissolving the thrombus. As the thrombus dissolves, blood flow resumes.

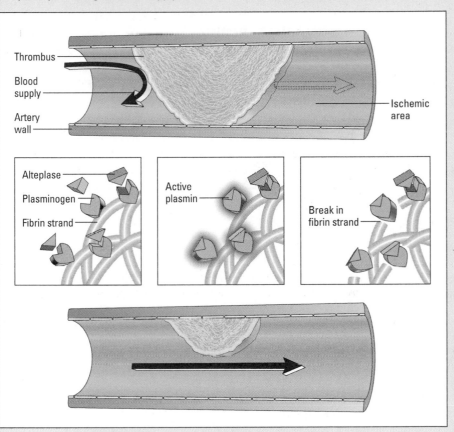

Here's the breakdown

Thrombolytic drugs are the drugs of choice to break down newly formed thrombi. They seem most effective when administered within 6 hours after the onset of symptoms.

To be more specific...

In addition, each drug has specific uses:

• Alteplase is used to treat acute MI, pulmonary embolism, acute ischemic stroke, and peripheral artery occlusion and to restore patency to clotted grafts and I.V. access devices.
• Streptokinase is used to treat acute MI, pulmonary embolism, and DVT.
• Reteplase and tenecteplase are used to treat acute MI.
• Urokinase is used to treat pulmonary embolism and coronary artery thrombosis and to clear catheters.

Drug interactions

These drug interactions can occur with thrombolytic drugs:
• Thrombolytic drugs interact with heparin, oral anticoagulants, antiplatelet drugs, and NSAIDs to increase the patient's risk of bleeding.
• Aminocaproic acid inhibits streptokinase and can be used to reverse its fibrinolytic effects.

Adverse reactions

The major reactions associated with the thrombolytic drugs are bleeding and allergic responses, especially with streptokinase.

Nursing process

These nursing process steps are appropriate for patients undergoing treatment with thrombolytic drugs.

Assessment

• Assess the patient's underlying condition before starting therapy.
• Monitor the patient closely for bleeding and other adverse reactions.
• Check PT, INR, and PTT.
• Monitor the patient's vital signs, hemoglobin level, hematocrit, and platelet count.
• Assess the patient's urine, stool, and emesis for blood.
• Assess the patient's cardiopulmonary status, including electrocardiogram and vital signs, before and during therapy.
• Monitor the patient for internal bleeding, and check puncture sites frequently.

Key nursing diagnoses

• Ineffective cardiopulmonary tissue perfusion related to the patient's underlying condition
• Risk for deficient fluid volume related to adverse effects of drug therapy

Prototype pro

Thrombolytic drugs: Streptokinase

Actions
• Dissolves clots by converting plasminogen to plasmin

Indications
• Deep vein thrombosis
• Pulmonary embolism
• Arterial thrombosis and embolism
• Acute myocardial infarction

Nursing considerations
• Monitor the patient for adverse effects, such as arrhythmias, bleeding, pulmonary edema, and hypersensitivity reactions.
• Monitor the patient's vital signs frequently.
• Monitor the patient frequently for bleeding.

• Deficient knowledge related to drug therapy

Planning outcome goals
• The patient's cardiopulmonary assessment findings will improve.
• The patient will maintain adequate fluid volume as evidenced by vital signs and laboratory studies.
• The patient and his family will demonstrate an understanding of drug therapy.

Implementation
• Notify the prescriber about serious or persistent adverse reactions.
• Maintain bleeding precautions throughout therapy.
• Administer I.V. solutions using an infusion pump as appropriate; reconstitute solutions according to facility protocol.
• Avoid excessive I.M., I.V., or subQ administration of other drugs to minimize the risk of hematoma.
• Administer heparin with thrombolytics according to facility protocol.
• Have antiarrhythmics available; monitor cardiac status closely.
• Avoid invasive procedures during thrombolytic therapy.

Evaluation
• Patient's cardiopulmonary assessment findings demonstrate improved perfusion.
• Patient has no evidence of bleeding or hemorrhaging.
• Patient and his family demonstrate an understanding of drug therapy.

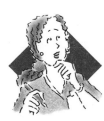

Quick quiz

1. Which administration method for parenteral iron helps avoid leakage into subQ tissue?
    A.   Z-track method
    B.   I.M. injection into the deltoid
    C.   subQ injection
    D.   Intradermal injection

Answer: A. The Z-track method helps to avoid leakage into subcutaneous tissue and staining of the skin.

2.   Which test should the nurse check in her assessment of a patient receiving heparin?

    A.   Complete blood count

    B.   PTT

    C.   Arterial blood gas levels

    D.   Hemoglobin level

Answer: B. PTT should be monitored to measure the effectiveness of heparin therapy.

3.   What's the most common adverse reaction experienced with I.V. antiplatelet drugs?

    A.   Nausea

    B.   Joint pain

    C.   Headache

    D.   Bleeding

Answer: D. Bleeding is the most common adverse effect of I.V. antiplatelet drugs.

Scoring

☆☆☆   If you answered all three questions correctly, magnificent! You're on top when it comes to managing clots.

  ☆☆   If you answered two questions correctly, way to go! You're in the know about drugs and blood flow.

    ☆   If you answered fewer than two questions correctly, stay calm. Another look at this chapter with efficiency should reverse any deficiencies.

Endocrine drugs

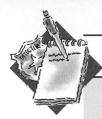

Just the facts

In this chapter, you'll learn:

♦ classes of drugs that affect the endocrine system

♦ uses and varying actions of these drugs

♦ absorption, distribution, metabolization, and excretion of these drugs

♦ drug interactions and adverse reactions to these drugs.

Drugs and the endocrine system

The endocrine system consists of glands, which are specialized cell clusters, and hormones, the chemical transmitters secreted by the glands in response to stimulation.

A delicate balance

Together with the central nervous system, the endocrine system regulates and integrates the body's metabolic activities and maintains homeostasis (the body's internal equilibrium). The drug types that treat endocrine system disorders include:
• natural hormones and their synthetic analogues, such as insulin and glucagon
• hormonelike substances
• drugs that stimulate or suppress hormone secretion.

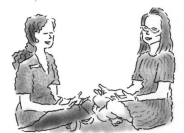

Ooooooooooom. The endocrine system, made up of glands and hormones, helps maintain the body's internal equilibrium.

Antidiabetic drugs and glucagon

Insulin, a pancreatic hormone, and oral antidiabetic drugs are classified as *hypoglycemic drugs* because they lower blood glucose levels. Glucagon, another pancreatic hormone, is classified as a *hyperglycemic drug* because it raises blood glucose levels.

Low insulin = high glucose

Diabetes mellitus, known simply as *diabetes*, is a chronic disease of insulin deficiency or resistance. It's characterized by disturbances in carbohydrate, protein, and fat metabolism. This leads to elevated levels of the sugar glucose in the body. The disease comes in two primary forms:

☝ type 1, previously referred to as *insulin-dependent diabetes mellitus*

✌ type 2, previously referred to as *non-insulin-dependent diabetes mellitus*.

Downward spiral

Situations that can decrease glucose levels too much in patients with diabetes include:
• an antidiabetic drug dosage that's too high
• an increase in activity (such as exercise)
• noncompliance with drug therapy (for example, taking an antidiabetic drug but not eating afterward).

Insulin

Patients with type 1 diabetes require an external source of insulin to control blood glucose levels. Insulin may also be given to patients with type 2 diabetes in certain situations.

Pick a rate, any rate

Types of insulin include:
• rapid-acting, such as lispro
• short-acting, such as regular insulin
• intermediate-acting, such as NPH
• long-acting, such as glargine.

Pharmacokinetics (how drugs circulate)

Insulin isn't effective when taken orally because the GI tract breaks down the protein molecule before it reaches the bloodstream.

Skin deep

All insulins, however, may be given by subcutaneous (subQ) injection. Absorption of subQ insulin varies according to the injection site, the blood supply, and the degree of tissue hypertrophy at the injection site.

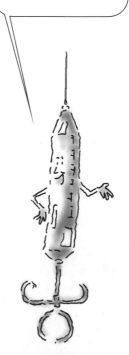

The amount of insulin absorbed depends on the injection site, the patient's blood supply, and the degree of tissue hypertrophy at the injection site.

In the I.V. league

Regular insulin may also be given I.V. as well as in dialysate fluid infused into the peritoneal cavity for patients on peritoneal dialysis therapy.

Far and wide

After absorption into the bloodstream, insulin is distributed throughout the body. Insulin-responsive tissues are located in the liver, adipose tissue, and muscle. Insulin is metabolized primarily in the liver and, to a lesser extent, in the kidneys and muscle. It's excreted in feces and urine.

Pharmacodynamics (how drugs act)

Insulin is an anabolic or building hormone that promotes:
- storage of glucose as glycogen (see *How insulin aids glucose uptake*, page 406.)
- an increase in protein and fat synthesis
- a deceleration of the breakdown of glycogen, protein, and fat
- a balance of fluids and electrolytes.

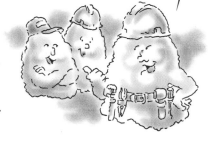

Okay, Team Insulin. Let's show this body what we building hormones can do!

Extracurricular activity

Although it has no antidiuretic effect, insulin can correct the polyuria (excessive urination) and polydipsia (excessive thirst) associated with the osmotic diuresis that can occur with hyperglycemia by decreasing the blood glucose level. Insulin also facilitates the movement of potassium from the extracellular fluid into the cell.

Pharmacotherapeutics (how drugs are used)

Insulin is indicated for:
- type 1 diabetes
- type 2 diabetes when other methods of controlling blood glucose levels have failed or are contraindicated
- type 2 diabetes when blood glucose levels are elevated during periods of emotional or physical stress (such as during infection, surgery, or medication therapy)
- type 2 diabetes when oral antidiabetic drugs are contraindicated because of pregnancy or hypersensitivity.

Calming complications

Insulin is also used to treat two complications of diabetes: diabetic ketoacidosis (DKA), which is more common with type 1 diabetes, and hyperosmolar hyperglycemic nonketotic syndrome, which is more common with type 2 diabetes.

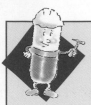

Pharm function

How insulin aids glucose uptake

These illustrations show how insulin allows a cell to use glucose for energy.

Glucose can't enter the cell without the aid of insulin.

Normally produced by the beta cells of the pancreas, insulin binds to the receptors on the surface of the target cell. Insulin and its receptor first move to the inside of the cell, which activates glucose transporter channels to move to the surface of the cell.

These channels allow glucose to enter the cell. The cell can then use the glucose for metabolism.

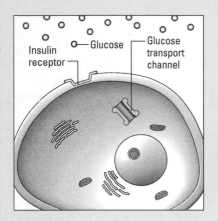

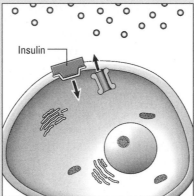

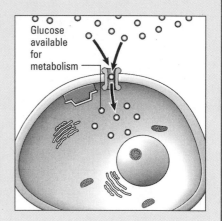

Nondiabetic duty

Insulin is also used to treat severe hyperkalemia (elevated serum potassium levels) in patients without diabetes. Potassium moves with glucose from the bloodstream into the cell, lowering serum potassium levels. (See *Hypoglycemic drugs: Insulin.*)

Drug interactions

Some drugs interact with insulin, altering its ability to decrease the blood glucose level; other drugs directly affect glucose levels:
• Anabolic steroids, salicylates, alcohol, sulfa drugs, angiotensin-converting enzyme inhibitors, propranolol, guanethidine, and monoamine oxidase (MAO) inhibitors may increase the hypoglycemic effect of insulin.

Insulin can be used in patients without diabetes to treat severe hyperkalemia.

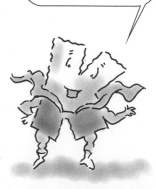

• Corticosteroids, sympathomimetic drugs, isoniazid, thyroid hormones, niacin, furosemide, and thiazide diuretics may reduce the effects of insulin, resulting in hyperglycemia.
• Beta-adrenergic blockers may prolong the hypoglycemic effect of insulin and may mask signs and symptoms of hypoglycemia.

Adverse reactions

Adverse reactions to insulin include:
• hypoglycemia (below-normal blood glucose levels)
• Somogyi effect (hypoglycemia followed by rebound hyperglycemia)
• hypersensitivity reactions
• lipodystrophy (disturbance in fat deposition)
• insulin resistance.

Nursing process

These nursing process steps are appropriate for patients undergoing treatment with insulin.

Assessment
• Assess the patient's glucose level before therapy and regularly thereafter. Monitor level more frequently if the patient is under stress, unstable, pregnant, recently diagnosed with diabetes, undergoing dietary changes, under orders to have nothing by mouth, experiencing nausea and vomiting, or taking drugs that can interact with insulin.
• Monitor the patient's glycosylated hemoglobin level regularly.
• Monitor the patient's urine ketone level when the glucose level is elevated.
• Assess for adverse reactions and drug interactions.
• Monitor injection sites for local reactions.
• Assess the patient's and family's knowledge of drug therapy.

Key nursing diagnoses
• Ineffective therapeutic regimen management related to inexpereince with treatment process and medication for hyperglycemia
• Risk for injury related to drug-induced hypoglycemia
• Deficient knowledge related to drug therapy

Planning outcome goals
• Blood glucose levels will be maintained within normal limits.
• The risk of injury to the patient will be minimized.

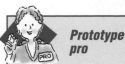

Prototype pro

Hypoglycemic drugs: Insulin

Actions
• Increases glucose transport across muscle and fat cell membranes to reduce blood glucose levels
• Promotes conversion of glucose to its storage form, glycogen
• Triggers amino acid uptake and conversion to protein in muscle cells and inhibits protein degradation
• Stimulates triglyoeride formation and inhibits the release of free fatty acids from adipose tissue
• Stimulates lipoprotein lipase activity, which converts circulating lipoproteins to fatty acids

Indications
• Type 1 diabetes
• Adjunct treatment in type 2 diabetes
• Diabetic ketoacidosis

Nursing considerations
• Monitor the patient for adverse effects, such as hypoglycemia and hypersensitivity reactions.

• The patient and his family will demonstrate an understanding of drug therapy.

Implementation

• Use regular insulin in patients with circulatory collapse, DKA, or hyperkalemia. Don't use regular insulin concentration (500 units/ml) I.V. Don't use intermediate- or long-acting insulins for a coma or other emergency that needs rapid drug action.
• Insulin resistance may develop; large insulin doses are needed to control signs and symptoms of diabetes in these cases. For severe insulin resistance, U-500 insulin is available as Regular (concentrated). Give the facility pharmacy sufficient notice before you need to refill an in-house prescription because every pharmacy may not stock it. Never store U-500 insulin in the same area as other insulin preparations because of the danger of severe overdose if given accidentally to other patients.

In the mix

• To mix the insulin suspension, swirl the vial gently or rotate it between your palms or between your palm and thigh. Don't shake the vial vigorously; doing so causes bubbling and creates air in the syringe.
• Lispro insulin has a rapid onset of action and should be given within 15 minutes before meals.
• Insulin glargine can't be diluted or mixed with any other insulin or solution.
• Regular insulin may be mixed with NPH or Lente insulins in any proportion. When mixing regular insulin with NPH insulin, always draw up regular insulin into the syringe first.
• Switching from separate injections to a prepared mixture may alter the patient's response.
• Whenever NPH or Lente is mixed with regular insulin in the same syringe, give the mixture immediately to avoid a loss of potency.
• Don't use insulin that has changed color or become clumped or granular.
• Check the expiration date on the vial before using.
• If administering I.V., use only regular insulin. Inject directly at the ordered rate into the vein, through an intermittent infusion device, or into a port close to the I.V. access site. If giving continuous infusion, infuse the drug diluted in normal saline solution at the prescribed rate.
• If administering subQ, pinch a fold of skin with the fingers starting at least 3″ (7.6 cm) apart and insert the needle at a 45- to 90-degree angle. Press but don't rub the site after injection. Rotate and chart injection sites to avoid overuse of one area. A patient with

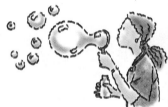

Shaking vials of insulin suspension causes bubbling and creates air in the syringe—and those are not the kind of bubbles you want to make!

diabetes may achieve better control if injection sites are rotated within the same anatomic region.

Highs and lows

• Ketosis-prone type 1, severely ill, and newly diagnosed diabetic patients with very high glucose levels may require hospitalization and I.V. treatment with regular fast-acting insulin.
• Notify the prescriber of sudden changes in glucose levels, dangerously high or low levels, or ketosis.
• Be prepared to provide supportive measures if the patient develops DKA or hyperglycemic nonketotic coma.

Sustaining snacks

• Treat hypoglycemic reactions with an oral form of rapid-acting glucose (if the patient can swallow) or with glucagon or I.V. glucose (if the patient can't be roused). Follow administration with a complex carbohydrate snack when the patient is awake, and then determine the cause of the reaction.
• Make sure that the patient is following an appropriate diet and exercise program. Expect to adjust the insulin dosage when other aspects of the regimen are altered.
• Discuss with the prescriber how to handle noncompliance.
• Teach the patient and his family how to monitor his glucose level and administer insulin. (See *Teaching about insulin.*)

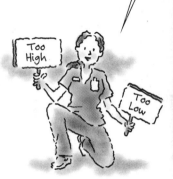

Notify the prescriber if your patient develops glucose levels that are dangerously high or low.

Education edge

Teaching about insulin

If insulin therapy is prescribed, review these points with the patient and his caregivers:
• Insulin relieves signs and symptoms but doesn't cure the disease; therapy is lifelong.
• Glucose monitoring is an essential guide to determining dosage and success of therapy; know the proper use of equipment for monitoring glucose level.
• Follow the prescribed therapeutic regimen; adhere to specific diet, weight reduction, exercise, and personal hygiene programs—including daily foot inspection—and consult with the prescriber about ways to avoid infection.
• Review the timing of injections and eating with the prescriber; don't skip meals.

• Accuracy of drug measurement is very important, especially with concentrated regular insulin. Aids, such as a magnifying sleeve or dose magnifier, may improve accuracy. Review with the prescriber and your family how to measure and give insulin.
• Don't alter the order in which insulin types are mixed or change the model or brand of the syringe or needle used.
• Learn to recognize signs and symptoms of hyperglycemia and hypoglycemia and what to do if they occur.
• Wear or carry medical identification at all times.
• Have carbohydrates (glucose tablets or candy) on hand for emergencies.

Evaluation
- Patient's glucose level is normal.
- Patient sustains no injury from drug-induced hypoglycemia.
- Patient and his family demonstrate an understanding of drug therapy.

Oral antidiabetic drugs

Types of oral antidiabetic drugs available include:
- first-generation sulfonylureas (such as acetohexamide, chlorpropamide, tolazamide, and tolbutamide)
- second-generation sulfonylureas (such as glimepiride, glipizide, and glyburide)
- thiazolidinedione drugs (pioglitazone and rosiglitazone)
- metformin (a biguanide drug)
- alpha-glucosidase inhibitors (acarbose and miglitol)
- meglitinides (such as repaglinide)
- nateglinide (an amino acid derivative)
- combination therapies (such as glipizide and metformin, glyburide and metformin, and rosiglitazone and metformin).

Pharmacokinetics

Oral antidiabetic drugs are absorbed well from the GI tract and distributed via the bloodstream throughout the body. They're metabolized primarily in the liver and are excreted mostly in urine, with some excreted in bile. Glyburide is excreted equally in urine and feces; rosiglitazone and pioglitazone are largely excreted in both. (See *Oral hypoglycemic drugs: Glyburide.*)

Pharmacodynamics

It's believed that oral antidiabetic drugs produce actions within and outside the pancreas (extrapancreatic) to regulate blood glucose.

To the pancreas...

Oral antidiabetic drugs probably stimulate pancreatic beta cells to release insulin in a patient with a minimally functioning pancreas. Within a few weeks to a few months of starting sulfonylureas, pancreatic insulin secretion drops to pretreatment levels but blood glucose levels remain normal or near normal. Most likely, it's the actions of the oral antidiabetic drugs outside of the pancreas that maintain this glucose control.

> If the pancreas isn't functioning properly, it's believed that oral antidiabetic drugs can temporarily stimulate it to release insulin.

Prototype pro

Oral hypoglycemic drugs: Glyburide

Actions
- Stimulates insulin release from the pancreatic beta cells and reduces glucose output by the liver
- Extrapancreatic effect increases peripheral sensitivity to insulin and causes mild diuretic effect

Indications
- Type 2 diabetes

Nursing considerations
- Monitor the patient for adverse effects, such as hypoglycemia, angioedema, and hematologic disorders.
- During times of stress, the patient may need insulin; monitor for hypoglycemia.

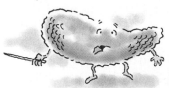

...and beyond!

Oral antidiabetic drugs provide several extrapancreatic actions to decrease and control blood glucose. They can go to work in the liver and decrease glucose production (gluconeogenesis) there. Also, by increasing the number of insulin receptors in the peripheral tissues, they provide more opportunities for the cells to bind sufficiently with insulin, initiating the process of glucose metabolism. Meglitinides have a short duration and are given preprandially for this reason.

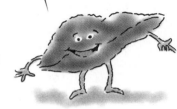

Oral antidiabetic drugs also work in the liver to decrease glucose production.

Let's get specific

These oral antidiabetic drugs produce specific actions:
• Pioglitazone and rosiglitazone improve insulin sensitivity.
• Metformin decreases liver production of glucose and intestinal absorption of glucose and improves insulin sensitivity.
• Acarbose and miglitol inhibit enzymes, delaying glucose absorption.

Pharmacotherapeutics

Oral antidiabetic drugs are indicated for patients with type 2 diabetes if diet and exercise can't control blood glucose levels. These drugs aren't effective in patients with type 1 diabetes because the pancreatic beta cells aren't functioning at a minimal level.

Calling all combos

Combinations of an oral antidiabetic drug and insulin therapy may be indicated for some patients who don't respond to either drug alone.

Drug interactions

Hypoglycemia and hyperglycemia are the main risks when oral antidiabetic drugs interact with other drugs.

Low blow

Hypoglycemia may occur when sulfonylureas are combined with alcohol, anabolic steroids, chloramphenicol, gemfibrozil, MAO inhibitors, salicylates, sulfonamides, fluconazole, cimetidine, warfarin, and ranitidine. It may also occur when metformin is combined with cimetidine, nifedipine, procainamide, ranitidine, and vancomycin. Hypoglycemia is less likely to occur when metformin is used as a single agent.

High fly

Hyperglycemia may occur when sulfonylureas are taken with corticosteroids, rifampin, sympathomimetics, and thiazide diuretics.

Metformin administration with iodinated contrast dyes can result in acute renal failure. Doses should be withheld in patients undergoing procedures that require I.V. contrast dyes.

Adverse reactions

Hypoglycemia is a major adverse reaction of oral antidiabetic drugs, especially when combination therapy is used.

Adverse reactions specific to sulfonylureas include:
- nausea
- epigastric fullness
- blood abnormalities
- water retention
- rash
- hyponatremia
- photosensitivity.

Adverse reactions to metformin include:
- metallic taste
- nausea and vomiting
- abdominal discomfort.

Acarbose may cause these reactions:
- abdominal pain
- diarrhea
- gas.

Thiazolidinediones may cause:
- weight gain
- swelling.

> Sun may not be fun for patients using sulfonylureas. Photosensitivity may occur.

Nursing process

These nursing process steps are appropriate for patients undergoing treatment with oral antidiabetic drugs.

Assessment
- Assess the patient's blood glucose level regularly.
- Keep in mind that the patient transferring from insulin therapy to oral antidiabetics needs glucose monitoring at least three times daily before meals.
- Assess for adverse reactions and drug interactions.
- Assess the patient's compliance with drug therapy and other aspects of treatment.
- Assess the patient's and family's knowledge of drug therapy.

Key nursing diagnoses
- Ineffective therapeutic regimen management related to inexperience with treatment process and medication for hyperglycemia.
- Risk for injury related to hypoglycemia
- Deficient knowledge related to drug therapy

Planning outcome goals

- Blood glucose level will be maintained within normal limits.
- The risk of injury to the patient will be minimized.
- The patient and his family will demonstrate an understanding of drug therapy.

Implementation

- Micronized glyburide has a smaller particle size and isn't bioequivalent to regular tablets. The dosage may need to be adjusted.

Timing is everything

- Give sulfonylureas 30 minutes before the morning meal (once-daily dosing) or 30 minutes before morning and evening meals (twice-daily dosing). Give metformin with morning and evening meals. Alpha-glucosidase inhibitors should be taken with the first bite of each main meal three times daily.
- A patient who takes a thiazolidinedione should have liver enzyme levels measured at the start of therapy, every 2 months for the first year of therapy, and periodically thereafter.
- A patient transferring from one oral hypoglycemic to another (except chlorpropamide) usually doesn't need a transition period.
- Although most patients take oral hypoglycemics once daily, patients taking increased doses may achieve better results with twice-daily dosage.
- Treat hypoglycemic reactions with an oral form of rapid-acting carbohydrates (if the patient can swallow) or with glucagon or I.V. glucose (if the patient can't swallow or is comatose). Follow up treatment with a complex carbohydrate snack when the patient is awake, and determine the cause of the reaction.
- Anticipate that the patient may need insulin therapy during periods of increased stress, such as with infection, fever, surgery, or trauma. Increase monitoring, especially for hyperglycemia, during these situations.
- Make sure that adjunct therapy, such as diet and exercise, is being used appropriately.
- Teach the patient how and when to monitor glucose levels and to recognize signs and symptoms of hyperglycemia and hypoglycemia. (See *Teaching about antidiabetic drugs,* page 414.)

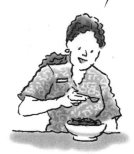

The first bite is just right. Alpha-glucosidase inhibitors should be taken with the first bite of each main meal three times daily.

Patients using oral antidiabetics may need insulin therapy during times of stress, such as when they have surgery.

Evaluation

- Patient maintains adequate hydration.
- Patient complies with therapy, as evidenced by a normal or near-normal glucose level.
- Patient sustains no injury.
- Patient and his family demonstrate an understanding of drug therapy.

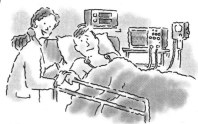

Education edge

Teaching about antidiabetic drugs

If antidiabetic drugs are prescribed, review these points with the patient and his caregivers:
• Therapy relieves signs and symptoms but doesn't cure the disease.
• Follow the prescribed therapeutic regimen; adhere to specific diet, weight reduction, exercise, and personal hygiene programs, and consult with the prescriber about ways to avoid infection.
• Know how and when to monitor glucose levels.

• Learn to recognize signs and symptoms of hyperglycemia and hypoglycemia and what to do if these occur.
• Don't change the dosage without the prescriber's consent.
• Report adverse reactions.
• Don't take other drugs, including over-the-counter drugs and herbal remedies, without first checking with the prescriber.
• Avoid consuming alcohol during drug therapy.
• Wear or carry medical identification at all times.

Glucagon

Glucagon, a hyperglycemic drug that raises blood glucose levels, is a hormone normally produced by the alpha cells of the islets of Langerhans in the pancreas. (See *How glucagon raises glucose levels*.)

Pharmacokinetics

After subQ, I.M., or I.V. injection, glucagon is absorbed rapidly. It's distributed throughout the body, although its effect occurs primarily in the liver.

Here, there, and (almost) everywhere

Glucagon is degraded extensively by the liver, kidneys, and plasma and at its tissue receptor sites in plasma membranes. It's removed from the body by the liver and kidneys.

Pharmacodynamics

Glucagon regulates the rate of glucose production through:
• glycogenolysis, the conversion of glycogen back into glucose by the liver
• gluconeogenesis, the formation of glucose from free fatty acids and proteins
• lipolysis, the release of fatty acids from adipose tissue for conversion to glucose.

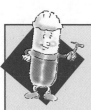

Pharm function

How glucagon raises glucose levels

When adequate stores of glycogen are present, glucagon can raise glucose levels in patients with severe hypoglycemia. Here's what happens:

• Initially, glucagon stimulates the formation of adenylate cyclase in the liver cell.

• Adenylate cyclase then converts adenosine triphosphate (ATP) to cyclic adenosine monophosphate (cAMP).

• This product initiates a series of reactions that result in an active phosphorylated glucose molecule.

• In this phosphorylated form, the large glucose molecule can't pass through the cell membrane.

• Through glycogenolysis (the breakdown of glycogen, the stored form of glucose), the liver removes the phosphate group and allows the glucose to enter the bloodstream, raising blood glucose levels for short-term energy needs.

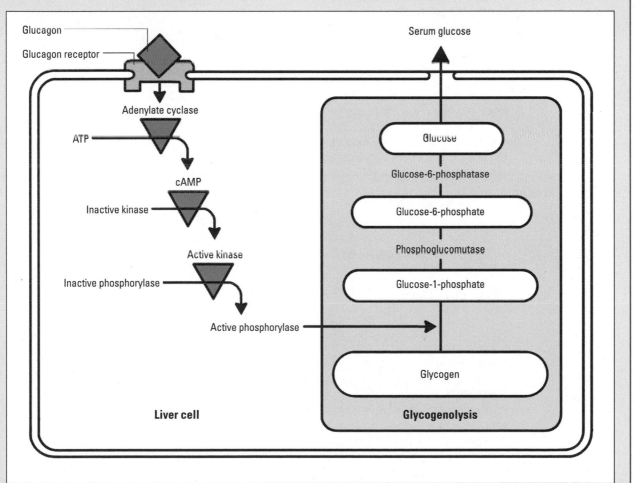

Pharmacotherapeutics

Glucagon is used for emergency treatment of severe hypoglycemia. It's also used during radiologic examination of the GI tract to reduce GI motility.

Drug interactions

Glucagon interacts adversely only with oral anticoagulants, increasing the tendency to bleed.

Adverse reactions

Adverse reactions to glucagon are rare.

Nursing process

These nursing process steps are appropriate for patients undergoing treatment with glucagon.

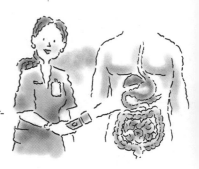

Glucagon is used during radiologic examination of the GI tract to reduce GI motility. How illuminating!

Assessment
• Assess the patient's blood glucose level regularly. Increase monitoring during periods of increased stress (infection, fever, surgery, or trauma).
• Assess for adverse reactions and drug interactions.
• Monitor the patient's hydration if vomiting occurs.
• Assess the patient's and family's knowledge of drug therapy.

Key nursing diagnoses
• Ineffective therapeutic regimen management related to inexperience with treatment process and medication for hyperglycemia
• Risk for injury related to hypoglycemia
• Deficient knowledge related to drug therapy

Planning outcome goals
• Blood glucose will remain within normal limits.
• The risk of injury to the patient will be reduced.
• The patient and his family will demonstrate an understanding of drug therapy.

Implementation
• For I.M. and subQ use, reconstitute the drug in a 1-unit vial with 1 ml of diluent; reconstitute the drug in a 10-unit vial with 10 ml of diluent.
• For I.V. administration, a drip infusion, such as dextrose solution, may be used, which is compatible with glucagon; the drug

forms precipitate in chloride solutions. Inject the drug over 2 to 5 minutes.
• Arouse the lethargic patient as quickly as possible. Give additional carbohydrates orally to prevent a secondary hypoglycemic episode, and then determine the cause of the reaction.
• Notify the prescriber that the patient's hypoglycemic episode required glucagon use.
• Be prepared to provide emergency intervention if the patient doesn't respond to glucagon administration. An unstable, hypoglycemic patient with diabetes may not respond to glucagon; give I.V. dextrose 50% instead.
• Notify the prescriber if the patient can't retain some form of sugar for 1 hour because of nausea or vomiting.

Evaluation

• Patient maintains normal glucose level.
• Patient sustains no injury.
• Patient and his family demonstrate an understanding of drug therapy.

> Inject the I.V. form of glucagon over 2 to 5 minutes.

Thyroid and antithyroid drugs

Thyroid and antithyroid drugs function to correct thyroid hormone deficiency (hypothyroidism) and thyroid hormone excess (hyperthyroidism).

Thyroid drugs

Thyroid drugs can be natural or synthetic hormones and may contain triiodothyronine (T_3), thyroxine (T_4), or both.

Nature's own

Natural thyroid drugs are made from animal thyroid and include:
• thyroid USP (desiccated), which contains T_3 and T_4
• thyroglobulin, which also contains T_3 and T_4.

Synthesized from sodium

Synthetic thyroid drugs actually are the sodium salts of the L-isomers of the hormones. These synthetic hormones include:
• levothyroxine sodium, which contains T_4
• liothyronine sodium, which contains T_3
• liotrix, which contains T_3 and T_4.

Pharmacokinetics

Thyroid hormones are absorbed variably from the GI tract, distributed in plasma, and bound to serum proteins. They're metabolized through deiodination, primarily in the liver, and excreted unchanged in feces.

Pharmacodynamics

The principal pharmacologic effect is an increased metabolic rate in body tissues. Thyroid hormones affect protein and carbohydrate metabolism and stimulate protein synthesis. They promote gluconeogenesis and increase the use of glycogen stores.

Taken to heart

Thyroid hormones increase heart rate and cardiac output (the amount of blood pumped by the heart each minute). They may even increase the heart's sensitivity to catecholamines and increase the number of beta-adrenergic receptors in the heart (stimulation of beta receptors in the heart increases heart rate and contractility).

More flow

Thyroid hormones may increase blood flow to the kidneys and increase the glomerular filtration rate (the amount of plasma filtered through the kidneys each minute) in patients with hypothyroidism, producing diuresis. (See *Thyroid hormones: Levothyroxine.*)

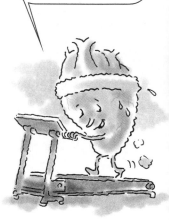

Talk about increasing productivity! Thyroid hormones increase my rate and output in addition to increasing the metabolic rate of body tissues.

Pharmacotherapeutics

Thyroid drugs act as replacement or substitute hormones in these situations:
• to treat the many forms of hypothyroidism
• with antithyroid drugs to prevent goiter formation (an enlarged thyroid gland) and hypothyroidism
• to differentiate between primary and secondary hypothyroidism during diagnostic testing
• to treat papillary or follicular thyroid carcinoma.

A winning choice

Levothyroxine is the drug of choice for thyroid hormone replacement and thyroid-stimulating hormone (TSH) suppression therapy.

Drug interactions

Thyroid drugs interact with several common drugs:
• They increase the effects of oral anticoagulants, increasing the tendency to bleed.

• Cholestyramine and colestipol reduce the absorption of thyroid hormones.
• Phenytoin may displace T_4 from plasma binding sites, temporarily increasing levels of free T_4.
• Taking thyroid drugs with digoxin may reduce serum digoxin levels, increasing the risk of arrhythmias or heart failure.
• Carbamazepine, phenytoin, phenobarbital, and rifampin increase thyroid hormone metabolism, reducing the effectiveness.
• Serum theophylline levels may increase when theophylline is administered with thyroid drugs.

Adverse reactions

Most adverse reactions to thyroid drugs result from toxicity.

Gut reactions

Adverse reactions in the GI system include diarrhea, abdominal cramps, weight loss, and increased appetite.

Cardiac concerns

Adverse reactions in the cardiovascular system include palpitations, sweating, rapid heart rate, increased blood pressure, angina, and arrhythmias.

Effects all around

General manifestations of toxic doses include:
• headache
• tremor
• insomnia
• nervousness
• fever
• heat intolerance
• menstrual irregularities.

Nursing process

These nursing process steps are appropriate for patients undergoing treatment with thyroid drugs.

Assessment

• Assess the patient's thyroid function test results regularly.
• Assess the patient's condition before therapy and regularly thereafter. Normal levels of T_4 should occur within 24 hours, followed by a threefold increase in the T_3 level in 3 days.
• Assess for adverse reactions and drug interactions.
• In a patient with coronary artery disease receiving thyroid hormone, watch for possible coronary insufficiency.

Thyroid hormones: Levothyroxine

Actions
• Stimulates metabolism of all body tissues by accelerating the rate of cellular oxidation

Indications
• Cretinism
• Myxedema coma
• Thyroid hormone replacement

Nursing considerations
• Monitor the patient for adverse effects, such as nervousness, insomnia, tremor, tachycardia, palpitations, angina, arrhythmias, and cardiac arrest.
• Use with extreme caution in elderly patients and in patients with cardiovascular disorders.

• Monitor the patient's pulse rate and blood pressure.
• Monitor the patient for signs of thyrotoxicosis or inadequate dosage, including diarrhea, fever, irritability, listlessness, rapid heartbeat, vomiting, and weakness.
• Monitor prothrombin time (PT) and International Normalized Ratio; a patient taking anticoagulants usually needs lower doses.
• Assess the patient's and family's knowledge of drug therapy.

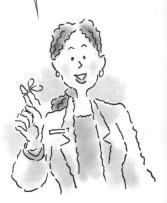

Don't forget: Patients are at risk for injury related to adverse reactions to thyroid drugs.

Key nursing diagnoses
• Ineffective health maintenance related to the presence of hypothyroidism
• Risk for injury related to drug-induced adverse reactions
• Deficient knowledge related to drug therapy

Planning outcome goals
• Thyroid levels will be within normal limits.
• The risk of injury to the patient will be minimized.
• The patient and his family will demonstrate an understanding of drug therapy.

Implementation
• Thyroid hormone dosages vary widely. Begin treatment at the lowest level, adjusting to higher doses according to the patient's symptoms and laboratory data, until a euthyroid state is reached.
• When changing from levothyroxine to liothyronine, stop levothyroxine and then start liothyronine. The dosage is increased in small increments after residual effects of levothyroxine disappear. When changing from liothyronine to levothyroxine, start levothyroxine several days before withdrawing liothyronine to avoid relapse.
• Give thyroid hormones at the same time each day, preferably in the morning, to prevent insomnia.
• Thyroid drugs may be supplied either in micrograms (mcg) or in milligrams (mg). Don't confuse these dose measurements.
• Thyroid hormones alter thyroid function test results. A patient taking levothyroxine who needs radioactive iodine uptake studies must discontinue the drug 4 weeks before the test.
• A patient taking a prescribed anticoagulant with thyroid hormones usually needs a reduced anticoagulant dosage.
• If the patient has diabetes, he may need an increased antidiabetic dosage when starting the thyroid hormone replacement.
• Instruct the patient never to stop the drug abruptly. Therapy is usually for life.

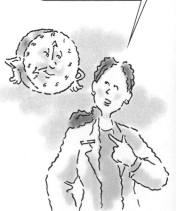

Give thyroid hormones at the same time each day, preferably in the morning, to prevent insomnia.

Evaluation
• Patient's thyroid hormone levels are normal.

• Patient sustains no injury from adverse reactions.
• Patient complies with therapy as evidenced by normal thyroid hormone levels and resolution of the underlying disorder.

Antithyroid drugs

A number of drugs act as antithyroid drugs, or *thyroid antagonists.* Used for patients with hyperthyroidism (thyrotoxicosis), these drugs include:
• thioamides, which include propylthiouracil and methimazole
• iodides, which include stable iodine and radioactive iodine.

Pharmacokinetics

Thioamides and iodides are absorbed through the GI tract, concentrated in the thyroid, and metabolized by conjugation. They are excreted in urine.

Pharmacodynamics

Drugs used to treat hyperthyroidism work in different ways.

Stopping synthesis

Thioamides block iodine's ability to combine with tyrosine, thereby preventing thyroid hormone synthesis.

Inhibited by iodine

Stable iodine inhibits hormone synthesis through the Wolff-Chaikoff effect, in which excess iodine decreases the formation and release of thyroid hormone.

Reduced by radiation

Radioactive iodine reduces hormone secretion by destroying thyroid tissue through induction of acute radiation thyroiditis (inflammation of the thyroid gland) and chronic gradual thyroid atrophy. Acute radiation thyroiditis usually occurs 3 to 10 days after administering radioactive iodine. Chronic thyroid atrophy may take several years to appear.

Pharmacotherapeutics

Antithyroid drugs commonly are used to treat hyperthyroidism, especially Graves' disease (hyperthyroidism caused by autoimmunity), which accounts for 85% of all cases.

Thioamides

Propylthiouracil, which lowers serum T_3 levels faster than methimazole, is usually used for rapid improvement of severe hyperthyroidism.

Good for gravidas

Propylthiouracil is preferred over methimazole in pregnant women because its rapid action reduces transfer across the placenta and because it doesn't cause aplasia cutis (a severe skin disorder) in the fetus.

Bad for breast-feeding

Propylthiouracil and methimazole are distributed in breast milk. Patients receiving these drugs shouldn't breast-feed. If nursing is absolutely necessary, propylthiouracil is the preferred drug.

Once a day

Because methimazole blocks thyroid hormone formation for a longer time, it's better suited for administration once per day to a patient with mild to moderate hyperthyroidism. Therapy may continue for 12 to 24 months before remission occurs.

Iodides

To treat hyperthyroidism, the thyroid gland may be removed by surgery or destroyed by radiation. Before surgery, stable iodine is used to prepare the gland for surgical removal by firming it and decreasing its vascularity. Stable iodine is also used after radioactive iodine therapy to control signs and symptoms of hyperthyroidism while the radiation takes effect.

Drug interactions

Iodide preparations may react synergistically with lithium, causing hypothyroidism. Other interactions with antithyroid drugs aren't clinically significant.

Adverse reactions

The most serious adverse reaction to thioamide therapy is granulocytopenia. Hypersensitivity reactions may also occur.

(Not) a spoonful of sugar

The iodides can cause an unpleasant brassy taste and burning sensation in the mouth, increased salivation, and painful swelling of the parotid glands.

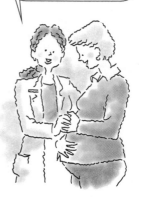

Propylthiouracil use is preferred in pregnant women because its rapid action reduces transfer of the drug across the placenta...

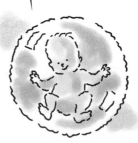

...and it doesn't put me at risk for aplasia cutis—although I am pretty cute!

Rare, but be aware

Rarely, I.V. iodine administration can cause an acute hypersensitivity reaction. Radioactive iodine also can cause a rare—but acute—reaction 3 to 14 days after administration.

Nursing process

These nursing process steps are appropriate for patients undergoing treatment with antithyroid drugs.

Assessment

• Assess the patient's condition and thyroid function test before therapy and regularly thereafter. Normal levels of T_4 should occur within 24 hours, followed by a threefold increase in the T_3 level in 3 days.
• Assess for adverse reactions and drug interactions.
• Watch for signs of hypothyroidism (depression; cold intolerance; hard, nonpitting edema); adjust the dosage as directed.
• Monitor complete blood count as directed to detect impending leukopenia, thrombocytopenia, and agranulocytosis.
• Monitor the patient's hydration status if adverse GI reactions occur.
• Assess the patient's and family's knowledge of drug therapy.

Key nursing diagnoses

• Ineffective health maintenance related to the presence of a thyroid condition
• Risk for injury related to drug-induced adverse reactions
• Deficient knowledge related to drug therapy

Planning outcome goals

• Thyroid levels will be within normal limits.
• The risk of injury to the patient will be minimized.
• The patient and his family will demonstrate an understanding of drug therapy.

Implementation

• Thyroid hormone dosages vary widely. Begin treatment at the lowest level, adjusting to higher doses according to the patient's symptoms and laboratory data until an euthyroid state is reached.
• Give thyroid hormones at the same time each day, preferably in the morning, to prevent insomnia.
• Give the drug with meals to reduce GI reactions.

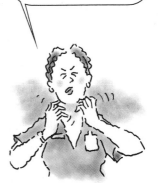

Stop the drug and notify the prescriber if a severe rash or enlarged cervical lymph nodes develop.

Education edge

Teaching about thyroid and antithyroid drugs

If thyroid or antithyroid drugs are prescribed, review these points with the patient and his caregivers:
• Take the drug exactly as prescribed. Take the dose at the same time each day, preferably in the morning before breakfast, to maintain constant hormone levels. Taking the drug in the morning prevents insomnia.
• Report signs and symptoms of thyroid hormone overdose (chest pain, palpitations, sweating, nervousness) or aggravated cardiovascular disease (chest pain, dyspnea, tachycardia).
• If taking antithyroid drugs, report skin eruptions (signs of hypersensitivity), fever, sore throat, or mouth sores (early signs of agranulocytosis).

• Ask the prescriber about using iodized salt and eating shellfish, especially if taking antithyroid medications, to avoid possible toxic levels of iodine.
• If a stable response has been achieved, don't change drug brands.
• Children may lose hair during the first months of therapy; this is a temporary reaction.
• Report unusual bleeding or bruising.
• Keep follow-up appointments, and have thyroid levels tested regularly.
• Don't use other drugs, over-the-counter products, or herbal remedies without first consulting with the prescriber or a pharmacist.

A rash decision

• Discontinue the drug and notify the prescriber if the patient develops a severe rash or enlarged cervical lymph nodes.
• Thyroid drugs may be supplied either in micrograms (mcg) or in milligrams (mg). Don't confuse these dose measurements.

Evaluation

• Patient's thyroid hormone levels are normal.
• Patient sustains no injury from adverse reactions.
• Patient complies with therapy as evidenced by normal thyroid hormone levels and resolution of the underlying disorder. (See *Teaching about thyroid and antithyroid drugs.*)

Pituitary drugs

Pituitary drugs are natural or synthetic hormones that mimic the hormones produced by the pituitary gland. The pituitary drugs consist of two groups:

Anterior pituitary drugs may be used diagnostically or therapeutically to control the function of other endocrine glands, such as the thyroid gland, adrenals, ovaries, and testes.

> Anterior pituitary drugs control the function of endocrine glands. Posterior pituitary drugs regulate fluid volume and stimulate smooth-muscle contraction.

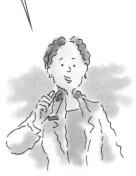

Posterior pituitary drugs may be used to regulate fluid volume and stimulate smooth-muscle contraction in selected clinical situations.

Anterior pituitary drugs

The protein hormones produced in the anterior pituitary gland regulate growth, development, and sexual characteristics by stimulating the actions of other endocrine glands. Anterior pituitary drugs include:
- adrenocorticotropics, which include corticotropin, corticotropin repository, and cosyntropin
- somatrem and somatropin, both growth hormones
- gonadotropics, which include chorionic gonadotropin and menotropins
- thyrotropics, which include TSH, thyrotropin alfa, and protirelin.

Pharmacokinetics

Anterior pituitary drugs aren't given orally because they're destroyed in the GI tract. Some of these hormones can be administered topically, but most require injection.

Sometimes slower than Mother Nature

Usually, natural hormones are absorbed, distributed, and metabolized rapidly. Some analogues, however, are absorbed and metabolized more slowly. Anterior pituitary hormone drugs are metabolized at the receptor site and in the liver and kidneys. The hormones are excreted primarily in urine.

Pharmacodynamics

Anterior pituitary drugs exert a profound effect on the body's growth and development. The hypothalamus controls secretions of the pituitary gland. In turn, the pituitary gland secretes hormones that regulate secretions or functions of other glands.

Production managers

The concentration of hormones in the blood helps determine the hormone production rate. Increased hormone levels inhibit hormone production; decreased levels raise production and secretion. Anterior pituitary drugs, therefore, control hormone production by increasing or decreasing the body's hormone levels.

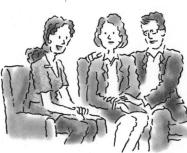

In women, chorionic gonadotropins and menotropins are used to help induce ovulation during infertility treatments.

Pharmacotherapeutics

The clinical indications for anterior pituitary hormone drugs are diagnostic and therapeutic:
• Corticotropin and cosyntropin are used diagnostically to differentiate between primary and secondary failure of the adrenal cortex.
• Corticotropin is also used to treat adrenal insufficiency.
• Somatrem is used to treat pituitary dwarfism.
• In males, chorionic gonadotropin is used to evaluate testosterone production, treat hypogonadism, and treat cryptorchidism (undescended testes).
• In women, chorionic gonadotropin and menotropins are used to help induce ovulation during infertility treatments.
• Thyrotropin alfa is a synthetic TSH used to treat thyroid cancer.

Drug interactions

Anterior pituitary drugs interact with several different types of drugs:
• Administering immunizations to a person receiving corticotropin increases the risk of neurologic complications and may reduce the antibody response.
• Corticotropin reduces salicylate levels.
• Enhanced potassium loss may occur when diuretics are taken with corticotropins.
• Barbiturates, phenytoin, and rifampin increase the metabolism of corticotropin, reducing its effects.
• Estrogen increases the effect of corticotropin.
• Taking estrogens, amphetamines, and lithium with cosyntropin can alter results of adrenal function tests.
• Amphetamines and androgens (concurrently) administered with somatrem may promote epiphyseal (cartilaginous bone growth plate) closure.
• Concurrent use of somatrem and corticosteroids inhibits the growth-promoting action of somatrem.

Adverse reactions

The major adverse reactions to pituitary drugs are hypersensitivity reactions. Long-term corticotropin use can cause Cushing's syndrome.

Nursing process

These nursing process steps are appropriate for patients undergoing treatment with anterior pituitary drugs.

Assessment

- Assess the patient's underlying condition before therapy and regularly during therapy.
- Assess the child's growth before therapy and regularly thereafter. Monitor the patient's height and blood with regular checkups; radiologic studies may also be needed.
- Assess for hypersensitivity and allergic reactions and have adrenal responsiveness verified before starting corticotropin treatment.
- Assess for adverse reactions and drug interactions.
- Note and record weight changes, fluid exchange, and resting blood pressures until the minimal effective dosage is achieved.
- Assess neonates of corticotropin-treated mothers for signs of hypoadrenalism.
- Monitor the patient for stress.
- With somatrem, observe the patient for signs of glucose intolerance, hyperglycemia, and hypothyroidism. Periodic thyroid function tests may be required.
- Assess the patient's and family's knowledge about the diagnostic test or drug therapy ordered.

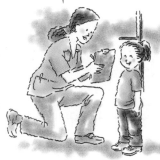

Children taking anterior pituitary drugs should have their growth assessed regularly.

Key nursing diagnoses

- Ineffective protection related to the underlying condition
- Risk for injury related to drug-induced adverse reactions
- Deficient knowledge related to drug test or therapy

Planning outcome goals

- The patient's underlying condition will improve.
- The risk of injury to the patient will be minimized.
- The patient and his family will demonstrate an understanding of the diagnostic test or drug therapy ordered.

Implementation

- Administer the drug as prescribed and monitor for effects.
- Corticotropin should be an adjunct, not the sole, therapy. The oral form is preferred for long-term therapy.
- If administering corticotropin I.V., dilute it in 500 ml of 5% dextrose in water and infuse over 8 hours.
- If administering corticotropin gel, warm it to room temperature and draw it into a large needle. Replace the needle with a 21G or 22G needle. Give slowly as a deep I.M. injection. Warn the patient that the injection is painful.
- Refrigerate reconstituted solution and use it within 24 hours.
- Counteract edema with a low-sodium, high-potassium diet; nitrogen loss with a high-protein diet; and psychotic changes with a reduction in corticotropin dosage or use of sedatives.

• Stress to the patient the importance of informing health care team members about corticotropin. Unusual stress may require additional use of rapidly acting corticosteroids. When possible, gradually reduce the corticotropin dosage to the smallest effective dosage to minimize induced adrenocortical insufficiency. Therapy can be restarted if a stressful situation, such as trauma, surgery, or severe illness, occurs shortly after stopping the drug.

Evaluation
• Patient's underlying condition improves with drug therapy.
• Patient doesn't experience injury as a result of drug-induced adverse reactions.
• Patient and his family demonstrate an understanding of the diagnostic test or drug therapy.

Posterior pituitary drugs

Posterior pituitary hormones are synthesized in the hypothalamus and stored in the posterior pituitary, which, in turn, secretes the hormones into the blood. Posterior pituitary drugs include:
• all forms of antidiuretic hormone (ADH), such as desmopressin acetate and vasopressin
• the oxytocic drug oxytocin.

Pharmacokinetics

Because enzymes in the GI tract can destroy all protein hormones, these drugs can't be given orally. Posterior pituitary drugs may be given by injection or intranasal spray.

ADH on the move

ADH is distributed throughout extracellular fluid and doesn't appear to bind with protein. Most of the drug is metabolized rapidly in the liver and kidneys. It's excreted in urine.

Slower (or maybe faster) by a nose

Like other natural hormones, oxytocin is absorbed, distributed, and metabolized rapidly. However, when oxytocin is administered intranasally, absorption is erratic.

Pharmacodynamics

Under neural control, posterior pituitary hormones affect:
• smooth-muscle contraction in the uterus, bladder, and GI tract
• fluid balance through kidney reabsorption of water
• blood pressure through stimulation of the arterial wall muscles.

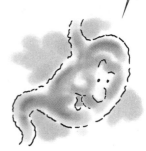

Posterior pituitary drugs can't be given orally because enzymes in the GI tract destroy protein hormones.

On the rise

ADH increases cyclic adenosine monophosphate, which increases the permeability of the tubular epithelium in the kidneys, promoting reabsorption of water. High dosages of ADH stimulate contraction of blood vessels, increasing blood pressure.

Less...and more

Desmopressin reduces diuresis and promotes clotting by increasing the plasma level of factor VIII (antihemophilic factor).

Mother's little helper

In a pregnant woman, oxytocin may stimulate uterine contractions by increasing the permeability of uterine cell membranes to sodium ions. It also can stimulate lactation through its effect on mammary glands.

Pharmacotherapeutics

ADH is prescribed for hormone replacement therapy in patients with neurogenic diabetes insipidus (an excessive loss of urine caused by a brain lesion or injury that interferes with ADH synthesis or release). However, it doesn't effectively treat nephrogenic diabetes insipidus (caused by renal tubular resistance to ADH).

The long and short of ADH therapy

Short-term ADH therapy is indicated for patients with transient diabetes insipidus after head injury or surgery; therapy may be lifelong for patients with idiopathic hormone deficiency.

The dirt on desmopressin

Desmopressin is the drug of choice for chronic ADH deficiency. It's also indicated for primary nocturnal enuresis. Desmopressin is administered intranasally. It has a long duration of action and a relative lack of adverse effects.

A lesson on vasopressin

Used for short-term therapy, vasopressin elevates blood pressure in patients with hypotension caused by lack of vascular tone. It also relieves postoperative gaseous distention. Additionally, vasopressin may be used for transient polyuria resulting from ADH deficiency related to neurosurgery or head injury.

Partum me, is this the OB?

Oxytocin is used to:
• induce labor and complete incomplete abortions
• treat preeclampsia, eclampsia, and premature rupture of the membranes

* control bleeding and uterine relaxation after delivery
* hasten uterine shrinking after delivery
* stimulate lactation.

It's a chore

Oxytocin is used to induce or reinforce labor only when:
* the mother's pelvis is known to be adequate
* vaginal delivery is indicated
* the fetus is mature
* the fetal position is favorable
* critical care facilities and an experienced clinician are immediately available.

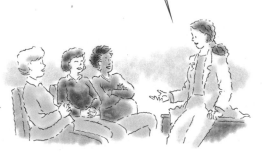

Oxytocin may be used under certain conditions to induce or reinforce labor.

Drug interactions

Various drugs may interact with posterior pituitary drugs:
* Alcohol, demeclocycline, and lithium may decrease ADH activity of desmopressin and vasopressin.
* Chlorpropamide, carbamazepine, and cyclophosphamide increase ADH activity.
* Synergistic effects may occur when barbiturates or cyclopropane anesthetics are used concurrently with ADH, leading to coronary insufficiency or arrhythmias.
* Cyclophosphamide may increase the effect of oxytocin.
* Concurrent use of vasopressors (anesthetics, ephedrine, methoxamine) and oxytocin increases the risk of hypertensive crisis and postpartum rupture of cerebral blood vessels.

Adverse reactions

Hypersensitivity reactions are the most common adverse reactions to posterior pituitary drugs. With natural ADH, anaphylaxis may occur after injection. Natural ADH can also cause:
* ringing in the ears
* anxiety
* hyponatremia (low serum sodium levels)
* proteins in the urine
* eclamptic attacks
* pupil dilation
* transient edema.
   Adverse reactions to synthetic ADH are rare.

"Expecting" some problems

Synthetic oxytocin can cause adverse reactions for pregnant women, including:

- bleeding after delivery
- GI disturbances
- sweating
- headache
- dizziness
- ringing in the ears
- severe water intoxication.

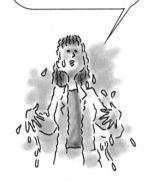

I know synthetic oxytoxin can cause severe water intoxication in pregnant women, but this is ridiculous!

Nursing process

These nursing process steps are appropriate for patients undergoing treatment with posterior pituitary hormones.

Assessment
- Obtain a history of the patient's underlying condition before therapy.
- Assess for adverse reactions and drug interactions.
- Assess the patient's and family's knowledge of drug therapy.

Key nursing diagnoses
- Deficient fluid volume related to underlying condition
- Risk for injury related to drug-induced adverse reactions
- Deficient knowledge related to drug therapy

Planning outcome goals
- The patient will maintain adequate fluid volume as evidenced by vital signs and urine output.
- The risk of injury to the patient will be minimized.
- The patient and his family will demonstrate an understanding of drug therapy.

Patients taking posterior pituitary drugs should be weighed daily.

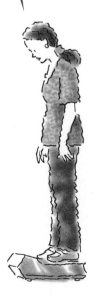

Implementation
- Administer the drug according to the prescriber's instructions, and monitor for effect.
- Assess the effectiveness of ADH by checking the patient's fluid intake and output, serum and urine osmolality, and urine specific gravity.
- Monitor the patient carefully for hypertension and water intoxication when giving ADH drugs. Seizures, coma, and death can occur from water intoxication. Watch for excessively elevated blood pressure or lack of response to the drug, which may be indicated by hypotension. Weigh the patient daily.
- Use a rectal tube to facilitate gas expulsion after vasopressin injection.

• Desmopressin injection shouldn't be used to treat severe cases of von Willebrand's disease or hemophilia A with factor VIII levels of 0% to 5%.
• When desmopressin is used to treat diabetes insipidus, the dosage or frequency of administration may be adjusted according to the patient's fluid output. Morning and evening doses are adjusted separately for adequate diurnal rhythm of water turnover.

Ban the bolus

• Oxytocin is administered only by I.V. infusion, not by I.V. bolus.
• When administering oxytocin, monitor and record uterine contractions, heart rate, blood pressure, intrauterine pressure, fetal heart rate, and blood loss every 15 minutes. Also monitor the patient's fluid intake and output. Antidiuretic effect may lead to fluid overload, seizures, and coma.
• Have magnesium sulfate (20% solution) available for relaxation of the myometrium when administering oxytocin.
• If contractions are less than 2 minutes apart, if they're above 50 mm Hg, or if they last 90 seconds or longer, stop oxytocin infusion, turn the patient on her left side, and notify the prescriber.
• Teach the patient and his caregivers how to properly measure and inhale the intranasal form of ADH. (See *Teaching about ADH*.)

Evaluation
• Patient achieves normal fluid and electrolyte balance.
• Patient is free from injury.
• Patient and his family demonstrate an understanding of drug therapy.

Estrogens

Estrogens mimic the physiologic effects of naturally occurring female sex hormones. They're used to correct estrogen-deficient states and, along with hormonal contraceptives, to prevent pregnancy.

Natural and synthetic estrogens

Estrogens that treat endocrine system disorders include:
• natural conjugated estrogenic substances (estradiol and estropipate)
• synthetic estrogens (esterified estrogens, estradiol cypionate, estradiol valerate, and ethinyl estradiol).

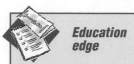

Education edge

Teaching about ADH

If an antidiuretic hormone (ADH) is prescribed, review these points with the patient and his caregivers:
• Clear the nasal passages before using the drug intranasally.
• Report such conditions as nasal congestion, allergic rhinitis, or upper respiratory tract infection; a dosage adjustment may be needed.
• If using subcutaneous desmopressin, rotate injection sites to avoid tissue damage.
• Drink only enough water to satisfy thirst.
• Monitor fluid intake and output.
• Wear or carry medical identification indicating that you're using ADH.

Prototype pro

Estrogens: Conjugated estrogenic substances

Actions
• Increases synthesis of deoxyribonucleic acid, ribonucleic acid, and protein in responsive tissues
• Reduces release of follicle-stimulating hormone and luteinizing hormone from the pituitary gland

Indications
• Abnormal uterine bleeding
• Palliative treatment of breast cancer at least 5 years after menopause
• Female castration
• Primary ovarian failure
• Osteoporosis
• Hypogonadism
• Vasomotor menopausal symptoms
• Atrophic vaginitis, kraurosis vulvae
• Palliative treatment of inoperable prostate cancer
• Vulvar and vaginal atrophy

Nursing considerations
• Monitor the patient for adverse reactions, such as seizures, thromboembolism and increased risk of stroke, pancreatitis, pulmonary embolism, myocardial infarction, endometrial cancer, hepatic adenoma, and breast cancer.
• Because of the risk of thromboembolism, therapy should be discontinued at least 1 month before procedures that may cause prolonged immobilization or thromboembolism, such as knee or hip surgery.
• Give oral forms at mealtime or at bedtime (if only one daily dose is required) to minimize nausea.

Pharmacokinetics

Estrogens are absorbed well and distributed throughout the body. Metabolism occurs in the liver, and the metabolites are excreted primarily by the kidneys.

Pharmacodynamics

The exact mechanism of action of estrogen isn't clearly understood. It's believed to increase synthesis of deoxyribonucleic acid, ribonucleic acid, and protein in estrogen-responsive tissues in the female breast, urinary tract, and genital organs. (See *Estrogens: Conjugated estrogenic substances.*)

Pharmacotherapeutics

Estrogens are prescribed:
• primarily for hormone replacement therapy in postmenopausal women to relieve symptoms caused by loss of ovarian function.
• less commonly for hormone replacement therapy in women with primary ovarian failure or female hypogonadism (reduced hormonal secretion by the ovaries) and in patients who have undergone surgical castration
• palliatively to treat advanced, inoperable breast cancer in postmenopausal women and prostate cancer in men.

> Want to provide some relief from those hot flashes? Try hormone replacement therapy with estrogen.

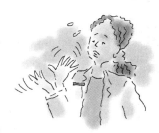

Drug interactions

Relatively few drugs interact with estrogens:
• Estrogens may decrease the effects of anticoagulants, increasing the risk of blood clots.
• Carbamazepine, barbiturates, antibiotics, phenytoin, primidone, and rifampin reduce estrogen's effectiveness.
• Estrogens interfere with the absorption of dietary folic acid, which may result in a folic acid deficiency.

Adverse reactions

Adverse reactions to estrogens include:
• hypertension
• thromboembolism (blood vessel blockage caused by a blood clot)
• thrombophlebitis (vein inflammation associated with clot formation).

Nursing process

These nursing process steps are appropriate for patients undergoing treatment with estrogens.

Assessment

• Obtain a history of the patient's underlying condition before therapy, and reassess regularly thereafter.
• Make sure that the patient has a thorough physical examination before starting estrogen therapy.

Year in, year out

• A patient receiving long-term therapy should have yearly examinations. Periodically monitor lipid levels, blood pressure, body weight, and liver function.
• Monitor the patient regularly to detect improvement or worsening of symptoms.
• Assess for adverse reactions and drug interactions.
• If the patient has diabetes mellitus, watch closely for loss of diabetes control.
• If the patient is also receiving a warfarin-type anticoagulant, monitor PT. If ordered, adjust the anticoagulant dosage.
• Assess the patient's and family's knowledge of drug therapy.

Key nursing diagnoses

• Ineffective health maintenance related to the underlying condition
• Risk of injury related to adverse effects
• Deficient knowledge related to drug therapy

Planning outcome goals

- The patient's underlying condition will improve.
- The risk for injury to the patient will be minimized.
- The patient and her family will demonstrate an understanding of drug therapy.

Implementation

- Notify the pathologist about the patient's estrogen therapy when sending specimens for evaluation.
- Keep in mind that estrogens usually are given cyclically (once daily for 3 weeks, followed by 1 week without drugs; repeated as needed).
- Administer the drug as prescribed and monitor for effects.
- Withhold the drug and notify the prescriber if a thromboembolic event is suspected; be prepared to provide supportive care as indicated.
- Teach the patient how to apply estrogen ointments or transdermal estrogen or how to insert an intravaginal estrogen suppository. Also inform the patient of the signs and symptoms that accompany a systemic reaction to ointments. (See *Teaching about estrogens.*)

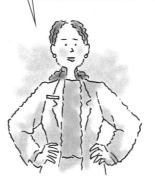

Stop estrogen therapy if a thromboembolic event is suspected.

Education edge

Teaching about estrogens

If estrogens are prescribed, review these points with the patient and her caregivers:

- Take the drug with meals or at bedtime to relieve nausea. Nausea usually disappears with continued therapy.
- Review with the prescriber how to apply estrogen ointments or transdermal estrogen.
- Be aware of signs and symptoms that accompany a systemic reaction to ointments.
- Use sanitary pads instead of tampons when using the suppository.
- Stop taking the drug immediately if pregnancy occurs because estrogens can harm the fetus.
- Don't breast-feed during estrogen therapy.
- If receiving cyclic therapy for postmenopausal symptoms, withdrawal bleeding may occur during the week off. However, fertility isn't restored and ovulation doesn't occur.

- Medical supervision is essential during prolonged therapy.
- Males on long-term therapy may experience temporary gynecomastia and impotence, which will disappear when therapy ends.
- Report abdominal pain; pain, numbness, or stiffness in the legs or buttocks; pressure or pain in the chest; shortness of breath; severe headaches; vision disturbances (such as blind spots, flashing lights, or blurriness); vaginal bleeding or discharge; breast lumps; swelling of hands or feet; yellow skin and sclera; dark urine; or light-colored stools to the prescriber immediately.
- If diabetic, report symptoms of hyperglycemia or glycosuria.
- Keep follow-up appointments for gynecologic examinations, clinical breast examinations, and mammography. Perform breast self-examinations as instructed.

Evaluation
- Patient's condition improves.
- Patient doesn't develop serious complications of estrogen therapy.
- Patient and her family understand drug therapy.

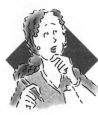

Quick quiz

1. Which type of insulin would the nurse expect to administer to a patient with DKA?
   A.   Regular
   B.   Intermediate-acting
   C.   Long-acting
   D.   Ultra-long-acting

Answer: A. Use regular insulin in a patient with circulatory collapse, DKA, or hyperkalemia.

2. Which drug or drug type would likely cause hyperglycemia if taken with glyburide?
   A.   Procainamide
   B.   Cimetidine
   C.   Warfarin
   D.   Thiazide diuretics

Answer: D. Hyperglycemia may occur if glyburide is taken with a thiazide diuretic.

3. Which drug is typically prescribed for a patient with diabetes insipidus?
   A.   ADH
   B.   Oxytocin
   C.   Pitocin
   D.   Corticotropin

Answer: A. ADH is prescribed for hormone replacement therapy in a patient with neurogenic diabetes insipidus.

Scoring

✰✰✰ If you answered all three questions correctly, perfect! There's no end to your endocrine drug knowledge!

✰✰ If you answered two questions correctly, marvelous! You've done your homework on homeostasis and hormones.

✰ If you answered fewer than two questions correctly, don't sink too low. You can always give the chapter another go.

Psychotropic drugs

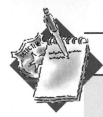

Just the facts

In this chapter, you'll learn:

♦ classes of drugs that alter psychogenic behavior and promote sleep

♦ uses and varying actions of these drugs

♦ absorption, distribution, metabolization, and excretion of these drugs

♦ drug interactions and adverse reactions to these drugs.

Drugs and psychiatric disorders

This chapter discusses drugs that are used to treat various sleep and psychogenic disorders, such as anxiety, depression, attention deficit hyperactivity disorder (ADIID), and psychotic disorders.

Sedative and hypnotic drugs

Sedatives reduce activity, tension, or excitement. Some degree of drowsiness commonly accompanies sedative use.

You're getting very sleepy...

When given in large doses, sedatives are considered *hypnotic drugs*, which induce a state resembling natural sleep. The three main classes of synthetic drugs used as sedatives and hypnotics are:

 benzodiazepines

 barbiturates

 nonbenzodiazepine-nonbarbiturate drugs.

Excuse me! When given in large doses, sedatives induce a state resembling natural sleep.

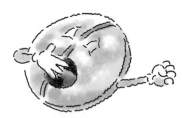

Benzodiazepines

Benzodiazepines produce many therapeutic effects, including some that aren't classified as sedative or hypnotic.

"Chill" pills

Benzodiazepines used primarily for their primary or secondary sedative or hypnotic effects include:
- alprazolam
- estazolam
- flurazepam
- lorazepam
- quazepam
- temazepam
- triazolam.

Pharmacokinetics (how drugs circulate)

Benzodiazepines are absorbed rapidly and completely from the GI tract and distributed widely in the body. Penetration into the brain is rapid. The rate of absorption determines how quickly the drug will work. Flurazepam and triazolam have the fastest onset.

Distribution determines duration

The duration of effect is determined by the extent of distribution. For example, triazolam is highly lipophilic and widely distributed; therefore, it has a short duration of effect.

The ins and outs

Benzodiazepines are usually given orally but may be given parenterally in certain situations, such as when a highly anxious patient needs sedation. All benzodiazepines are metabolized in the liver and excreted primarily in urine. Some benzodiazepines have active metabolites, which may give them a longer action.

Pharmacodynamics (how drugs act)

Researchers believe that benzodiazepines work by stimulating gamma-aminobutyric acid (GABA) receptors in the ascending reticular activating system (RAS) of the brain. This RAS is associated with wakefulness and attention and includes the cerebral cortex and limbic, thalamic, and hypothalamic levels of the central nervous system (CNS). (See *How benzodiazepines work.*)

Snooze inducer

When given in higher dosages, benzodiazepines induce sleep, probably because they depress the RAS of the brain. Benzodi-

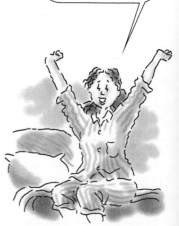

Benzodiazepines increase total sleep time and decrease the number of awakenings.

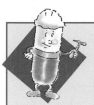

Pharm function

How benzodiazepines work

These illustrations show how benzodiazepines work at the cellular level.

Speed and passage

The speed of impulses from a presynaptic neuron across a synapse is influenced by the amount of chloride in the post-synaptic neuron. The passage of chloride ions into the postsynaptic neuron depends on the inhibitory neurotransmitter called *gamma-aminobutyric acid, or GABA.*

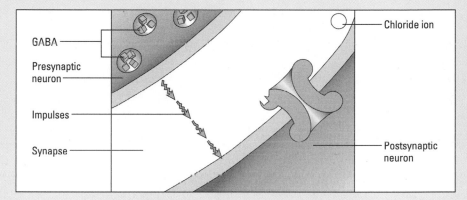

It binds

When GABA is released from the presynaptic neuron, it travels across the synapse and binds to GABA receptors on the postsynaptic neuron. This binding opens the chloride channels, allowing chloride ions to flow into the postsynaptic neuron and causing the nerve impulses to slow down.

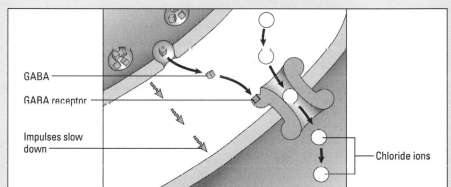

The result is another kind of depression

Benzodiazepines bind to receptors on or near the GABA receptor, enhancing the effect of GABA and allowing more chloride ions to flow into the postsynaptic neuron. This depresses the nerve impulses, causing them to slow down or stop.

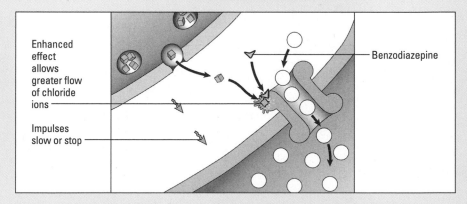

azepines increase total sleep time and produce a reduced number of awakenings.

(Not) a real eye opener

In most cases, benzodiazepines don't decrease the time spent in rapid eye movement sleep (the state of sleep in which brain activity resembles the activity it shows when awake; the body's muscles relax, and the eyes move rapidly). This gives benzodiazepines a significant advantage over barbiturates. (See *Benzodiazepines: Alprazolam.*)

Pharmacotherapeutics (how drugs are used)

Clinical indications for benzodiazepines include:
- relaxing the patient before surgery
- treating insomnia
- producing I.V. anesthesia
- treating alcohol withdrawal symptoms
- treating anxiety and seizure disorders
- producing skeletal muscle relaxation.

Drug interactions

Except for other CNS depressants such as alcohol, few drugs interact with benzodiazepines. Triazolam may be affected by drugs that inhibit the cytochrome P450 3A4 system, such as erythromycin and ketoconazole.

A lethal combination

When benzodiazepines are taken with other CNS depressants (including alcohol and anticonvulsants), the result is enhanced sedative and CNS depressant effects, including reduced level of consciousness (LOC), reduced muscle coordination, respiratory depression, and death.

Hormonal contraceptives may reduce the metabolism of flurazepam, increasing the risk of toxicity.

Adverse reactions

Benzodiazepines may cause:
- amnesia
- fatigue
- muscle weakness
- mouth dryness
- nausea and vomiting
- dizziness
- ataxia (impaired ability to coordinate movement).

Prototype pro

Benzodiazepines: Alprazolam

Actions
- Enhances or facilitates the action of gamma-aminobutyric acid, an inhibitory neurotransmitter in the central nervous system (CNS)
- Acts at the limbic, thalamic, and hypothalamic levels of the CNS
- Produces anxiolytic, sedative, hypnotic, skeletal muscle relaxant, and anticonvulsant effects
- Produces CNS depression

Indications
- Anxiety
- Panic disorders

Nursing considerations
- Monitor the patient for adverse reactions, such as drowsiness, dry mouth, diarrhea, and constipation.
- The drug isn't recommended for long-term use.
- Don't withdraw the drug abruptly; seizures may occur.

Feeling a little out of it?

Unintentional daytime sedation, hangover effect (residual drowsiness and impaired reaction time on awakening), and rebound insomnia may also occur. Additionally, benzodiazepines have a potential for abuse, tolerance, and physical dependence.

Senior alert!

Benzodiazepines with a long half-life or active metabolites may accumulate and cause adverse effects in elderly patients and should be avoided. If they must be used, start the patient at a lower dosage and gradually increase it.

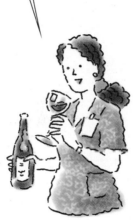

Be careful! Taking benzodiazepines with other CNS depressants such as alcohol enhances sedative and CNS depressant effects.

Nursing process

These nursing process steps are appropriate for patients undergoing treatment with benzodiazepines.

Assessment

• Assess the patient's anxiety before therapy and frequently thereafter.
• In the patient receiving repeated or prolonged therapy, monitor liver, renal, and hematopoietic function test results periodically.
• Assess for adverse reactions and drug interactions.
• Assess the patient's and family's knowledge of drug therapy.

Key nursing diagnoses

• Anxiety related to the patient's underlying condition
• Risk for injury related to drug-induced reactions
• Deficient knowledge related to drug therapy

Planning outcome goals

• The patient will state that his anxiety is reduced.
• The risk of injury to the patient will be minimized.
• The patient and his family will demonstrate an understanding of drug therapy.

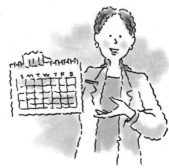

Benzodiazepines shouldn't be given for more than 4 months.

Implementation

• Don't give benzodiazepines for everyday stress or use them for long-term therapy (more than 4 months).
• Check to see that the patient has swallowed tablets before leaving his room.
• Expect to give lower doses at longer intervals in an elderly or a debilitated patient.
• Don't withdraw benzodiazepines abruptly after long-term use; withdrawal symptoms may occur. Abuse or addiction is possible.

Evaluation
• Patient reports decreased anxiety.
• Patient doesn't experience injury from adverse CNS reactions.
• Patient and his family demonstrate an understanding of drug therapy.

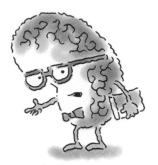

Are you paying attention? Barbiturates reduce overall CNS alertness.

Barbiturates

The major pharmacologic action of barbiturates is to reduce overall CNS alertness. Barbiturates used primarily as sedatives and hypnotics include:
• amobarbital
• butabarbital
• mephobarbital
• pentobarbital
• phenobarbital
• secobarbital.

The highs and lows

Low doses of barbiturates depress the sensory and motor cortex in the brain, causing drowsiness. High doses may cause respiratory depression and death because of their ability to depress all levels of the CNS.

Pharmacokinetics

Barbiturates are absorbed well from the GI tract. They're distributed rapidly, metabolized by the liver, and excreted in urine.

Pharmacodynamics

As sedatives and hypnotics, barbiturates depress the sensory cortex of the brain, decrease motor activity, alter cerebral function, and produce drowsiness, sedation, and hypnosis. These drugs appear to act throughout the CNS; however, the RAS of the brain, which is responsible for wakefulness, is a particularly sensitive site. (See *Barbiturates: Phenobarbital*.)

Pharmacotherapeutics

Barbiturates have many clinical indications, some of which go beyond sedative and hypnotic uses. They're used for:
• daytime sedation (for short periods only, typically less than 2 weeks)
• relief from insomnia
• preoperative sedation and anesthesia
• relief from anxiety
• anticonvulsant effects.

Prototype pro

Barbiturates: Phenobarbital

Actions
• Induces an imbalance in central inhibitory and facilitatory mechanisms, which influence cerebral cortex and reticular formation
• Decreases presynaptic and postsynaptic membrane excitability
• Produces all levels of central nervous system (CNS) depression (mild sedation to coma to death)
• Facilitates the action of gamma-aminobutyric acid, an inhibitory neurotransmitter in the CNS
• Exerts a central effect, which depresses respiration and GI motility
• Reduces nerve transmission and decreases excitability of the nerve cell as its principal anticonvulsant mechanism of action

• Raises the seizure threshold

Indications
• Epilepsy
• Febrile seizures
• Need for sedation

Nursing considerations
• Monitor the patient for adverse reactions, such as drowsiness, lethargy, hangover, respiratory depression, apnea, Stevens-Johnson syndrome, and angioedema.
• Don't withdraw the drug abruptly; seizures may worsen.
• Watch for signs of toxicity: coma, asthmatic breathing, clammy skin, and cyanosis.

A little too good

Tolerance to barbiturates occurs more rapidly than tolerance to benzodiazepines. Physical dependence may occur even with a small daily dosage. In comparison, benzodiazepines are relatively effective and safe and, for these reasons, have replaced barbiturates as the sedatives and hypnotics of choice.

Drug interactions

Barbiturates may interact with many other drugs:
• They may reduce the effects of beta-adrenergic blockers (such as metoprolol and propranolol), chloramphenicol, corticosteroids, doxycycline, oral anticoagulants, hormonal contraceptives, quinidine, tricyclic antidepressants, metronidazole, theophylline, and cyclosporine.
• Hydantoins, such as phenytoin, reduce the metabolism of phenobarbital, resulting in increased toxic effects.
• Methoxyflurane, when taken with barbiturates, may stimulate production of metabolites that are toxic to the kidneys.
• Barbiturate use with other CNS depressants may cause excessive CNS depression.
• Valproic acid may increase barbiturate levels.
• Monoamine oxidase (MAO) inhibitors slow down barbiturate metabolism, increasing sedative effects.
• When taken with acetaminophen, an increased risk of liver toxicity results.

Yikes! It says here that using methoxyflurane and barbiturates together may stimulate production of metabolites that are toxic to the kidneys.

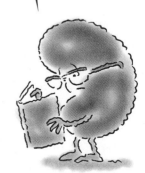

Adverse reactions

Barbiturates may have widespread adverse effects.

Draining the brain

CNS reactions include:
- drowsiness
- lethargy
- headache
- depression.

"Heart-y" responses

Cardiovascular effects include:
- mild bradycardia
- hypotension.

"Air" ways

Respiratory effects include:
- hypoventilation
- spasm of the larynx (voice box) and bronchi
- reduced rate of breathing
- severe respiratory depression.

And the rest of the story

Other reactions include:
- vertigo
- nausea and vomiting
- diarrhea
- epigastric pain
- allergic reactions.

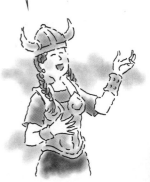

Barbiturates can cause spasm of the voice box—but I need to keep my voice box spasm-free. LAAA!

Nursing process

These nursing process steps are appropriate for patients undergoing treatment with barbiturates.

Assessment

- Assess the patient's condition before therapy and regularly thereafter.
- Assess the patient's LOC and sleeping patterns before and during therapy to evaluate the drug's effectiveness. Monitor his neurologic status for alteration or deterioration.
- Assess the patient's vital signs frequently, especially during I.V. administration.
- Assess for adverse reactions and drug interactions.

Key nursing diagnoses
- Risk for injury related to adverse drug reaction
- Risk for trauma related to the underlying condition
- Deficient knowledge related to drug therapy

Planning outcome goals
- The risk of injury to the patient will be minimized.
- The risk of trauma to the patient will be minimized.
- The patient and his family will demonstrate an understanding of drug therapy.

Implementation
- When giving parenteral forms, avoid extravasation, which may cause local tissue damage and tissue necrosis; inject I.V. or deep I.M. only. Don't exceed 5 ml for any I.M. injection site to avoid tissue damage.
- Be prepared to resuscitate. Too-rapid I.V. administration may cause respiratory depression, apnea, laryngospasm, or hypotension.
- Take seizure precautions as necessary. Monitor seizure character, frequency, and duration for changes, as indicated.

Safety first

- Institute safety measures to prevent patient falls and injury. Raise side rails, assist the patient out of bed, and keep the call light within easy reach.
- Monitor blood levels of the drug closely. Therapeutic levels range from 15 to 40 mcg/ml.
- Observe the patient to prevent hoarding or self-dosing, especially if he's depressed, suicidal, or drug dependent.
- Stop the drug slowly. Abrupt discontinuation may cause withdrawal symptoms or worsen seizures.

Evaluation
- Patient sustains no injury from sedation.
- Patient sustains no trauma during therapy.
- Patient and his family demonstrate an understanding of drug therapy. (See *Teaching about barbiturates*, page 446.)

Nonbenzodiazepines-nonbarbiturates

Nonbenzodiazepines-nonbarbiturates act as hypnotics for short-term treatment of simple insomnia. These drugs, which offer no special advantages over other sedatives, include:
- chloral hydrate
- eszopiclone

Teaching about barbiturates

If barbiturates are prescribed, review these points with the patient and his caregivers:
• Barbiturates can cause physical or psychological dependence.
• Take the drug exactly as prescribed. Don't change the dosage or take other drugs, including over-the-counter drugs or herbal remedies, without the prescriber's approval.
• A morning hangover is common after therapeutic use of barbiturates.

• Avoid hazardous tasks, driving a motor vehicle, or operating machinery while taking the drug. Review other safety measures with your health care provider to prevent injury.
• The drug's full effects don't occur for 2 to 3 weeks, except when a loading dose is used.
• Don't stop taking the drug abruptly.
• If using hormonal contraceptives, consider using other birth control methods such as condoms.
• Report skin eruptions or other significant adverse effects.

> • zaleplon
> • zolpidem.

Shoring up sleep for the short term

With the exception of zolpidem, which may be effective for up to 35 days, nonbenzodiazepines-nonbarbiturates are for short-term use only.

Pharmacokinetics

Nonbenzodiazepines-nonbarbiturates are absorbed rapidly from the GI tract. They're metabolized in the liver and excreted in urine.

Pharmacodynamics

The mechanism of action for nonbenzodiazepines-nonbarbiturates isn't fully known. They produce depressant effects similar to barbiturates.

Pharmacotherapeutics

Nonbenzodiazepines-nonbarbiturates are typically used for:
• short-term treatment of simple insomnia
• sedation before surgery
• sedation before EEG studies.

Drug interactions

Drug interactions involving nonbenzodiazepines-nonbarbiturates primarily occur when they're used with other CNS depressants, causing additive CNS depression resulting in drowsiness, respiratory depression, stupor, coma, and death.

These mixes don't match

Chloral hydrate may increase the risk of bleeding in patients taking oral anticoagulants. Use with I.V. furosemide may produce sweating, flushing, variable blood pressure, and uneasiness.

Adverse reactions

The most common dose-related adverse reactions involving nonbenzodiazepines-nonbarbiturates include:
• nausea and vomiting
• gastric irritation
• hangover effects (possibly leading to respiratory depression or even respiratory failure).

Nursing process

These nursing process steps are appropriate for patients undergoing treatment with nonbenzodiazepines-nonbarbiturates.

Assessment
• Assess the patient's underlying condition.
• Evaluate the drug's effectiveness after administration.
• Assess for adverse reactions and drug interactions.
• Assess the patient's and family's knowledge of drug therapy.

Key nursing diagnoses
• Insomnia related to patient's underlying condition
• Risk for injury related to adverse CNS reactions
• Deficient knowledge related to drug therapy

Planning outcome goals
• The patient's insomnia will improve.
• The risk of injury to the patient will be minimized.
• The patient and his family will demonstrate an understanding of drug therapy.

Implementation
• Administer the drug as ordered and monitor for its effects.
• To minimize the unpleasant taste of liquid forms, dilute or give the drug with liquid.
• Administer the drug immediately before bedtime.
• Refrigerate rectal suppositories.
• Long-term use isn't recommended; nonbenzodiazepines-nonbarbiturates lose their efficacy in promoting sleep after 14

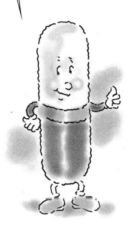

Nonbenzodiazepines-nonbarbiturates are used for short-term treatment of insomnia and for sedation before surgery or EEG studies.

days of continued use. Long-term use may cause drug dependence. The patient may experience withdrawal symptoms if the drug is suddenly stopped.

• Caution the patient about performing activities that require mental alertness or physical coordination. For an inpatient, supervise walking and raise bed rails, particularly for an elderly patient.

• Tell the patient to report adverse effects, such as severe hangover or feelings of oversedation, so the prescriber can be consulted to adjust the dosage or change the drug.

Evaluation

• Patient states drug effectively induced sleep.
• Patient's safety is maintained.
• Patient and his family demonstrate an understanding of drug therapy.

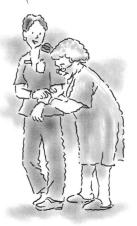

Supervise patients taking nonbenzodiazepines-nonbarbiturates when they're walking, especially if they're elderly.

Antianxiety drugs

Antianxiety drugs, also called *anxiolytics,* include some of the most commonly prescribed drugs in the United States. They're used primarily to treat anxiety disorders. The three main types of antianxiety drugs are:

• benzodiazepines
• barbiturates
• buspirone.

Experiencing drug déjà vu?

Benzodiazepines and barbiturates were discussed earlier in this chapter in regard to their sedative and hypnotic use, but they're also used to treat anxiety.

Anxiety "it" list

Benzodiazepines used primarily to treat anxiety include:

• alprazolam
• chlordiazepoxide
• clonazepam
• clorazepate
• diazepam
• halazepam
• lorazepam
• oxazepam.

Taking the edge off

When given in low dosages, these benzodiazepines decrease anxiety by acting on the limbic system and other areas of the brain that help regulate emotional activity. The drugs can usually calm the patient without causing drowsiness.

Back to the barbiturates

Barbiturates used to treat anxiety include:
• amobarbital
• mephobarbital
• pentobarbital
• secobarbital.

The difference is in the dosage

Benzodiazepines and barbiturates act the same way as when they're used as sedatives and hypnotics. However, the dosages may vary.

Addendum for anxiolytic use

When these drugs are used to treat anxiety, the nursing process steps are generally the same as when they're used as sedative hypnotics. However, keep these additional points in mind:
• Benzodiazepines and barbiturates are generally prescribed for short-term use. Patients undergoing long-term therapy should be referred to psychiatric counseling.
• The patient will need to identify and examine the source of his anxiety in order to reduce or eliminate it.
• Teach the patient various relaxation techniques, such as deep breathing and meditation, to help reduce anxiety. (See *Teaching about antianxiety drugs*, page 450.)

Buspirone

Buspirone is the first antianxiety drug in a class of drugs known as *azaspirodecanedione derivatives*. This drug's structure and mechanism of action differ from those of other antianxiety drugs.

Advantage, buspirone

Buspirone has several advantages, including:
• less sedation
• no increase in CNS depressant effects when taken with alcohol or sedative-hypnotics
• lower abuse potential.

Pharmacokinetics

Buspirone is absorbed rapidly, undergoes extensive first-pass effect, and is metabolized in the liver to at least one active metabolite. The drug is eliminated in urine and feces.

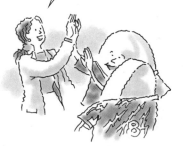

Buspirone has less sedation and a lower abuse potential. Now that's a winning combination!

Education edge

Teaching about antianxiety drugs

If antianxiety drugs are prescribed, review these points with the patient and his caregivers:

• These drugs help relieve symptoms temporarily but don't cure or solve the underlying problem. Counseling or psychotherapy may help find ways to decrease nervousness and assist with sleep.

• Use other methods to promote relaxation, such as physical exercise, stress-management techniques, and relaxation techniques.

• Identify factors that cause symptoms. Avoiding such products as caffeine, cold medications, and appetite suppressants can help reduce symptoms of nervousness and insomnia.

• Tell other health care providers what drugs you're using to avoid being prescribed other drugs with similar effects.

• Avoid hazardous activities that require alertness and psychomotor coordination until the central nervous system effects of the drug are known.

• Avoid alcohol consumption and smoking while taking the drug.

• Don't take other drugs, over-the-counter products, or herbal remedies without first consulting the prescriber or a pharmacist.

• Take the drug as prescribed; don't stop taking it without the prescriber's approval.

• Dependence on the drug may occur if it's taken longer than directed.

• Take the drug later in the day or at night as indicated to help decrease daytime drowsiness.

Pharmacodynamics

Although buspirone's mechanism of action remains unknown, it's clear that buspirone doesn't affect GABA receptors like benzodiazepines. Buspirone seems to produce various effects in the midbrain and acts as a midbrain modulator, possibly due to its high affinity for serotonin receptors.

Pharmacotherapeutics

Buspirone is used to treat generalized anxiety states. Patients who haven't received benzodiazepines seem to respond better to buspirone.

Slow as a tortoise

Because of its slow onset of action, buspirone is ineffective when quick relief from anxiety is needed.

Not for simple stress

Although buspirone hasn't shown potential for abuse and hasn't been classified as a controlled substance, it isn't recommended for relief of everyday stress.

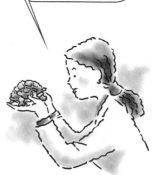

No, you've got buspione beat. Your onset of action is just a little bit slower!

Drug interactions

Unlike other antianxiety drugs, buspirone doesn't interact with alcohol or other CNS depressants. However, when buspirone is given with MAO inhibitors, hypertensive reactions may occur.

Adverse reactions

The most common reactions to buspirone include:
- dizziness
- light-headedness
- insomnia
- rapid heart rate
- palpitations
- headache.

Nursing process

These nursing process steps are appropriate for patients undergoing treatment with buspirone.

Assessment
- Obtain a history of the patient's anxiety before therapy, and reassess regularly thereafter.
- Assess for adverse reactions and drug interactions.
- Assess the patient's and family's understanding of drug therapy.

Key nursing diagnoses
- Anxiety related to the underlying condition
- Fatigue related to drug-induced adverse reactions
- Deficient knowledge related to drug therapy

Planning outcome goals
- The patient will state that his anxiety is reduced.
- The patient won't experience fatigue.
- The patient and his family will demonstrate an understanding of drug therapy.

Implementation
- Before starting therapy in the patient already being treated with a benzodiazepine, make sure that he doesn't stop the benzodiazepine abruptly; a withdrawal reaction may occur.
- Give the drug with food or milk.
- The dosage may be increased in 2- to 4-day intervals as ordered.
- Warn the patient to avoid hazardous activities that require alertness and psychomotor coordination until the CNS effects of the drug are known.

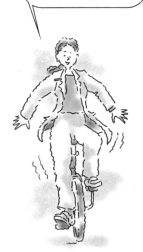

Tell the patient to avoid activities that require alertness and psychomotor coordination until the CNS effects of buspirone are known.

• Signs of improvement usually appear within 7 to 10 days; optimal results occur after 3 to 4 weeks of therapy.

Evaluation

• Patient's anxiety is relieved.
• Patient's fatigue is decreased.
• Patient and his family demonstrate an understanding of drug therapy.

Antidepressant and mood stabilizer drugs

Antidepressant and mood stabilizer drugs are used to treat affective disorders—disturbances in mood, characterized by depression or elation.

One pole

Unipolar disorders, characterized by periods of clinical depression, are treated with:
• selective serotonin reuptake inhibitors (SSRIs)
• MAO inhibitors
• tricyclic antidepressants (TCAs)
• other antidepressants.

Two poles

Lithium is used to treat bipolar disorders, characterized by alternating periods of manic behavior and clinical depression.

SSRIs

Developed to treat depression with fewer adverse effects, SSRIs are chemically different from TCAs and MAO inhibitors. Some of the SSRIs currently available are:
• citalopram
• escitalopram
• fluoxetine
• fluvoxamine
• paroxetine
• sertraline.

Pharmacokinetics

SSRIs are absorbed almost completely after oral administration and are highly protein bound. They're primarily metabolized in the liver and excreted in urine.

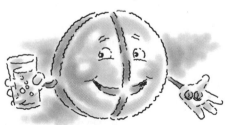

Good news! SSRIs treat depression with fewer adverse effects.

Pharmacodynamics

SSRIs inhibit the neuronal reuptake of the neurotransmitter serotonin. (See *Selective serotonin reuptake inhibitors: Fluoxetine.*)

Pharmacotherapeutics

SSRIs are used to treat major depressive episodes. They have the same degree of effectiveness as TCAs.

Here's the (SSRI) scoop

SSRIs may also be useful in treating panic disorders, eating disorders, personality disorders, impulse control disorders, and anxiety disorders. For example, paroxetine is indicated for social anxiety disorder. Fluoxetine is approved for the treatment of bulimia. Fluoxetine and sertraline are approved for the treatment of premenstrual (dysphoric) disorder. Fluvoxamine, fluoxetine, sertraline, and paroxetine are also used to treat obsessive-compulsive disorder, and paroxetine and sertraline are used for posttraumatic stress disorder.

Drug interactions

Drug interactions with SSRIs are associated with their ability to competitively inhibit a liver enzyme that's responsible for oxidation of numerous drugs, including TCAs; antipsychotics, such as clozapine and thioridazine; carbamazepine; metoprolol; flecainide; and encainide.

Danger ahead!

Using SSRIs with MAO inhibitors can cause serious, potentially fatal reactions. Individual SSRIs also have their own particular interactions:
- Using citalopram and paroxetine with warfarin may lead to increased bleeding.
- Carbamazepine may increase the clearance of citalopram.
- Fluoxetine increases the half-life of diazepam and displaces highly protein-bound drugs, leading to toxicity.
- Fluvoxamine use with diltiazem may cause bradycardia.
- Paroxetine shouldn't be used with tryptophan because this combination can cause headache, nausea, sweating, and dizziness.
- Paroxetine may increase procyclidine levels, causing increased anticholinergic effects.
- Cimetidine, phenobarbital, and phenytoin may reduce paroxetine metabolism by the liver, increasing the risk of toxicity.
- Paroxetine and sertraline may interact with other highly protein-bound drugs, causing adverse reactions to either drug.

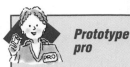

Prototype pro

Selective serotonin reuptake inhibitors: Fluoxetine

Actions
- Presumed to be linked to the inhibition of central nervous system (CNS) neuronal uptake of serotonin

Indications
- Depression
- Treatment of binge eating and vomiting behaviors in patients with moderate to severe bulimia nervosa
- Premenstrual dysphoric disorder
- Anorexia nervosa
- Panic disorder
- Alcohol dependence

Nursing considerations
- Monitor the patient for adverse reactions, such as anxiety, insomnia, drowsiness, nausea, diarrhea, dry mouth.
- Give the drug in the morning to prevent insomnia.
- Warn the patient to avoid hazardous activities that require alertness and psychomotor coordination until the CNS effects of the drug are known.

SSRI discontinuation syndrome

Abrupt discontinuation of selective serotonin reuptake inhibitors (SSRIs) may result in a condition called *SSRI discontinuation syndrome.* This syndrome is characterized by dizziness, vertigo, ataxia, nausea, vomiting, muscle pains, fatigue, tremor, and headache. The patient may also experience psychological symptoms, such as anxiety, crying spells, irritability, sad feelings, memory problems, and vivid dreams.

The half-life of it

SSRI discontinuation syndrome occurs in up to one-third of patients taking SSRIs. It's more common in patients who are stopping SSRIs with a short half-life, such as paroxetine. Fluoxetine is the least likely to cause this problem because of its extremely long half-life.

How to deal

This syndrome is self-limited. With treatment, it usually resolves within 2 to 3 weeks. Tapering the drug dosage slowly over several weeks can help prevent it.

Adverse reactions

Anxiety, insomnia, somnolence, and palpitations may occur with the use of an SSRI. Sexual dysfunction (anorgasm and delayed ejaculation) and various skin rashes have been reported. Decreased glucose concentrations in plasma can occur with fluoxetine. Orthostatic hypotension may occur with citalopram and paroxetine use.

Suicide watch

SSRIs have been linked with increased suicidal ideation and aggression. More research is needed to prove a direct association between SSRIs and these thoughts and behaviors.

Stopping...may be starting

Other symptoms may develop when a patient stops taking an SSRI. (See *SSRI discontinuation syndrome.*)

Nursing process

These nursing process steps are appropriate for patients undergoing treatment with SSRIs.

Assessment

• Assess the patient's condition before therapy, and reassess regularly throughout therapy.
• Assess for adverse reactions and drug interactions.
• Assess the patient's and family's knowledge of drug therapy.

Key nursing diagnoses
- Ineffective coping related to the underlying condition
- Insomnia related to drug therapy
- Deficient knowledge related to drug therapy

Planning outcome goals
- The patient's ability to cope will improve.
- The patient's insomnia will improve.
- The patient and his family will demonstrate an understanding of drug therapy.

Implementation
- Elderly or debilitated patients and patients with renal or hepatic dysfunction may need lower dosages or less frequent dosing.
- Give SSRIs in the morning to prevent insomnia.
- Give antihistamines or topical corticosteroids to treat rashes or pruritus.
- Lower-weight children may need several weeks between dosage increases.

> Elderly or debilitated patients and patients with renal or hepatic dysfunction may need lower dosages of SSRIs or less frequent dosing.

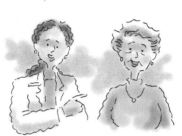

Evaluation
- Patient behavior and communication indicate an improvement of depression with drug therapy.
- Patient has no insomnia with drug use.
- Patient and his family demonstrate an understanding of drug therapy. (See *Teaching about SSRIs.*)

Education edge

Teaching about SSRIs

If selective serotonin reuptake inhibitors (SSRIs) are prescribed, review these points with the patient and his caregivers:
- Take the drug as directed; don't alter the dose, even when symptoms subside. SSRIs are usually given for several months — sometimes longer.
- Relief from symptoms may not occur until 2 to 4 weeks after the drug is started; don't stop taking the drug prematurely.
- Don't take other drugs, over-the-counter products, or herbal remedies without first consulting with the prescriber. Serious drug interactions may occur.
- Tell other health care providers that you're taking an SSRI to avoid drug interactions.

- Avoid activities that require alertness and psychomotor coordination until the drug's effects on the central nervous system are known.
- SSRIs may be taken without regard to food.
- Take the drug in the morning to help avoid insomnia or nervousness, unless otherwise directed.
- Report excessive drowsiness, dizziness, difficulty breathing, or other adverse reactions to the prescriber.
- Don't stop taking the drug without first consulting with the prescriber.
- Counseling, support groups, stress management techniques, and relaxation techniques may be helpful in addition to drug therapy.

MAO inhibitors

MAO inhibitors are divided into two classifications based on their chemical structure:

  hydrazines, which include phenelzine

  nonhydrazines, consisting of a single drug, tranylcypromine.

Pharmacokinetics

MAO inhibitors are absorbed rapidly and completely from the GI tract and are metabolized in the liver to inactive metabolites. These metabolites are excreted mainly by the GI tract and, to a lesser degree, by the kidneys.

Pharmacodynamics

MAO inhibitors appear to work by inhibiting monoamine oxidase, the widely distributed enzyme that normally metabolizes many neurotransmitters, including norepinephrine and serotonin. This action makes more norepinephrine, dopamine, and serotonin available to the receptors, thereby relieving the symptoms of depression.

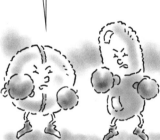

We MAO inhibitors don't play well with others.

Pharmacotherapeutics

Indications for MAO inhibitors are similar to those for other antidepressants. They're particularly effective in panic disorder with agoraphobia, eating disorders, posttraumatic stress syndrome, and pain disorder.

Not a typical depression

MAO inhibitors are also thought to be effective in atypical depression. Atypical depression produces signs opposite of those of typical depression. For example, the patient gains weight, sleeps more, and has a higher susceptibility to rejection.

Battling the blues

MAO inhibitors may be used to treat typical depression resistant to other therapies or when other therapies are contraindicated. Other uses include the treatment of:
• phobic anxieties
• neurodermatitis (an itchy skin disorder seen in some anxious people)
• hypochondriasis (abnormal concern about health)
• refractory narcolepsy (sudden sleep attacks).

Drug interactions

MAO inhibitors interact with many drugs:
• Taking MAO inhibitors with amphetamines, methylphenidate, levodopa, sympathomimetics, or nonamphetamine appetite suppressants may increase catecholamine release, causing hypertensive crisis.
• Using MAO inhibitors with fluoxetine, tricyclic antidepressants, citalopram, clomipramine, trazodone, sertraline, paroxetine, and fluvoxamine may result in an elevated body temperature, excitation, and seizures. (See *Stopping MAO inhibitors*.)
• When taken with doxapram, MAO inhibitors may cause hypertension and arrhythmias and may increase the adverse reactions to doxapram.
• MAO inhibitors may enhance the hypoglycemic effects.
• Administering MAO inhibitors with meperidine may result in excitation, hypertension or hypotension, extremely elevated body temperature, and coma.

Eat, drink and...be careful

Certain foods can interact with MAO inhibitors and produce severe reactions. The most serious reactions involve tyramine-rich foods, such as red wine, aged cheese, and fava beans. Foods with moderate tyramine contents—for example, yogurt and ripe bananas—may be eaten occasionally, but with care. Caffeine may also interact with MAO inhibitors, but the reactions aren't as serious as with tyramine-rich foods.

Adverse reactions

Administering MAO inhibitors in small, divided doses may relieve some of the following adverse reactions:
• hypertensive crisis (when taken with tyramine-rich foods)
• orthostatic hypotension
• restlessness, drowsiness, dizziness, and insomnia
• headache
• constipation, anorexia, and nausea and vomiting
• weakness and joint pain
• dry mouth
• blurred vision
• peripheral edema
• urine retention and transient impotence
• rash
• skin and mucous membrane hemorrhage.

Stopping MAO inhibitors

Monoamine oxidase (MAO) inhibitors should be discontinued 2 weeks before starting an alternative antidepressant. If a patient is switching from another antidepressant to an MAO inhibitor, a waiting period of 2 weeks (5 weeks for fluoxetine) is recommended before starting the MAO inhibitor.

Patients taking MAO inhibitors need to watch what they eat. Tyramine-rich foods—such as aged cheese—can interact with these drugs and produce hypertensive crisis.

Nursing process

These nursing process steps are appropriate for patients undergoing treatment with MAO inhibitors.

Assessment

• Assess the patient's condition before therapy and regularly thereafter.
• Assess the patient for risk of self-harm.
• Obtain baseline blood pressure, heart rate, complete blood count (CBC), and liver function test results before beginning therapy; monitor these throughout treatment.
• Assess for adverse reactions and drug interactions.
• Assess the patient's and family's knowledge of drug therapy.

Key nursing diagnoses

• Disturbed thought processes related to presence of depression
• Risk for injury related to drug-induced adverse CNS reactions
• Deficient knowledge related to drug therapy

Planning outcome goals

• The patient will exhibit improved thought processes.
• The risk of injury to the patient will be minimized.
• The patient and his family will demonstrate an understanding of drug therapy.

Implementation

• The dosage is usually reduced to a maintenance level as soon as possible.
• Don't withdraw the drug abruptly.
• Discontinue MAO inhibitors 14 days before elective surgery as indicated to avoid interaction with anesthetics.
• If the patient develops symptoms of overdose (such as palpitations, severe hypotension, or frequent headaches), withhold the dose and notify the prescriber.
• Have phentolamine available to combat severe hypertension.
• Continue precautions for 10 days after stopping the drug because it has long-lasting effects.

Signs of MAO inhibitor overdose include palpitations, severe hypotension, and frequent headaches.

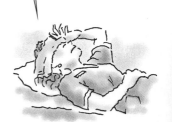

Evaluation

• Patient's behavior and communication exhibit improved thought processes.
• Patient doesn't experience injury from adverse CNS reactions.
• Patient and his family demonstrate an understanding of drug therapy. (See *Teaching about MAO inhibitors.*)

Education edge

Teaching about MAO inhibitors

If monoamine oxidase (MAO) inhibitors are prescribed, review these points with the patient and his caregivers:
• Avoid foods high in tyramine (such as aged cheese, red wine, beer, avocados, chocolate, and meat tenderizers) as well as large amounts of caffeine. Tranylcypromine is the MAO inhibitor most commonly reported to cause hypertensive crisis with ingestion of foods high in tyramine.

• Sit up for 1 minute before getting out of bed to avoid dizziness.
• Avoid overexertion because MAO inhibitors may suppress angina.
• Consult the prescriber before taking other prescription or over-the-counter drugs. Severe adverse effects can occur if MAO inhibitors are taken with cold, hay fever, or diet aids.
• Don't stop taking the drug suddenly.

TCAs

TCAs are used to treat depression. They include:
• amitriptyline hydrochloride
• amoxapine
• clomipramine
• desipramine
• doxepin
• imipramine hydrochloride
• imipramine pamoate
• nortriptyline
• protriptyline
• trimipramine.

Pharmacokinetics

All of the TCAs are active pharmacologically, and some of their metabolites are also active. They're absorbed completely when taken orally but undergo first-pass effect.

Passing it on

With first-pass effect, a drug passes from the GI tract to the liver, where it's partially metabolized before entering the circulation. TCAs are metabolized extensively in the liver and eventually excreted in urine as inactive compounds. Only small amounts of active drug are excreted in urine.

Oh-so-soluble

The extreme fat solubility of these drugs accounts for their wide distribution throughout the body, slow excretion, and long half-lives.

Pharmacodynamics

Researchers believe that TCAs increase the amount of norepinephrine, serotonin, or both in the CNS by preventing their reuptake (reentry) into the storage granules in the presynaptic nerves. Preventing reuptake results in increased levels of these neurotransmitters in the synapses, relieving depression. TCAs also block acetylcholine and histamine receptors.

Pharmacotherapeutics

TCAs are used to treat episodes of major depression. They're especially effective in treating depression of insidious onset accompanied by weight loss, anorexia, or insomnia. Physical signs and symptoms may respond after 1 to 2 weeks of therapy; psychological symptoms, after 2 to 4 weeks.

Working together

TCAs may be helpful when used with a mood stabilizer in treating acute episodes of depression in patients with type 1 bipolar disorder.

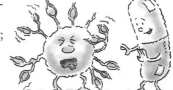

Now, just relax. I'm here to prevent your reuptake of norepinephrine and serotonin, which should help you feel less depressed.

Additional assistance

TCAs are also used to prevent migraine headaches and treat:
- panic disorder with agoraphobia
- urinary incontinence
- ADHD
- obsessive-compulsive disorder
- diabetic neuropathy
- enuresis. (See *Tricyclic antidepressants: Imipramine.*)

Prototype pro

Tricyclic antidepressants: Imipramine

Actions
- May inhibit the reuptake of norepinephrine and serotonin in central nervous system (CNS) nerve terminals (presynaptic neurons), thus enhancing the concentration and activity of neurotransmitters in the synaptic cleft
- Exerts antihistaminic, sedative, anticholinergic, vasodilatory, and quinidine-like effects

Indications
- Depression

- Enuresis in children older than age 6

Nursing considerations
- Monitor the patient for adverse reactions, such as sedation, anticholinergic effects, and orthostatic hypotension.
- Don't withdraw the drug abruptly; gradually reduce the dosage over several weeks.
- Warn the patient to avoid hazardous activities that require alertness and psychomotor coordination until the CNS effects of the drug are known.

Drug interactions

TCAs interact with several commonly used drugs:
• TCAs increase the catecholamine effects of amphetamines and sympathomimetics, leading to hypertension.
• Barbiturates increase the metabolism of TCAs and decrease their blood levels.
• Cimetidine impairs the metabolism of TCAs by the liver, increasing the risk of toxicity.

Temperature's rising

• Using TCAs concurrently with MAO inhibitors may cause an extremely elevated body temperature, excitation, and seizures.
• An increased anticholinergic effect, such as dry mouth, urine retention, and constipation, is seen when anticholinergic drugs are taken with TCAs.
• TCAs reduce the antihypertensive effects of clonidine and guanethidine.

Adverse reactions

Adverse reactions to TCAs include:
• orthostatic hypotension
• sedation
• jaundice
• rashes and photosensitivity reactions
• resting tremor
• decreased sexual desire and inhibited ejaculation
• transient eosinophilia
• reduced white blood cell (WBC) count
• manic episodes (in patients with or without bipolar disorder)
• exacerbation of psychotic symptoms in susceptible patients.

On the rare side

Although rare, TCA therapy may also lead to:
• granulocytopenia
• palpitations
• conduction delays
• rapid heartbeat
• impaired cognition and cardiovascular effects.

Deadly desipramine?

Sudden death has occurred in children and adolescents taking desipramine. Obtain a baseline electrocardiogram (ECG) in these patients before giving a TCA.

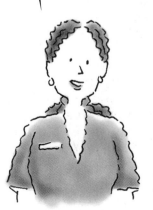

TCAs increase the effects of anticholinergic drugs, which can result in dry mouth, urine retention, and constipation.

Education edge

Teaching about TCAs

If tricyclic antidepressants (TCAs) are prescribed, review these points with the patient and his caregivers:
• Know the risks and benefits of therapy. The full therapeutic effect may not occur for several weeks.
• Take the drug exactly as prescribed. Don't increase the dosage, stop the drug, or take another drug (including over-the-counter drugs and herbal remedies) without medical approval.
• Because an overdose with TCAs is commonly fatal, entrust a reliable family member with the drug and warn him to store it safely away from children.

• Avoid alcohol while taking TCAs.
• Avoid hazardous tasks that require mental alertness until the drug's full effects are known.
• Excessive exposure to sunlight, heat lamps, or tanning beds may cause burns and abnormal hyperpigmentation.
• If you have diabetes, monitor your glucose level carefully because the drug may alter it.
• Chew sugarless gum, suck on hard candy or ice chips, or use artificial saliva to relieve dry mouth.
• Report adverse reactions promptly.

Nursing process

These nursing process steps are appropriate for patients undergoing treatment with TCAs.

Assessment

• Check an ECG in patients older than age 40 before starting therapy.
• Observe the patient for mood changes to monitor drug effectiveness; benefits may not appear for 2 to 4 weeks.
• Assess the patient's vital signs regularly for decreased blood pressure or tachycardia (fast heart rate); observe him carefully for other adverse reactions, and report changes. In particular, assess him for anticholinergic adverse reactions (dry mouth, urine retention, or constipation), which may require a dosage reduction.

Key nursing diagnoses

• Disturbed thought processes related to adverse effects
• Risk for injury related to sedation and orthostatic hypotension
• Noncompliance related to long-term therapy

Planning outcome goals

• The patient will exhibit improved thought processes.
• The risk of injury to the patient will be minimized.
• The patient will comply with therapy.

Implementation
• Make sure that the patient swallows each dose; a depressed patient may hoard pills for a suicide attempt, especially when symptoms begin to improve.
• Don't withdraw the drug abruptly; gradually reduce the dosage over several weeks to avoid a rebound effect or other adverse reactions.
• Follow the manufacturer's instructions for reconstitution, dilution, and storage of drugs.

Evaluation
• Patient regains normal thought processes.
• Patient sustains no injury from adverse reactions.
• Patient complies with therapy. (See *Teaching about TCAs.*)

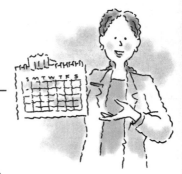

> Withdraw TCAs gradually over several weeks to avoid a rebound effect or other adverse reactions.

Miscellaneous antidepressants

Other antidepressants in use today include:
• maprotiline and mirtazapine, tetracyclic antidepressants
• bupropion, a dopamine reuptake blocking drug
• venlafaxine and duloxetine, serotonin-norepinephrine reuptake inhibitor
• trazodone, a triazolopyridine drug
• nefazodone, a phenyl piperazine drug.

Pharmacokinetics

The paths these antidepressants take through the body may vary:
• Maprotiline and mirtazapine are absorbed from the GI tract, distributed widely in the body, metabolized by the liver, and excreted by the kidneys.
• Bupropion is well absorbed from the GI tract and metabolized by the liver. Its metabolites are excreted by the kidneys. It appears to be highly bound to plasma proteins.
• Venlafaxine and duloxetine are rapidly absorbed after oral administration, metabolized in the liver, and excreted in urine.
• Venlafaxine is partially bound to plasma proteins; in contrast, duloxetine is highly bound to albumin.
• Trazodone is well absorbed from the GI tract, distributed widely in the body, and metabolized by the liver. About 75% is excreted in urine. The rest is excreted in feces.
• Nefazodone is rapidly and completely absorbed but, because of extensive metabolism, only about 20% of the drug is available. The drug is almost completely bound to plasma proteins and is excreted in urine.

Pharmacodynamics

Much about how these drugs work has yet to be fully understood:
• Maprotiline and mirtazapine probably increase the amount of norepinephrine, serotonin, or both in the CNS by blocking their reuptake by presynaptic neurons (nerve terminals).

Rethinking reuptake

• Bupropion was once thought to inhibit the reuptake of the neurotransmitter dopamine; however, its action is more likely on nonadrenergic receptors.
• Venlafaxine and duloxetine are thought to potentiate neurotransmitter activity in the CNS by inhibiting the neural reuptake of serotonin and norepinephrine.
• Trazodone, although its effect is unknown, is thought to exert antidepressant effects by inhibiting the reuptake of norepinephrine and serotonin in the presynaptic neurons.
• Nefazodone's action isn't precisely defined. It inhibits neuronal uptake of serotonin and norepinephrine. It's also a serotonin antagonist, which explains its effectiveness in treating anxiety.

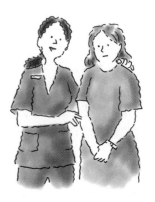

Nefazodone is effective in treating both anxiety and depression.

Pharmacotherapeutics

These miscellaneous drugs are all used to treat depression. Trazodone may also be effective in treating aggressive behavior and panic disorder. Nefazodone is sometimes used to treat anxiety.

Drug interactions

All of these antidepressants may have serious, potentially fatal reactions when combined with MAO inhibitors. Each of these drugs also carries individual, specific risks when used with other drugs:
• Maprotiline and mirtazapine interact with CNS depressants, resulting in additive effects.
• Bupropion, when combined with levodopa, phenothiazines, or TCAs, increases the risk of adverse reactions, including seizures.
• Trazodone may increase serum levels of digoxin and phenytoin. Its use with antihypertensive drugs may cause increased hypotensive effects. CNS depression may be enhanced if trazodone is administered with other CNS depressants.
• Nefazodone may increase the digoxin level if administered with digoxin, and it increases CNS depression when combined with CNS depressants.

Adverse reactions

Adverse reactions to maprotiline include:
• seizures
• orthostatic hypotension

- tachycardia
- ECG changes.

Mirtazapine maladies

Mirtazapine may cause:
- tremors
- confusion
- nausea
- constipation.

Bupropion blues

These adverse reactions may occur with bupropion:
- headache
- confusion
- tremor
- agitation
- tachycardia
- anorexia
- nausea and vomiting.

Venlafaxine, duloxetine, and nefazodone negatives

Adverse reactions to venlafaxine, duloxetine, and nefazodone include:
- headache
- somnolence
- dizziness
- nausea.

Trazodone trouble

Trazodone may cause:
- drowsiness
- dizziness.

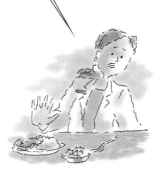

Several of the antidepressants can cause nausea. No, thank you!

Nursing process

These nursing process steps are appropriate for patients undergoing treatment with miscellaneous antidepressants.

Assessment

- Assess the patient's condition before therapy and regularly thereafter.
- Assess for adverse reactions and drug interactions.
- Assess the patient's and family's knowledge of drug therapy.

Key nursing diagnoses

- Ineffective coping related to the underlying condition
- Insomnia related to drug therapy
- Deficient knowledge related to drug therapy

Planning outcome goals
- The patient's ability to cope will improve.
- The patient's insomnia will improve.
- The patient and his family will demonstrate an understanding of drug therapy.

Implementation
- Elderly or debilitated patients and patients with renal or hepatic dysfunction may need lower dosages or less frequent dosing.
- Give these drugs in the morning to prevent insomnia, unless otherwise directed.
- Administer the drugs as prescribed.
- Monitor the patient for effects of drug therapy.

Evaluation
- Patient's behavior and communication indicate improvement of depression with drug therapy.
- Patient has no insomnia with drug use.
- Patient and his family demonstrate an understanding of drug therapy.

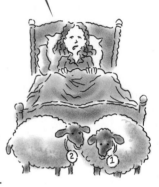

Antidepressants such as bupropion should be taken in the morning. Otherwise, insomnia may result—and I'm tired of counting sheep.

Lithium

Lithium carbonate and lithium citrate are mood stabilizers used to prevent or treat mania. The discovery of lithium was a milestone in treating mania and bipolar disorders.

Pharmacokinetics

When taken orally, lithium is absorbed rapidly and completely and is distributed to body tissues. An active drug, lithium isn't metabolized and is excreted from the body unchanged.

Pharmacodynamics

In mania, one theory is that the patient experiences excessive catecholamine stimulation. In bipolar disorder, the patient is affected by swings between the excessive catecholamine stimulation of mania and the diminished catecholamine stimulation of depression.

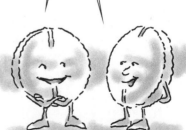

I hear excessive catecholamine stimulation results in mania, and diminished catecholamine stimulation causes depression.

Yes, but we lithium tablets may regulate catecholamine release to treat mania and bipolar disorders. Pretty cool, eh?

Curbing catecholamines

Lithium's exact mechanism is unknown. A few of the ways it may regulate catecholamine release in the CNS are by:
• increasing norepinephrine and serotonin uptake
• reducing the release of norepinephrine from the synaptic vesicles (where neurotransmitters are stored) in the presynaptic neuron
• inhibiting norepinephrine's action in the postsynaptic neuron.

Under study

Researchers are also examining lithium's effects on electrolyte and ion transport. It may also modify actions of second messengers, such as cyclic adenosine monophosphate.

Pharmacotherapeutics

Lithium is used primarily to treat acute episodes of mania and to prevent relapses of bipolar disorders. Other uses of lithium being researched include preventing unipolar depression and migraine headaches and treating depression, alcohol dependence, anorexia nervosa, syndrome of inappropriate antidiuretic hormone, and neutropenia.

Drug interactions

Lithium has a narrow therapeutic margin of safety. A blood level that's even slightly higher than the therapeutic level can be dangerous. Serious interactions with other drugs can occur because of this narrow therapeutic range:
• The risk of lithium toxicity increases when lithium is taken with thiazide and loop diuretics and nonsteroidal anti-inflammatory drugs.
• Administration of lithium with haloperidol, phenothiazines, and carbamazepine may produce an increased risk of neurotoxicity.
• Lithium may increase the hypothyroid effects of potassium iodide.
• Sodium bicarbonate may increase lithium excretion, reducing its effects.
• Lithium's effects are reduced when taken with theophylline.

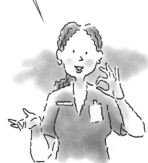

Lithium has a narrow therapeutic margin. A blood level even a little higher than the therapeutic level can be dangerous.

Salt at fault?

• A patient on a severe salt-restricted diet is susceptible to lithium toxicity. On the other hand, an increased intake of sodium may reduce the therapeutic effects of lithium.

Adverse reactions

Common adverse reactions to lithium include:
- reversible ECG changes
- thirst
- polyuria
- elevated WBC count.

Toxic times

Toxic blood levels of lithium may produce:
- confusion
- lethargy
- slurred speech
- increased reflex reactions
- seizures.

Nursing process

These nursing process steps are appropriate for patients undergoing treatment with lithium.

Assessment

- Assess the patient's condition before therapy and regularly thereafter. Expect a delay of 1 to 3 weeks before the drug's beneficial effects are noticed.
- Obtain a baseline ECG, thyroid and kidney studies, and electrolyte levels. Monitor lithium blood levels 8 to 12 hours after the first dose, usually before the morning dose, two or three times weekly in the first month, and then weekly to monthly during maintenance therapy.
- Perform outpatient follow-up of thyroid and kidney function every 6 to 12 months. Palpate the thyroid to check for enlargement.
- Assess for adverse reactions and drug interactions.

Key nursing diagnoses

- Disturbed thought processes related to manic disorder
- Ineffective health maintenance related to drug-induced endocrine dysfunction
- Deficient knowledge related to drug therapy

Planning outcome goals

- The patient's behavior and thought processes will improve.
- The patient's health status will improve.
- The patient and his family will demonstrate an understanding of drug therapy.

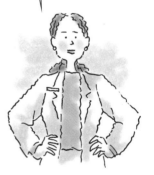

Remember: It may take 1 to 3 weeks to notice lithium's beneficial effects.

Education edge

Teaching about lithium

If lithium is prescribed, review these points with the patient and his caregivers:
• Take the drug with plenty of water and after meals to minimize GI upset.
• Lithium has a narrow therapeutic margin of safety. A blood level that's even slightly high can be dangerous.
• Watch for signs and symptoms of toxicity, such as diarrhea, vomiting, tremor, drowsiness, muscle weakness, and ataxia. Withhold one dose of the drug and call the prescriber if toxic symptoms appear. Don't stop the drug abruptly.

• Expect transient nausea, polyuria, thirst, and discomfort during the first few days of therapy.
• Avoid activities that require alertness and good psychomotor coordination until the drug's central nervous system effects are known.
• Don't switch brands or take other prescription or over-the-counter drugs without the prescriber's approval.
• Wear or carry medical identification.

Implementation
• Determination of lithium blood levels is crucial to safe use of the drug. Lithium shouldn't be used in a patient who can't have his blood levels checked regularly.
• Give the drug with plenty of water and after meals to minimize GI reactions.
• Before leaving the bedside, make sure that the patient has swallowed the drug.
• Notify the prescriber if the patient's behavior hasn't improved in 3 weeks or if it worsens.
• Adverse reactions usually are mild when the blood level of lithium remains below 1.5 mEq/L.
• If the patient has diuresis, check his urine specific gravity and report a level below 1.005, which may indicate diabetes insipidus.
• Lithium may alter glucose tolerance in a patient with diabetes. Monitor his glucose level closely.

Evaluation
• Patient exhibits improved behavior and thought processes.
• Patient maintains normal endocrine function throughout therapy.
• Patient and his family demonstrate an understanding of drug therapy. (See *Teaching about lithium.*)

Antipsychotic drugs

Antipsychotic drugs can control psychotic symptoms (delusions, hallucinations, and thought disorders) that can occur with schizophrenia, mania, and other psychoses.

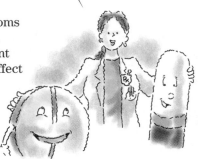

Antipsychotic drugs can control psychotic symptoms, such as delusions, hallucinations, and thought disorders.

The name game

Drugs used to treat psychoses have several different names, including:
• antipsychotic, because they can eliminate signs and symptoms of psychoses
• major tranquilizer, because they can calm an agitated patient
• neuroleptic, because they have an adverse neurobiologic effect that causes abnormal body movements.

One...or the other

Regardless of what they're called, all antipsychotic drugs belong to one of two major groups:

  atypical antipsychotics

  typical antipsychotics.

Atypical antipsychotics

Atypical antipsychotics are drugs designed to treat schizophrenia. They include:
• clozapine
• olanzapine
• risperidone
• quetiapine
• ziprasidone
• aripiprazole.

Pharmacokinetics

Atypical antipsychotics are absorbed after oral administration. They're metabolized by the liver. Metabolites of clozapine, quetiapine, ziprasidone, and olanzapine are inactive, whereas risperidone has an active metabolite. They're highly plasma protein–bound and eliminated in urine, with a small portion eliminated in feces.

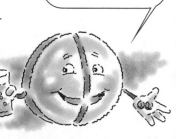

I'm not your run-of-the-mill antipsychotic. I block the activity of two receptors, dopamine and serotonin, to treat schizophrenia.

Pharmacodynamics

Atypical antipsychotics typically block the dopamine receptors, but to a lesser extent than the typical antipsychotics, resulting in far fewer extrapyramidal adverse effects. Additionally, atypical antipsychotics block serotonin receptor activity. These combined actions account for the effectiveness of atypical antipsychotics against the positive and negative symptoms of schizophrenia.

Pharmacotherapeutics

Atypical antipsychotics are considered the first line of treatment for patients with schizophrenia because of equal or improved effectiveness and improved tolerability. They're commonly used to treat behavioral and psychotic symptoms in patients with dementia, but dosages are significantly lower.

Drug interactions

Drugs that alter the P450 enzyme system will alter the metabolism of some atypical antipsychotics.

The straight "dopa"

Atypical antipsychotics counteract the effects of levodopa and other dopamine agonists.

And the rest of the story...

Several drug interactions may occur:
• Atypical antipsychotics taken with antihypertensives may potentiate hypotensive effects.
• Atypical antipsychotics taken with benzodiazepines or CNS depressants may enhance CNS depression.
• Clozapine combined with anticholinergics may increase anticholinergic effects.
• When clozapine is taken with citalopram, fluoroquinolones, fluoxetine, fluvoxamine, paroxetine, sertraline, or risperidone, increased clozapine levels may occur, resulting in toxicity.
• Clozapine combined with digoxin or warfrain may increase levels of these drugs.
• Clozapine taken with phenytoin can decrease clozapine levels.
• Clozapine taken with drugs that cause bone marrow depression (such as cancer drugs) can increase bone marrow depression.
• Olanzapine taken with ciprofloxacin, fluoxetine, or fluvoxamine may increase olanzapine levels.
• Risperidone combined with ziprasidone or carbamazepine may decrease the effectiveness of risperidone.
• Taking erythromycin, fluconazole, intraconazole, or ketoconazole with quetiapine decreases quetiapine clearance.

• Quetiapine clearance is increased when taken with carbamazepine, glucocorticoids, phenobarbital, phenytoin, rifampin, or thioridazine.
• Ziprasidone taken with antiarrhythmics, arsenic trioxide, cisapride, dolasetron, droperidol, levomethadyl, mefloquine, pentamidine, phenothiazines, pimozide, quinolones, tacrolimus, or diuretics can cause life-threatening arrhythmias.
• Ziprasidone and itraconazole or ketoconazole may increase ziprasidone levels.
• Aripiprazole taken with ketoconazole, fluoxetine, paroxetine, or quinidine may increase aripiprazole levels and result in toxicity.
• Aripiprazole combined with carbamazepine may decrease aripiprazole levels, decreasing effectiveness.

Adverse reactions

Atypical antipsychotics have fewer extrapyramidal effects than typical antipsychotics and a minimal risk of seizures (except for clozapine). Clozapine is associated with agranulocytosis. Weight gain is also common, and seizures may occur.

Extra! Extra!

Olanzapine places the patient at minimal risk for extrapyramidal effects, but weight gain is common. Risperidone has a higher risk for extrapyramidal effects than other atypical antipsychotics if it's prescribed at doses higher than 6 mg/day.

Quetiapine and aripiprazole (a newer atypical antipsychotic) are associated with sedation. Ziprasidone isn't recommended for patients with heart problems because it can cause ECG changes.

Nursing process

These nursing process steps are appropriate for patients undergoing treatment with atypical antipsychotics.

Assessment

• Assess the patient's disorder before therapy and regularly thereafter.
• Assess for adverse reactions and drug interactions.
• Monitor the patient for tardive dyskinesia (involuntary movements). It may occur after prolonged use. This sign may not appear until months or years later, and it may disappear spontaneously or persist for life despite stopping the drug.
• Assess the patient's and family's knowledge of drug therapy.

Key nursing diagnoses

• Disturbed thought processes related to the underlying condition

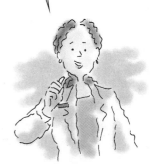

Tardive dyskinesia can occur after prolonged use of atypical antipsychotics. It may persist even after the drug is stopped.

- Impaired physical mobility related to extrapyramidal effects
- Deficient knowledge related to drug therapy

Planning outcome goals
- The patient will exhibit improved thought processes.
- The patient will exhibit adequate physical mobility.
- The patient and his family will demonstrate an understanding of drug therapy.

Implementation
- Administer the drug as prescribed and monitor for its effect.
- When changing forms of the drug, the dosage will change to meet the patient's needs.
- Protect the drug from light as indicated. Discard the drug if it's markedly discolored.
- Don't stop the drug abruptly unless severe adverse reactions occur.
- Acute dystonic reactions may be treated with diphenhydramine.
- Warn the patient to avoid activities that require alertness and psychomotor coordination until the drug's CNS effects are known.
- Advise the patient to avoid alcohol while taking atypical antipsychotics.
- Tell the patient to chew sugarless gum or suck hard candy to help relieve dry mouth.

Evaluation
- Patient demonstrates decreased psychotic behavior and agitation.
- Patient maintains physical mobility.
- Patient and his family demonstrate an understanding of drug therapy.

Typical antipsychotics

Typical antipsychotics, which include phenothiazines and non-phenothiazines, can be broken down into smaller classifications.

A sorted affair

Many clinicians believe that the phenothiazines should be treated as three distinct drug classes because of the differences in the adverse reactions they cause:
- *Aliphatics* primarily cause sedation and anticholinergic effects and are low-potency drugs. They include drugs such as chlorpromazine.

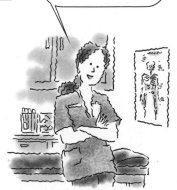

Now, that's so typical! Typical antipsychotics, which include phenothiozines, can be broken down into smaller classifications.

• *Piperazines* primarily cause extrapyramidal reactions and include fluphenazine decanoate, fluphenazine hydrochloride, perphenazine, and trifluoperazine.

• *Piperidines* primarily cause sedation and anticholinergic and cardiac effects and include mesoridazine besylate and thioridazine.

By chemical structure

Based on their chemical structure, nonphenothiazine antipsychotics can be divided into several drug classes, including:

• butyrophenones, such as haloperidol and haloperidol decanoate
• dibenzoxazepines, such as loxapine succinate
• dihydroindolones, such as molindone
• diphenylbutylpiperidines, such as pimozide
• thioxanthenes, such as thiothixene and thiothixene hydrochloride.

Pharmacokinetics

Although typical antipsychotics are absorbed erratically, they're very lipid-soluble and highly protein-bound. Therefore, they're distributed to many tissues and are highly concentrated in the brain. All typical antipsychotics are metabolized in the liver and excreted in urine and bile.

Effects keep going and going and going and going

Because fatty tissues slowly release accumulated phenothiazine metabolites into the plasma, phenothiazines may produce effects up to 3 months after they're stopped.

Pharmacodynamics

Although the mechanism of action of typical antipsychotics isn't understood fully, researchers believe that these drugs work by blocking postsynaptic dopaminergic receptors in the brain.

Blocking...

The antipsychotic effect of phenothiazines and nonphenothiazines comes about from a receptor blockade in the limbic system. Their antiemetic effects result from the receptor blockade in the chemoreceptor trigger zone located in the brain's medulla.

...and stimulating

Phenothiazines also stimulate the extrapyramidal system (motor pathways that connect the cerebral cortex with the spinal nerve pathways). (See *Phenothiazines: Chlorpromazine.*)

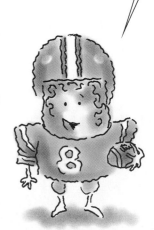

When typical antipsychotics come into play, they block postsynaptic dopaminergic receptors in the brain. Let's see if you can tackle that concept!

Prototype pro

Phenothiazines: Chlorpromazine

Actions
• Functions as a dopamine antagonist by blocking postsynaptic dopamine receptors in various parts of the central nervous system (CNS)
• Produces antiemetic effects by blocking the chemoreceptor trigger zone
• Produces varying degrees of anticholinergic and alpha-adrenergic receptor blocking actions

Indications
• Agitated psychotic state, hallucinations, manic-depressive illness, excessive motor and autonomic activity
• Severe nausea and vomiting induced by CNS disturbances
• Moderate anxiety
• Behavioral problems caused by chronic organic mental syndrome, tetanus, acute intermittent porphyria, intractable hiccups, itching, and symptomatic rhinitis

Nursing considerations
• Monitor the patient for adverse reactions and extrapyramidal symptoms (ranging from akathisia during early treatment to tardive dyskinesia after long-term use).
• A neuroleptic malignant syndrome resembling severe parkinsonism may occur.
• Elevated liver enzyme levels that progress to obstructive jaundice usually indicate an allergic reaction.
• Don't withdraw the drug abruptly; gradually reduce the dosage over several weeks.
• Warn the patient to avoid hazardous activities that require alertness and psychomotor coordination until the drug's CNS effects are known.

Pharmacotherapeutics

Phenothiazines are used primarily to:
• treat schizophrenia
• calm anxious or agitated patients
• improve a patient's thought processes
• alleviate delusions and hallucinations.

Even more uses

Other therapeutic uses have been found for phenothiazines:
• They're administered to treat other psychiatric disorders, such as brief reactive psychosis, atypical psychosis, schizoaffective psychosis, autism, and major depression with psychosis.
• In combination with lithium, they're used in the treatment of patients with bipolar disorder, until the slower-acting lithium produces its therapeutic effect.
• They're prescribed to quiet mentally challenged children and agitated geriatric patients, particularly those with dementia.
• They may be given to boost the preoperative effects of analgesics.

• They help manage pain, anxiety, and nausea in patients with cancer.

Group dynamics

As a group, nonphenothiazines are used to treat psychotic disorders. Thiothixene is also used to control acute agitation. In addition, haloperidol and pimozide may be used to treat Tourette syndrome.

Drug interactions

Phenothiazines and nonphenothiazines have different drug interactions.

Serious business

Phenothiazines interact with many different types of drugs and may have serious effects:
• Increased CNS depressant effects, such as stupor, may occur when they're taken with CNS depressants.
• CNS depressants may reduce phenothiazine effectiveness, resulting in increased psychotic behavior or agitation.
• Taking anticholinergic drugs with phenothiazines may result in increased anticholinergic effects, such as dry mouth and constipation. By increasing phenothiazine metabolism, anticholinergic drugs may also reduce the antipsychotic effects of phenothiazines.
• Phenothiazines may reduce the antiparkinsonian effects of levodopa.
• Concurrent use with lithium increases the risk of neurotoxicity.
• Concurrent use with droperidol increases the risk of extrapyramidal effects.
• The threshold for seizures is lowered when phenothiazines are used with anticonvulsants.
• Phenothiazines may increase the serum levels of TCAs and beta-adrenergic blockers. Thioridazine can cause serious, fatal cardiac arrhythmias when combined with fluvoxamine, propranolol, pindolol, fluoxetine, drugs that inhibit the cytochrome P-450 2D6 isoenzyme, and drugs known to prolong the QTc interval.

Voted less likely to interact

Nonphenothiazines interact with fewer drugs than phenothiazines. Their dopamine-blocking activity can inhibit levodopa and may cause disorientation in patients receiving both drugs. Haloperidol may boost the effects of lithium, producing encephalopathy (brain dysfunction).

Adverse reactions

Neurologic reactions are the most common and serious adverse reactions associated with phenothiazines. Extrapyramidal symptoms may appear after the first few days of therapy; tardive dyskinesia may occur after several years of treatment.

Going to extremes

Neuroleptic malignant syndrome is a potentially fatal condition that produces muscle rigidity, extreme extrapyramidal symptoms, severely elevated body temperature, hypertension, and rapid heart rate. If left untreated, it can result in respiratory failure and cardiovascular collapse.

Shared traits

Most nonphenothiazines cause the same adverse reactions as phenothiazines.

Nursing process

These nursing process steps are appropriate for patients undergoing treatment with typical antipsychotics.

Assessment
• Assess the patient's vital signs regularly for decreased blood pressure (especially before and after parenteral therapy) or tachycardia; observe him carefully for other adverse reactions.
• Assess intake and output, watching for urine retention or constipation, which may require a dosage reduction.
• Monitor bilirubin levels weekly for the first 4 weeks. Obtain baseline CBC, ECG (for quinidine-like effects), liver and renal function test results, electrolyte levels (especially potassium), and eye examination findings. Monitor these findings periodically thereafter, especially in the patient receiving long-term therapy.
• Assess the patient for mood changes, and monitor his progress.
• Monitor the patient for involuntary movements. Check the patient receiving prolonged treatment at least once every 6 months.

Key nursing diagnoses
• Risk for injury related to adverse reactions
• Impaired mobility related to extrapyramidal symptoms
• Noncompliance related to long-term therapy

Planning outcome goals
• The risk of injury to the patient will be minimized.
• The patient will maintain mobility.
• The patient will comply with drug therapy.

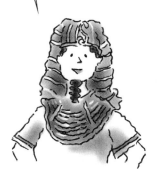

Watch closely for extrapyramidal symptoms, which may appear after the first few days of phenothiazine therapy. I think I see an extra pyramid off in the distance...

Education edge

Teaching about antipsychotic drugs

If antipsychotic drugs are prescribed, review these points with the patient and his caregivers:
• Take the drug as prescribed. Don't increase the dosage or discontinue the drug without the prescriber's approval.
• Take the full dose at bedtime if daytime sedation occurs.
• The drug's full therapeutic effect may not occur for several weeks.
• Watch for adverse reactions and report unusual effects, especially involuntary movements.
• Avoid alcohol while taking this drug.

• Don't take other drugs, including over-the-counter or herbal products, without the prescriber's approval.
• Avoid hazardous tasks until the drug's full effects are established. Sedative effects will lessen after several weeks.
• Excessive exposure to sunlight, heat lamps, or tanning beds may cause photosensitivity reactions.
• Avoid exposure to extreme heat or cold.
• Phenothiazines may cause pink or brown discoloration of urine.

Implementation
• Don't withdraw the drug abruptly. Although physical dependence doesn't occur with antipsychotic drugs, rebound worsening of psychotic symptoms may occur and many drug effects may persist.
• Follow the manufacturer's guidelines for reconstitution, dilution, administration, and storage of drugs; slightly discolored liquids may or may not be acceptable for use. Check with the pharmacist.

Evaluation
• Patient remains free from injury.
• Extrapyramidal symptoms don't develop.
• Patient complies with therapy as evidenced by improved thought processes. (See *Teaching about antipsychotic drug.*)

Stimulants

Stimulants, another type of psychotropic drug, are used to treat ADHD, a condition characterized by inattention, impulsiveness, and hyperactivity. Examples of stimulants include:
• dextroamphetamine
• methylphenidate
• mixed amphetamine salts.

Pharmacokinetics

Stimulants, another type of psychotropic drug, are absorbed well from the GI tract and are distributed widely in the body. Methylphenidate, however, undergoes significant first-pass effect. Stimulants are metabolized in the liver and excreted primarily in urine.

Pharmacodynamics

Stimulants are believed to work by increasing levels of dopamine and norepinephrine, either by blocking the reuptake of dopamine and norepinephrine, by enhancing the presynaptic release, or by inhibiting MAO.

Pharmacotherapeutics

Stimulants are the treatment of choice for ADHD. They're helpful in improving attention span, leading to improved school or work performance and decreasing impulsiveness and hyperactivity.

Wake-up call

Dextroamphetamine and methylphenidate are also used in the treatment of narcolepsy.

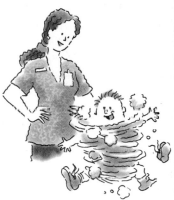

Stimulants are the treatment of choice for ADHD, helping to decrease impulsiveness and hyperactivity.

Drug interactions

Stimulants shouldn't be used within 14 days of discontinuing an MAO inhibitor. Also, methylphenidate may decrease the effect of guanethidine and increase the effects of TCAs, warfarin, and some anticonvulsants.

Adverse reactions

Stimulants are highly abused substances. Close monitoring of the patient is required. Although controversial, some prescribers recommend stopping the drug for a brief period, such as when children are on summer break from school, to reassess the need for therapy. Stimulants may affect growth. Monitor children closely for height and weight changes.

Dextroamphetamine downers

Adverse reactions specific to dextroamphetamine include:
- restlessness
- tremor
- insomnia
- tachycardia
- palpitations

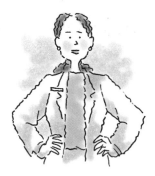

Stimulants are highly abused drugs. Monitor the patient closely.

- arrhythmias
- dry mouth
- unpleasant taste
- diarrhea.

Methylphenidate misfortune

Methylphenidate may cause:
- dizziness
- insomnia
- seizures
- palpitations
- arrhythmias
- abdominal pain
- rash
- thrombocytopenia.

Nursing process

These nursing process steps are appropriate for patients undergoing treatment with stimulants.

Assessment

- Obtain a history of the patient's underlying condition before therapy, and reassess regularly throughout therapy.
- Assess for adverse reactions and drug interactions.
- Monitor the patient's sleeping pattern, and observe him for signs of excessive stimulation.
- Assess the patient's and family's knowledge of drug therapy.

Key nursing diagnoses

- Ineffective health maintenance related to underlying condition
- Insomnia related to drug therapy
- Deficient knowledge related to drug therapy

Planning outcome goals

- The patient's underlying condition will improve.
- The patient's insomnia will improve.
- The patient and his family will demonstrate an understanding of drug therapy.

Implementation

- Give the drug at least 6 hours before bedtime to avoid sleep interference.
- Prolonged use may cause psychological dependence or habituation, especially in a patient with a history of drug addiction.

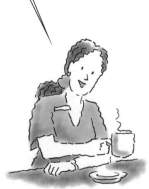

Hold the lattes for patients taking stimulants! Caffeine increases the effects of these drugs.

• After prolonged use, reduce the dosage gradually to prevent acute rebound depression.
• Advise the patient to avoid hazardous activities until the drug's CNS effects are known.
• Tell the patient to avoid drinks containing caffeine, which increases the effects of amphetamines and related amines.
• Report adverse effects, such as excess stimulation, tolerance to effect, or decreased effectiveness, to the prescriber.

Evaluation

• Patient maintains improvement in underlying condition.
• Patient experiences no insomnia with drug use.
• Patient and family demonstrate an understanding of drug therapy.

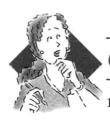

Quick quiz

1. Which benzodiazepine is used primarily to treat anxiety?
   A. Lorazepam
   B. Temazepam
   C. Triazolam
   D. Flurazepam

Answer: A. Benzodiazepines used to treat anxiety include lorazepam, alprazolam, chlordiazepoxide hydrochloride, clonazepam, clorazepate dipotassium, diazepam, halazepam, and oxazepam.

2. Which adverse reaction is common in the patient taking buspirone?
   A. Nausea
   B. Diarrhea
   C. Constipation
   D. Headache

Answer: D. Common reactions to buspirone include headache, dizziness, light-headedness, insomnia, rapid heart rate, and palpitations.

3. Which food should the patient taking an MAO inhibitor avoid?
   A. Cheese
   B. Apples
   C. Bananas
   D. Beer

Answer: A. Certain foods can interact with MAO inhibitors and produce severe reactions. The most serious reactions involve tyramine-rich foods, such as red wine, aged cheese, and fava beans. Foods with moderate tyramine contents, such as ripe bananas, may be eaten occasionally.

Scoring

☆☆☆   If you answered all three questions correctly, great job! You're solid with the psychotropics.

☆☆   If you answered two questions correctly, you did just fine! There's no reason for you to be depressed.

☆   If you answered only one question correctly, stay calm. A quick review of the chapter may help relieve your anxiety.

Anti-infective drugs

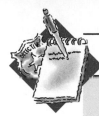

Just the facts

In this chapter, you'll learn:

♦ classes of drugs that act as anti-infectives

♦ uses and varying actions of these drugs

♦ absorption, distribution, metabolization, and excretion of these drugs

♦ drug interactions and adverse reactions to these drugs.

Drugs and infection

When infection attacks the body, anti-infective drugs can help turn the tide of battle. Four types of anti-infective drugs exist: antibacterial, antiviral, antitubercular, and antifungal.

Selecting an anti-infective drug

Selecting an appropriate anti-infective drug to treat a specific infection involves several important factors:

First, the microorganism must be isolated and identified—generally through growing a culture.

Then its susceptibility to various drugs must be determined. Because culture and sensitivity results take 48 hours, treatment typically starts at assessment and is then reevaluated when test results are obtained.

The location of the infection must be considered. For therapy to be effective, an adequate concentration of the anti-infective drug must be delivered to the infection site.

When infection attacks, anti-infective drugs can help you win the battle. Get back!

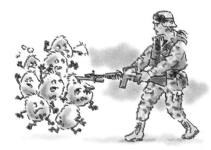

The rise of the resistance movement

Indiscriminate use of anti-infective drugs has serious consequences. Unnecessary exposure of organisms to these drugs encourages the emergence of resistant strains. These resistant strains are likely to do far more damage than their predecessors.

Make reservations

Use of anti-infective drugs should be reserved for patients with infections caused by susceptible organisms and should be used in high enough doses and for an appropriate period. New anti-infective drugs should be reserved for severely ill patients with serious infections that don't respond to conventional drugs.

Finally, the cost of the drug as well as its potential adverse effects and the possibility of patient allergies must be considered.

Preventing pathogen resistance

The usefulness of anti-infective drugs is limited by the pathogens that may develop resistance to a drug's action.

The mutants strike back

Resistance is the ability of a microorganism to live and grow in the presence of an anti-infective drug. Resistance usually results from genetic mutation of the microorganism. (See *The rise of the resistance movement*.)

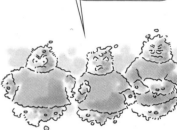

When anti-infective drugs are used indiscriminately, our resistance grows.

Antibacterial drugs

Antibacterial drugs, also known as *antibiotics*, are drugs that either kill bacteria or inhibit the growth of bacteria. They're mainly used to treat systemic (involving the whole body rather than a localized area) bacterial infections. Antibacterial drugs include:
- aminoglycosides
- penicillins
- cephalosporins
- tetracyclines
- clindamycin
- macrolides
- vancomycin
- carbapenems
- monobactams
- fluoroquinolones
- sulfonamides
- nitrofurantoin.

Aminoglycosides

Aminoglycosides are bactericidal (they destroy bacteria). They're effective against:
- gram-negative bacilli
- some aerobic gram-positive bacteria
- mycobacteria
- some protozoa.

Naming names

Aminoglycosides currently in use include:
- amikacin sulfate
- gentamicin sulfate
- kanamycin sulfate
- neomycin sulfate
- netilmicin sulfate
- paromomycin sulfate
- streptomycin sulfate
- tobramycin sulfate.

Pharmacokinetics (how drugs circulate)

Because aminoglycosides are absorbed poorly from the GI tract, they're usually given parenterally. After I.V. or I.M. administration, aminoglycoside absorption is rapid and complete.

Flowing with extracellular fluid

Aminoglycosides are distributed widely in extracellular fluid. They readily cross the placental barrier but don't cross the blood-brain barrier.

You're kidney-ing me!

Aminoglycosides aren't metabolized. They're excreted primarily by the kidneys.

Pharmacodynamics (how drugs act)

Aminoglycosides act as bactericidal drugs against susceptible organisms by binding to the bacteria's 30S subunit, a specific ribosome in the microorganism, thereby interrupting protein synthesis and causing the bacteria to die.

Reasons behind resistance

Bacterial resistance to aminoglycosides may be related to:
- failure of the drug to cross the cell membrane
- altered binding to ribosomes
- destruction of the drug by bacterial enzymes.

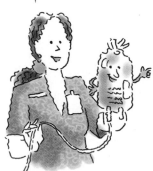

Aminoglycosides kill bacteria by binding to their 30S subunit ribosomes.

Prototype pro

Aminoglycosides: Gentamicin

Actions
• Inhibits protein synthesis by binding directly to the 30S ribosomal subunit; usually bactericidal

Indications
• Serious infections caused by susceptible organisms
• Prevention of endocarditis during GI and genitourinary procedures or surgery

Nursing considerations
• Monitor the patient for adverse effects, such as ototoxicity, nephrotoxicity, anaphylaxis, thrombocytopenia, and agranulocytosis.
• Peak gentamicin levels occur 1 hour after I.M. injection and 30 minutes after I.V. infusion; check trough levels before the next dose.

Penetration power provided by penicillin

Some gram-positive enterococci resist aminoglycoside transport across the cell membrane. When penicillin is used with aminoglycoside therapy, the cell wall is altered, allowing the aminoglycoside to penetrate the bacterial cell. (See *Aminoglycosides: Gentamicin.*)

Pharmacotherapeutics (how drugs are used)

Aminoglycosides are most useful in treating:
• infections caused by gram-negative bacilli
• serious nosocomial (hospital-acquired) infections, such as gram-negative bacteremia (abnormal presence of microorganisms in the bloodstream), peritonitis (inflammation of the peritoneum, the membrane that lines the abdominal cavity), and pneumonia in critically ill patients
• urinary tract infections (UTIs) caused by enteric bacilli that are resistant to less-toxic antibacterial drugs, such as penicillins and cephalosporins
• infections of the central nervous system (CNS) and the eye (treated with local instillation).

Combo care

Aminoglycosides are used in combination with penicillins to treat infections caused by gram-positive organisms, such as staphylococci and enterococci. Combination therapy increases the drugs' effectiveness.

Taming strains

Individual aminoglycosides may have their own particular usefulness:

• Streptomycin is active against many strains of mycobacteria, including *Mycobacterium tuberculosis*, and against the gram-positive bacteria *Nocardia* and *Erysipelothrix*.

• Amikacin, gentamicin, and tobramycin are active against *Acinetobacter*, *Citrobacter*, *Enterobacter*, *Escherichia coli*, *Klebsiella*, *Proteus* (indole-positive and indole-negative), *Providencia*, *Pseudomonas aeruginosa*, and *Serratia*.

• Neomycin is given orally to suppress intestinal bacteria before surgery and is active against *E. coli* infectious diarrhea.

When the drug's a dud

Aminoglycosides are inactive against anaerobic bacteria.

Drug interactions

Carbenicillin and ticarcillin reduce the effects of amikacin, gentamicin, kanamycin, neomycin, streptomycin, and tobramycin. This is especially true if the penicillin and aminoglycoside are mixed in the same container or I.V. line.

Amplified effects

Amikacin, gentamicin, kanamycin, neomycin, streptomycin, and tobramycin administered with neuromuscular blockers increase neuromuscular blockade, resulting in increased muscle relaxation and respiratory distress.

Toxic mix

Toxicity to the kidneys may result in renal failure, and toxicity to the neurologic system results in peripheral neuropathy with numbness and tingling of the extremities. The risk of renal toxicity also increases when amikacin, gentamicin, kanamycin, or tobramycin is taken with cyclosporine, amphotericin B, or acyclovir.

Oh dear, those poor ears

The symptoms of ototoxicity (damage to the ear) caused by aminoglycosides may be masked by antiemetic drugs. Loop diuretics taken with aminoglycosides increase the risk of ototoxicity. Hearing loss may occur in varying degrees and may be irreversible.

Adverse reactions

Serious adverse reactions limit the use of aminoglycosides and include:

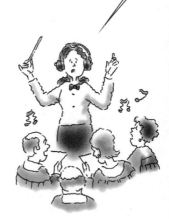

Some drugs taken with aminoglycosides increase the risk of ototoxicity. I have to say, that isn't sounding so bad to me right now!

• neuromuscular reactions, ranging from peripheral nerve toxicity to neuromuscular blockade
• ototoxicity
• renal toxicity.

Oral report

Adverse reactions to oral aminoglycosides include:
• nausea
• vomiting
• diarrhea.

Nursing process

These nursing process steps are appropriate for patients undergoing treatment with aminoglycosides.

Assessment
• Obtain the patient's allergy history.
• Obtain culture and sensitivity tests before giving the first dose; therapy may begin pending test results. Check these tests periodically to assess the drug's efficacy.
• Assess vital signs, electrolyte levels, hearing ability, and renal function studies before and during therapy.
• Weigh the patient and review baseline renal function studies before therapy and then regularly during therapy. Notify the prescriber of changes so that the dosage may be adjusted.
• Assess for drug interactions and adverse reactions.
• Assess the patient's and family's knowledge of drug therapy.

Key nursing diagnoses
• Risk for injury related to adverse effects of drug
• Risk for infection related to drug-induced superinfection
• Risk for deficient fluid volume related to adverse GI reactions

Planning outcome goals
• The patient's risk of injury will be minimized.
• The patient's risk of superinfection will be minimized.
• The patient's fluid volume will remain within normal limits as evidenced by vital signs and intake and output.

Implementation
• Keep the patient well hydrated to minimize chemical irritation of the renal tubules.
• Don't add or mix other drugs with I.V. infusions, particularly penicillins, which inactivate aminoglycosides. If other drugs must be given I.V., temporarily stop infusion of the primary drug.

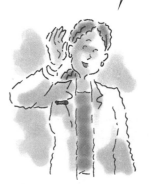

Because of the potential for ototoxicity, make sure you assess the patient's hearing ability before and during therapy with aminoglycosides.

- Follow the manufacturer's instructions for reconstitution, dilution, and storage of drugs; check expiration dates.
- Shake oral suspensions well before administering them.

Muscling in

- Administer an I.M. dose deep into a large muscle mass (gluteal or midlateral thigh); rotate injection sites to minimize tissue injury. Apply ice to the injection site to relieve pain.
- Because too-rapid I.V. administration may cause neuromuscular blockade, infuse an I.V. drug continuously or intermittently over 30 to 60 minutes for adults and over 1 to 2 hours for infants; dilution volume for children is determined individually.

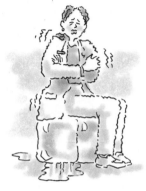

Brrr! Applying ice can help relieve pain at an I.M. injection site.

Peak experience

- With gentamicin, draw blood to check for the peak level 1 hour after I.M. injection (30 minutes to 1 hour after I.V. infusion); for the trough level, draw a sample just before the next dose. Peak gentamicin levels above 12 mcg/ml and trough levels above 2 mcg/ml may increase the risk of toxicity. Time and date all blood samples. Don't use a heparinized tube to collect blood samples because it interferes with results.
- Be aware that hemodialysis (8 hours) removes up to 50% of gentamicin from blood. Scheduling dosages may need to be adjusted accordingly.
- Notify the prescriber about signs and symptoms of decreasing renal function or changes in hearing.
- Be aware that therapy usually continues for 7 to 10 days. If no response occurs in 3 to 5 days, therapy may be stopped and new specimens obtained for culture and sensitivity testing.
- Encourage adequate fluid intake; the patient should be well hydrated while taking the drug to minimize chemical irritation of the renal tubules.

Evaluation

- Patient maintains pretreatment renal function and hearing levels.
- Patient is free from infection.
- Patient maintains adequate hydration.

Penicillins

Penicillins remain one of the most important and useful antibacterial drugs, despite the availability of numerous others. The penicillins can be divided into four groups:

- natural penicillins (penicillin G benzathine, penicillin G potassium, penicillin G procaine, penicillin G sodium, penicillin V potassium)
- penicillinase-resistant penicillins (dicloxacillin sodium, cloxacillin sodium, nafcillin sodium)
- aminopenicillins (amoxicillin, ampicillin, amoxicillin-clavulanate potassium)
- extended-spectrum penicillins (carbenicillin indanyl sodium, ticarcillin disodium).

Pharmacokinetics

After oral administration, penicillins are absorbed mainly in the duodenum and the upper jejunum of the small intestine.

Affecting absorption

Absorption of oral penicillin varies and depends on such factors as:
- particular penicillin used
- pH of the patient's stomach and intestine
- presence of food in the GI tract.

Food factors

Most penicillins should be given on an empty stomach (1 hour before or 2 hours after a meal) to enhance absorption. Penicillins that can be given without regard to meals include amoxicillin, penicillin V, and amoxicillin-clavulanate potassium.

Well traveled

Penicillins are distributed widely to most areas of the body, including the lungs, liver, kidneys, muscle, bone, and placenta. High concentrations also appear in urine, making penicillins useful in treating UTIs.

Exit route

Penicillins are metabolized to a limited extent in the liver to inactive metabolites. Most penicillins are excreted 60% unchanged by the kidneys. Nafcillin and oxacillin, however, are excreted in bile.

Pharmacodynamics

Penicillins are usually bactericidal in action. They bind reversibly to several enzymes outside the bacterial cytoplasmic membrane. These enzymes, known as *penicillin-binding proteins* (PBPs), are involved in cell-wall synthesis and cell division. Interference with these processes inhibits cell-wall synthesis, causing rapid destruction of the cell.

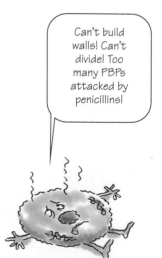

Can't build walls! Can't divide! Too many PBPs attacked by penicillins!

Prototype pro

Natural penicillins: Penicillin G sodium

Actions
• Inhibits cell wall synthesis during microorganism multiplication
• Resists penicillinase enzymes produced by bacteria that convert penicillins to inactive penicilloic acid

Indications
• Bacterial infection caused by non-penicillinase-producing strains of gram-positive and gram-negative aerobic cocci, spirochetes, or certain gram-positive aerobic and anaerobic bacilli

Nursing considerations
• Monitor the patient for adverse effects, such as seizures, anaphylaxis, leukopenia, and thrombocytopenia.
• Obtain a specimen for culture and sensitivity tests before giving the first dose. Therapy may begin pending results.

Pharmacotherapeutics

No other class of antibacterial drugs provides as wide a spectrum of antimicrobial activity as the penicillins. As a class, they cover gram-positive, gram-negative, and anaerobic organisms, although specific penicillins are more effective against specific organisms.

I.M.: A solution for the insoluble

Penicillin is given by I.M. injection when oral administration is inconvenient or a patient's compliance is questionable. Because long-acting preparations of penicillin G (penicillin G benzathine and penicillin G procaine) are relatively insoluble, they must be administered by the I.M. route. (See *Natural penicillins: Penicillin G sodium.*)

> Penicillin can be given I.M. when oral administration is inconvenient or a patient's compliance is in question.

Drug interactions

Penicillins may interact with various drugs:
• Probenecid increases the plasma concentration of penicillins.
• Penicillins reduce tubular secretion of methotrexate in the kidneys, increasing the risk of methotrexate toxicity.
• Tetracyclines and chloramphenicol reduce the bactericidal action of penicillins.
• Neomycin decreases the absorption of penicillin V.
• The effectiveness of hormonal contraceptives is reduced when they're taken with penicillin V or ampicillin. If applicable, advise the patient to use a reliable alternative method of contraception in addition to hormonal contraceptives during penicillin therapy.
• Large doses of I.V. penicillins can increase the bleeding risks of anticoagulants by prolonging bleeding time. Nafcillin and dicloxacillin have been implicated in warfarin resistance.

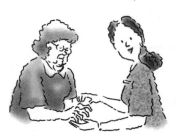

• High dosages of penicillin G and extended-spectrum penicillins (carbenicillin, ticarcillin) inactivate aminoglycosides.

Adverse reactions

Hypersensitivity reactions are the major adverse reactions to penicillins, including:
• anaphylactic reactions
• serum sickness (a hypersensitivity reaction occurring 1 to 2 weeks after injection of a foreign serum)
• drug fever
• various skin rashes.

GI didn't know this could happen

Adverse GI reactions associated with oral penicillins include:
• tongue inflammation
• nausea and vomiting
• diarrhea.

I'm all nerves

CNS reactions may include:
• lethargy
• hallucinations
• anxiety or depression
• confusion
• seizures.

Dangerous diarrhea

The aminopenicillins and extended-spectrum penicillins can produce pseudomembranous colitis (diarrhea caused by a change in the flora of the colon or an overgrowth of a toxin-producing strain of *Clostridium difficile*).

Nursing process

These nursing process steps are appropriate for patients undergoing treatment with penicillins.

Assessment

• Obtain a history of the patient's infection before therapy; reassess for improvement regularly thereafter.
• Assess the patient's allergy history. Try to find out whether previous reactions were true hypersensitivity reactions or adverse reactions (such as GI distress) that the patient interpreted as an allergy.

- Obtain culture and sensitivity tests before giving the first dose; therapy may begin pending test results. Repeat these tests periodically to assess the drug's effectiveness.
- Monitor vital signs, electrolytes, and renal function studies.
- Assess the patient's consciousness and neurologic status when giving high doses; CNS toxicity can occur.
- Because coagulation abnormalities, even frank bleeding, can follow high doses, especially of extended-spectrum penicillins, monitor prothrombin time (PT), International Normalized Ratio, and platelet counts, and assess the patient for signs of occult or frank bleeding.
- Assess for adverse reactions and drug interactions.
- Assess the patient's and family's knowledge of drug therapy.

Key nursing diagnoses
- Risk for infection related to altered immune status
- Risk for deficient fluid volume related to adverse GI reactions
- Deficient knowledge related to drug therapy

Planning outcome goals
- The patient's infection will resolve as evidenced by negative cultures, normal temperature, and normal white blood cell (WBC) counts.
- The patient will maintain adequate fluid hydration.
- The patient and his family will demonstrate an understanding of drug therapy.

Implementation
- Give penicillins at least 1 hour before bacteriostatic antibacterial drugs (tetracyclines, erythromycins, and chloramphenicol); these drugs inhibit bacterial cell growth and decrease the rate of penicillin uptake by bacterial cell walls.
- Follow the manufacturers' directions for reconstituting, diluting, and storing drugs; check expiration dates.
- Give oral penicillins at least 1 hour before or 2 hours after meals to enhance GI absorption.
- Refrigerate oral suspensions (stable for 14 days); shake well before administering to ensure the correct dosage.
- Give an I.M. dose deep into a large muscle mass (gluteal or mid-lateral thigh), rotate injection sites to minimize tissue injury, and apply ice to the injection site to relieve pain. Don't inject more than 2 g of drug per injection site.
- With I.V. infusions, don't add or mix another drug, especially an aminoglycoside, which becomes inactive if mixed with a penicillin. If other drugs must be given I.V., temporarily stop infusion of the primary drug.

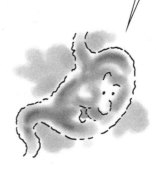

Oral penicillins should be given 1 hour before or 2 hours after meals to enhance GI absorption.

Education edge

Teaching about anti-infective therapy

If anti-infective therapy is prescribed, review these points with the patient and his caregivers:
• Take this drug exactly as prescribed. Complete the entire prescribed regimen, comply with instructions for around-the-clock scheduling, and keep follow-up appointments.
• Report unusual reactions, such as a rash, fever, or chills. These may be signs and symptoms of hypersensitivity to the drug.
• Check the drug's expiration date before taking it. Discard unused drug after the prescribed therapeutic regimen is taken.
• If using hormonal contraceptives, use an additional form of contraception during drug therapy.

• Don't stop taking the drug, even if symptoms are relieved. The symptoms of the current infection may recur or a new infection may develop.
• Don't take drugs left over from a previous illness or take someone else's drugs.
• Don't take other drugs, over-the-counter products, or herbal remedies without first consulting with the prescriber.
• Take the drug on an empty stomach and 1 hour before or 2 hours after meals. Food may decrease drug absorption.
• Take the drug with a full glass of water.
• Store the drug appropriately; some drugs may need refrigeration.

• Infuse an I.V. drug continuously or intermittently (over 30 minutes). Rotate the infusion site every 48 hours. An intermittent I.V. infusion may be diluted in 50 to 100 ml of sterile water, normal saline solution, dextrose 5% in water (D_5W), D_5W and half-normal saline, or lactated Ringer's solution.
• Monitor the patient continuously for possible allergic reactions. A patient who has never had a penicillin hypersensitivity reaction may still have future allergic reactions.
• Monitor patients (especially elderly patients, debilitated patients, and patients receiving immunosuppressants or radiation) receiving long-term therapy for possible superinfection.
• Monitor the patient's hydration status if adverse GI reactions occur.

Evaluation
• Patient is free from infection.
• Patient maintains adequate hydration.
• Patient and family demonstrate an understanding of drug therapy. (See *Teaching about anti-infective therapy.*)

Just because a patient hasn't had an allergic reaction to penicillin before doesn't mean he won't have one in the future. Make sure you monitor for possible allergic reactions during penicillin therapy.

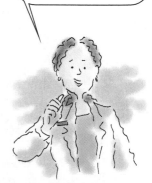

Cephalosporins

Many antibacterial drugs introduced for clinical use in recent years have been cephalosporins.

Therapy that spans generations

Cephalosporins are grouped into generations according to their effectiveness against different organisms, their characteristics, and their development:
• First generation cephalosporins include cefadroxil, cefazolin sodium, and cephalexin hydrochloride monohydrate. (See *First-generation cephalosporins: Cefazolin.*)
• Second-generation cephalosporins include cefaclor, cefotetan, cefprozil, ceftibuten, cefoxitin, cefuroxime axetil, and cefuroxime sodium.
• Third-generation cephalosporins include cefdinir, cefoperazone sodium, cefotaxime sodium, cefpodoxime proxetil, ceftazidime, ceftizoxime sodium, and ceftriaxone sodium.
• Fourth-generation cephalosporins include cefditoren pivoxil and cefepime hydrochloride.

Similar components = similar reactions

Because penicillins and cephalosporins are chemically similar (they both have what's called a *beta-lactam* molecular structure), cross-sensitivity occurs in 3% to 16% of patients. This means that someone who has had a reaction to penicillin is also at risk for a reaction to cephalosporins.

Pharmacokinetics

Many cephalosporins are administered parenterally because they aren't absorbed from the GI tract. Some cephalosporins are absorbed from the GI tract and can be administered orally, but food usually decreases their absorption rate, although not the amount absorbed. Two cephalosporins (oral cefuroxime and cefpodoxime) actually have increased absorption when given with food.

No service to the CNS

After absorption, cephalosporins are distributed widely, although most aren't distributed in the CNS.

First-generation cephalosporins: Cefazolin

Actions
• Inhibits cell wall synthesis promoting osmotic instability
• Usually are bactericidal

Indications
• Infection caused by susceptible organisms

Nursing considerations
• Obtain a specimen for culture and sensitivity tests before giving the first dose. Therapy may begin pending results.
• Monitor the patient for adverse effects, such as diarrhea, hematologic disorders, rash, and hypersensitivity reactions.
• With large doses or prolonged treatment, monitor the patient for superinfections.

I'm proud to be part of four generations of infection-fighting cephalosporins!

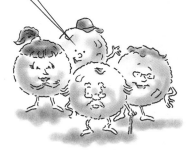

Crossing the line

Cefuroxime (second-generation) and the third-generation drugs cefotaxime, ceftizoxime, ceftriaxone, and ceftazidime cross the blood-brain barrier. Cefepime (fourth-generation) also crosses the blood-brain barrier, but the extent to which it does isn't known.

Much ado about metabolism

Many cephalosporins aren't metabolized at all. Cefotaxime is metabolized to the nonacetyl form, which provides less antibacterial activity than the parent compound. To a small extent, ceftriaxone is metabolized in the intestines to inactive metabolites, which are excreted via the biliary system.

Making an exit

All cephalosporins are excreted primarily unchanged by the kidneys with the exception of cefoperazone and ceftriaxone, which are excreted in feces via bile.

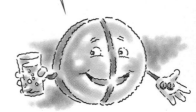

There's always an exception to the rule! Although the absorption of oral cephalosporins usually decreases when given with food, the absorption of oral cefuroxime and cefpodoxime increases with food.

Pharmacodynamics

Like penicillins, cephalosporins inhibit cell-wall synthesis by binding to the bacterial PBP enzymes located on the cell membrane. After the drug damages the cell wall by binding with the PBPs, the body's natural defense mechanisms destroy the bacteria. (See *How cephalosporins attack bacteria.*)

Pharmacotherapeutics

The four generations of cephalosporins have particular therapeutic uses:
• First-generation cephalosporins, which act primarily against gram-positive organisms, may be used as alternative therapy in a patient who's allergic to penicillin, depending on how sensitive to penicillin the person is. They're also used to treat staphylococcal and streptococcal infections, including pneumonia, cellulitis (skin infection), and osteomyelitis (bone infection).
• Second-generation cephalosporins act against gram-negative bacteria. Cefoxitin and cefotetan are the only cephalosporins effective against anaerobes (organisms that live without oxygen).
• Third-generation cephalosporins, which act primarily against gram-negative organisms, are the drugs of choice for infections caused by *Enterobacter, P. aeruginosa,* and anaerobic organisms.
• Fourth-generation cephalosporins are active against a wide range of gram-positive and gram-negative bacteria.

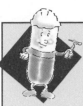

Pharm function

How cephalosporins attack bacteria

The antibacterial action of cephalosporins depends on their ability to penetrate the bacterial wall and bind with proteins on the cytoplasmic membrane, as shown below.

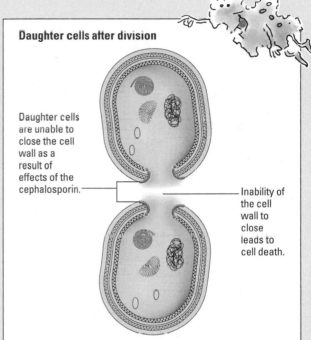

Cephalosporins penetrate and bind. That's how they wipe me out!

Mature bacterial cell

- Capsule
- Cytoplasmic membrane
- Chromosomes
- Ribosome
- Cephalosporin incorporates itself into the cell wall of a susceptible, mature gram-positive or gram-negative bacterium.
- Inclusion body

Daughter cells after division

Daughter cells are unable to close the cell wall as a result of effects of the cephalosporin.

Inability of the cell wall to close leads to cell death.

Drug interactions

Patients receiving cephalosporins who drink alcoholic beverages with or up to 72 hours after taking a dose may experience acute alcohol intolerance, with such signs and symptoms as headache, flushing, dizziness, nausea, vomiting, or abdominal cramps within 30 minutes of alcohol ingestion. This reaction can occur up to 3 days after discontinuing the antibiotic.

Cephalosporins and alcohol don't mix. Acute alcohol intolerance can occur, even 3 days after stopping the drug.

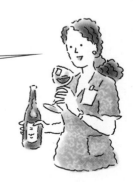

Advantageous interaction

Uricosurics (drugs to relieve gout), such as probenecid and sulfinpyrazone, can reduce kidney excretion of some cephalosporins.

Sometimes, probenecid is used therapeutically to increase and prolong plasma cephalosporin concentrations.

Adverse reactions

Adverse reactions to cephalosporins include:
- confusion
- seizures
- bleeding
- nausea
- vomiting
- diarrhea.

Bleed, indeed

Cefoperazone, cefotetan, and ceftriaxone in particular may be associated with a decrease in PT and partial thromboplastin time, leading to an increased risk of bleeding. Populations at risk include elderly, debilitated, malnourished, and immunocompromised patients and those with renal impairment, hepatic disease, or impaired vitamin K synthesis or storage.

Systemically speaking

Hypersensitivity reactions are the most common systemic adverse reactions to cephalosporins and include:
- hives
- itching
- rash that appears like the measles
- serum sickness (reaction after injection of a foreign serum characterized by edema, fever, hives, and inflammation of the blood vessels and joints)
- anaphylaxis (in rare cases).

Nursing process

These nursing process steps are appropriate for patients undergoing treatment with cephalosporins.

Assessment

- Review the patient's allergy history. Try to determine whether previous reactions were true hypersensitivity reactions or adverse effects (such as GI distress) that the patient interpreted as an allergy.
- Assess the patient continuously for possible hypersensitivity reactions or other adverse effects.
- Obtain a culture and sensitivity specimen before administering the first dose; therapy may begin pending test results. Check test results periodically to assess the drug's effectiveness.

> Attention, all history buffs! Review the patient's allergy history to help determine if previous reactions to cephalosporins were true hypersensitivity reactions.

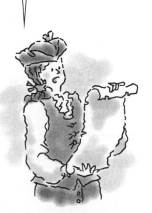

Key nursing diagnoses
- Risk for infection related to superinfection
- Risk for deficient fluid volume related to adverse GI reactions
- Deficient knowledge related to drug therapy

Planning outcome goals
- The patient's infection will resolve as evidenced by culture reports, temperature, and WBC counts.
- The patient will maintain adequate fluid volume.
- The patient and his family will demonstrate an understanding of drug therapy.

Implementation
- Administer cephalosporins at least 1 hour before bacteriostatic antibacterial drugs (tetracyclines, erythromycins, and chloramphenicol); by decreasing cephalosporin uptake by bacterial cell walls, the antibacterial drugs inhibit bacterial cell growth.

Keeping cool

- Refrigerate oral suspensions (stable for 14 days); shake well before administering to ensure the correct dosage.
- Follow the manufacturers' directions for reconstitution, dilution, and storage of drugs; check expiration dates.
- Administer an I.M. dose deep into a large muscle mass (gluteal or midlateral thigh); rotate injection sites to minimize tissue injury.
- Don't add or mix other drugs with I.V. infusions, particularly aminoglycosides, which are inactivated if mixed with cephalosporins. If other drugs must be given I.V., temporarily stop infusion of the primary drug.
- Ensure adequate dilution of the I.V. infusion and rotate injection sites every 48 hours to help minimize local vein irritation; using a small-gauge needle in a larger available vein may be helpful.
- Monitor renal function studies; dosages of certain cephalosporins must be lowered in patients with severe renal impairment. In patients with decreased renal function, monitor blood urea nitrogen (BUN) and creatinine levels and urine output for significant changes.
- Monitor PT and platelet counts, and assess the patient for signs of hypoprothrombinemia, which may occur (with or without bleeding) during therapy with cefoperazone, cefotetan, or ceftriaxone.
- Monitor patients on long-term therapy for possible bacterial and fungal superinfection, especially elderly and debilitated patients and those receiving immunosuppressants or radiation therapy.

Teaching about cephalosporins

If cephalosporins are prescribed, review these points with the patient and his caregivers:
• Take the drug exactly as prescribed for as long as prescribed. Follow the prescriber's instructions for maintaining an around-the-clock dosage.
• Take the oral form with food if GI irritation occurs.
• Review proper storage and disposal of the drug, and check the drug's expiration date before use.

• Watch for signs and symptoms of hypersensitivity (such as hives, itching, or rash) and other adverse reactions. Report any unusual effects.
• Report signs and symptoms of bacterial or fungal superinfection promptly.
• Don't consume alcohol in any form within 72 hours of treatment with cephalosporins.
• Eat yogurt or drink buttermilk to prevent intestinal superinfection resulting

from the drug's suppression of normal intestinal flora.
• If diabetic and required to monitor urine glucose, use Diastix. Don't use Clinitest because results may be incorrect.
• Keep all follow-up appointments.
• Don't take other drugs, over-the-counter preparations, or herbal remedies without first consulting with the prescriber.

Signs and symptoms include fever, malaise, muscular aches and pains, and oral ulcerations.
• Monitor susceptible patients receiving sodium salts of cephalosporins for possible fluid retention.

Evaluation
• Patient is free from infection.
• Patient maintains adequate hydration.
• Patient and family demonstrate an understanding of drug therapy. (See *Teaching about cephalosporins*.)

Tetracyclines

Tetracyclines are broad-spectrum antibacterial drugs. They may be classified as:
• intermediate-acting compounds, such as demeclocycline hydrochloride and tetracycline hydrochloride
• long-acting compounds, such as doxycycline hyclate and minocycline hydrochloride.

Pharmacokinetics

Tetracyclines are absorbed from the duodenum when taken orally. They're distributed widely into body tissues and fluids and concentrated in bile.

The way out

Tetracyclines are excreted primarily by the kidneys. Doxycycline is also excreted in feces. Minocycline undergoes enterohepatic recirculation.

Pharmacodynamics

All tetracyclines are primarily bacteriostatic, meaning they inhibit the growth or multiplication of bacteria. They penetrate the bacterial cell by an energy-dependent process. Within the cell, they bind primarily to a subunit of the ribosome, inhibiting the protein synthesis required for maintaining the bacterial cell. (See *Tetracyclines: Tetracycline hydrochloride.*)

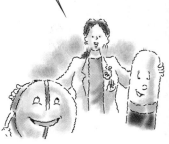

Tetracyclines inhibit bacteria growth or multiplication.

Packing more bacteriostatic action

The long-acting compounds doxycycline and minocycline provide more action against various organisms than other tetracyclines.

Pharmacotherapeutics

Tetracyclines provide a broad spectrum of activity, which means they cover a wide range of organisms, including:
- gram-positive and gram-negative aerobic and anaerobic bacteria
- spirochetes
- mycoplasmas
- rickettsiae
- chlamydiae
- gonorrhea
- some protozoa.
  Tetracyclines are used to treat:

Prototype pro

Tetracyclines: Tetracycline hydrochloride

Actions
- Is bacteriostatic but may be bactericidal against certain organisms
- Binds reversibly to 30S and 50S ribosomal subunits, inhibiting bacterial protein synthesis

Indications
- Infection caused by susceptible organisms
- Gonorrhea

Nursing considerations
- Obtain a specimen for culture and sensitivity tests before giving the first dose. Therapy may begin pending results.
- Monitor the patient for adverse effects, such as nausea, diarrhea, hematologic disorders, Stevens-Johnson syndrome, rash, photosensitivity, and hypersensitivity reactions.
- With large doses or prolonged treatment, monitor the patient for superinfections.

- Rocky Mountain spotted fever
- Q fever
- Lyme disease
- nongonococcal urethritis caused by *Chlamydia* and *Ureaplasma urealyticum*.

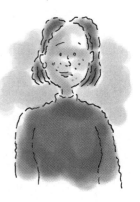

Low dosages of tetracyclines are used to treat acne.

Two-timing

Combination therapy with a tetracycline and streptomycin is the most effective treatment for brucellosis.

Faces are gonna clear up

Tetracyclines in low dosages effectively treat acne because they decrease the fatty acid content of sebum.

Drug interactions

Tetracyclines can reduce the effectiveness of hormonal contraceptives, which may result in breakthrough bleeding or ineffective contraception. Patients taking hormonal contraceptives should use a reliable, secondary method of contraception. Tetracyclines may also decrease the bactericidal action of penicillin.

Creating new pharmacodynamics

Other interactions commonly affect the ability of tetracyclines to move through the body:
- Aluminum, calcium, and magnesium antacids reduce the absorption of oral tetracyclines.
- Iron salts, bismuth subsalicylate, and zinc sulfate reduce the absorption of doxycycline and tetracycline. Reduced absorption can be prevented by separating doses of tetracyclines and these agents by 2 to 3 hours.
- Barbiturates, carbamazepine, and phenytoin increase the metabolism and reduce the antibiotic effect of doxycycline.

Be wary of dairy

Tetracyclines, with the exception of doxycycline and minocycline, may also interact with milk and milk products, which bind with the drugs and prevent their absorption. To prevent decreased absorption, administer the tetracycline 1 hour before or 2 hours after meals.

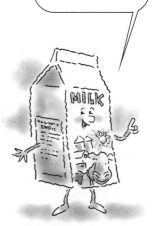

Tetracyclines can also interact with milk!

Adverse reactions

Tetracyclines produce many of the same adverse reactions as other antibacterials, including:
- superinfection
- nausea

- vomiting
- abdominal distress and distention
- diarrhea.
  Other adverse reactions include:
- photosensitivity reactions (red rash on areas exposed to sunlight)
- hepatic toxicity
- renal toxicity.

Nursing process

These nursing process steps are appropriate for patients undergoing treatment with tetracyclines.

Assessment
- Assess the patient's allergy history.
- Assess the patient for adverse reactions.
- Obtain a specimen for culture and sensitivity tests before giving the first dose; therapy may begin pending test results. Check cultures periodically to assess the drug's effectiveness.

Key nursing diagnoses
- Risk for infection related to altered immune status
- Risk for deficient fluid volume related to adverse GI reactions
- Deficient knowledge related to drug therapy

Planning outcome goals
- The patient's infection will resolve as evidenced by culture reports, temperature, and WBC counts.
- The patient's fluid volume will remain within normal limits as evidenced by intake and output.
- The patient and his family will demonstrate an understanding of drug therapy.

Implementation
- Give all oral tetracyclines (except doxycycline and minocycline) 1 hour before or 2 hours after meals for maximum absorption; don't give tetracyclines with food, milk or other dairy products, sodium bicarbonate, iron compounds, or antacids, which may impair absorption.

Water, water, everywhere...
- Give water with and after the patient takes the oral drug to promote passage to the stomach. Incomplete swallowing can cause severe esophageal irritation.

• Don't give the drug within 1 hour of bedtime to prevent esophageal reflux.
• Follow the manufacturer's directions for reconstituting and storing the drug; keep the drug refrigerated and away from light.
• Check the drug's expiration date before administration. Outdated tetracyclines may cause nephrotoxicity.
• Monitor the patient for bacterial and fungal superinfection, especially he's elderly, debilitated, or receiving immunosuppressants or radiation therapy. Watch especially for oral candidiasis.
• Monitor I.V. injection sites and rotate them routinely to minimize local irritation. I.V. administration may cause severe phlebitis.

Evaluation

• Patient is free from infection.
• Patient maintains adequate hydration.
• Patient and family demonstrate an understanding of drug therapy. (See *Teaching about tetracyclines*.)

Clindamycin

Clindamycin is a derivative of another drug, lincomycin. Because of its high potential for causing serious adverse effects, clindamycin is prescribed only when there's no therapeutic alternative. It's used for various gram-positive and anaerobic organisms.

Pharmacokinetics

When taken orally, clindamycin is absorbed well and distributed widely in the body. It's metabolized by the liver and excreted by the kidneys and biliary pathways.

Pharmacodynamics

Clindamycin inhibits bacterial protein synthesis and may also inhibit the binding of bacterial ribosomes. At therapeutic concentrations, clindamycin is primarily bacteriostatic against most organisms.

Pharmacotherapeutics

Because of its potential for causing serious toxicity and pseudomembranous colitis (characterized by severe diarrhea, abdominal pain, fever, and mucus and blood in feces), clindamycin is limited to a few clinical situations in which safer alternative antibacterials aren't available:

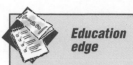

Education edge

Teaching about tetracyclines

If tetracyclines are prescribed, review these points with the patient and his caregivers:
• Take the drug exactly as prescribed for as long as prescribed.
• Keep all follow-up appointments.
• Don't take the drug with food, milk or other dairy products, sodium bicarbonate, or iron compounds because they may interfere with absorption.
• Wait 3 hours after taking a tetracycline before taking an antacid.
• Check the drug's expiration date before using and discard expired drug.
• Report adverse reactions promptly.
• Avoid direct exposure to sunlight and use a sunscreen to help prevent photosensitivity reactions.

• It's potent against most aerobic gram-positive organisms, including staphylococci, streptococci (except *Enterococcus faecalis*), and pneumococci.

• It's effective against most of the clinically important anaerobes and is used primarily to treat anaerobic intra-abdominal, pleural, or pulmonary infections caused by *Bacteroides fragilis*. It's also used as an alternative to penicillin in treating *Clostridium perfringens* infections.

• It may be used as an alternative to penicillin in treating staphylococcal infections in patients who are allergic to penicillin.

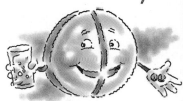

Because of its high potential for causing serious adverse effects, clindamycin is a last resort, of sorts.

Drug interactions

Clindamycin has neuromuscular blocking properties and may enhance the blocking action of neuromuscular blockers. This can lead to profound respiratory depression.

Adverse reactions

Pseudomembranous colitis may occur with clindamycin use. This syndrome can be fatal and requires prompt discontinuation of the drug as well as aggressive fluid and electrolyte management. Although this is the most serious reaction to clindamycin and limits its use, other reactions may also occur, such as:

• diarrhea
• stomatitis (mouth inflammation)
• nausea
• vomiting
• hypersensitivity reactions.

Nursing process

These nursing process steps are appropriate for patients undergoing treatment with clindamycin.

Assessment

• Assess the patient's infection before therapy and regularly throughout therapy.
• Obtain a specimen for culture and sensitivity tests before giving the first dose. Therapy may begin pending results.
• Monitor renal, hepatic, and hematopoietic functions during prolonged therapy.
• Assess for adverse reactions and drug interactions.
• Monitor the patient's hydration status if adverse GI reactions occur.
• Assess the patient's and family's knowledge about drug therapy.

Key nursing diagnoses
• Risk for infection related to altered immune status
• Risk for deficient fluid volume related to adverse GI reactions
• Deficient knowledge related to drug therapy

Planning outcome goals
• The patient's infection will resolve as evidenced by culture reports, temperature, and WBC counts.
• The patient's fluid volume will remain within normal limits as evidenced by intake and output.
• The patient and his family will demonstrate an understanding of drug therapy.

Implementation
• Don't refrigerate a reconstituted oral solution because it will thicken. The drug is stable for 2 weeks at room temperature.
• Give the capsule form with a full glass of water to prevent dysphagia.
• Check the I.V. site daily for phlebitis and irritation. Follow the drug's dilution protocol and administer as directed.
• Inject the drug deeply I.M. and rotate sites. Warn the patient that I.M. injections may be painful. Doses over 600 mg per injection aren't recommended.
• Be aware that I.M. injections may raise creatine kinase levels in response to muscle irritation.
• Don't give opioid antidiarrheals to treat drug-induced diarrhea; they may prolong and worsen diarrhea.

Evaluation
• Patient is free from infection.
• Patient maintains adequate hydration.
• Patient and family demonstrate an understanding of drug therapy.

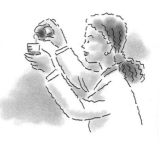

Don't refrigerate reconstituted oral clindamycin because it will thicken.

Macrolides

Macrolides are used to treat many common infections. They include erythromycin and its derivatives, such as:
• erythromycin estolate
• erythromycin ethylsuccinate
• erythromycin lactobionate
• erythromycin stearate.
    Other macrolides include:
• azithromycin
• clarithromycin.

Pharmacokinetics

Because erythromycin is acid-sensitive, it must be buffered or have an enteric coating to prevent destruction by gastric acid. Erythromycin is absorbed in the duodenum. It's distributed to most tissues and body fluids except, in most cases, cerebrospinal fluid (CSF). However, as a class, macrolides can enter the CSF when meninges are inflamed.

Following many paths

Erythromycin is metabolized by the liver and excreted in bile in high concentrations; small amounts are excreted in urine. It also crosses the placental barrier and is secreted in breast milk.

Something in common

Azithromycin is rapidly absorbed by the GI tract and is distributed throughout body. It readily penetrates cells but doesn't readily enter the CNS. Like erythromycin, azithromycin is excreted mostly in bile; small amounts are excreted in urine.

Wide ranging

Clarithromycin is rapidly absorbed and widely distributed and is excreted in urine.

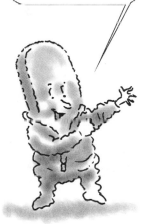

Being the acid-sensitive erythromycin I am, I must be buffered or have an enteric coating to prevent being destroyed by gastric acid.

Pharmacodynamics

Macrolides inhibit ribonucleic acid (RNA)–dependent protein synthesis by acting on a small portion of the ribosome, much like clindamycin.

Pharmacotherapeutics

Erythromycin has a range of therapeutic uses.
• It provides a broad spectrum of antimicrobial activity against gram-positive and gram-negative bacteria, including *Mycobacterium*, *Treponema*, *Mycoplasma*, and *Chlamydia*.
• It's effective against pneumococci and group A streptococci.
• *Staphylococcus aureus* is sensitive to erythromycin; however, resistant strains may appear during therapy.
• It's the drug of choice for treating *Mycoplasma pneumoniae* infections as well as pneumonia caused by *Legionella pneumophila*.

More tolerable

In patients who are allergic to penicillin, erythromycin is effective for infections produced by group A beta-hemolytic streptococci or *Streptococcus pneumoniae*. It may also be used to treat gonorrhea and syphilis in patients who can't tolerate penicillin G or the tetracyclines. Erythromycin may also be used to treat minor staphylococcal infections of the skin.

Applaud for the broads (spectrums, that is)

Each of these broad-spectrum antibacterial drugs (drugs that cover a wide range of organisms) has its own therapeutic actions:
• Azithromycin provides a broad spectrum of antimicrobial activity against gram-positive and gram-negative bacteria, including *Mycobacterium*, *S. aureus*, *Haemophilus influenzae*, *Moraxella catarrhalis*, and *Chlamydia*.
• Azithromycin is also effective against pneumococci and groups C, F, and G streptococci.
• Clarithromycin is active against gram-positive aerobes, such as *Staphylococcus aureus*, *Streptococcus pneumoniae*, and *Streptococcus pyogenes*; gram-negative aerobes, such as *H. influenzae* and *Moraxella catarrhalis*; and other aerobes such as *Mycoplasma pneumoniae*.
• Clarithromycin has been used in combination with antacids, histamine-2 (H_2) receptor antagonists, and proton pump inhibitors to treat *Helicobacter pylori*–induced duodenal ulcer disease.

Drug interactions

Macrolides may cause these drug interactions:
• Erythromycin, azithromycin, and clarithromycin can increase theophylline levels in patients receiving high dosages of theophylline, increasing the risk of theophylline toxicity.
• Clarithromycin may increase the concentration of carbamazepine when the drugs are used together.

Adverse reactions

Although macrolides have few adverse effects, they may produce:
• epigastric distress
• nausea and vomiting
• diarrhea (especially with large doses)
• rashes
• fever
• eosinophilia (an increase in the number of eosinophils, a type of WBC)
• anaphylaxis.

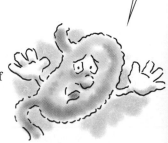

Why me? Epigastric distress is an adverse effect of macrolides.

Nursing process

These nursing process steps are appropriate for patients undergoing treatment with macrolides.

Assessment

• Assess the patient's infection before therapy and regularly throughout therapy.
• Obtain a specimen for culture and sensitivity tests before giving the first dose. Therapy may begin pending results.
• Assess for adverse reactions and drug interactions.
• Assess the patient's and family's knowledge about drug therapy.

Key nursing diagnoses

• Risk for infection related to altered immune status
• Risk for deficient fluid volume related to adverse GI reactions
• Deficient knowledge related to drug therapy

Planning outcome goals

• The patient's infection will resolve as evidenced by culture reports, temperature, and WBC counts.
• The patient's fluid volume will remain within normal limits as evidenced by intake and output.
• The patient and his family will demonstrate an understanding of drug therapy.

Implementation

• When giving the suspension, note the concentration.
• For best absorption, give the oral form with a full glass of water 1 hour before or 2 hours after meals.
• Coated tablets may be taken with meals.
• Tell the patient not to drink fruit juice with the drug.
• Chewable erythromycin tablets shouldn't be swallowed whole.
• Coated tablets or encapsulated pellets cause less GI upset; they may be more tolerable in patients who have trouble tolerating erythromycin.
• Reconstitute the drug according to the manufacturer's directions, and dilute each 250 mg in at least 100 ml of normal saline solution. Infuse over 1 hour.
• Don't give erythromycin lactobionate with other drugs.
• Monitor hepatic function (increased levels of alkaline phosphatase, alanine aminotransferase, aspartate aminotransferase, and bilirubin may occur). Be aware that erythromycin estolate may cause serious hepatotoxicity in adults (reversible cholestatic jaundice). Other erythromycin derivatives cause hepatotoxicity to a lesser degree. Patients who develop hepatotoxicity from erythromycin estolate may react similarly to treatment with other erythromycin preparations.
• Monitor the patient's hydration status if adverse GI reactions occur.

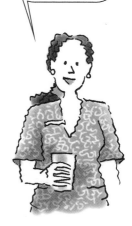

Withhold the fruit juice when giving a patient macrolides.

Evaluation
- Patient is free from infection.
- Patient maintains adequate hydration.
- Patient and family demonstrate an understanding of drug therapy.

Vancomycin

Vancomycin hydrochloride is used increasingly to treat methicillin-resistant *S. aureus*, which has become a major concern in the United States and other parts of the world. Because of the emergence of vancomycin-resistant enterococci, vancomycin must be used judiciously. As a rule of thumb, it should be used only when culture and sensitivity test results confirm the need for it.

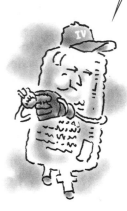

Let me pitch out this bit of news: Vancomycin must be given I.V. to treat systemic infections because it's absorbed poorly from the GI tract.

Pharmacokinetics

Because vancomycin is absorbed poorly from the GI tract, it must be given I.V. to treat systemic infections. An oral form of vancomycin is used to treat pseudomembranous colitis. Remember, however, that I.V. vancomycin can't be used in place of oral vancomycin and vice versa. The two forms aren't interchangeable.

Flowing with fluids

Vancomycin diffuses well into pleural (around the lungs), pericardial (around the heart), synovial (joint), and ascitic (in the peritoneal cavity) fluids.

And then what happens?

The metabolism of vancomycin is unknown. Approximately 85% of the dose is excreted unchanged in urine within 24 hours. A small amount may be eliminated through the liver and biliary tract.

Pharmacodynamics

Vancomycin inhibits bacterial cell-wall synthesis, damaging the bacterial plasma membrane. When the bacterial cell wall is damaged, the body's natural defenses can attack the organism.

Pharmacotherapeutics

Vancomycin has several therapeutic uses:
- It's active against gram-positive organisms, such as *Staphylococcus aureus*, *Staphylococcus epidermidis*, *Streptococcus pyogenes*, *Enterococcus*, and *Streptococcus pneumoniae*.

Staving off staph

• The I.V. form is the therapy of choice for patients with serious resistant staphylococcal infections who are hypersensitive to penicillins.

Coping with colitis

• The oral form is used for patients with antibiotic-associated *C. difficile* colitis who can't take or have responded poorly to metronidazole.

Alternative for allergies

• When used with an aminoglycoside, vancomycin is also the treatment of choice for *E. faecalis* endocarditis in patients who are allergic to penicillin.

Drug interactions

Vancomycin may increase the risk of toxicity when administered with other drugs toxic to the kidneys and organs of hearing, such as aminoglycosides, amphotericin B, cisplatin, bacitracin, colistin, and polymyxin B.

Adverse reactions

Adverse reactions to vancomycin, although rare, include:
• hypersensitivity and anaphylactic reactions
• drug fever
• eosinophilia
• neutropenia (reduced number of neutrophils, a type of WBC)
• hearing loss (transient or permanent), especially in excessive doses, such as when it's given with other ototoxic drugs.

Slow it down!

Severe hypotension may occur with rapid I.V. administration of vancomycin and may be accompanied by a red rash with flat and raised lesions on the face, neck, chest, and arms (red man's syndrome). Doses of less than or equal to 1 g should be given over 1 hour and doses greater than 1 g over 1½ to 2 hours.

Nursing process

These nursing process steps are appropriate for patients undergoing treatment with vancomycin.

Assessment

• Assess the patient's infection before therapy and regularly throughout therapy.

• Obtain a specimen for culture and sensitivity tests before giving the first dose. Therapy may begin pending results.
• Obtain hearing evaluation and kidney function studies before therapy and repeat during therapy.
• Monitor serum levels regularly, especially in elderly patients, premature neonates, and those with decreased renal function.
• Assess for adverse reactions and drug interactions.
• Assess the patient's and family's knowledge of drug therapy.

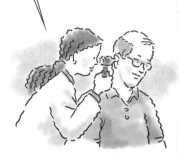

You'll need to obtain a hearing evaluation before and during vancomycin therapy.

Key nursing diagnoses

• Risk for infection related to altered immune status
• Risk for deficient fluid volume related to adverse GI reactions
• Deficient knowledge related to drug therapy

Planning outcome goals

• The patient's infection will resolve as evidenced by culture reports, temperature, and WBC counts.
• The patient's fluid volume will remain within normal limits as evidenced by intake and output.
• The patient and his family will demonstrate an understanding of drug therapy.

Implementation

• Adjust the dosage for a patient with renal dysfunction.
• Know that the oral form of the drug is stable for 2 weeks if refrigerated.
• For I.V. infusion, dilute in 200 ml of D_5W and infuse over 60 minutes.
• Check the I.V. site daily for phlebitis and irritation. Report the presence of pain at the infusion site. Watch for irritation and infiltration; extravasation can cause tissue damage and necrosis.
• Don't give the drug I.M.
• If red-neck or red man's syndrome occurs because the drug is infused too rapidly, stop the infusion and report this finding to the prescriber.
• Refrigerate an I.V. solution after reconstitution and use it within 96 hours.
• When using vancomycin to treat staphylococcal endocarditis, give it for at least 4 weeks.

Evaluation

• Patient is free from infection.
• Patient maintains adequate hydration.
• Patient and family demonstrate an understanding of drug therapy.

Carbapenems

Carbapenems are a class of beta-lactam antibacterials that includes:
- imipenem-cilastatin sodium (a combination drug)
- meropenem
- ertapenem.

Super-sized spectrum of activity

The antibacterial spectrum of activity for imipenem-cilastatin is broader than that of other antibacterial drugs studied to date. Because of this broad spectrum of activity, it's used for serious or life-threatening infection, especially gram-positive and gram-negative nosocomial infections.

Pharmacokinetics

The pharmacokinetic properties of carbapenems vary slightly.

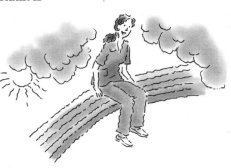

Because of its broad spectrum of activity, imipenem-cilastatin is used for serious or life-threatening infection.

Enabling imipenem's effects

Imipenem is given with cilastatin because imipenem alone is rapidly metabolized in the tubules of the kidneys, rendering it ineffective. After parenteral administration, imipenem-cilastatin is distributed widely. It's metabolized by several mechanisms and excreted primarily in urine.

Follow the ertapenem road

Ertapenem is completely absorbed after I.V. administration and is more highly protein-bound than the other two carbapenems. It's metabolized by hydrolysis and excreted mainly in urine.

Sights on the CNS and elsewhere

After parenteral administration, meropenem is distributed widely, including to the CNS. Metabolism is insignificant; 70% of the drug is excreted unchanged in urine.

Pharmacodynamics

Imipenem-cilastatin, ertapenem, and meropenem are usually bactericidal. They exert antibacterial activity by inhibiting bacterial cell-wall synthesis.

Pharmacotherapeutics

Imipenem-cilastatin has the broadest spectrum of activity of currently available beta-lactam antibacterial drugs:
• It's effective against aerobic gram-positive species, such as *Streptococcus*, *Staphylococcus aureus*, and *Staphylococcus epidermidis*.
• It inhibits most *Enterobacter* species.
• It inhibits *P. aeruginosa* (including strains resistant to piperacillin and ceftazidime) and most anaerobic species, including *B. fragilis*.
• It may be used to treat serious nosocomial infections and infections in immunocompromised patients caused by mixed aerobic and anaerobic organisms.

Meropenem marvels

Meropenem is indicated for treatment of intra-abdominal infections as well as for management of bacterial meningitis caused by susceptible organisms.

Enter ertapenem

Ertapenem's spectrum of activity includes intra-abdominal, skin, urinary tract, and gynecologic infections as well as community-acquired pneumonias caused by various gram-positive, gram-negative, and anaerobic organisms.

Drug interactions

These drug interactions may occur with carbapenems:
• Taking probenecid with imipenem-cilastatin increases the serum concentration of cilastatin and slightly increases the serum concentration of imipenem.
• Probenecid may cause meropenem and ertapenem to accumulate to toxic levels.
• The combination of imipenem-cilastatin and an aminoglycoside acts synergistically against *E. faecalis*.

Adverse reactions

Common adverse reactions to imipenem-cilastatin, ertapenem, and meropenem include:
• nausea and vomiting
• diarrhea
• hypersensitivity reactions such as rashes (particularly in patients with known hypersensitivity to penicillins).

Ertapenem extras

Ertapenem may also cause:
- seizures
- hypotension
- hyperkalemia
- respiratory distress
- death.

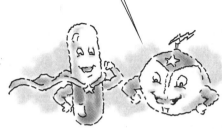

What a pair! Imipenem-cilastatin is used with an aminoglycoside to fight *E. faecalis.*

Nursing process

These nursing process steps are appropriate for patients undergoing treatment with carbapenems.

Assessment
- Assess the patient's infection before therapy and regularly throughout therapy.
- Obtain a specimen for culture and sensitivity tests before giving the first dose. Therapy may begin pending results.
- Assess for adverse reactions and drug interactions.
- Assess the patient's and family's knowledge of drug therapy.

Key nursing diagnoses
- Risk for infection related to altered immune status
- Risk for deficient fluid volume related to adverse GI reactions
- Deficient knowledge related to drug therapy

Planning outcome goals
- The patient's infection will resolve as evidenced by culture reports, temperature, and WBC counts.
- The patient's fluid volume will remain within normal limits as evidenced by intake and output.
- The patient and his family will demonstrate an understanding of drug therapy.

Implementation
- Don't give the drug by direct I.V. bolus injection; reconstitute it as directed. Infuse over 40 to 60 minutes. If nausea occurs, slow the infusion.
- When reconstituting the powder form, shake it until the solution is clear. Solutions may range from colorless to yellow; variations of color within this range don't affect the drug's potency. After reconstitution, the solution is stable for 10 hours at room temperature and for 48 hours when refrigerated.
- Reconstitute the drug for an I.M. injection with 1% lidocaine hydrochloride (without epinephrine) as directed.

• If seizures develop and persist despite using anticonvulsants, notify the prescriber, who may discontinue the drug and institute seizure precautions and protocols.
• Monitor the patient's hydration status if adverse GI reactions occur.
• In a patient with decreased or impaired renal function, the dosage of carbapenems may need to be adjusted.

Evaluation

• Patient is free from infection.
• Patient maintains adequate hydration.
• Patient and family demonstrate an understanding of drug therapy.

Monobactams

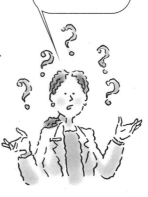

What do you do when a patient is allergic to penicillin?

Monobactams are used when a patient is allergic to penicillin. They bind and inhibit enzymes like other antibacterial drugs, but their composition is slightly different. Aztreonam is the first member in this class of antibacterial drugs and the only one currently available. It's a synthetic monobactam with a narrow spectrum of activity that includes many gram-negative aerobic bacteria.

Pharmacokinetics

After parenteral administration, aztreonam is rapidly and completely absorbed and widely distributed. It's metabolized partially and excreted primarily in urine as unchanged drug.

Pharmacodynamics

Aztreonam's bactericidal activity results from inhibition of bacterial cell-wall synthesis. It binds to the PBP-3 of susceptible gram-negative bacteria, inhibiting cell-wall division and resulting in lysis.

Use a monobactam instead!

Pharmacotherapeutics

Aztreonam is indicated in a range of therapeutic situations:
• It's effective against a variety of gram-negative aerobic organisms, including *P. aeruginosa*.
• It's effective against most strains of *E. coli, Enterobacter, Klebsiella pneumoniae, K. oxytoca, Proteus mirabilis, Serratia marcescens, H. influenzae,* and *Citrobacter*.
• It's used to treat complicated and uncomplicated UTIs, septicemia, and lower respiratory tract, skin and skin-structure, intra-

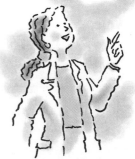

abdominal, and gynecologic infections caused by susceptible gram-negative aerobic bacteria.

• It's usually active against gram-negative aerobic organisms that are resistant to antibiotics hydrolyzed by beta-lactamases. (Beta-lactamase is an enzyme that makes an antibacterial drug ineffective.)

When experience doesn't count

Aztreonam shouldn't be used alone as empiric therapy (treatment based on clinical experience rather than on medical data) in seriously ill patients who may have a gram-positive bacterial infection or a mixed aerobic-anaerobic bacterial infection.

Drug interactions

Aztreonam may interact with several other drugs:

• Probenecid increases serum levels of aztreonam by prolonging the tubular secretion rate of aztreonam in the kidneys.

• Synergistic or additive effects occur when aztreonam is used with aminoglycosides or other antibiotics, such as cefoperazone, cefotaxime, clindamycin, and piperacillin.

• Potent inducers of beta-lactamase production (such as cefoxitin and imipenem) may inactivate aztreonam. Concomitant use isn't recommended.

• Taking aztreonam with clavulanic acid–containing antibiotics may produce synergistic or antagonistic effects, depending on the organism involved.

Adverse reactions

Adverse reactions to aztreonam include:

• diarrhea
• hypersensitivity and skin reactions
• hypotension
• nausea and vomiting
• transient electrocardiogram (ECG) changes (including ventricular arrhythmias)
• transient increases in serum liver enzymes.

Nursing process

These nursing process steps are appropriate for patients undergoing treatment with monobactams.

Assessment

• Assess the patient's infection before therapy and regularly throughout therapy.

- Obtain a specimen for culture and sensitivity tests before giving the first dose. Therapy may begin pending results.
- Assess for adverse reactions and drug interactions.
- Assess the patient's and family's knowledge of drug therapy.

Key nursing diagnoses
- Risk for infection related to altered immune status
- Risk for deficient fluid volume related to adverse GI reactions
- Deficient knowledge related to drug therapy

Planning outcome goals
- The patient's infection will resolve as evidenced by culture reports, temperature, and WBC counts.
- The patient's fluid volume will remain within normal limits as evidenced by intake and output.
- The patient and his family will demonstrate an understanding of drug therapy.

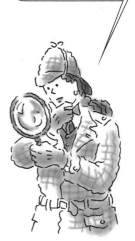

Evidence of infection can be found in the patient's culture reports, temperature, and WBC counts.

Implementation
- Although patients who are allergic to penicillins or cephalosporins may not be allergic to aztreonam, closely monitor patients who have had an immediate hypersensitivity reaction to these antibacterial drugs.
- To give an I.V. bolus dose, inject the drug slowly over 3 to 5 minutes directly into a vein or I.V. tubing.
- Give infusions over 20 minutes to 1 hour.
- Give I.M. injections deep into a large muscle mass, such as the upper, outer quadrant of the gluteus maximus or the lateral aspect of the thigh.
- Give doses larger than 1 g by the I.V. route.
- Warn the patient receiving the drug I.M. that pain and swelling may develop at the injection site.

Evaluation
- Patient is free from infection.
- Patient maintains adequate hydration.
- Patient and family demonstrate an understanding of drug therapy.

Fluoroquinolones

Fluoroquinolones are structurally similar synthetic antibacterial drugs. They're primarily administered to treat UTIs, upper respiratory tract infections, pneumonia, and gonorrhea. Examples of fluoroquinolones include:
- ciprofloxacin

- levofloxacin
- moxifloxacin hydrochloride
- norfloxacin
- ofloxacin.

Pharmacokinetics

After oral administration, fluoroquinolones are absorbed well. They aren't highly protein-bound, are minimally metabolized in the liver, and are excreted primarily in urine.

Pharmacodynamics

Fluoroquinolones interrupt deoxyribonucleic acid (DNA) synthesis during bacterial replication by inhibiting DNA gyrase, an essential enzyme of replicating DNA. As a result, the bacteria can't reproduce.

Pharmacotherapeutics

Fluoroquinolones can be used to treat a wide variety of UTIs. Each drug in this class also has specific indications:
• Ciprofloxacin is used to treat lower respiratory tract infections, infectious diarrhea, and skin, bone, and joint infections.
• Levofloxacin is indicated for treatment of lower respiratory tract infections, skin infections, and UTIs.
• Moxifloxacin is used to treat acute bacterial sinusitis and mild to moderate community-acquired pneumonia.
• Norfloxacin is used to treat UTIs and prostatitis.
• Ofloxacin is used to treat selected sexually transmitted diseases, lower respiratory tract infections, skin and skin-structure infections, and prostatitis (inflammation of the prostate gland).

Drug interactions

Several drug interactions may occur with the fluoroquinolones:
• Administration with antacids that contain magnesium or aluminum hydroxide results in decreased absorption of the fluoroquinolone.
• Some fluoroquinolones, such as ciprofloxacin, norfloxacin, and ofloxacin, interact with xanthine derivatives, such as aminophylline and theophylline, increasing the plasma theophylline concentration and the risk of theophylline toxicity.
• Giving ciprofloxacin or norfloxacin with probenecid results in decreased kidney elimination of these fluoroquinolones, increasing their serum concentrations and half-lives.

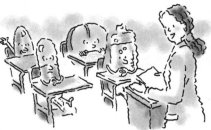

Fluoroquinolones are at the head of the class when it comes to treating UTIs!

• Drugs that prolong the QT interval, such as antiarrhythmics, should be used cautiously during moxifloxacin therapy.

Adverse reactions

Fluoroquinolones are well tolerated by most patients, but some adverse effects may occur, including:
• dizziness
• nausea and vomiting
• diarrhea
• abdominal pain.

Blister in the sun

Moderate to severe phototoxic reactions have occurred with direct and indirect sunlight and with artificial ultraviolet lights, both with and without sunscreen. These types of light should be avoided while the patient is on fluoroquinolone therapy and for several days after cessation of therapy.

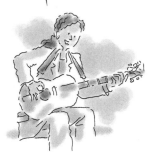

I haven't got time for the pain...abdominal pain, that is—an adverse effect of fluoroquinolones.

Nursing process

These nursing process steps are appropriate for patients undergoing treatment with fluoroquinolones.

Assessment

• Assess the patient's infection before therapy and regularly throughout therapy.
• Obtain a specimen for culture and sensitivity tests before giving the first dose. Therapy may begin pending results.
• Assess for adverse reactions and drug interactions.
• Assess the patient's and family's knowledge of drug therapy.

Education edge

Teaching about fluoroquinolones

If fluoroquinolones are prescribed, review these points with the patient and his caregivers:
• Take the oral form 2 hours before or after meals.
• Take prescribed antacids at least 2 hours after taking the drug.

• Drink plenty of fluids to reduce the risk of crystalluria.
• Avoid hazardous tasks that require alertness, such as driving, until the drug's central nervous system effects are known.
• Hypersensitivity reactions may occur even after the first dose. If a rash or oth-

er allergic reactions develop, stop the drug immediately and notify the prescriber.
• Stop breast-feeding during treatment or consult with the prescriber about taking a different drug.

Key nursing diagnoses
- Risk for infection related to altered immune status
- Risk for deficient fluid volume related to adverse GI reactions
- Deficient knowledge related to drug therapy

Planning outcome goals
- The patient's infection will resolve as evidenced by culture reports, temperature, and WBC counts.
- The patient's fluid volume will remain within normal limits as evidenced by intake and output.
- The patient and his family will demonstrate an understanding of drug therapy.

Implementation
- Oral forms may be given 2 hours after meals, 2 hours before meals, or 6 hours after taking antacids, sucralfate, or products that contain iron (such as vitamins with mineral supplements).
- Dilute the drug for I.V. use as directed and monitor for adverse effects. Infuse slowly over 1 hour into a large vein.
- Adjust the dosage as necessary in a patient with impaired renal function.
- Monitor the patient's hydration status if adverse GI reactions occur.

Evaluation
- Patient is free from infection.
- Patient maintains adequate hydration.
- Patient and family demonstrate an understanding of drug therapy. (See *Teaching about fluoroquinolones.*)

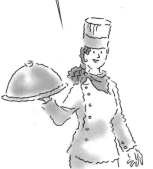

Oral forms of fluoroquinolones may be given 2 hours before or after—not with—meals.

Sulfonamides

Sulfonamides were the first effective systemic antibacterial drugs. They include:
- co-trimoxazole (sulfamethoxazole and trimethoprim)
- sulfadiazine
- sulfasalazine
- sulfisoxazole.

Pharmacokinetics
Most sulfonamides are well absorbed and widely distributed in the body. They're metabolized in the liver to inactive metabolites and excreted by the kidneys.

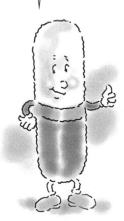

Sulfonamides were the first effective systemic antibacterial drugs.

A fluid situation

Because crystalluria and subsequent stone formation may occur during the metabolic excretory phase, adequate fluid intake is highly recommended during oral sulfonamide therapy.

Pharmacodynamics

Sulfonamides are bacteriostatic drugs that prevent the growth of microorganisms by inhibiting folic acid production. The decreased folic acid synthesis decreases the number of bacterial nucleotides and inhibits bacterial growth.

Pharmacotherapeutics

Sulfonamides are commonly used to treat acute UTIs. With recurrent or chronic UTIs, the infecting organism may not be susceptible to sulfonamides. Therefore, the choice of therapy should be based on bacteria susceptibility tests.

Other targets

Sulfonamides also are used to treat infections caused by *Nocardia asteroides* and *Toxoplasma gondii*. In addition, sulfonamides exhibit a wide spectrum of activity against gram-positive and gram-negative bacteria.

Winning combination

Co-trimoxazole (a combination of a sulfa drug and a folate antagonist) is used for various other infections, such as *Pneumocystis carinii* pneumonia, acute otitis media (due to *H. influenzae* and *S. pneumoniae*), and acute exacerbations of chronic bronchitis (due to *H. influenzae* and *S. pneumoniae*). (See *Sulfonamides: Co-trimoxazole.*)

Drug interactions

Sulfonamides have few significant interactions:
• They increase the hypoglycemic effects of the sulfonylureas (oral antidiabetic drugs), which may decrease blood glucose levels.
• When taken with methenamine, they may lead to the development of crystals in the urine.
• Co-trimoxazole may increase the anticoagulant effect of coumarin anticoagulants.
• Co-trimoxazole plus cyclosporine increases the risk of kidney toxicity.

Prototype pro

Sulfonamides: Co-trimoxazole

Actions
• Is bacteriostatic (mechanism of action correlates directly with the structural similarities it shares with para-aminobenzoic acid)
• Inhibits biosynthesis of folic acid, thus inhibiting susceptible bacteria that synthesize folic acid

Indications
• Infection of the urinary tract, respiratory tract, and ear caused by susceptible organisms
• Chronic bacterial prostatitis
• Prevention of recurrent urinary tract infection in women and of "traveler's diarrhea"

Nursing considerations
• Obtain a specimen for culture and sensitivity tests before giving the first dose. Therapy may begin pending results.
• Monitor the patient for adverse effects, such as seizures, nausea, vomiting, diarrhea, hematologic disorders, Stevens-Johnson syndrome, toxic nephrosis, and hypersensitivity reactions.
• Reduced dosages are needed in patients with renal and hepatic impairment.
• With large dosages or prolonged treatment, monitor the patient for superinfections.

Adverse reactions

These adverse reactions may occur with sulfonamides:
• Excessively high doses of less water-soluble sulfonamides can produce crystals in the urine and deposits of sulfonamide crystals in the renal tubules; however, this complication isn't a problem with the newer water-soluble sulfonamides.
• Hypersensitivity reactions may occur and appear to increase as the dosage increases.
• A reaction that resembles serum sickness may occur, producing fever, joint pain, hives, bronchospasm, and leukopenia (reduced WBC count).
• Photosensitivity may occur.

Nursing process

These nursing process steps are appropriate for patients undergoing treatment with sulfonamides.

Assessment
• Assess the patient's infection before therapy and regularly thereafter.

Patients with diabetes need to watch their glucose levels when taking sulfonamides. Sulfonamides increase the hypoglycemic effects of oral antidiabetic drugs.

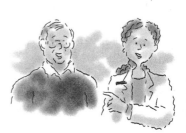

The sulfur situation

• Assess the patient's history of allergies, especially to sulfonamides or to drugs containing sulfur (such as thiazides, furosemide, and oral sulfonylureas).
• Assess the patient for adverse reactions and drug interactions; patients with acquired immunodeficiency syndrome (AIDS) have a much higher risk of adverse reactions.
• Obtain a specimen for culture and sensitivity tests before giving the first dose; treatment may begin pending test results. Check test results periodically to assess the drug's effectiveness.
• Monitor intake and output.
• Monitor urine cultures, complete blood count (CBC), and urinalysis before and during therapy.

Key nursing diagnoses

• Risk for infection related to superinfection
• Risk for deficient fluid volume related to adverse GI reactions
• Deficient knowledge related to drug therapy

Planning outcome goals

• The patient's infection will resolve as evidenced by culture reports, temperature, and WBC counts.
• The patient's fluid volume will remain within normal limits as evidenced by intake and output.
• The patient and his family will demonstrate an understanding of drug therapy.

Implementation

• Give an oral dose with 8 oz (240 ml) of water. Give 3 to 4 L of fluids daily, depending on the drug. Urine output should be at least 1,500 ml daily to ensure proper hydration. Inadequate urine output can lead to crystalluria or tubular deposits of the drug.
• Follow the manufacturers' directions for reconstituting, diluting, and storing drugs; check expiration dates.
• Shake oral suspensions well before administration to ensure the correct dosage.
• During long-term therapy, monitor the patient for possible superinfection.

Evaluation

• Patient is free from infection.
• Patient maintains adequate hydration.
• Patient and family demonstrate an understanding of drug therapy. (See *Teaching about sulfonamides*.)

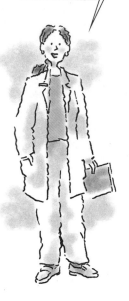

Before giving sulfonamides, confirm that the patient isn't allergic to drugs containing sulfur.

Education edge

Teaching about sulfonamides

If sulfonamides are prescribed, review these points with the patient and his caregivers:
• Take the drug exactly as prescribed, complete the prescribed regimen, and keep follow-up appointments.
• Take the oral form with a full glass of water, and drink plenty of fluids. The tablet may be crushed and swallowed with water to ensure maximal absorption.
• Report signs and symptoms of hypersensitivity and other adverse reactions, such as bloody urine, difficulty breathing, rash, fever, chills, or severe fatigue.

• Avoid direct sun exposure, and use a sunscreen to help prevent photosensitivity reactions.
• Sulfonamides may increase the effects of oral hypoglycemic drugs. Don't use Clinitest to monitor urine glucose levels.
• Sulfasalazine may cause an orange-yellow discoloration of urine or the skin and may permanently stain soft contact lenses yellow.

Nitrofurantoin

Nitrofurantoin is a drug that has higher antibacterial activity in acid urine. It's commonly used to treat acute and chronic UTIs.

Pharmacokinetics

After oral administration, nitrofurantoin is absorbed rapidly and well from the GI tract. Taking the drug with food enhances its bioavailability.

Form facts

Nitrofurantoin is available in a microcrystalline form and a macrocrystalline form. The microcrystalline form is absorbed more slowly because of slower dissolution and thus causes less GI distress.

Oh where oh where does nitrofurantoin go?

Nitrofurantoin is 20% to 60% protein-bound. It crosses the placental barrier and is secreted in breast milk. It's also distributed in bile. Nitrofurantoin is partially metabolized by the liver, and 30% to 50% is excreted unchanged in urine.

Pharmacodynamics

Usually bacteriostatic, nitrofurantoin may become bactericidal, depending on its urinary concentration and the susceptibility of the infecting organisms.

Zapping bacterial energy

Although its exact mechanism of action is unknown, nitrofurantoin appears to inhibit the formation of acetyl coenzyme A from pyruvic acid, thereby inhibiting the energy production of the infecting organism. Nitrofurantoin also may disrupt bacterial cell-wall formation.

Pharmacotherapeutics

Because the absorbed drug concentrates in urine, nitrofurantoin is used to treat UTIs. Nitrofurantoin isn't effective against systemic bacterial infections.

Can't handle the kidneys

Nitrofurantoin isn't useful in treating pyelonephritis or perinephric (around the kidney) diseases.

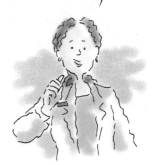

Fortunately, nitrofurantoin has few significant drug interactions.

Drug interactions

Nitrofurantoin has few significant interactions:
• Probenecid and sulfinpyrazone inhibit the excretion of nitrofurantoin by the kidneys, reducing its efficacy and increasing its toxic potential.
• Magnesium salts and antacids containing magnesium can decrease the extent and rate of nitrofurantoin absorption.
• Nitrofurantoin may decrease the antibacterial activity of norfloxacin and nalidixic acid.

Adverse reactions

Adverse reactions to nitrofurantoin include:
• GI irritation
• anorexia
• nausea and vomiting
• diarrhea
• dark yellow or brown urine
• abdominal pain
• chills
• fever
• joint pain
• anaphylaxis
• hypersensitivity reactions involving the skin, lungs, blood, and liver.

Nursing process

These nursing process steps are appropriate for patients undergoing treatment with nitrofurantoin.

Assessment

- Assess the patient's infection before therapy and regularly thereafter.
- Assess the patient's allergy history, especially allergies to sulfonamides or to drugs containing sulfur (such as thiazides, furosemide, and oral sulfonylureas).
- Assess the patient for adverse reactions and drug interactions.
- Obtain a specimen for culture and sensitivity tests before giving the first dose; treatment may begin pending results. Check these test results periodically to assess the drug's effectiveness.
- Assess the patient's and family's knowledge of drug therapy.

Key nursing diagnoses

- Risk for infection related to superinfection
- Risk for deficient fluid volume related to adverse GI reactions
- Deficient knowledge related to drug therapy

Planning outcome goals

- The patient's infection will resolve as evidenced by culture reports, temperature, and WBC counts.
- The patient's fluid volume will remain within normal limits as evidenced by intake and output.
- The patient and his family will demonstrate an understanding of drug therapy.

Implementation

- Give the drug with food or milk to minimize GI distress.
- Monitor the patient for hypersensitivity, which can develop during drug therapy.
- Monitor urine cultures; treatment continues for 3 days after urine specimens become sterile.
- Monitor the patient's hydration status if adverse GI reactions occur.
- Monitor CBC and pulmonary status regularly.
- Monitor intake and output. This drug may turn urine brown or dark yellow.

Evaluation

- Patient is free from infection.
- Patient maintains adequate hydration.
- Patient and family demonstrate an understanding of drug therapy.

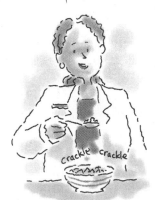

Give nitrofurantoin with food or milk to minimize GI distress.

crackle crackle

Antiviral drugs

Antiviral drugs are used to prevent or treat viral infections ranging from influenza to human immunodeficiency virus (HIV). The major antiviral drug classes used to treat systemic infections include:
- synthetic nucleosides
- pyrophosphate analogues
- influenza A and syncytial virus drugs
- nucleoside analogue reverse transcriptase inhibitors (NRTIs)
- non-nucleoside reverse transcriptase inhibitors (NNRTIs)
- nucleotide analogue reverse transcriptase inhibitors
- protease inhibitors.

Synthetic nucleosides

Synthetic nucleosides are a group of drugs used to treat various viral syndromes that can occur in immunocompromised patients, including herpes simplex virus (HSV) and cytomegalovirus (CMV). Drugs in this class include:
- acyclovir
- famciclovir
- ganciclovir
- valacyclovir hydrochloride
- valganciclovir hydrochloride.

Pharmacokinetics

Each of these synthetic nucleosides travels its own route through the body:
- When given orally, acyclovir absorption is slow and only 15% to 30% complete. It's distributed throughout the body and metabolized primarily inside the infected cells; most of the drug is excreted in urine.
- Famciclovir is less than 20% bound to plasma proteins. It's extensively metabolized in the liver and excreted in urine.
- Ganciclovir is administered I.V. because it's absorbed poorly from the GI tract. More than 90% of ganciclovir isn't metabolized and is excreted unchanged by the kidneys.

A true convert

- Valacyclovir is converted to acyclovir during its metabolism and has pharmacokinetic properties similar to those of acyclovir.
- Valganciclovir is metabolized in the intestinal wall and liver to ganciclovir; however, interchanging the two drugs isn't effective.

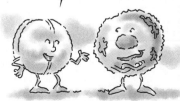

So I'll need to be metabolized inside you to do my job.

As long as it gets rid of the infection!

Pharmacodynamics

The actions of these drugs also varies:
• Acyclovir enters virus-infected cells, where it's changed through a series of steps to acyclovir triphosphate. Acyclovir triphosphate inhibits virus-specific DNA polymerase, an enzyme necessary for viral growth, thus disrupting viral replication.
• On entry into virus-infected cells, ganciclovir is converted to ganciclovir triphosphate, which is thought to produce its antiviral activity by inhibiting viral DNA synthesis.
• Famciclovir enters viral cells (HSV types 1 and 2, varicella zoster), where it inhibits DNA polymerase, viral DNA synthesis and, thus, viral replication.
• Valacyclovir rapidly converts to acyclovir, and acyclovir then becomes incorporated into viral DNA and inhibits viral DNA polymerase, thus inhibiting viral multiplication.
• Valganciclovir is converted to ganciclovir, which inhibits replication of viral DNA synthesis of CMV.

Pharmacotherapeutics

Acyclovir is an effective antiviral drug that causes minimal toxicity to cells. Oral acyclovir is used primarily to treat initial and recurrent HSV type 2 infections. (See *Antivirals: Acyclovir*.)

I.V. instances

I.V. acyclovir is used to treat:
• severe initial HSV type 2 infections in patients with normal immune systems
• initial and recurrent skin and mucous membrane HSV type 1 and 2 infections in immunocompromised patients
• herpes zoster infections (shingles) caused by the varicella-zoster virus in immunocompromised patients
• disseminated varicella-zoster virus in immunocompromised patients
• varicella infections (chickenpox) caused by the varicella-zoster virus in immunocompromised patients.

Rounding out the group

Other synthetic nucleosides have their own therapeutic uses:
• Ganciclovir is used to treat CMV retinitis in immunocompromised patients, including those with AIDS, other CMV infections (such as encephalitis), and HSV.
• Famciclovir is used to treat acute herpes zoster, genital herpes, and recurrent herpes simplex in HIV-infected patients.
• Valacyclovir is effective against herpes zoster, genital herpes, and herpes labialis.
• Valganciclovir is used to treat CMV retinitis in AIDS patients.

Prototype pro

Antivirals: Acyclovir

Actions
• Interferes with deoxyribonucleic acid synthesis and inhibits viral multiplication

Indications
• Herpes simplex virus types 1 and 2
• Varicella

Nursing considerations
• Monitor the patient for adverse effects, such as malaise, headache, encephalopathy, renal failure, thrombocytopenia, and pain at the injection site.

Drug interactions

These drug interactions may occur with synthetic nucleosides:
• Probenecid reduces kidney excretion and increases blood levels of ganciclovir, valganciclovir, valacyclovir, famciclovir, and acyclovir, increasing the risk of toxicity.

Tearing into tissue cells

• Taking ganciclovir with drugs that are damaging to tissue cells, such as dapsone, pentamidine isethionate, flucytosine, vincristine, vinblastine, doxorubicin, amphotericin B, and co-trimoxazole, inhibits replication of rapidly dividing cells in the bone marrow, GI tract, skin, and sperm-producing cells.
• Imipenem-cilastatin increases the risk of seizures when taken with ganciclovir or valganciclovir.
• Zidovudine increases the risk of granulocytopenia (reduced number of granulocytes, a type of WBC) when taken with ganciclovir.

Adverse reactions

Treatment with synthetic nucleosides may cause these adverse reactions:
• Reversible kidney impairment may occur with rapid I.V. injection or infusion of acyclovir.
• Headache, nausea, vomiting, and diarrhea are common reactions to oral acyclovir.
• Hypersensitivity reactions may occur with acyclovir.
• Granulocytopenia and thrombocytopenia are the most common adverse reactions to ganciclovir.
• Famciclovir and valacyclovir may cause headache and nausea.
• Valganciclovir may cause seizures, retinal detachment, neutropenia, and bone marrow suppression.

Nursing process

These nursing process steps are appropriate for patients undergoing treatment with synthetic nucleosides.

Assessment

• Obtain a baseline assessment of the patient's viral infection; reassess regularly to monitor the drug's effectiveness.
• Assess for adverse reactions and drug interactions.
• Assess the patient's and family's knowledge of drug therapy.

Key nursing diagnoses

• Ineffective protection related to adverse hematologic reactions
• Risk for deficient fluid volume related to adverse GI reactions

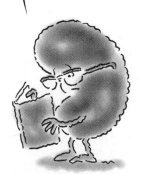

Says here that rapid I.V. infusion or injection of acyclovir can cause kidney impairment. Thank goodness it's reversible!

• Deficient knowledge related to drug therapy

Planning outcome goals
• The patient won't incur injury while receiving drug therapy.
• The patient's fluid volume will remain within normal limits as evidenced by intake and output.
• The patient and his family will demonstrate an understanding of drug therapy.

Implementation
• Monitor renal and hepatic function, CBC, and platelet count regularly.
• Monitor the patient's mental status when giving the drug I.V. Encephalopathic changes are more likely in patients with neurologic disorders or in those who have had neurologic reactions to cytotoxic drugs.
• Monitor the patient's hydration status if adverse GI reactions occur.
• Follow the manufacturers' guidelines for reconstituting and administering these drugs.
• Obtain an order for an antiemetic or antidiarrheal drug if needed.

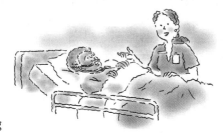

If a patient has adverse CNS reactions to an antiviral drug, take safety precautions such as raising the bed rails.

Safety first

• Take safety precautions if the patient has adverse CNS reactions. For example, place the bed in a low position, raise the bed rails, and supervise ambulation and other activities.
• Notify the prescriber about serious or persistent adverse reactions.
• Instruct the patient on how to prevent spreading the infection.

Evaluation
• Patient doesn't incur injury while receiving drug therapy.
• Patient maintains adequate hydration.
• Patient and family demonstrate an understanding of drug therapy. (See *Teaching about antiviral drug therapy*, page 532.)

Pyrophosphate analogues

Pyrophosphate analogues target pyrophosphate-binding sites of certain viruses. Foscarnet sodium is one such drug that's used to treat CMV retinitis in patients with AIDS. It's also used to treat acyclovir-resistant HSV infections in immunocompromised patients.

Education edge

Teaching about antiviral drug therapy

If antiviral drug therapy is prescribed, review these points with the patient and his caregivers:
• Take the drug exactly as prescribed, even if signs and symptoms improve.
• Notify the prescriber promptly about severe or persistent adverse reactions.
• Keep appointments for follow-up care.
• The drug effectively manages viral infection but may not eliminate it or cure it.
• Report early signs and symptoms of infection, such as fever, pain, and itching.
• Maintain immunizations against viral infections as indicated.
• The drug won't prevent the infection from spreading to others. Use proper techniques to prevent the spread of infection. For example, avoid sexual intercourse when visible lesions are present, always wash hands after touching lesions, practice safer sex by using a condom, and avoid sharing I.V. needles.
• Maintain an adequate diet.
• Be sure to get adequate amounts of rest and exercise.

How retro
If the patient is taking antiretroviral drugs, review these additional points:
• Effective treatment of human immunodeficiency virus (HIV) requires drug therapy with several drugs and daily doses. Missing doses decreases blood levels of the drugs and results in increased HIV replication. This can result in drug-resistant viral strains.
• Don't take other drugs, over-the-counter products, or herbal preparations without first consulting the prescriber. They may make anti-HIV drugs less effective or more toxic.
• Adverse effects may vary depending on the specific drugs used; request information about the adverse effects and what to do if they occur.
• Have regular tests, such as viral load, CD4+ cell count, complete blood count, and renal and hepatic function, as indicated.

Pharmacokinetics

Foscarnet is poorly bound to plasma proteins. In patients with normal kidney function, the majority of foscarnet is excreted unchanged in urine.

Pharmacodynamics

Foscarnet prevents viral replication by selectively inhibiting DNA polymerase.

Pharmacotherapeutics

Foscarnet's primary therapeutic use is treating CMV retinitis in patients with AIDS. It's also used in combination with ganciclovir for patients who have relapsed with either drug.

Drug interactions

Foscarnet has few drug interactions:
• Foscarnet and pentamidine together increase the risk of hypocalcemia and toxicity to the kidneys.

• Using foscarnet along with other drugs that alter serum calcium levels may result in hypocalcemia.
• The risk of kidney impairment increases when drugs toxic to the kidneys, such as amphotericin B and aminoglycosides, are taken with foscarnet. Because of the risk of kidney toxicity, patients should be aggressively hydrated during treatment.

Adverse reactions

Adverse reactions to foscarnet may include:
• fatigue
• depression
• fever
• confusion
• headache
• numbness and tingling
• dizziness
• seizures
• nausea and vomiting
• diarrhea
• abdominal pain
• granulocytopenia
• leukopenia
• involuntary muscle contractions
• neuropathy
• difficulty breathing
• rash
• altered kidney function.

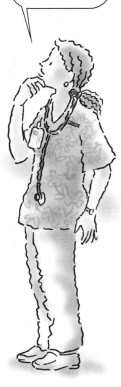

That's quite a list of adverse reactions...

Nursing process

These nursing process steps are appropriate for patients undergoing treatment with pyrophosphate analogs.

Assessment
• Obtain a baseline assessment of the patient's viral infection; reassess regularly to monitor the drug's effectiveness.
• Assess for adverse reactions and drug interactions.
• Assess the patient's and family's knowledge of drug therapy.

Key nursing diagnoses
• Ineffective protection related to adverse hematologic reactions
• Risk for deficient fluid volume related to adverse GI reactions
• Deficient knowledge related to drug therapy

Planning outcome goals
• The patient won't incur injury while receiving drug therapy.

• The patient's fluid volume will remain within normal limits as evidenced by intake and output.
• The patient and his family will demonstrate an understanding of drug therapy.

Implementation
• Give the drug over at least 1 hour using an infusion pump. To minimize renal toxicity, ensure adequate hydration before and during the infusion.
• Monitor renal and hepatic function, CBC, and platelet count regularly.
• Monitor electrolyte levels (calcium, phosphate, magnesium, and potassium).
• Monitor creatinine clearance two to three times weekly during induction and at least once every 1 to 2 weeks during maintenance.

Eying electrolyte levels
• Monitor for tetany and seizures with abnormal electrolyte levels; the drug may cause a dose-related transient decrease in ionized serum calcium, which may not be reflected in laboratory values.
• Monitor the patient's mental status. Encephalopathic changes are more likely in patients with neurologic disorders or in those who have had neurologic reactions to cytotoxic drugs.
• Follow the manufacturer's guidelines for reconstituting and administering the drug.
• Obtain an order for an antiemetic or antidiarrheal drug if needed.
• Take safety precautions if the patient has adverse CNS reactions. For example, place the bed in a low position, raise the bed rails, and supervise ambulation and other activities.
• Notify the prescriber about serious or persistent adverse reactions.

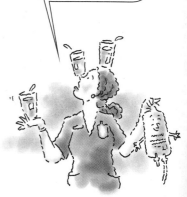

To minimize renal toxicity, ensure adequate hydration before and during foscarnet infusion. It's trickier than it looks!

Evaluation
• Patient doesn't incur injury while receiving therapy.
• Patient maintains adequate hydration.
• Patient and family demonstrate an understanding of drug therapy.

Influenza A and syncytial virus drugs
Influenza A and syncytial virus drugs include:
• amantadine hydrochloride
• rimantadine hydrochloride (an amantadine derivative)
• ribavirin.

Pharmacokinetics

After oral administration, amantadine and rimantadine are well absorbed in the GI tract and widely distributed throughout the body. Amantadine is eliminated primarily in urine; rimantadine is extensively metabolized and then excreted in urine.

Take a deep breath

Ribavirin may be administered by nasal inhalation or by aerosol inhalation with a small-particle aerosol generator. The drug is well absorbed, but it has a limited, specific distribution, with the highest concentrations found in the respiratory tract and in red blood cells (RBCs).

Ribavirin may be administered by nasal or aerosol inhalation.

Swallow this

Ribavirin capsules are rapidly absorbed after administration and are distributed in plasma. Ribavirin is metabolized in the liver and by RBCs, and then excreted primarily by the kidneys, with some excreted in feces.

Pharmacodynamics

Influenza A and syncytial virus drugs act in various ways:
• Although its exact mechanism of action is unknown, amantadine appears to inhibit an early stage of viral replication.
• Rimantadine inhibits viral RNA and protein synthesis.
• The mechanism of action of ribavirin isn't known completely, but the drug's metabolites inhibit viral DNA and RNA synthesis, subsequently halting viral replication.

Pharmacotherapeutics

Amantadine and rimantadine are used to prevent and treat respiratory tract infections caused by strains of the influenza A virus. They can reduce the severity and duration of fever and other symptoms in patients already infected with influenza A.

Offering some protection

Amantadine and rimantadine also protect patients who have received the influenza vaccine during the 2 weeks needed for immunity to develop as well as patients who can't take the influenza vaccine because of hypersensitivity.

Tremor tamer

Amantadine is also used to treat parkinsonism and drug-induced extrapyramidal reactions (abnormal involuntary movements).

Amantadine and rimantadine can reduce the severity of symptoms in patients infected with influenza A. That's nothing to sneeze at!!

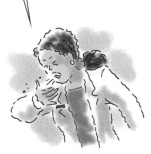

Ribavirin remedy

Ribavirin is used to treat respiratory syncytial virus in children as well as in combination with interferon alfa 2B to treat chronic hepatitis C in adults.

Drug interactions

These drug interactions may occur with amantadine:
• Taking anticholinergics with amantadine increases adverse anticholinergic effects.
• Amantadine given with the combination drug hydrochlorothiazide and triamterene results in decreased urine excretion of amantadine, resulting in increased amantadine levels.
• Amantadine and trimethoprim (co-trimoxazole) levels are increased when used together.

Not a troublemaker

No clinically significant drug interactions have been documented with rimantadine.

Intoxicating

Ribavirin has few interactions with other drugs:
• Ribavirin reduces the antiviral activity of zidovudine; using these drugs together may cause blood toxicity.
• Taking ribavirin and digoxin together can cause digoxin toxicity, producing such effects as GI distress, CNS abnormalities, and cardiac arrhythmias.

Adverse reactions

Rimantadine and amantadine share similar adverse reactions; however, those resulting from rimantadine tend to be less severe. Adverse reactions include:
• anorexia
• anxiety
• confusion
• depression
• fatigue
• forgetfulness
• hallucinations
• hypersensitivity reactions
• insomnia
• irritability
• nausea
• nervousness
• psychosis.

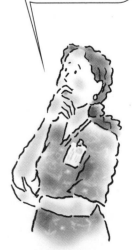

What was it? It was just on the tip of my tongue... something about amantadine and rimantadine causing forgetfulness...

Ribavirin reactions

Adverse reactions to ribavirin include:
- apnea (lack of breathing)
- cardiac arrest
- hypotension
- pneumothorax (air in the pleural space, causing the lung to collapse)
- worsening of respiratory function.

Nursing process

These nursing process steps are appropriate for patients undergoing treatment with influenza A and syncytial virus drugs.

Assessment

- Obtain a baseline assessment of the patient's viral infection; re-assess regularly to monitor the drug's effectiveness.
- Assess for adverse reactions and drug interactions.
- Assess the patient's and family's knowledge of drug therapy.

Key nursing diagnoses

- Ineffective protection related to adverse hematologic reactions
- Risk for deficient fluid volume related to adverse GI reactions
- Deficient knowledge related to drug therapy

Planning outcome goals

- The patient won't incur injury while receiving drug therapy.
- The patient's fluid volume will remain within normal limits as evidenced by intake and output.
- The patient and his family will demonstrate an understanding of drug therapy.

Implementation

- Monitor renal and hepatic function, CBC, and platelet count regularly.
- Monitor the patient's hydration status if adverse GI reactions occur.
- If the patient has a history of heart failure, watch closely for exacerbation or recurrence during amantadine therapy.
- Follow the manufacturers' guidelines for reconstituting and administering these drugs.
- Obtain an order for an antiemetic or antidiarrheal drug if needed.
- Take safety precautions if adverse CNS reactions occur. For example, place the bed in a low position, raise the bed rails, and supervise ambulation and other activities.

Patients with a history of heart failure should be watched for exacerbation or recurrence of the condition during amantadine therapy.

Well, of course!

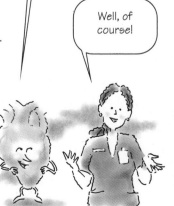

• Notify the prescriber about serious or persistent adverse reactions.
• Warn the patient with parkinsonism not to stop the drug abruptly; doing so could cause a parkinsonian crisis.

Evaluation
• Patient doesn't incur injury while receiving drug therapy.
• Patient maintains adequate hydration.
• Patient and family demonstrate an understanding of drug therapy.

NRTIs

NRTIs are used to treat advanced HIV infections. Drugs in this class include:
• zidovudine
• didanosine
• zalcitabine
• abacavir sulfate
• lamivudine
• stavudine
• emtricitabine.

Pharmacokinetics
Each of the NRTIs has its own pharmacokinetic properties.

A familiar path
Zidovudine is well absorbed from the GI tract, widely distributed throughout the body, metabolized by the liver, and excreted by the kidneys.

Buffed up
Because didanosine is degraded rapidly in gastric acid, didanosine tablets and powder contain a buffering drug to increase pH. The exact route of metabolism isn't fully understood. Approximately one-half of an absorbed dose is excreted in urine.

Food for thought
Oral zalcitabine is well absorbed from the GI tract when administered on an empty stomach. Absorption is reduced when the drug is given with food. Zalcitabine penetrates the blood-brain barrier.

Abracad-abacavir
Abacavir is rapidly and extensively absorbed after oral administration. It's distributed in the extravascular space, and about 50%

binds with plasma proteins. Abacavir is metabolized by the cytosolic enzymes and excreted primarily in urine with the remainder excreted in feces.

Ride the rapids

Lamivudine and stavudine are both rapidly absorbed after administration and are excreted by the kidneys. Emtricitabine is rapidly and extensively absorbed after oral administration. It's also excreted by the kidneys.

Pharmacodynamics

NRTIs must undergo conversion to their active metabolites to produce their action:
• Zidovudine is converted by cellular enzymes to an active form, zidovudine triphosphate, which prevents viral DNA from replicating. (See *How zidovudine works*, page 540.)
• Didanosine and zalcitabine undergo cellular enzyme conversion to their active antiviral metabolites to block HIV replication.
• Zalcitabine is converted to its active metabolite and inhibits replication of HIV by blocking viral DNA synthesis.
• Abacavir is converted to an active metabolite that inhibits the activity of HIV-1 transcriptase by competing with a natural component and incorporating into viral DNA.
• Lamivudine and stavudine are converted in the cells to their active metabolites, which inhibit viral DNA replication.
• Emtricitabine inhibits the enzyme reverse transcriptase and thus inhibits viral DNA replication.

Pharmacotherapeutics

NRTIs are used to treat HIV and AIDS.

Common combinations

Zalcitabine, lamivudine, stavudine, emtricitabine, and abacavir are used in combination with other antiretrovirals to treat HIV infection. For example, Combivir is a combination therapy that includes lamivudine and zidovudine. Trizivir is a combination therapy that includes abacavir, lamivudine, and zidovudine.

The vein game

The I.V. form of zidovudine is used as part of a multidrug regimen in hospitalized patients who can't take oral drugs. It's also used to prevent transmission of HIV from mother to fetus and to treat AIDS-related dementia.

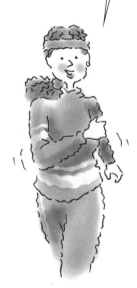

NRTIs must undergo conversion to their active metabolites to produce their action. Talk about keeping active!

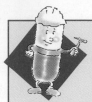

Pharm function

How zidovudine works

Zidovudine inhibits replication of human immunodeficiency virus (HIV). The first two illustrations show how HIV invades cells and then replicates itself. The bottom illustration shows how zidovudine blocks viral transformation.

Invade and replicate

HIV particle enters cell.

HIV uses reverse transcriptase to change its own ribonucleic acid (RNA) into deoxyribonucleic acid (DNA).

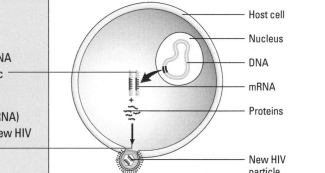

HIV particle

Host cell

DNA

Reverse transcriptase

RNA

Nucleus

Virus-constructed DNA takes over cellular genetic mechanism.

Messenger RNA (mRNA) and other proteins form new HIV particle.

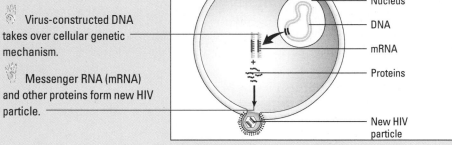

Host cell

Nucleus

DNA

mRNA

Proteins

New HIV particle

Blocked transformation

HIV particle enters cell.

Zidovudine mimics structure of reverse transcriptase so it can block viral transformation of RNA to DNA.

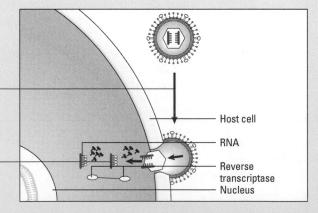

Host cell

RNA

Reverse transcriptase

Nucleus

Another option

Didanosine, in combination with other antiretrovirals, is an alternative initial treatment for HIV infection.

Drug interactions

NRTIs may be responsible for a number of drug interactions:

• Potentially fatal lactic acidosis (increased lactic acid production in the blood) and severe hepatomegaly (enlargement of liver) with steatosis (accumulation of fat) have occurred in patients taking NRTIs alone or with other antiretrovirals such as tenofovir. Most of these patients were women. Obesity and prolonged NRTI exposure may be additional risk factors.

• An increased risk of cellular and kidney toxicity occurs when zidovudine is taken with such drugs as dapsone, pentamidine isethionate, flucytosine, vincristine, vinblastine, doxorubicin, interferon, and ganciclovir.

• Taking zidovudine with probenecid, aspirin, acetaminophen, indomethacin, cimetidine, or lorazepam increases the risk of toxicity of either drug.

• Zidovudine plus acyclovir may produce profound lethargy and drowsiness.

• Didanosine may reduce the absorption of tetracyclines, delavirdine, and fluoroquinolones.

• The risk of peripheral neuropathy (nerve degeneration or inflammation) increases when zalcitabine is taken with didanosine, cimetidine, chloramphenicol, cisplatin, ethionamide, gold salts, hydralazine, iodoquinol, isoniazid, metronidazole, nitrofurantoin, or vincristine.

• Zalcitabine plus pentamidine isethionate increases the risk of pancreatitis.

• Absorption of zalcitabine is reduced when taken with antacids that contain magnesium or aluminum.

• Abacavir levels increase with alcohol consumption.

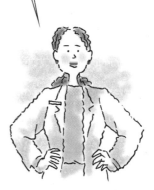

Lactic acidosis and severe hepatomegaly with steatosis can occur in patients taking NRTIs.

Bad combinations

Because of the inhibition of phosphorylation (the process needed to form the active DNA-inhibiting metabolite), lamivudine shouldn't be given in combination with zalcitabine, and stavudine shouldn't be given in combination with zidovudine.

Plays well with others

Emtricitabine has no clinically significant drug interactions when used in combination with indinavir, stavudine, famciclovir, and tenofovir.

Adverse reactions

Adverse reactions to zidovudine and lamivudine include:
- blood-related reactions
- headache and fever
- dizziness
- muscle pain
- rash
- nausea and vomiting
- abdominal pain and diarrhea.

Details on didanosine

Didanosine may cause:
- nausea and vomiting
- abdominal pain and constipation or diarrhea
- stomatitis
- unusual taste or loss of taste
- dry mouth
- pancreatitis
- headache, peripheral neuropathy, or dizziness
- muscle weakness or pain
- rash and itchiness
- hair loss.

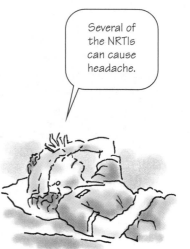

Several of the NRTIs can cause headache.

Zee zalcitabine and stavudine story

Zalcitabine and stavudine may cause:
- peripheral neuropathy
- mouth ulcers
- nausea
- rash
- headache
- muscle pain
- fatigue.

Abacavir may cause potentially fatal hypersensitivity reactions. Emtricitabine may cause severe hepatomegaly and lactic acidosis.

Nursing process

These nursing process steps are appropriate for patients undergoing treatment with NRTIs.

Assessment

- Obtain a baseline assessment of the patient's viral infection; reassess regularly to monitor the drug's effectiveness.
- Assess for adverse reactions and drug interactions.
- Assess the patient's and family's knowledge of drug therapy.

Key nursing diagnoses

- Ineffective protection related to adverse hematologic reactions
- Risk for deficient fluid volume related to adverse GI reactions
- Deficient knowledge related to drug therapy

Planning outcome goals

- The patient won't incur injury while receiving drug therapy.
- The patient's fluid volume will remain within normal limits as evidenced by intake and output.
- The patient and his family will demonstrate an understanding of drug therapy.

Implementation

- Monitor renal and hepatic function, CBC, and platelet count regularly.
- Monitor the patient's mental status when giving drugs I.V. Encephalopathic changes are more likely in patients with neurologic disorders or in those who have had neurologic reactions to cytotoxic drugs.
- Monitor the patient's hydration status if adverse GI reactions occur.
- Follow the manufacturers' guidelines for reconstituting and administering these drugs.
- Obtain an order for an antiemetic or antidiarrheal drug if needed.

Better safe than sorry

- Take safety precautions if adverse CNS reactions occur. For example, place the bed in a low position, raise the bed rails, and supervise ambulation and other activities.
- Notify the prescriber about serious or persistent adverse reactions.
- Dosages may need to be adjusted in a patient with kidney or liver disease.

Evaluation

- Patient doesn't incur injury while receiving drug therapy.
- Patient maintains adequate hydration.
- Patient and family demonstrate an understanding of drug therapy. (See *Teaching about zidovudine therapy*.)

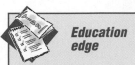

Education edge

Teaching about zidovudine therapy

If zidovudine therapy is prescribed, review these points with the patient and his caregivers:

- Blood transfusions may be needed during treatment because the drug commonly causes a low red blood cell count.
- Compliance with the every-4-hour dosage schedule is important. Use reminders, such as an alarm clock, to avoid missing doses.
- Don't take other drugs (including illicit drugs) without first consulting the prescriber. Other drugs, including other acquired immunodeficiency syndrome drugs, may interfere with zidovudine's effectiveness.
- For pregnant women infected with human immunodeficiency virus (HIV), drug therapy only reduces the risk of HIV transmission to neonates. Long-term risks to infants are unknown.

NNRTIs

NNRTIs are used in combination with other antiretrovirals to treat HIV infection. The three drugs in this class include:
- nevirapine
- delavirdine mesylate
- efavirenz.

Pharmacokinetics

Efavirenz and delavirdine are highly protein-bound after absorption and distribution. Nevirapine is widely distributed throughout the body. All three drugs are metabolized by the cytochrome P450 liver enzyme system and excreted in urine and feces.

Pharmacodynamics

Nevirapine and delavirdine bind to the reverse transcriptase enzyme, preventing it from exerting its effect. This prevents HIV replication.

Healthy competition

Efavirenz competes for the enzyme through noncompetitive inhibition.

Pharmacotherapeutics

NNRTIs are used in combination with other antiretrovirals in HIV treatment; nevirapine is specifically indicated for patients whose clinical condition and immune status have deteriorated.

Drug interactions

These drug interactions may occur with NNRTIs:
- Nevirapine may decrease the activity of protease inhibitors and hormonal contraceptives; don't use these drugs together.

Drop that dosage!

- Delavirdine may increase concentrations of benzodiazepines, clarithromycin, rifabutin, saquinavir, and warfarin; it may also significantly increase concentrations of indinavir, requiring the indinavir dosage to be decreased.
- Indinavir levels are decreased when administered with efavirenz.

Adverse reactions

Adverse reactions to NNRTIs include:

- headache
- dizziness
- asthenia
- nausea and vomiting
- diarrhea.

Rash response

In addition, nevirapine has been associated with a severe rash that may be life-threatening. If a rash occurs, discontinue the drug.

Nursing process

These nursing process steps are appropriate for patients undergoing treatment with NNRTIs.

Assessment
- Obtain a baseline assessment of the patient's viral infection; reassess regularly to monitor the drug's effectiveness.
- Assess for adverse reactions and drug interactions.
- Assess the patient's and family's knowledge of drug therapy.

Key nursing diagnoses
- Ineffective protection related to adverse hematologic reactions
- Risk for deficient fluid volume related to adverse GI reactions
- Deficient knowledge related to drug therapy

Planning outcome goals
- The patient won't incur injury while receiving drug therapy.
- The patient's fluid volume will remain within normal limits as evidenced by intake and output.
- The patient and his family will demonstrate an understanding of drug therapy.

Implementation
- Monitor renal and hepatic function, CBC, and platelet count regularly.
- Monitor the patient's mental status when giving the drug I.V. Encephalopathic changes are more likely in patients with neurologic disorders or in those who have had neurologic reactions to cytotoxic drugs.
- Monitor the patient's hydration status if adverse GI reactions occur.
- Follow the manufacturers' guidelines for reconstituting and administering these drugs.
- Obtain an order for an antiemetic or antidiarrheal drug if needed.

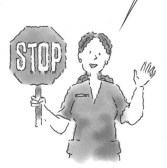

Patients taking nevirapine may develop a severe, life-threatening rash. If this happens, stop the drug.

• Take safety precautions if adverse CNS reactions occur. For example, place the bed in a low position, raise the bed rails, and supervise ambulation and other activities.
• Notify the prescriber about serious or persistent adverse reactions.

Evaluation
• Patient doesn't incur injury while receiving drug therapy.
• Patient maintains adequate hydration.
• Patient and family demonstrate an understanding of drug therapy.

Nucleotide analogue reverse transcriptase inhibitors

The only drug in this class approved for HIV treatment is tenofovir. It works similarly to the NRTIs.

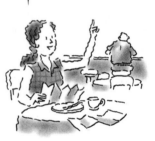

Tenofovir is absorbed better after a high-fat meal. Waiter! I'll have sour cream with that baked potato.

Pharmacokinetics

Tenofovir is absorbed better after a high-fat meal. It's then distributed in small amounts into plasma and serum proteins. Metabolism isn't thought to be mediated by cytochrome P450 liver enzymes, and the drug is excreted by the kidneys.

Pharmacodynamics

Tenofovir competes with substrates and is subsequently incorporated into the DNA chain, thus halting HIV replication.

Pharmacotherapeutics

Tenofovir is used to treat HIV infection in combination with other drugs.

Drug interactions

These drug interactions may occur with tenofovir:
• Drugs that are eliminated through the kidneys or that decrease renal function may increase levels of tenofovir when given concurrently.
• Didanosine concentrations increase when given with tenofovir; watch for didanosine-based adverse effects.

Adverse reactions

Adverse reactions to tenofovir include:
• nausea and vomiting
• diarrhea

- anorexia
- abdominal pain.

Handle with care

Potentially fatal lactic acidosis and severe hepatomegaly with steatosis have occurred in patients taking tenofovir alone or with other antiretrovirals. Most patients were women. Obesity and previous NRTI exposure may also be risk factors. Patients with preexisting liver disease should take this drug with caution. Suspend treatment if hepatotoxicity is suspected.

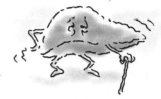

Patients with preexisting liver disease should take tenofovir with caution.

Nursing process

These nursing process steps are appropriate for patients undergoing treatment with nucleotide analogue reverse transcriptase inhibitors.

Assessment

- Obtain a baseline assessment of the patient's viral infection; reassess regularly to monitor the drug's effectiveness.
- Assess for adverse reactions and drug interactions.
- Assess the patient's and family's knowledge of drug therapy.

Key nursing diagnoses

- Ineffective protection related to adverse hematologic reactions
- Risk for deficient fluid volume related to adverse GI reactions
- Deficient knowledge related to drug therapy

Planning outcome goals

- The patient won't incur injury while receiving drug therapy.
- The patient's fluid volume will remain within normal limits as evidenced by intake and output.
- The patient and his family will demonstrate an understanding of drug therapy.

Implementation

- Monitor renal and hepatic function, CBC, and platelet count regularly. Monitor for body changes in fat as well as for bone abnormalities and renal toxicity.
- Monitor the patient's mental status when giving the drug I.V. Encephalopathic changes are more likely in patients with neurologic disorders or in those who have had neurologic reactions to cytotoxic drugs.
- Monitor the patient's hydration status if adverse GI reactions occur.

- Follow the manufacturer's guidelines for reconstituting and administering antiviral drugs.
- Obtain an order for an antiemetic or antidiarrheal drug if needed.
- Take safety precautions if adverse CNS reactions occur. For example, place the bed in a low position, raise the bed rails, and supervise ambulation and other activities.
- Notify the prescriber about serious or persistent adverse reactions.

Evaluation

- Patient doesn't incur injury while receiving drug therapy.
- Patient maintains adequate hydration.
- Patient and family demonstrate an understanding of drug therapy.

Protease inhibitors

Protease inhibitors are drugs that act against the HIV enzyme protease, preventing it from dividing a larger viral precursor protein into the active smaller enzymes that the HIV virus needs to fully mature. The result is an immature, noninfectious cell. Drugs in this group include:
- saquinavir mesylate
- nelfinavir mesylate
- ritonavir
- indinavir sulfate
- lopinavir
- amprenavir
- atazanavir sulfate.

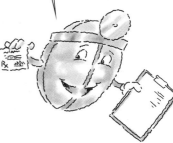

Protease inhibitors prevent the HIV virus from fully maturing.

Pharmacokinetics

Protease inhibitors have different pharmacokinetic properties.

Saquinavir's story

Saquinavir mesylate is poorly absorbed from the GI tract. It's widely distributed, highly bound to plasma proteins, metabolized by the liver, and excreted mainly by the kidneys.

Nelfinavir notables

Nelfinavir's bioavailability (the degree to which it becomes available to target tissue after administration) isn't known. Food increases its absorption. It's highly protein-bound, metabolized in the liver, and excreted primarily in feces.

Ritonavir review

Ritonavir is well absorbed, metabolized by the liver, and broken down into at least five metabolites. It's mainly excreted in feces, with some elimination through the kidneys.

Inside indinavir

Indinavir sulfate is rapidly absorbed and moderately bound to plasma proteins. It's metabolized by the liver into seven metabolites. The drug is excreted mainly in feces.

One boosts the other

Lopinavir is extensively metabolized by the liver's cytochrome P450 system. Lopinavir and ritonavir are used in combination because of their positive effects on HIV RNA levels and CD4+ counts. When given together, ritonavir inhibits the metabolism of lopinavir, leading to increased plasma lopinavir levels.

All about amprenavir

Amprenavir is metabolized in the liver to active and inactive metabolites and is minimally excreted in urine and feces.

At last, atazanavir

Atazanavir is rapidly absorbed and is metabolized in the liver by the cytochrome P450 3A (CYP3A) pathway. The drug is excreted mainly in feces and urine.

Pharmacodynamics

All of these drugs inhibit the activity of HIV protease and prevent the cleavage (division) of viral polyproteins.

Pharmacotherapeutics

Protease inhibitors are used in combination with other antiretroviral agents to treat HIV infection. (See *Raltegravir and maraviroc: Two new HIV drugs*, page 550.)

Drug interactions

Protease inhibitors may interact with many drugs. Here are some common interactions:
• Saquinavir mesylate may decrease the effectiveness of hormonal contraceptives.

On the increase

• Ritonavir may increase the effects of alpha-adrenergic blockers, antiarrhythmics, antidepressants, antiemetics, antifungals, an-

Raltegravir and maraviroc: Two new HIV drugs

Two drugs have recently been approved for treatment of human immunodeficiency virus (HIV): raltegravir, an integrase inhibitor, and maraviroc, a CCR5 blocking entry inhibitor. Both are indicated for patients who have strains of HIV that are resistant to multiple antiretroviral drugs. However, to work effectively, they must be combined with other HIV drugs.

Raltegravir's role

Raltegravir blocks the activity of integrase, an enzyme that hides HIV's deoxyribonucleic acid (DNA). When integrase is blocked, the HIV's DNA can't combine with the healthy cell's DNA.

So far, raltegravir seems to have few interactions with other drugs, although plasma levels of raltegravir are decreased when it's taken with rifampin. Adverse effects include diarrhea, nausea, headache, and an elevated creatine kinase level. Raltegravir also increases the risk of opportunistic infections; monitor the patient for indications of such an infection.

Maraviroc moves in

Maraviroc works by binding to a protein on the membrane of CD4 cells called *CCR5*, which blocks HIV from attaching to CD4 cells. When maraviroc instead of HIV is bound to CD4 cells, HIV can't infect these cells.

Maraviroc interacts with some drugs: Anticonvulsants and rifampin can decrease levels of maraviroc in the bloodstream. Conversely, clarithromycin, ketoconazole, and itraconazole can increase maraviroc levels. Maraviroc can also interact with other HIV medications, so dosages must be adjusted accordingly.

Adverse effects include cough, fever, respiratory tract infections, rash, muscle and joint pain, stomach pain, and diarrhea. Some patients have experienced systemic allergic reactions and, later, liver toxicity. Keep in mind that maraviroc should be used cautiously in patients at risk for cardiovascular events such as myocardial infarction. Patients are also at increased risk for developing opportunistic infections and malignancies.

tilipemics, antimalarials, antineoplastics, beta-adrenergic blockers, calcium channel blockers, cimetidine, corticosteroids, erythromycin, immunosuppressants, methylphenidate, pentoxifylline, phenothiazines, and warfarin.

• Indinavir sulfate inhibits the metabolism of midazolam and triazolam, increasing the risk of potentially fatal events such as cardiac arrhythmias.

• Didanosine decreases gastric absorption of indinavir; give these drugs at least 1 hour apart.

• Rifampin markedly reduces plasma concentrations of most protease inhibitors, including atazanavir.

• Nelfinavir may greatly increase plasma levels of amiodarone, ergot derivatives, midazolam, rifabutin, quinidine, and triazolam.

• Carbamazepine, phenobarbital, and phenytoin may reduce the effectiveness of nelfinavir.

• Protease inhibitors may increase sildenafil concentrations and result in sildenafil-associated adverse reactions, including hypotension, vision changes, and priapism (a persistent, possibly painful erection).

• Atazanavir shouldn't be given with other drugs metabolized by the CYP3A pathway, such as HMG-CoA reductase inhibitors. Concurrent use may increase the risk of myopathy and rhabdomyolysis.

Interval increaser

• Atazanavir may prolong the PR interval. Drugs that prolong the PR interval, such as calcium channel blockers (diltiazem, for example) and beta-adrenergic blockers (atenolol, for example), should be used cautiously with atazanavir.

• Atazanavir shouldn't be administered with such benzodiazepines as midazolam and triazolam because of the potential for increased sedation or respiratory depression.

• Atazanavir shouldn't be administered with ergot derivatives, such as ergotamine and dihydroergotamine, because life-threatening ergot toxicity can result, causing peripheral vasospasm and ischemia of the extremities.

• St. John's wort may reduce plasma concentrations of atazanavir.

• Indinavir and ritonavir may increase plasma nelfinavir levels.

Adverse reactions

Adverse reactions depend on the type of protease inhibitor used:

• Saquinavir mesylate may cause dizziness, an increase in triglyceride and lipid levels, changes in body fat, anxiety, blurred vision, diarrhea, constipation or abdominal discomfort, night sweats, sleeplessness, or bleeding gums.

• Ritonavir's adverse reactions include muscle weakness, nausea, diarrhea, vomiting, anorexia, abdominal pain, and taste perversion.

• Adverse reactions to indinavir include abdominal pain, muscle weakness, fatigue, flank pain, nausea, diarrhea, vomiting, acid reflux, anorexia, dry mouth, headache, insomnia, dizziness, taste perversion, and back pain.

• Nelfinavir may cause seizures, suicidal ideation, diarrhea, pancreatitis, hepatitis, hypoglycemia, or allergic reactions.

• Amprenavir may cause paresthesia, nausea, vomiting, loose stools, hyperglycemia, and rash.

• Reactions to combination therapy with lopinavir and ritonavir include encephalopathy, deep vein thrombosis, diarrhea, nausea, hemorrhagic colitis, and pancreatitis.

• Atazanavir may cause hepatotoxicity, arrhythmias, or lactic acidosis.

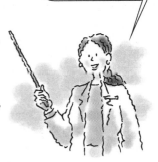

Adverse reactions to protease inhibitors vary from drug to drug. Make sure you familiarize yourself with the specific reactions of the drug your patient is taking.

Nursing process

These nursing process steps are appropriate for patients undergoing treatment with protease inhibitors.

Assessment

- Obtain a baseline assessment of the patient's viral infection; reassess regularly to monitor the drug's effectiveness.
- Assess for adverse reactions and drug interactions.
- Assess the patient's and family's knowledge of drug therapy.

Key nursing diagnoses

- Ineffective protection related to adverse hematologic reactions
- Risk for deficient fluid volume related to adverse GI reactions
- Deficient knowledge related to drug therapy

Planning outcome goals

- The patient won't incur injury while receiving drug therapy.
- The patient's fluid volume will remain within normal limits as evidenced by intake and output.
- The patient and his family will demonstrate an understanding of drug therapy.

Implementation

- Monitor renal and hepatic function, CBC, and platelet count regularly.
- Monitor the patient's mental status when giving the drug I.V. Encephalopathic changes are more likely in patients with neurologic disorders or in those who have had neurologic reactions to cytotoxic drugs.
- Monitor the patient's hydration status if adverse GI reactions occur.

Sugar, sugar

- Check the blood sugar levels of diabetic patients taking saquinavir mesylate.
- Follow the manufacturer's guidelines for reconstituting and administering antiviral drugs.
- Obtain an order for an antiemetic or antidiarrheal drug if needed.
- Take safety precautions if adverse CNS reactions occur. For example, place the bed in a low position, raise the bed rails, and supervise ambulation and other activities.
- Notify the prescriber about serious or persistent adverse reactions.

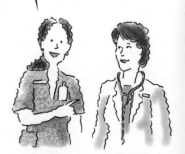

Notify the prescriber if the patient develops serious or persistent adverse reactions to a protease inhibitor.

Evaluation

- Patient doesn't incur injury while receiving drug therapy.
- Patient maintains adequate hydration.
- Patient and family demonstrate an understanding of drug therapy.

Antitubercular drugs

Antitubercular drugs are used to treat tuberculosis (TB), which is caused by *M. tuberculosis*. These drugs also are effective against less common mycobacterial infections caused by *M. kansasii, M. avium-intracellulare, M. fortuitum,* and related organisms. Although not always curative, these drugs can halt the progression of a mycobacterial infection.

Compliance can get complicated

Unlike most antibacterials, antitubercular drugs may need to be administered over many months. This creates such problems as patient noncompliance, the development of bacterial resistance, and drug toxicity. (See *Directly observable therapy for TB*.)

Tag team therapy

Traditionally, isoniazid, rifampin, and ethambutol hydrochloride were the mainstays of multidrug TB therapy and successfully prevented the emergence of drug resistance.

Because of the current incidence of drug-resistant TB strains, however, a four-drug regimen is now recommended for initial treatment:
- isoniazid
- rifampin
- pyrazinamide
- streptomycin sulfate or ethambutol.

Directly observable therapy for TB

Among infectious diseases, tuberculosis (TB) remains a frequent killer worldwide. Treatment is difficult because it requires long-term medical therapy—often as long as 6 to 9 months. The length of treatment commonly creates problems with patient compliance, and poor compliance contributes to reactivation of the disease and development of drug-resistant TB.

DOT on the spot

Directly observable therapy (DOT) was developed to combat these treatment issues. DOT requires that a health care worker observe a patient take every dose of the drug for the duration of therapy. A controversy exists over whether every individual with TB should be observed, called *universal DOT,* or whether only those at risk for poor compliance should be observed *(selective DOT).*

Who fails to comply?

Patients at risk for poor compliance include those with a previous history of poor compliance, an inability or unwillingness to follow a treatment plan, and a recent history of drug or alcohol abuse, mental illness, homelessness, incarceration, or residence in a homeless shelter. Some areas, such as Mississippi and New York City, practice universal DOT; other areas, including Massachusetts, first evaluate a patient's ability and willingness to comply.

Times to modify

The antitubercular regimen should be modified if local testing shows resistance to one or more of these drugs. If local outbreaks of TB resistant to isoniazid and rifampin are occurring in institutions (for example, health care or correctional facilities), then five-drug or six-drug regimens are recommended as initial therapy.

Pharmacokinetics

Most antitubercular drugs are administered orally. When given orally, these drugs are well absorbed from the GI tract and widely distributed throughout the body. They're metabolized primarily in the liver and excreted by the kidneys.

Pharmacodynamics

Antitubercular drugs are specific for mycobacteria. At usual dosages, ethambutol and isoniazid are tuberculostatic, meaning that they inhibit the growth of *M. tuberculosis*. In contrast, rifampin is tuberculocidal, meaning that it destroys the mycobacteria. Because bacterial resistance to isoniazid and rifampin can develop rapidly, they should always be used with other antitubercular drugs.

Mysterious ways

The exact mechanism of action of ethambutol remains unclear, but it may be related to inhibition of cell metabolism, arrest of multiplication, and cell death. Ethambutol acts only against replicating bacteria.

Wall buster

Although isoniazid's exact mechanism of action isn't known, the drug is believed to inhibit the synthesis of mycolic acids, important components of the mycobacterium cell wall. This inhibition disrupts the cell wall. Only replicating, not resting, bacteria appear to be inhibited. (See *Antitubercular drugs: Isoniazid*.)

RNA repressor

Rifampin inhibits RNA synthesis in susceptible organisms. The drug is effective primarily in replicating bacteria but may have some effect on resting bacteria as well.

Acid wash

The exact mechanism of action of pyrazinamide isn't known, but the antimycobacterial activity appears to be linked to the drug's conversion to the active metabolite pyrazinoic acid. Pyrazinoic acid, in turn, creates an acidic environment where mycobacteria can't replicate.

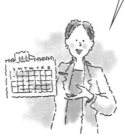

Antitubercular drugs may need to be administered over many months.

Prototype pro

Antitubercular drugs: Isoniazid

Actions
• Appears to inhibit cell wall biosynthesis by interfering with lipid and deoxyribonucleic acid synthesis

Indications
• Tuberculosis

Nursing considerations
• Monitor the patient for adverse effects, such as peripheral neuropathy, seizures, hematologic disorders, hepatitis, and hypersensitivity reactions.
• Always give isoniazid with other antitubercular drugs to prevent the development of resistant organisms.

Pharmacotherapeutics

Isoniazid is usually used with ethambutol, rifampin, or streptomycin. This is because combination therapy for TB and other mycobacterial infections can prevent or delay the development of resistance.

For simpler times

Ethambutol is used with isoniazid and rifampin to treat patients
with uncomplicated pulmonary TB. It's also used to treat infections resulting from *M. bovis* and most strains of *M. kansasii*.

Preventive power

Although isoniazid is the most important drug for treating TB, bacterial resistance develops rapidly if it's used alone. However, resistance doesn't pose a problem when isoniazid is used alone to prevent TB in individuals who have been exposed to the disease, and
no evidence exists of cross-resistance between isoniazid and other antitubercular drugs. Isoniazid is typically given orally but may
be given I.V. if necessary.

Rapid resistance

Rifampin is used to treat pulmonary TB with other antitubercular
drugs. It combats many gram-positive and some gram-negative
bacteria but is seldom used for nonmycobacterial infections because bacterial resistance develops rapidly. It's used to treat
asymptomatic carriers of *Neisseria meningitidis* when the risk of
meningitis is high, but it isn't used to treat *N. meningitidis* infections because of the potential for bacterial resistance.

First in line

Pyrazinamide is currently recommended as a first-line TB drug in
combination with ethambutol, rifampin, and isoniazid. Pyrazinamide is a highly specific drug that's active only against *M. tuberculosis*. Resistance to pyrazinamide may develop rapidly when it's
used alone.

Drug interactions

Antitubercular drugs may interact with a number of other drugs:
• Cycloserine and ethionamide may produce additive CNS effects,
such as drowsiness, dizziness, headache, lethargy, depression,
tremor, anxiety, confusion, and tinnitus, when administered with
isoniazid.
• Isoniazid may increase levels of phenytoin, carbamazepine, diazepam, ethosuximide, primidone, theophylline, and warfarin.

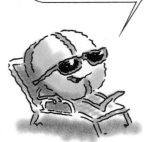

Isoniazid is the
most important
drug for treating
TB. It's nice to get
the recognition I
deserve!

• When corticosteroids and isoniazid are taken together, the effectiveness of isoniazid is reduced, whereas the effects of corticosteroids are increased.
• Isoniazid may reduce the plasma concentration of ketoconazole, itraconazole, and oral antidiabetic drugs.
• When given together, the combination of rifampin, isoniazid, ethionamide, and pyrazinamide increases the risk of hepatotoxicity.
• Pyrazinamide combined with phenytoin may increase phenytoin levels.

Adverse reactions

Adverse reactions to antitubercular drugs vary:
• Ethambutol may cause itching, joint pain, GI distress, malaise, leukopenia, headache, dizziness, numbness and tingling of the extremities, and confusion. Although rare, hypersensitivity reactions to ethambutol may produce rash and fever. Anaphylaxis may also occur.
• Peripheral neuropathy is the most common adverse reaction to isoniazid. Severe and occasionally fatal hepatitis associated with isoniazid may occur even many months after treatment has stopped. Patients must be monitored carefully.
• The most common adverse reactions to rifampin include epigastric pain, nausea, vomiting, abdominal cramps, flatulence, anorexia, and diarrhea.
• Liver toxicity is the major limiting adverse reaction to pyrazinamide. GI disturbances include nausea, vomiting, and anorexia.

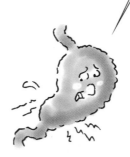

Common adverse reactions to rifampin include—ouch—epigastric pain and abdominal cramps.

Nursing process

These nursing process steps are appropriate for patients undergoing treatment with antitubercular drugs.

Assessment
• Assess the patient's infection before therapy.
• Monitor the patient for improvement, and evaluate culture and sensitivity tests.
• Assess for adverse reactions and drug interactions.
• Assess the patient's and family's knowledge of drug therapy.

Key nursing diagnoses
• Risk for infection related to the underlying process
• Disturbed sensory perception (tactile) related to drug-induced peripheral neuropathy
• Deficient knowledge related to drug therapy

Planning outcome goals

• The patient will be free from infection as evidenced by negative cultures and normal WBC counts.
• The patient will state that tactile sensations are normal.
• The patient and his family will demonstrate an understanding of drug therapy.

Implementation

• Administer oral doses 1 hour before or 2 hours after meals to avoid decreased absorption.
• Follow the protocol for I.M. dosage. Switch to the oral form as soon as possible.
• Monitor the patient for paresthesia of the hands and feet, which usually precedes peripheral neuropathy, especially in patients who are malnourished, alcoholic, or diabetic.
• Monitor hepatic function closely for changes.

Evaluation

• Patient is free from infection.
• Patient maintains normal peripheral nervous system function.
• Patient and family demonstrate an understanding of drug therapy. (See *Teaching about antitubercular drugs.*)

Antifungal drugs

Antifungal, or antimycotic, drugs are used to treat fungal infections. They include:
• polyenes
• flucytosine
• ketoconazole
• synthetic triazoles
• glucan synthesis inhibitors. (See *Other antifungal drugs*, page 558.)

Polyenes

The polyenes include amphotericin B and nystatin. The potency of amphotericin B has made it the most widely used antifungal drug for severe systemic fungal infections. Nystatin is used only topically or orally to treat local fungal infections because it's extremely toxic when administered parenterally.

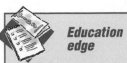

Education edge

Teaching about antitubercular drugs

If antitubercular drugs are prescribed, review these points with the patient and his caregivers:
• Take the drug as prescribed; don't stop the drug without the prescriber's consent. Treatment may last for several months.
• Take the drug with food if GI irritation occurs.
• Avoid alcohol during drug therapy.
• Avoid certain foods, including fish (such as tuna) and products containing tyramine (such as aged cheese, beer, and chocolate), because the drug has some monoamine-oxidase inhibitor activity.
• Notify the prescriber immediately if signs and symptoms of liver impairment occur (loss of appetite, fatigue, malaise, jaundice, or dark urine).

Other antifungal drugs

Several other antifungal drugs offer alternative forms of treatment for topical fungal infections.

Clotrimazole

An imidazole derivative, clotrimazole is used:
- topically to treat dermatophyte and *Candida albicans* infections
- orally to treat oral candidiasis
- vaginally to treat vaginal candidiasis.

Griseofulvin

Griseofulvin is used to treat fungal infections of the:
- skin (tinea corporis)
- feet (tinea pedis)
- groin (tinea cruris)
- beard area of the face and neck (tinea barbae)
- nails (tinea unguium)
- scalp (tinea capitis).

No relapse allowed

To prevent a relapse, griseofulvin therapy must continue until the fungus is eradicated and the infected skin or nails are replaced.

Miconazole

Available as miconazole or miconazole nitrate, this imidazole derivative is used to treat local fungal infections, such as vaginal and vulvar candidiasis, and topical fungal infections such as chronic candidiasis of the skin and mucous membranes.

Delivery options

Miconazole may be administered:
- I.V. or intrathecally (into the subarachnoid space) to treat fungal meningitis
- I.V. or in bladder irrigations to treat fungal bladder infections
- locally to treat vaginal infections
- topically to treat topical infections.

Other topical antimycotic drugs

Ciclopirox, econazole nitrate, butoconazole nitrate, naftifine, tioconazole, terconazole, tolnaftate, butenafine hydrochloride, sulconazole nitrate, oxiconazole nitrate, triacetin, and undecylenic acid are available only as topical drugs.

Pharmacokinetics

After I.V. administration, amphotericin B is distributed throughout the body and excreted by the kidneys. Its metabolism isn't well defined.

Not much circulation

Oral nystatin undergoes little or no absorption, distribution, or metabolism. It's excreted unchanged in feces. Topical nystatin isn't absorbed through intact skin or mucous membranes.

Pharmacodynamics

Amphotericin B works by binding to sterol (a lipid) in the fungal cell membrane, altering cell permeability and allowing intracellular components to leak out.

Fungi town

Amphotericin B usually acts as a fungistatic drug (inhibiting fungal growth and multiplication) but can become fungicidal (destroying fungi) if it reaches high concentrations in the fungi.

Manipulating membranes

Nystatin binds to sterols in fungal cell membranes and alters the permeability of the membranes, leading to loss of cell components. Nystatin can act as a fungicidal or fungistatic drug, depending on the organism present.

Pharmacotherapeutics

Amphotericin B is usually administered to treat severe systemic fungal infections and meningitis caused by fungi sensitive to the drug. It's never used for noninvasive forms of fungal disease because it's highly toxic. It's usually the drug of choice for severe infections caused by *Candida*, *Paracoccidioides brasiliensis*, *Blastomyces dermatitidis*, *Coccidioides immitis*, *Cryptococcus neoformans*, and *Sporothrix schenckii*. It's also effective against *Aspergillus fumigatus*, *Microsporum audouinii*, *Rhizopus*, *Trichophyton*, and *Rhodotorula*.

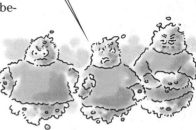

Amphotericin B comes along and thinks it can just end me and all my friends parking!

Know the limits

Because amphotericin B is highly toxic, its use is limited to patients who have a definitive diagnosis of life-threatening infection and are under close medical supervision.

Canning candidal infections

Different forms of nystatin are available for treating different types of candidal infections:
• Topical nystatin is used to treat candidal skin or mucous membrane infections, such as oral thrush, diaper rash, vaginal and vulvar candidiasis, and candidiasis between skin folds.
• Oral nystatin is used to treat GI infections.

Drug interactions

Amphotericin B may have significant interactions with many drugs:
• Because of the synergistic effects between flucytosine and amphotericin B, these two drugs are commonly combined in therapy for candidal or cryptococcal infections, especially for cryptococcal meningitis.
• The risk of kidney toxicity increases when amphotericin B is taken with aminoglycosides, cyclosporine, or acyclovir.
• Corticosteroids, extended-spectrum penicillins, and digoxin may worsen hypokalemia (low blood potassium levels) produced by amphotericin B, possibly leading to heart problems. Moreover, the risk of digoxin toxicity is increased.
• Amphotericin B increases muscle relaxation when given with nondepolarizing skeletal muscle relaxants (such as pancuronium bromide).

• Electrolyte solutions may inactivate amphotericin B when diluted in the same solution. Amphotericin B preparations must be mixed with D$_5$W; they can't be mixed with saline solutions.

A wallflower

Nystatin doesn't interact significantly with other drugs.

Adverse reactions

Almost all patients receiving I.V. amphotericin B, particularly at the beginning of low-dose therapy, experience:
• chills
• fever
• nausea and vomiting
• anorexia
• muscle and joint pain
• indigestion.

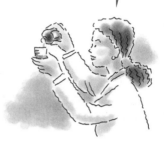

Don't mix amphotericin B preparations with saline solutions! They must be mixed with D$_5$W.

Watch those RBCs

Most patients also develop normochromic (adequate hemoglobin in each RBC) or normocytic anemia (too few RBCs) that significantly decreases hematocrit.

Altered electrolytes

Hypomagnesemia and hypokalemia may occur, causing ECG changes requiring replacement electrolyte therapy. Magnesium and potassium levels and renal function must be monitored frequently in patients receiving amphotericin.

Losing concentration

Up to 80% of patients may develop some degree of kidney toxicity, causing the kidneys to lose their ability to concentrate urine.

The higher the dosage, the harder they react

Reactions to nystatin seldom occur, but high dosages may produce:
• diarrhea
• nausea and vomiting
• abdominal pain
• a bitter taste
• hypersensitivity reactions
• skin irritation (topical form).

Nursing process

These nursing process steps are appropriate for patients undergoing treatment with polyenes.

Assessment

- Obtain a history of the fungal infection as well as a specimen for culture and sensitivity tests before giving the first dose. Reevaluate the patient's condition during therapy.
- Assess for adverse reactions and drug interactions.
- Assess the patient's and family's knowledge of drug therapy.

Key nursing diagnoses

- Risk for infection related to the underlying condition
- Risk for injury related to drug-induced adverse reactions
- Deficient knowledge related to drug therapy

Planning outcome goals

- The patient's infection will resolve as evidenced by culture reports, temperature, and WBC counts.
- The patient won't incur injury while receiving drug therapy.
- The patient and his family will demonstrate an understanding of drug therapy.

Implementation

- The lozenge form of the drug should be dissolved slowly.
- Parenteral I.V. use is for hospitalized patients only after diagnosis of potentially fatal fungal infection is confirmed. The initial dose is usually a test dose and administered over 20 to 30 minutes.
- Use an infusion pump and in-line filter with a mean pore diameter larger than 1 micron. Infuse over 2 to 6 hours; rapid infusion may cause cardiovascular collapse.
- Give antibacterials separately; don't mix them or give them piggyback with other drugs.
- Monitor the patient's pulse, respiratory rate, temperature, and blood pressure every 30 minutes for at least 4 hours after giving the drug I.V.; fever, shaking chills, anorexia, nausea, vomiting, headache, tachypnea, and hypotension may appear 1 to 3 hours after the start of an I.V. infusion. Signs and symptoms are usually more severe with initial doses.
- Monitor BUN, creatinine (or creatinine clearance), and electrolyte levels; CBC; and liver function test results at least weekly. If the BUN level exceeds 40 mg/dl or if the creatinine level exceeds 3 mg/dl, the prescriber may reduce or stop the drug until renal function improves.
- Monitor for rhinocerebral phycomycosis, especially in a patient with uncontrolled diabetes. Leukoencephalopathy may also occur. Monitor pulmonary function. Acute reactions are characterized by dyspnea, hypoxemia, and infiltrates.
- If the patient has severe adverse infusion reactions to the initial dose, stop the infusion and notify the prescriber, who may pre-

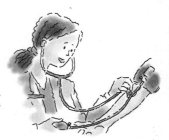

Take the patient's blood pressure every 30 minutes for at least 4 hours after giving polyenes I.V.

scribe antipyretics, antihistamines, antiemetics, or small doses of corticosteroids. To prevent reactions during subsequent infusions, premedicate with these drugs or give amphotericin B on an alternate-day schedule.

Evaluation
- Patient is free from fungal infection.
- Patient doesn't experience injury as a result of drug-induced adverse reactions.
- Patient and family demonstrate an understanding of drug therapy.

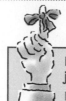

Memory jogger

If a drug is fungicidal, it destroys the fungus—*cidus* is a Latin term for "killing." If it's fungistatic, it prevents fungal growth and multiplication—*stasis* is a Greek term for "halting."

Flucytosine

Flucytosine, a fluorinated pyrimidine analogue, is the only antimetabolite (a substance that closely resembles one required for normal physiologic functioning and that exerts its effect by interfering with metabolism) that acts as an antifungal. Flucytosine is a purine and pyrimidine inhibitor.

Pharmacokinetics

After oral administration, flucytosine is well absorbed from the GI tract and widely distributed. It undergoes little metabolism and is excreted primarily by the kidneys.

Pharmacodynamics

Flucytosine penetrates fungal cells, where it's converted to its active metabolite fluorouracil. Fluorouracil is then incorporated into the RNA of the fungal cells, altering their protein synthesis and causing cell death.

Pharmacotherapeutics

Flucytosine is used primarily with another antifungal drug such as amphotericin B to treat systemic fungal infections. For example, although amphotericin B is effective in treating candidal and cryptococcal meningitis alone, flucytosine is given with it to reduce the dosage and the risk of toxicity. This combination therapy is the treatment of choice for cryptococcal meningitis.

Drug interactions

Cytarabine may antagonize the antifungal activity of flucytosine, possibly by competitive inhibition. Hemato-

Flucytosine reduces the risk of amphotericin B toxicity when the drugs are given together.

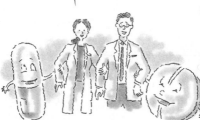

logic, kidney, and liver function must be closely monitored during flucytosine therapy because of the drug's serious risk of toxicity.

Adverse reactions

Flucytosine may produce unpredictable adverse reactions, including:
- confusion
- headache
- drowsiness
- vertigo
- hallucinations
- difficulty breathing
- respiratory arrest
- rash
- nausea and vomiting
- abdominal distention
- diarrhea
- anorexia.

Nursing process

These nursing process steps are appropriate for patients undergoing treatment with flucytosine.

Assessment
- Assess the patient's fungal infection before therapy and regularly throughout therapy.
- Before therapy, obtain hematologic tests and renal and liver function studies. Make sure susceptibility tests showing that the organism is flucytosine-sensitive are included on the chart.
- Assess for adverse reactions and drug interactions.
- Assess the patient's and family's knowledge of drug therapy.

Key nursing diagnoses
- Risk for infection related to the underlying condition
- Risk for deficient fluid volume related to adverse GI reactions
- Deficient knowledge related to drug therapy

Planning outcome goals
- The patient's infection will resolve as evidenced by culture reports, temperature, and WBC counts.
- The patient's fluid volume will remain within normal limits as evidenced by intake and output.
- The patient and his family will demonstrate an understanding of drug therapy.

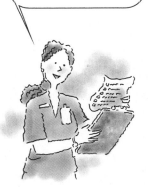

Before starting therapy, make sure susceptibility tests showing that the organism is flucytosine-sensitive are included on the patient's chart.

Implementation

- Give capsules over 15 minutes to reduce adverse GI reactions.
- Monitor the patient for adverse CNS reactions.
- Monitor blood, liver, and renal function studies frequently; obtain susceptibility tests weekly to monitor drug resistance.
- If possible, regularly perform blood level assays of the drug to maintain flucytosine at therapeutic levels (25 to 120 mcg/ml). Higher blood levels may be toxic.
- Monitor the patient's hydration status if adverse GI reactions occur.

Evaluation

- Patient is free from infection.
- Patient maintains adequate hydration.
- Patient and family demonstrate an understanding of drug therapy.

Ketoconazole

Ketoconazole, a synthetic imidazole derivative, is an effective oral antifungal drug with a broad spectrum of activity.

Pharmacokinetics

When given orally, ketoconazole is absorbed variably and distributed widely. It undergoes extensive liver metabolism and is excreted in bile and feces.

Pharmacodynamics

Within the fungal cells, ketoconazole interferes with sterol synthesis, damaging the cell membrane and increasing its permeability. This leads to a loss of essential intracellular elements and inhibition of cell growth.

Fungicidal tendencies

Ketoconazole usually produces fungistatic effects but can also produce fungicidal effects under certain conditions.

Pharmacotherapeutics

Ketoconazole is used to treat topical and systemic infections caused by susceptible fungi, which include dermatophytes and most other fungi.

Drug interactions

Ketoconazole may have significant interactions with other drugs:
• Ketoconazole use with drugs that decrease gastric acidity, such as cimetidine, ranitidine, famotidine, nizatidine, antacids, and anticholinergic drugs, may decrease absorption of ketoconazole and reduce its antimycotic effects. If the patient must take these drugs, delay administration of ketoconazole by at least 2 hours.
• Taking ketoconazole with phenytoin may alter metabolism and increase blood levels of both drugs.
• When taken with theophylline, ketoconazole may decrease the serum theophylline level.
• Use with other hepatotoxic drugs may increase the risk of liver disease.
• Combined with cyclosporine therapy, ketoconazole may increase cyclosporine and serum creatinine levels.
• Ketoconazole increases the effect of oral anticoagulants and can cause hemorrhage.

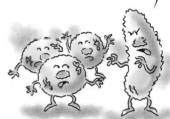

Help! We need antifungal activity!

Feeling a bit inhibited

• Ketoconazole can inhibit metabolism (and possibly increase concentrations) of quinidine, sulfonylureas, carbamazepine, and protease inhibitors.
• Ketoconazole shouldn't be given with rifampin because serum ketoconazole concentrations may decrease.

Adverse reactions

The most common adverse reactions to ketoconazole are nausea and vomiting. Less frequent reactions include:
• anaphylaxis
• joint pain
• chills
• fever
• tinnitus
• impotence
• photophobia
• hepatotoxicity (rare; reversible when the drug is stopped).

Nursing process

These nursing process steps are appropriate for patients undergoing treatment with ketoconazole.

Assessment

• Assess the patient's fungal infection before therapy and regularly throughout therapy.
• Assess for adverse reactions and drug interactions.

• Assess the patient's and family's knowledge of drug therapy.

Key nursing diagnoses
• Risk for infection related to the underlying condition
• Risk for deficient fluid volume related to adverse GI reactions
• Deficient knowledge related to drug therapy

Planning outcome goals
• The patient's infection will resolve as evidenced by culture reports, temperature, and WBC counts.
• The patient's fluid volume will remain within normal limits as evidenced by intake and output.
• The patient and his family will demonstrate an understanding of drug therapy.

Implementation
• Because of the risk of serious hepatotoxicity, the drug shouldn't be used for less serious conditions, such as fungal infections of the skin or nails.
• To minimize nausea, divide the daily amount into two doses and give the drug with meals.
• Monitor the patient's hydration status if adverse GI reactions occur.

Evaluation
• Patient is free from infection.
• Patient maintains adequate hydration.
• Patient and family demonstrate an understanding of drug therapy.

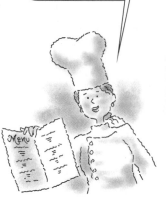

To minimize nausea, divide the daily amount into two doses and give the drug with meals. So that'll be a glass of OJ, a bowl of corn flakes, and a side of ketoconazole?

Synthetic triazoles

The synthetic triazoles include fluconazole, itraconazole, and voriconazole.

Pharmacokinetics

After oral administration, fluconazole is about 90% absorbed. It's distributed into all body fluids, and more than 80% of the drug is excreted unchanged in urine.

With and without food

Oral bioavailability is greatest when itraconazole is taken with food; voriconazole is more effective if taken 1 hour before or after a meal. Both itraconazole and voriconazole are bound to plasma proteins and extensively metabolized in the liver into a large number of metabolites. They're minimally excreted in feces.

Pharmacodynamics

Fluconazole inhibits fungal cytochrome P450, an enzyme responsible for fungal sterol synthesis, causing fungal cell walls to weaken.

The wall comes tumbling down

Itraconazole and voriconazole interfere with fungal cell-wall synthesis by inhibiting the formation of ergosterol and increasing cell-wall permeability, making the fungus susceptible to osmotic instability.

Pharmacotherapeutics

The synthetic triazoles treat various infections:
• Fluconazole is used to treat mouth, throat, and esophageal candidiasis and serious systemic candidal infections, including UTIs, peritonitis, and pneumonia. It's also used to treat cryptococcal meningitis.
• Itraconazole is used to treat blastomycosis, nonmeningeal histoplasmosis, candidiasis, aspergillosis, and fungal nail disease.
• Voriconazole is used to treat invasive aspergillosis and serious fungal infections caused by *Scedosporium apiospermum* and *Fusarium* species.

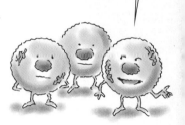

So here's how it works, guys. Synthetic triazoles either cause fungal cell walls to weaken or interfere with cell wall synthesis. Got it?

Drug interactions

Fluconazole may have these drug interactions:
• Use with warfarin may increase the risk of bleeding.
• It may increase levels of phenytoin and cyclosporine.
• It may increase the plasma concentration of oral antidiabetic drugs, such as glyburide, tolbutamide, and glipizide, increasing the risk of hypoglycemia.
• Rifampin and cimetidine enhance the metabolism of fluconazole, reducing its plasma level.
• It may increase the activity of zidovudine.

And the interactions just keep coming...

Itraconazole and voriconazole have these drug interactions:
• Both may increase the risk of bleeding when combined with oral anticoagulants.
• Antacids, H_2-receptor antagonists, phenytoin, and rifampin lower plasma itraconazole levels.
• Voriconazole may inhibit the metabolism of phenytoin, benzodiazepines, calcium channel blockers, sulfonylureas, and tacrolimus.
• Voriconazole is contraindicated with sirolimus and ergot alkaloids because voriconazole may increase plasma concentrations of these drugs.

• Voriconazole is contraindicated with quinidine and pimozide because of the risk of prolonged QT intervals and, rarely, torsades de pointes.

Adverse reactions

Adverse reactions to fluconazole and voriconazole include:
• abdominal pain
• diarrhea
• dizziness
• headache
• increase in liver enzymes
• nausea and vomiting
• rash.
  Adverse reactions to itraconazole include:
• dizziness
• headache
• hypertension
• impaired liver function
• nausea.

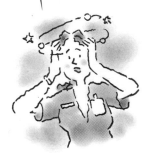

This list of adverse reactions makes me dizzy—just one of the possible side effects of synthetic triazoles.

Nursing process

These nursing process steps are appropriate for patients undergoing treatment with synthetic triazoles.

Assessment
• Assess the patient's fungal infection before therapy and regularly throughout therapy.
• Periodically monitor liver function during prolonged therapy. Although adverse hepatic effects are rare, they can be serious.
• Assess for adverse reactions and drug interactions.
• Assess the patient's and family's knowledge of drug therapy.

Key nursing diagnoses
• Risk for infection related to the underlying condition
• Risk for deficient fluid volume related to adverse GI reactions
• Deficient knowledge related to drug therapy

Planning outcome goals
• The patient's infection will resolve as evidenced by culture reports, temperature, and WBC counts.
• The patient's fluid volume will remain within normal limits as evidenced by intake and output.
• The patient and his family will demonstrate an understanding of drug therapy.

Implementation

• Don't remove protective overwraps from I.V. bags of fluconazole until just before use to ensure product sterility.
• Give by continuous infusion with an infusion pump at a rate of no more than 200 mg/hour. To prevent air embolism, don't give the drug in a series with other infusions.
• Don't add other drugs to the solution.
• If the patient develops a mild rash, monitor him closely. Stop the drug if lesions progress, and notify the prescriber.
• Monitor the patient's hydration status if adverse GI reactions occur.

Evaluation

• Patient is free from infection.
• Patient maintains adequate hydration.
• Patient and family demonstrate an understanding of drug therapy.

Glucan synthesis inhibitors

Caspofungin acetate is a drug in a class known as *glucan synthesis inhibitors* (also known as *echinocandins*). Caspofungin is primarily used when other antifungal therapies haven't been successful.

Pharmacokinetics

Given I.V., caspofungin is highly protein-bound, with little distribution into RBCs. The drug is slowly metabolized and excreted in urine and feces.

Pharmacodynamics

Caspofungin inhibits the synthesis of beta (1,3)-D-glucan, an integral component of the fungal cell wall.

Pharmacotherapeutics

Caspofungin is used to treat invasive aspergillosis in patients who have failed to respond to, or can't tolerate, other antifungals, such as amphotericin B or itraconazole. It hasn't been studied as an initial treatment for invasive aspergillosis.

Drug interactions

Caspofungin is known to cause these drug interactions:

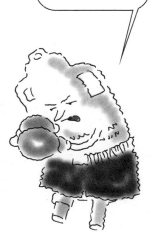

Caspofungin is called into the ring when other antifungal therapies have failed.

• Patients taking caspofungin and tacrolimus may need higher doses of tacrolimus because caspofungin decreases the blood tacrolimus level.

All clear

• Inducers of drug clearance, such as phenytoin, carbamazepine, efavirenz, nevirapine, and nelfinavir, may lower caspofungin clearance.
• Concurrent use of caspofungin and cyclosporine may result in elevated liver enzyme levels and decreased caspofungin clearance; their use together isn't recommended.

Adverse reactions

Adverse reactions to caspofungin include:
• paresthesia
• tachycardia
• tachypnea
• nausea and vomiting
• diarrhea
• rash
• facial swelling.

Nursing process

These nursing process steps are appropriate for patients undergoing treatment with glucan synthesis inhibitors.

Assessment
• Assess the patient's hepatic function before starting drug therapy.
• Observe the patient for histamine-mediated reactions (rash, facial swelling, pruritus, sensation of warmth).
• Assess the patient's and family's knowledge of drug therapy.

Key nursing diagnoses
• Risk for infection related to adverse effects of I.V. drug administration
• Ineffective health maintenance related to the underlying disease process and immunocompromised state
• Deficient knowledge related to aspergillosis infection and drug therapy

Planning outcome goals
• The patient's infection will resolve as evidenced by culture reports, temperature, and WBC counts.

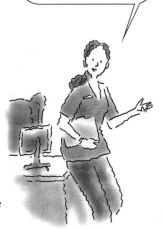

Patients taking caspofungin may experience histamine-mediated reactions, including rash, facial swelling, pruritus, and a sensation of warmth.

• The patient will maintain adequate health status throughout drug therapy.
• The patient and his family will demonstrate an understanding of drug therapy.

Implementation

• Dilute drugs as directed and administer slowly via I.V. infusion over 1 hour.
• Keep in mind that the dosage may need to be adjusted if the patient has hepatic insufficiency.
• Monitor the I.V. site carefully for phlebitis.
• Monitor the patient's laboratory test results carefully for an increase in liver function test values.

Evaluation

• Patient is free from infection.
• Patient responds positively to antifungal drug therapy.
• Patient and family demonstrate an understanding of drug therapy.

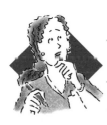

Quick quiz

1. What's an adverse reaction to aminoglycosides?
   A.   Peripheral nerve toxicity
   B.   Cardiotoxicity
   C.   Hepatic toxicity
   D.   Toxic megacolon

Answer: A. Adverse reactions to aminoglycosides include neuromuscular reactions, ranging from peripheral nerve toxicity to neuromuscular blockade, ototoxicity, and renal toxicity.

2. Which food should the patient receiving isoniazid therapy avoid?
   A.   Red wine
   B.   Chocolate
   C.   Coffee
   D.   Eggs

Answer: B. The patient taking isoniazid should avoid fish (such as tuna) and products containing tyramine (such as aged cheese, beer, and chocolate) because the drug has some monoamine oxidase inhibitor activity.

3. Which implementation step is appropriate for a patient who's taking zidovudine for an HIV infection?

    A.   Anticipate the need for dosage adjustment for impaired hepatic function.

    B.   Administer the drug every 4 hours, around the clock.

    C.   Administer one dose daily.

    D.   Monitor the patient's cardiac status.

Answer: B. Zidovudine is usually administered over 1 hour at a constant rate and is given every 4 hours around the clock.

Scoring

☆☆☆   If you answered all three questions correctly, impeccable! You're privy to the pills that pounce those pesky pathogens.

  ☆☆   If you answered two questions correctly, magnificent! Those malicious microorganisms are marked now that you're on the scene.

    ☆   If you answered fewer than two questions correctly, don't get in a funk. You'll be fluent in antifungals and all the rest before you know it.

Anti-inflammatory, antiallergy, and immunosuppressant drugs

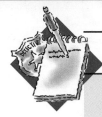

Just the facts

In this chapter, you'll learn:

♦ classes of drugs that modify immune or inflammatory responses

♦ uses and varying actions of these drugs

♦ absorption, distribution, metabolization, and excretion of these drugs

♦ drug interactions and adverse reactions to these drugs.

Drugs and the immune system

Immune and inflammatory responses protect the body from invading foreign substances. Certain classes of drugs can modify these responses:

• *Antihistamines* block the effects of histamine on target tissues.
• *Corticosteroids* suppress immune responses and reduce inflammation.
• *Immunosuppressants (noncorticosteroids)* prevent rejection of transplanted organs and can be used to treat autoimmune disease.
• *Uricosurics* control the occurrence of gouty arthritis attacks.

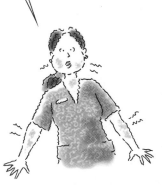

I think I need an antihistamine—right now!

Antihistamines

Antihistamines primarily act to block histamine effects that occur in an immediate (type I) hypersensitivity reaction, commonly called an *allergic reaction*. They're available alone or in combination products and may be obtained by prescription or over the counter.

Histamine-1 receptor antagonists

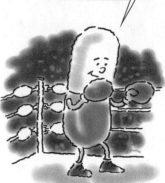

Come on, histamine! I can take you on.

The term *antihistamine* refers to drugs that act as histamine-1 (H_1) receptor antagonists; that is, they compete with histamine for H_1-receptor sites throughout the body. However, they don't displace histamines already bound to receptors.

It's all about chemistry

Antihistamines are categorized into major classes based on their chemical structures:
• *Ethanolamines* include clemastine fumarate, dimenhydrinate, and diphenhydramine hydrochloride.
• *Alkylamines* include brompheniramine, chlorpheniramine, and dexchlorpheniramine.
• *Phenothiazines* include promethazine hydrochloride.
• *Piperidines* include azatadine maleate, cetirizine, cyproheptadine hydrochloride, desloratadine, fexofenadine, loratadine, and meclizine hydrochloride.
• Miscellaneous drugs, such as hydroxyzine hydrochloride and hydroxyzine pamoate, also act as antihistamines.

Pharmacokinetics (how drugs circulate)

H_1-receptor antagonists are absorbed well after oral or parenteral administration. Some can also be given rectally. With the exception of loratadine and desloratadine, antihistamines are distributed widely throughout the body and central nervous system (CNS).

On the alert

Fexofenadine, desloratadine, and loratadine are nonsedating antihistamines. Because these drugs only minimally penetrate the blood-brain barrier, they aren't widely distributed throughout the CNS. As a result, they produce fewer sedative effects than other antihistamines.

Antihistamines are metabolized by liver enzymes and excreted in urine, with small amounts secreted in breast milk. Fexofenadine, mainly excreted in feces, is an exception. Cetirizine undergoes hepatic metabolism.

Pharmacodynamics (how drugs act)

H_1-receptor antagonists compete with histamine for H_1 receptors on effector cells (the cells that cause allergic signs and symp-

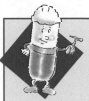

Pharm function

How chlorpheniramine stops allergic response

Although chlorpheniramine can't reverse an allergic response, it can stop its progression. Here's what happens.

Release the mediators
When sensitized to an antigen, a mast cell reacts to repeated antigen exposure by releasing chemical mediators. One of these mediators, histamine, binds to histamine-1 (H_1) receptors found on effector cells (the cells responsible for allergic signs and symptoms). This initiates the allergic response that typical-ly affects the respiratory, cardiovascular, GI, endocrine, and integumentary systems.

The first one there wins
Chlorpheniramine acts by competing with histamine for H_1 receptor sites on the effector cells. By attaching to these sites first, the drug prevents histamine from binding to the effector cells, inhibiting additional systemic responses, as shown below.

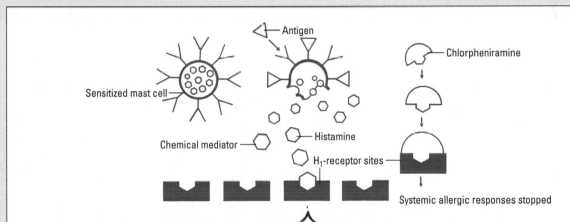

Antigen

Chlorpheniramine

Sensitized mast cell

Chemical mediator

Histamine

H_1-receptor sites

Systemic allergic responses stopped

Effector cells

Respiratory responses
• Bronchial constric-tion and broncho-spasm
• Decreased vital capacity
• Itchy nose and throat
• Rhinorrhea (runny nose)
• Sneezing

Cardiovascular responses
• Decreased blood pressure
• Elevated heart rate
• Increased vasodila-tion
• Increased capillary permeability

GI responses
• Increased parietal cell secretion
• Increased smooth-muscle contraction

Endocrine responses
• Increased release of epinephrine and norepinephrine

Integumentary responses
• Angioedema (hives and swelling of skin, mucous membranes, or internal organs)
• Flushing
• Itching

toms), blocking histamine from producing its effects. (See *How chlorpheniramine stops allergic response.*)

Antagonizing line of attack

H_1-receptor antagonists produce their effects by:
• blocking the action of histamine on small blood vessels
• decreasing arteriole dilation and tissue engorgement
• reducing leakage of plasma proteins and fluids out of the capillaries (capillary permeability), thereby lessening edema
• inhibiting most smooth-muscle responses to histamine (in particular, blocking the constriction of bronchial, GI, and vascular smooth muscle)
• relieving symptoms by acting on the terminal nerve endings in the skin that flare and itch when stimulated by histamine
• suppressing adrenal medulla stimulation, autonomic ganglia stimulation, and exocrine gland secretion, such as lacrimal and salivary secretion.

It's all in your head

Several antihistamines have a high affinity for H_1 receptors in the brain and are used for their CNS effects. These drugs include diphenhydramine, dimenhydrinate, promethazine, and various piperidine derivatives. (See *Antihistamines: Diphenhydramine.*)

H_1-receptor antagonists don't affect parietal cell secretion in the stomach because the receptors of these cells are H_2 receptors, not H_1 receptors.

Pharmacotherapeutics (how drugs are used)

Antihistamines are used to treat signs and symptoms of type I hypersensitivity reactions, such as:
• allergic rhinitis (runny nose and itchy eyes caused by a local sensitivity reaction)
• vasomotor rhinitis (rhinitis not caused by allergy or infection)
• allergic conjunctivitis (inflammation of the eye membranes)
• urticaria (hives)
• angioedema (submucosal swelling in the hands, face, and feet).

Beyond the obvious

Antihistamines have other therapeutic uses. Many are used primarily as antiemetics (to control nausea and vomiting). They can also be used as adjunctive therapy to treat an anaphylactic reaction after serious signs and symptoms are controlled. Diphenhydramine can be used to help treat Parkinson's disease and drug-induced extrapyramidal reactions (abnormal involuntary movements). Because of its antiserotonin qualities, cyproheptadine

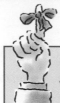

Memory jogger

Anti- is a familiar prefix that means opposing. And that's exactly what antihistamines do: they oppose histamine effects (or allergic reactions).

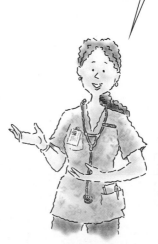

Antihistamines relieve the signs and symptoms of an allergic reaction. However, they don't give the body immunity to the allergy itself.

Prototype pro

Antihistamines: Diphenhydramine

Actions
• Competes with histamine for histamine-1 receptor sites on the smooth muscle of the bronchi, GI tract, uterus, and large blood vessels, binding to the cellular receptors and preventing access and subsequent activity of histamine
• Antagonizes the action of histamine that causes increased capillary permeability and resultant edema and suppresses flare and pruritus associated with endogenous release of histamine (doesn't directly alter histamine or prevent its release)

Indications
• Rhinitis
• Allergy symptoms
• Motion sickness
• Parkinson's disease

Nursing considerations
• Monitor for adverse effects, such as drowsiness, sedation, seizures, nausea, dry mouth, thrombocytopenia, agranulocytosis, thickening of secretions, and anaphylactic shock.
• Use with extreme caution in patients with prostatic hyperplasia, asthma, chronic obstructive pulmonary disease, hyperthyroidism, cardiovascular disease, or hypertension.

may be used to treat Cushing's disease, serotonin-associated diarrhea, vascular cluster headaches, and anorexia nervosa.

Drug interactions

Antihistamines interact with many other drugs, sometimes with life-threatening consequences. Here are a few examples:
• Antihistamines may block or reverse the vasopressor effects of epinephrine, producing vasodilation, increased heart rate, and dangerously low blood pressure.
• Antihistamines may mask toxic signs and symptoms of ototoxicity (a detrimental effect on hearing) associated with aminoglycosides or large doses of salicylates.
• Antihistamines may increase the sedative and respiratory depressant effects of CNS depressants, such as tranquilizers and alcohol.
• Loratadine may cause serious cardiac effects when taken with macrolide antibiotics (such as erythromycin), fluconazole, ketoconazole, itraconazole, miconazole, cimetidine, ciprofloxacin, and clarithromycin.

Adverse reactions

The most common adverse reaction to antihistamines (with the exception of fexofenadine, loratadine, and desloratadine) is CNS depression. Other CNS reactions include:
• dizziness
• fatigue

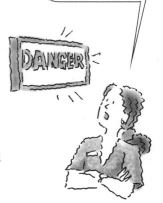

Beware of the potentially dangerous drug interactions that may occur when giving antihistamines.

- disturbed coordination
- muscle weakness.

Gut reactions

GI reactions may include:
- epigastric distress
- loss of appetite
- nausea and vomiting
- constipation
- diarrhea
- dryness of the mouth, nose, and throat.

Cardiac concerns

Cardiovascular reactions may include:
- hypotension
- hypertension
- rapid heart rate
- arrhythmias.

A sensitive issue

Sensitivity reactions can also occur.

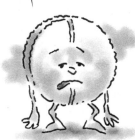

Sigh. I guess I'm just feeling a bit sensitive about the sensitivity reactions I can sometimes cause.

Nursing process

These nursing process steps are appropriate for patients undergoing treatment with antihistamines.

Assessment
- Obtain a history of the patient's underlying condition before therapy and reassess regularly thereafter.
- Monitor the patient for adverse reactions and drug interactions.
- Monitor blood counts during long-term therapy; watch for signs of blood dyscrasia.
- Evaluate the patient's and family's knowledge of drug therapy.

Key nursing diagnoses
- Ineffective health maintenance related to the underlying condition
- Risk for injury related to drug-induced adverse CNS reactions
- Deficient knowledge related to drug therapy

Planning outcome goals
- The patient will exhibit an improvement in the underlying condition.
- The risk of injury to the patient will be minimized.
- The patient and his family will demonstrate an understanding of drug therapy.

Education edge

Teaching about antihistamines

If antihistamine therapy is prescribed, review these points with the patient and his caregivers:

• Take the drug with meals or snacks to prevent GI upset.

• Drinking coffee or tea may reduce drowsiness.

• Use warm water rinses, artificial saliva, ice chips, or sugarless gum or candy to relieve dry mouth. Avoid overuse of mouthwash, which may worsen dryness and destroy normal flora.

• If you're using the medication to prevent motion sickness, take the drug 30 minutes before travel.

• Avoid hazardous activities such as driving until the full central nervous system effects of the drug are known.

• Seek medical approval before using alcohol, tranquilizers, sedatives, pain relievers, or sleeping medications.

• Stop taking antihistamines 4 days before diagnostic skin tests to preserve the accuracy of test results.

• Notify your prescriber if tolerance develops because a different antihistamine may need to be prescribed.

• Be aware that the drug may cause photosensitivity. Use sunblock or wear protective clothing.

• Avoid using other products containing diphenhydramine, including topical forms, because of the risk of adverse reactions.

Implementation

• Reduce GI distress by giving antihistamines with food.

• Follow the manufacturer's guidelines for I.V. administration.

• If administering the drug I.M., alternate injection sites to prevent irritation. Give I.M. injections into large muscles.

• Provide sugarless gum, hard candy, or ice chips to relieve dry mouth.

• Increase the patient's fluid intake (if allowed) or humidify the air to decrease thickened secretions.

• Notify the prescriber if tolerance is observed because the patient may require a substitute antihistamine.

Evaluation

• Patient shows an improvement in the underlying condition.

• Patient sustains no injury from result of therapy.

• Patient and family demonstrate an understanding of drug therapy. (See *Teaching about antihistamines*.)

Corticosteroids

Corticosteroids suppress immune responses and reduce inflammation. They're available as natural or synthetic steroids.

Nature's bounty

Natural corticosteroids are hormones produced by the adrenal cortex; most corticosteroid drugs are synthetic forms of these hormones.

Natural and synthetic corticosteroids are classified according to their biological activities:
- *Glucocorticoids*, such as cortisone acetate and dexamethasone, affect carbohydrate and protein metabolism.
- *Mineralocorticoids*, such as aldosterone and fludrocortisone acetate, regulate electrolyte and water balance.

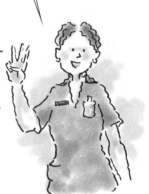

Glucocorticoids work in three ways, exerting anti-inflammatory, metabolic, and immunosuppressant effects.

Glucocorticoids

Most glucocorticoids are synthetic analogues of hormones secreted by the adrenal cortex. They exert anti-inflammatory, metabolic, and immunosuppressant effects. Drugs in this class include:
- beclomethasone
- betamethasone
- cortisone
- dexamethasone
- hydrocortisone
- methylprednisolone
- prednisolone
- prednisone
- triamcinolone.

Pharmacokinetics

Glucocorticoids are well absorbed when administered orally. After I.M. administration, they're completely absorbed.

Glucocorticoids are bound to plasma proteins and distributed through the blood. They're metabolized in the liver and excreted by the kidneys.

Pharmacodynamics

Glucocorticoids suppress hypersensitivity and immune responses through a process that isn't entirely understood.

The research suggests...

Researchers believe that glucocorticoids inhibit immune responses by:
- suppressing or preventing cell-mediated immune reactions
- reducing levels of leukocytes, monocytes, and eosinophils
- decreasing the binding of immunoglobulins to cell surface receptors
- inhibiting interleukin synthesis.

Oh so soothing

Glucocorticoids suppress the redness, edema, heat, and tenderness associated with the inflammatory response. They start on the cellular level by stabilizing the lysosomal membrane (a structure within the cell that contains digestive enzymes) so that it doesn't release its store of hydrolytic enzymes into the cells. (See *Corticosteroids: Prednisone.*)

A job well done

Glucocorticoids prevent leakage of plasma from capillaries, suppress the migration of polymorphonuclear leukocytes (cells that kill and digest microorganisms), and inhibit phagocytosis (cellular ingestion and destruction of solid substances).

To ensure a job well done, glucocorticoids decrease antibody formation in injured or infected tissues and disrupt histamine synthesis, fibroblast development, collagen deposition, capillary dilation, and capillary permeability. (See *How methylprednisolone works*, page 582.)

Pharmacotherapeutics

Glucocorticoids are used as replacement therapy for patients with adrenocortical insufficiency. They're also prescribed for immunosuppression (such as in allergic reactions) and disorders requiring treatment by reduction of inflammation (such as arthritis). They're also prescribed for their effects on the blood and lymphatic systems.

Drug interactions

These drug interactions can occur with glucocorticoids:
• Barbiturates, phenytoin, rifampin, and aminoglutethimide may reduce the effects of glucocorticoids.
• Amphotericin B, chlorthalidone, ethacrynic acid, furosemide, and thiazide diuretics may enhance glucocorticoids' potassium-wasting effects.
• Erythromycin and troleandomycin may increase the effects of glucocorticoids by reducing their metabolism.
• Glucocorticoids reduce the serum concentration and effects of salicylates.
• The risk of peptic ulcers associated with nonsteroidal anti-inflammatory drugs and salicylates is increased when these agents are taken with corticosteroids.
• The response to vaccines and toxoids may be reduced in a patient taking glucocorticoids.
• Estrogen and hormonal contraceptives that contain estrogen increase the effects of glucocorticoids.

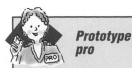

Prototype pro

Corticosteroids: Prednisone

Actions
• Decreases inflammation by stabilizing leukocyte lysosomal membranes, suppressing immune response, stimulating bone marrow, and influencing protein, fat, and carbohydrate metabolism

Indications
• Severe inflammation
• Immunosuppression

Nursing considerations
• Monitor for adverse effects, such as euphoria, insomnia, heart failure, thromboembolism, peptic ulcers, and acute adrenal insufficiency.
• Monitor for cushingoid effects, such as moon face, buffalo hump, central obesity, thinning hair, and increased susceptibility to infection.
• Monitor the patient's weight, blood pressure, and serum electrolytes.
• The drug may mask signs of infection.
• The dosage must be gradually reduced after long-term therapy.

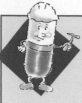

Pharm function

How methylprednisolone works

Tissue trauma normally leads to tissue irritation, edema, inflammation, and production of scar tissue. Methylprednisolone counteracts the initial effects of tissue trauma, promoting healing.

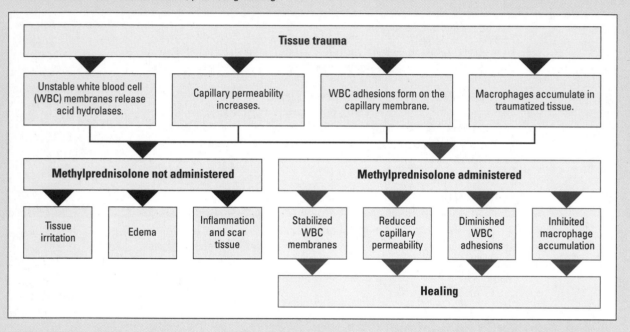

• The effects of antidiabetic drugs may be reduced, resulting in increased blood glucose levels.

Adverse reactions

Glucocorticoids affect almost all body systems. Their widespread adverse effects include:
• insomnia
• increased sodium and water retention
• increased potassium excretion
• suppressed immune and inflammatory responses
• osteoporosis
• intestinal perforation
• peptic ulcers
• impaired wound healing.

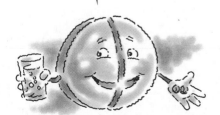

Glucocorticoids affect almost all body systems. You might say we're all-inclusive.

Endocrine system

Endocrine system reactions may include:
- diabetes mellitus
- hyperlipidemia
- adrenal atrophy
- hypothalamic-pituitary axis suppression
- cushingoid signs and symptoms (such as buffalo hump, moon face, and elevated blood glucose levels).

Nursing process

These nursing process steps are appropriate for patients undergoing treatment with glucocorticoids.

Assessment

- Assess the patient's condition before therapy and regularly thereafter.
- Establish baseline blood pressure, fluid and electrolyte status, and weight; reassess regularly.
- Watch for depression or psychotic episodes, especially at high dosages.
- Monitor the glucose levels of a patient with diabetes closely; increased insulin may be needed.
- Monitor the patient's stress level; dosage adjustment may be needed.
- Closely monitor the patient for adverse reactions and drug interactions.
- Evaluate the drug's effectiveness at regular intervals.
- Evaluate the patient's and family's knowledge of drug therapy.

Key nursing diagnoses

- Ineffective protection related to drug-induced adverse reactions
- Risk for infection related to immunosuppression
- Deficient knowledge related to drug therapy

Planning outcome goals

- The patient won't experience adverse reactions.
- The patient will be free from infection as evidenced by normal temperature, cultures, and white blood cell (WBC) counts.
- The patient and his family will demonstrate an understanding of drug therapy.

Implementation

- Give the drug early in the day to mimic circadian rhythm.
- Give the drug with food to prevent GI irritation.
- Take precautions to avoid exposing the patient to infection.

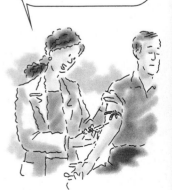

Glucocorticoids can reduce the effects of antidiabetic drugs. Monitor glucose levels of a patient with diabetes closely.

• Expect to increase the drug dosage during times of physiologic stress, such as surgery, trauma, or infection.
• Don't stop the drug abruptly. (See *Pitfalls of abrupt withdrawal.*)
• Avoid prolonged use of corticosteroids, especially in children.
• Notify the prescriber of severe or persistent adverse reactions.

Please pass the potassium...

• Unless contraindicated, offer a low-sodium diet that's high in potassium and protein. Administer potassium supplements as needed.

Evaluation

• Patient shows no evidence of adrenal insufficiency.
• Patient is free from infection.
• Patient and family demonstrate an understanding of drug therapy. (See *Teaching about corticosteroid therapy.*)

Mineralocorticoids

Mineralocorticoids affect electrolyte and water balance. One mineralocorticoid is fludrocortisone acetate, a synthetic analogue of hormones secreted by the adrenal cortex.

Pharmacokinetics

Fludrocortisone acetate is absorbed well and distributed to all parts of the body. It's metabolized in the liver to inactive metabolites and excreted by the kidneys.

Pharmacodynamics

Fludrocortisone acetate affects fluid and electrolyte balance by acting on the distal renal tubule to increase sodium reabsorption and potassium and hydrogen secretion.

Pharmacotherapeutics

Fludrocortisone acetate is used as replacement therapy for patients with adrenocortical insufficiency (reduced secretion of glucocorticoids, mineralocorticoids, and androgens).

Keeping things in balance

Fludrocortisone acetate may also be used to treat salt-losing congenital adrenogenital syndrome (characterized by a lack of cortisol and deficient aldosterone production) after the patient's electrolyte balance has been restored.

Pitfalls of abrupt withdrawal

If corticosteroids are rapidly withdrawn, abrupt withdrawal signs and symptoms can occur. These include rebound inflammation, fatigue, weakness, arthralgia, fever, dizziness, lethargy, depression, fainting, orthostatic hypotension, dyspnea, anorexia, and hypoglycemia. After long-term therapy, increased stress or abrupt withdrawal may cause acute adrenal insufficiency. Sudden withdrawal after prolonged therapy can be fatal.

Education edge

Teaching about corticosteroid therapy

If corticosteroid therapy is prescribed, review these points with the patient and his caregivers:

• Take the drug exactly as prescribed, and never stop the drug suddenly. If you miss a dose, don't double the next dose. Continue with your regular dosing schedule and follow up with your prescriber. Missed doses or suddenly stopping the drug may result in complications (especially if you're on long-term corticosteroid therapy). It's important to notify your prescriber of a change in your regular dosing schedule.

• Notify your prescriber if your stress level increases; the dosage may need to be temporarily adjusted.

• Take the oral form of the drug with food.

• Report sudden weight gain, swelling, slow healing, black tarry stools, bleeding, bruising, blurred vision, emotional changes, or other unusual effects.

• If receiving long-term therapy, ask your prescriber about vitamin D or calcium supplements and have periodic eye examinations.

• Wear or carry medical identification at all times indicating the need for systemic glucocorticoids during stress.

• If receiving long-term therapy, watch for cushingoid signs and symptoms (weight gain, swelling of the face) and report them immediately.

• Be aware of early signs and symptoms of adrenal insufficiency, including fatigue, muscular weakness, joint pain, fever, anorexia, nausea, dyspnea, dizziness, and fainting.

• Keep regular medical checkups to help detect early adverse reactions, evaluate disease status, and assess drug response. Dosage adjustments may be needed.

• Don't take other medications, over-the-counter preparations, or herbal remedies without first consulting your prescriber.

• Ask your physician about activity or exercise needed to help prevent or delay osteoporosis, a common adverse reaction.

• Report signs and symptoms of infection to your prescriber.

Drug interactions

The drug interactions associated with mineralocorticoids are similar to those associated with glucocorticoids.

Adverse reactions

The adverse reactions associated with mineralocorticoids are similar to those associated with glucocorticoids.

Nursing process

These nursing process steps are appropriate for patients undergoing treatment with mineralocorticoids.

Assessment

• Assess the patient's condition before therapy and regularly thereafter.

• Establish baseline blood pressure, fluid and electrolyte status, and weight; reassess regularly.

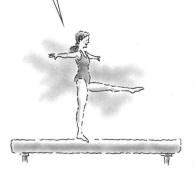

After a patient's electrolyte balance has been restored, fludrocortisone acetate may be used to treat salt-losing congenital adrenogenital syndrome.

- Monitor the patient closely for adverse reactions and drug interactions.
- Evaluate the drug's effectiveness at regular intervals.
- Evaluate the patient's and family's knowledge of drug therapy.

Key nursing diagnoses

- Risk for injury related to drug-induced adverse reactions
- Excess fluid volume related to drug-induced adverse effects
- Deficient knowledge related to drug therapy

Planning outcome goals

- The patient won't experience adverse reactions.
- The patient's fluid volume status will remain within normal limits as evidenced by intake and output and vital signs.
- The patient and his family will demonstrate an understanding of drug therapy.

Implementation

- Administer the drug as prescribed, and monitor for adverse reactions and drug interactions.
- Notify the prescriber of severe or persistent adverse reactions.
- Notify the prescriber if hypertension occurs.
- Monitor the patient's electrolyte levels; potassium supplements may be needed. Assess for indications of hypokalemia, such as muscle cramps and electrocardiogram changes.

Evaluation

- Patient's health is improved.
- Patient doesn't develop sodium and water insufficiency.
- Patient and family demonstrate an understanding of drug therapy.

Immunosuppressants

Several drugs used for their immunosuppressant effects in patients undergoing allograft transplantation (a transplant between two people who aren't identical twins) are also used experimentally to treat autoimmune diseases (diseases resulting from an inappropriate immune response directed against the self). They include:

- anakinra
- azathioprine
- basiliximab
- cyclosporine
- daclizumab

- lymphocyte immune globulin (ATG [equine])
- muromonab-CD3
- mycophenolate mofetil
- sirolimus
- tacrolimus
- thymoglobulin (antithymocyte globulin [rabbit]).

Pharmacokinetics

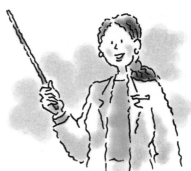

Immunosuppressants take different paths through the body:
- When administered orally, azathioprine is absorbed readily from the GI tract, whereas absorption of cyclosporine and sirolimus is varied and incomplete.
- ATG, muromonab-CD3, anakinra, basiliximab, daclizumab, and thymoglobulin are administered only by I.V. injection.
- The distributions of azathioprine, daclizumab, and basiliximab aren't fully understood.
- Cyclosporine and muromonab-CD3 are distributed widely throughout the body.
- Azathioprine and cyclosporine cross the placental barrier.
- The distribution of ATG isn't clear, but it may be distributed to breast milk.
- Distribution of tacrolimus depends on several factors, with 75% to 99% being protein bound. Sirolimus is 97% protein bound.

How it all adds up...

Azathioprine and cyclosporine are metabolized in the liver. Muromonab-CD3 is consumed by T cells circulating in the blood. The metabolism of ATG is unknown. Mycophenolate is metabolized in the liver to mycophenolate acid, an active metabolite, and then further metabolized to an inactive metabolite, which is excreted in urine and bile. The mycophenolate concenration may be increased in the presence of nephrotoxicity.

...and out

Azathioprine, anakinra, and ATG are excreted in urine; cyclosporine is excreted principally in bile. The excretion route of muromonab-CD3 is unknown. Tacrolimus is extensively metabolized and primarily excreted in bile; less than 1% is excreted unchanged in urine. Sirolimus is metabolized by a mixed function oxidase system, primarily cytochrome P450 3A4; 91% is excreted in feces and 2.2% in urine. Metabolism and excretion of basiliximab and daclizumab isn't understood.

Pharmacodynamics

It's unknown how certain immunosuppressants achieve their desired effects.

The jury's still out...

For example, the exact mechanisms of action of azathioprine, cyclosporine, and ATG are unknown; however, these drugs may undergo these processes:

• Azathioprine antagonizes the metabolism of the amino acid purine and, therefore, inhibits ribonucleic acid and deoxyribonucleic acid structure and synthesis. It may also inhibit coenzyme formation and function.

• Cyclosporine is thought to inhibit helper T cells and suppressor T cells.

• ATG may eliminate antigen-reactive T cells in the blood, alter T-cell function, or both.

...but this much is known

In a patient receiving a kidney allograft, azathioprine suppresses cell-mediated hypersensitivity reactions and produces various alterations in antibody production. Muromonab-CD3, a monoclonal antibody, is understood to block T cells' function.

Anakinra, basiliximab, and daclizumab block the activity of interleukin. Mycophenolate inhibits responses of T- and B-lymphocytes, suppresses antibody formation by B-lymphocytes, and may inhibit the recruitment of leukocytes into sites of inflammation and graft rejection. Sirolimus is an immunosuppressant that inhibits T-lymphocyte activation and proliferation that occurs in response to antigenic and cytokine stimulation; it also inhibits antibody formation.

Pharmacotherapeutics

Immunosuppressants are mainly used to prevent rejection in patients undergoing organ transplantation.

Crusader against cancer

Cyclophosphamide, classified as an alkylating drug, is primarily used to treat cancer. However, it can also be used as an immunosuppressant.

Anakinra is indicated for adults with moderate to severely active rheumatoid arthritis who have taken at least one disease-modifying antirheumatic drug.

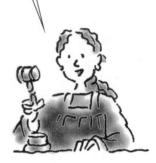

In my judgment, the jury's still out on the exact mechanism of action of several immunosuppressants. But let's hear from my colleagues below about their involvement...

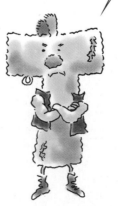

I'd say we're definitely involved in the action...

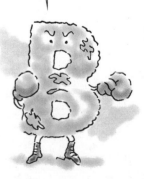

Absolutely! Like that mycophenolate. It's always trying to inhibit our responses, no matter what kind of fight I put up!

Drug interactions

Drug interactions with this class commonly involve other immunosuppressant and anti-inflammatory drugs or various antibiotic and antimicrobial drugs:

• Allopurinol increases the blood levels of azathioprine.
• Verapamil increases the blood levels of sirolimus.
• Levels of cyclosporine may be increased by ketoconazole, calcium channel blockers, cimetidine, anabolic steroids, hormonal contraceptives, erythromycin, and metoclopramide.
• Coadministration of voriconazole and sirolimus is contraindicated because of the inhibition of cytochrome P450 3A4 enzymes by voriconazole, which increase sirolimus levels.
• The absorption of mycophenolate is decreased when taken with antacids or cholestyramine. Coadministration of mycophenolate with acyclovir may increase concentrations of both drugs, especially in a patient with renal impairment.

Kidney concerns

• The risk of toxicity to the kidneys increases when cyclosporine is taken with acyclovir, aminoglycosides, or amphotericin B.
• The risk of infection and lymphoma (neoplasm of the lymph tissue, most likely malignant) is increased when cyclosporine or sirolimus is taken with other immunosuppressants (except corticosteroids).
• Barbiturates, rifampin, phenytoin, sulfonamides, and trimethoprim decrease plasma cyclosporine and sirolimus levels.
• Serum digoxin levels may be increased when cyclosporine is taken with digoxin.
• Taking ATG, muromonab-CD3, anakinra, basiliximab, daclizumab, and thymoglobulin with other immunosuppressant drugs increases the risk of infection and lymphoma. Anakinra therapy shouldn't be initiated in a patient with an active infection or neutropenia.

Adverse reactions

All immunosuppressants can cause hypersensitivity reactions. Listed here are adverse reactions to individual drugs.

Azathioprine

Adverse reactions to azathioprine include:
• bone marrow suppression
• nausea and vomiting
• liver toxicity.

Cyclosporine

Adverse reactions to cyclosporine include:

- kidney toxicity
- hyperkalemia
- infection
- liver toxicity
- nausea and vomiting.

Daclizumab

Adverse reactions to daclizumab include:

- GI disorders
- hypertension or hypotension
- chest pain
- tachycardia
- edema
- dyspnea
- pulmonary edema
- thrombosis
- bleeding
- renal tubular necrosis.

ATG and thymoglobulin

Adverse reactions to ATG and thymoglobulin include:

- fever
- chills
- reduced WBC or platelet count
- infection
- nausea and vomiting.
    Additional adverse reactions to thymoglobulin include:
- headache
- abdominal pain
- diarrhea
- dyspnea
- systemic infections
- dizziness.

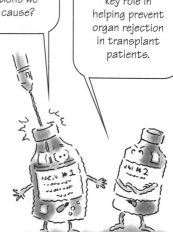

Wait! What about all these adverse reactions we can cause?

Come on! You know we play a key role in helping prevent organ rejection in transplant patients.

Muromonab-CD3

Adverse reactions to muromonab-CD3 include:

- fever
- chills
- nausea and vomiting
- tremors
- pulmonary edema
- infection.

Mycophenolate

Adverse reactions to mycophenolate include:

- nausea
- diarrhea
- leukopenia
- headache
- tremors
- weakness
- chest pain
- urinary tract infection
- liver function test abnormalities
- skin rash.

Sirolimus

Adverse reactions to sirolimus include:

- tremors
- anemia
- leukopenia
- thrombocytopenia
- hyperlipidemia
- hypertension
- arthralgia
- myalgia
- urinary frequency.

Tacrolimus

Adverse reactions to tacrolimus include:

- nausea and vomiting
- diarrhea or constipation
- tremors
- leukopenia
- hypertension
- nephrotoxicity
- hepatotoxicity.

Nursing process

These nursing process steps are appropriate for patients undergoing treatment with immunosuppressants.

Assessment

- Obtain a history of the patient's immune status before therapy.
- Monitor the drug's effectiveness by observing the patient for signs of organ rejection. Therapeutic response usually occurs within 8 weeks.
- Watch for adverse reactions and drug interactions.

• Monitor hemoglobin, hematocrit, and WBC and platelet counts at least once monthly; monitor them more often at the beginning of treatment.
• Evaluate the patient's and family's knowledge of drug therapy.

Key nursing diagnoses
• Ineffective protection related to threat of organ rejection
• Risk for infection related to drug-induced immunosuppression
• Deficient knowledge related to drug therapy

Planning outcome goals
• The patient's vital signs will be within normal limits and assessment findings will be normal.
• The patient will show no signs of infection as evidenced by normal WBC and temperature and negative culture results.
• The patient and his family will demonstrate an understanding of drug therapy.

Implementation
• Administer the medication as prescribed; reconstitute according to policy and procedure.
• Monitor the patient's reaction to the medication and watch for adverse reactions.
• Monitor WBC counts; the medication may need to be stopped if the patient's WBC count is less than 3,000/mm^3. Notify the prescriber.
• To prevent bleeding, avoid I.M. injections when the patient's platelet count is below 100,000/mm^3.

You give me fever...

• Monitor the patient for signs of infection and report fever, sore throat, and malaise because the drug is a potent immunosuppressant.
• Instruct a female patient to avoid conception during therapy and for 4 months after stopping therapy.
• Warn the patient that hair thinning may occur.
• Tell the patient that medication can take up to 12 weeks to be effective.

Evaluation
• Patient exhibits no signs of organ rejection.
• Patient demonstrates no signs and symptoms of infection.
• Patient and family demonstrate an understanding of drug therapy.

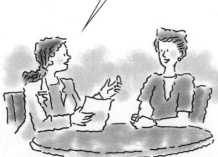

You shouldn't become pregnant while taking immunosuppressant drugs and for 4 months after stopping therapy.

Uricosurics

Uricosurics and other antigout drugs exert their anti-inflammatory actions through their effects on uric acid. Increased uric acid in the blood (hyperuricemia) results in gout, a specific form of acute arthritis.

Uricosuric drugs

The two major uricosurics are probenecid and sulfinpyrazone.

Out with the gout

Uricosurics act by increasing uric acid excretion in urine. The primary goal in using uricosurics is to prevent or control the frequency of gouty arthritis attacks.

Pharmacokinetics

Uricosurics are absorbed from the GI tract. Distribution of the two drugs is similar, with 75% to 95% of probenecid and 98% of sulfinpyrazone being protein bound. Metabolism of the drugs occurs in the liver, and excretion occurs primarily through the kidneys. Only small amounts of these drugs are excreted in feces.

Pharmacodynamics

Probenecid and sulfinpyrazone reduce the reabsorption of uric acid at the proximal convoluted tubules of the kidneys. This results in excretion of uric acid in urine, reducing serum urate levels.

Pharmacotherapeutics

Probenecid and sulfinpyrazone are indicated for the treatment of:
• chronic gouty arthritis
• tophaceous gout (the deposition of tophi or urate crystals under the skin and into joints).

Outbound action

Probenecid is also used to promote uric acid excretion in patients experiencing hyperuricemia.

When acute, substitute

Probenecid and sulfinpyrazone shouldn't be given during an acute gouty attack. If taken at that time, these drugs prolong inflammation. Because these drugs may increase the chance of an acute gouty attack when therapy begins and whenever the serum urate level changes rapidly, colchicine is administered during the first 3 to 6 months of therapy.

Drug interactions

Many drug interactions, some potentially serious, can occur with uricosuric drugs:
• Probenecid can significantly increase and prolong the effects of cephalosporins, penicillins, and sulfonamides.
• Serum urate levels may be increased when probenecid is taken with antineoplastic drugs.

Kicking up concentrations

• Probenecid increases the serum concentration of dapsone, aminosalicylic acid, and methotrexate, causing toxic reactions.
• Sulfinpyrazone increases the effectiveness of warfarin, increasing the risk of bleeding.
• Salicylates reduce the effects of sulfinpyrazone.
• Sulfinpyrazone may increase the effects of oral antidiabetic agents, increasing the risk of hypoglycemia.

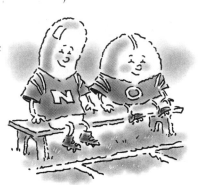

During an acute gouty attack, probenecid and sulfinpyrazone shouldn't be "in the game" because they can prolong inflammation and the duration of the attack.

Adverse reactions

Adverse reactions to uricosurics include uric acid stone formation and blood abnormalities.

Probenecid

Additional adverse reactions to probenecid include:
• headache
• anorexia
• nausea and vomiting
• hypersensitivity reactions.

Sulfinpyrazone

Additional adverse reactions to sulfinpyrazone include:
• nausea
• indigestion
• GI pain
• GI blood loss.

Nursing process

These nursing process steps are appropriate for patients undergoing treatment with uricosurics.

Assessment

- Assess the patient's condition before therapy and regularly thereafter.
- Periodically monitor blood urea nitrogen levels and renal function tests in long-term therapy. Note that the drug is ineffective in patients with chronic renal insufficiency (glomerular filtration rate of less than 30 ml/minute).
- Be alert for adverse reactions and drug interactions.
- Monitor the patient's hydration status if adverse GI reactions occur.
- Evaluate the patient's and family's knowledge of drug therapy.

Key nursing diagnoses

- Ineffective health maintenance related to the underlying condition
- Risk for deficient fluid volume related to adverse GI reactions
- Deficient knowledge related to drug therapy

Planning outcome goals

- Assessment parameters will be within normal limits.
- The patient will exhibit adequate hydration as demonstrated by intake and output.
- The patient and his family will demonstrate an understanding of drug therapy.

Implementation

- Give the medication with milk, food, or antacids to minimize GI distress. Continued disturbances may indicate a need to lower the dosage.

Drink up!

- Encourage the patient to drink fluids to maintain a minimum daily output of 2 L of water per day. Sodium bicarbonate or potassium citrate may be needed to alkalinize urine. These measures prevent hematuria, renal colic, urate stone development, and costovertebral pain.
- Begin therapy when an acute attack subsides. Keep in mind that the drug contains no analgesic or anti-inflammatory agents and isn't useful during acute gout attacks.
- Be aware that the drug may increase the frequency, severity, and duration of acute gout attacks during the first 12 months of therapy. Prophylactic colchicine or another anti-inflammatory is given during the first 3 to 6 months.
- Instruct the patient to avoid drugs that contain aspirin, which may precipitate gout.

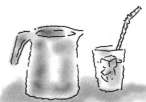

• Tell the patient to avoid alcohol during drug therapy because it increases the urate level.
• Advise the patient to limit intake of foods high in purine, such as anchovies, liver, sardines, kidneys, sweetbreads, peas, and lentils.

Evaluation

• Patient responds positively to therapy.
• Patient maintains adequate hydration.
• Patient and family demonstrate an understanding of drug therapy.

Other antigout drugs

Other antigout drugs include allopurinol and colchicine. Allopurinol is used to reduce uric acid production, preventing gouty attacks, and colchicine is used to treat acute gouty attacks.

Pharmacokinetics

Allopurinol and colchicine take somewhat different paths through the body.

All aboard allopurinol

When given orally, allopurinol is absorbed from the GI tract. Allopurinol and its metabolite oxypurinol are widely distributed throughout the body except in the brain, where drug concentrations are less than those found in the rest of the body. It's metabolized by the liver and excreted in urine.

"Tracting" colchicine's course

Colchicine is also absorbed from the GI tract. It's partially metabolized in the liver. The drug and its metabolites then reenter the intestinal tract through biliary secretions. After reabsorption from the intestines, colchicine is distributed to various tissues. The drug is excreted primarily in feces and to a lesser degree in urine.

Pharmacodynamics

Allopurinol and its metabolite oxypurinol inhibit xanthine oxidase, the enzyme responsible for the production of uric acid. By reducing uric acid formation, allopurinol eliminates the hazards of hyperuricosuria.

WBCs, don't go there!

Colchicine appears to reduce the inflammatory response to monosodium urate crystals deposited in joint tissues. Colchicine

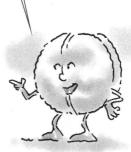

Other antigout drugs include allopurinol and colchicine.

may produce its effects by inhibiting migration of WBCs to the inflamed joint. This reduces phagocytosis and lactic acid production by WBCs, decreasing urate crystal deposits and reducing inflammation.

Pharmacotherapeutics

Allopurinol treats primary gout, hopefully preventing acute gouty attacks. It can be prescribed with uricosurics when smaller dosages of each drug are directed. It's used to:
• treat gout or hyperuricemia that may occur with blood abnormalities and during treatment of tumors or leukemia
• treat primary or secondary uric acid nephropathy (with or without the accompanying signs and symptoms of gout)
• treat and prevent recurrent uric acid stone formation
• treat patients who respond poorly to maximum dosages of uricosurics or who have allergic reactions or intolerance to uricosurics.

What a relief!

Colchicine is used to relieve the inflammation of acute gouty arthritis attacks. If given promptly, it's especially effective in relieving pain. Also, giving colchicine during the first several months of allopurinol, probenecid, or sulfinpyrazone therapy may prevent the acute gouty attacks that sometimes accompany the use of these drugs.

Drug interactions

Colchicine doesn't interact significantly with other drugs. When allopurinol is used with other drugs, the resulting interactions can be serious:
• Allopurinol potentiates the effects of oral anticoagulants.
• Allopurinol increases the serum concentrations of mercaptopurine and azathioprine, increasing the risk of toxicity.
• Angiotensin-converting enzyme inhibitors increase the risk of hypersensitivity reactions to allopurinol.
• Allopurinol increases serum theophylline levels.
• The risk of bone marrow depression increases when cyclophosphamide is taken with allopurinol.

Adverse reactions

The most common adverse reaction to allopurinol is a rash. Prolonged administration of colchicine may cause bone marrow suppression.
Allopurinol and colchicine commonly cause:

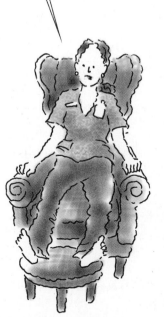

Colchicine relieves the inflammation of acute gouty arthritis attacks. Now, that feels better!

• nausea and vomiting
• diarrhea
• intermittent abdominal pain.

Nursing process

These nursing process steps are appropriate for patients undergoing treatment with other antigout drugs.

Assessment

• Assess the patient's condition before therapy and regularly thereafter.

Worth the wait

• Assess the patient's uric acid level, joint stiffness, and pain before and during therapy. Optimal benefits may require 2 to 6 weeks of therapy.
• Monitor the patient's complete blood count and hepatic and renal function at the start of therapy and periodically during therapy.
• Be alert for adverse reactions and drug interactions.
• Monitor the patient's fluid intake and output. Daily urine output of at least 2 L and maintenance of neutral or slightly alkaline urine are desirable.
• Evaluate the patient's and family's knowledge of drug therapy.

Key nursing diagnoses

• Acute pain related to the underlying condition
• Risk for infection related to drug-induced agranulocytosis
• Deficient knowledge related to drug therapy

Planning outcome goals

• The patient will state that pain is decreased.
• The patient will show no signs and symptoms of infection.
• The patient and his family will demonstrate an understanding of drug therapy.

Implementation

• Give the medication with meals or immediately after to minimize GI distress.
• Encourage the patient to drink fluids while taking the drug unless contraindicated.
• Notify the prescriber if renal insufficiency occurs during treatment; this usually warrants a dosage reduction.

• Give colchicine with allopurinol if ordered. This combination prophylactically treats acute gout attacks that may occur in the first 6 weeks of therapy.
• Advise the patient to refrain from driving or performing hazardous tasks requiring mental alertness until the CNS effects of the drug are known.
• Advise the patient taking allopurinol for treatment of recurrent calcium oxalate stones to reduce intake of animal protein, sodium, refined sugars, oxalate-rich foods, and calcium.
• Stop the drug at the first sign of a rash, which may precede a severe hypersensitivity or another adverse reaction. A rash is more common in patients taking diuretics and those with renal disorders. Tell the patient to report all adverse reactions immediately.
• Tell the patient to avoid alcohol during drug therapy because it increases the urate level.

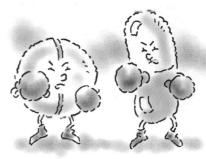

Give colchicine with allopurinol for a 1-2 punch against gout.

Evaluation

• Patient expresses relief from joint pain.
• Patient is free from infection.
• Patient and family demonstrate an understanding of drug therapy.

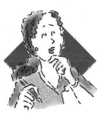

Quick quiz

1. During the nursing assessment, the patient states that he's taking digoxin, furosemide, a tranquilizer, and amoxicillin. Which medication would cause a drug interaction with the antihistamine the practitioner prescribed?

    A.   Digoxin
    B.   Furosemide
    C.   Tranquilizer
    D.   Amoxicillin

Answer: C. Antihistamines can interact with many drugs, sometimes with life-threatening consequences. They may increase the sedative and respiratory depressant effects of CNS depressants, such as tranquilizers and alcohol.

2. The nurse is monitoring a patient receiving prednisone. For which adverse reaction should the nurse monitor the patient?

    A.   Somnolence
    B.   Hyperglycemia
    C.   Hyperkalemia
    D.   Hypoglycemia

Answer: B. Corticosteroids affect almost all body systems. Endocrine system reactions may include decreased glucose tolerance, resulting in hyperglycemia and possibly precipitating diabetes mellitus.

3. Which medication interacts with allopurinol?
   A. Oral anticoagulants
   B. Antihistamines
   C. Cardiac glycosides
   D. Antidiabetic agents

Answer: A. Allopurinol potentiates the effects of oral anticoagulants.

Scoring

☆☆☆ If you answered all three questions correctly, extraordinary! You certainly aren't allergic to smarts!

☆☆ If you answered two questions correctly, congratulations! You're taking the sting out of learning!

☆ If you answered fewer than two questions correctly, keep trying! With continued improvement, the next chapter should have you feeling better!

Antineoplastic drugs

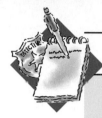

Just the facts

In this chapter, you'll learn:

♦ classes of drugs used to treat cancer

♦ uses and varying actions of these drugs

♦ absorption, distribution, metabolization, and excretion of these drugs

♦ drug interactions and adverse reactions to these drugs.

Drugs and cancer

In the 1940s, antineoplastic (chemotherapeutic) drugs were developed to treat cancer. However, these agents commonly caused serious adverse reactions.

A change for the better

Today, many of these drugs have lower toxicity levels so they aren't as devastating to the patient. With modern chemotherapy, childhood malignancies such as acute lymphoblastic leukemia and adult cancers such as testicular cancer are curable in most cases. Novel therapeutic strategies, such as using monoclonal antibodies or targeting specific proteins, are further improving the time that a patient's cancer can remain in remission. In addition, other drugs such as interferons are being used to treat patients with cancer. Specific types of antineoplastic agents include:

• alkylating drugs
• antimetabolite drugs
• antibiotic antineoplastic drugs
• hormonal antineoplastic drugs and hormone modulators
• natural antineoplastic drugs
• monoclonal antibodies
• topoisomerase I inhibitors
• targeted therapies
• unclassified antineoplastic drugs.

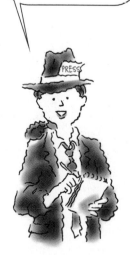

Newsflash! Antineoplastic drugs were developed to treat cancer in the 1940s.

Alkylating drugs

Alkylating drugs, either given alone or with other drugs, effectively act against various malignant neoplasms. These drugs are categorized into one of six classes:
- nitrogen mustards
- alkyl sulfonates
- nitrosoureas
- triazenes
- ethylenimines
- alkylating-like drugs.

Unfazed at any phase

Alkylating drugs produce their antineoplastic effects by damaging deoxyribonucleic acid (DNA). They halt DNA's replication process by cross-linking its strands so that amino acids don't pair up correctly. Alkylating drugs are cell cycle–phase nonspecific. This means that their alkylating actions may take place at any phase of the cell cycle.

Nitrogen mustards

Nitrogen mustards represent the largest group of alkylating drugs. They include:
- chlorambucil
- cyclophosphamide
- estramustine
- ifosfamide
- mechlorethamine hydrochloride
- melphalan.

The opening act

Mechlorethamine hydrochloride was the first nitrogen mustard introduced and is rapid acting.

Pharmacokinetics (how drugs circulate)

As with most alkylating drugs, the absorption and distribution of nitrogen mustards vary widely. Nitrogen mustards are metabolized in the liver and excreted by the kidneys.

Before you can say 1-2-3

Mechlorethamine undergoes metabolism so rapidly that, after a few minutes, no active drug remains. Most nitrogen mustards possess more intermediate half-lives than mechlorethamine.

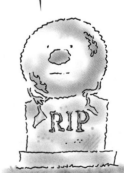

Alkylating drugs deactivate my DNA, cutting my life short.

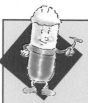

Pharm function

How alkylating drugs work

Alkylating drugs can attack deoxyribonucleic acid (DNA) in two ways, as shown in the illustrations below.

Bifunctional alkylation
Some drugs become inserted between two base pairs in the DNA chain, forming an irreversible bond between them. This is called *bifunctional alkylation,* which causes cytotoxic effects capable of destroying or poisoning cells.

Monofunctional alkylation
Other drugs react with just one part of a pair, separating it from its partner and eventually causing it and its attached sugar to break away from the DNA molecule. This is called *monofunctional alkylation,* which eventually may cause permanent cell damage.

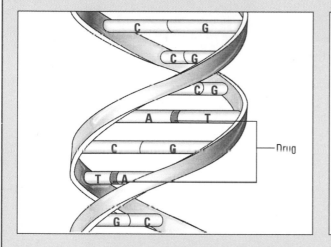

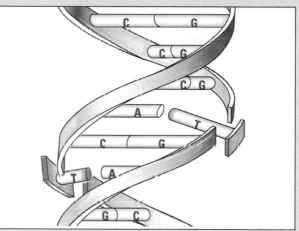

Pharmacodynamics (how drugs act)

Nitrogen mustards form covalent bonds with DNA molecules in a chemical reaction known as alkylation. Alkylated DNA can't replicate properly, thereby resulting in cell death. Unfortunately, cells may develop resistance to the cytotoxic effects of nitrogen mustards. (See *How alkylating drugs work.*)

Pharmacotherapeutics (how drugs are used)

Because they produce leukopenia (a reduced number of white blood cells [WBCs]), nitrogen mustards are effective in treating malignant neoplasms, such as Hodgkin's disease (cancer that causes painless enlargement of the lymph nodes, spleen, and lymphoid tissues) and leukemia (cancer of the blood-forming tissues), that can have an associated elevated WBC count.

Nitrogen bomb

Nitrogen mustards also prove effective against malignant lymphoma (cancer of the lymphoid tissue), multiple myeloma (cancer of the marrow plasma cells), melanoma (malignancy that arises from melanocytes), and cancer of the breast, ovaries, uterus, lung, brain, testes, bladder, prostate, and stomach.

Drug interactions

Nitrogen mustards interact with several other drugs:
• Calcium-containing drugs and foods, such as antacids and dairy products, reduce absorption of estramustine.
• Taking cyclophosphamide with cardiotoxic drugs produces additive cardiac effects.
• Cyclophosphamide can reduce serum digoxin levels.
• An increased risk of ifosfamide toxicity exists when the drug is taken with allopurinol, barbiturates, chloral hydrate, or phenytoin.
• Corticosteroids reduce the effects of ifosfamide.
• The lung toxicity threshold of carmustine may be reduced when taken with melphalan.
• Interferon alpha may reduce the serum concentration of melphalan.

Adverse reactions

Many patients experience fatigue during nitrogen mustard therapy. Other adverse reactions include:
• bone marrow suppression, leading to severe leukopenia and thrombocytopenia
• nausea and vomiting from central nervous system (CNS) irritation
• stomatitis
• reversible hair loss.

Handle with care

Because nitrogen mustards are powerful local vesicants (blistering drugs), direct contact with these drugs or their vapors can cause severe reactions, especially to the skin, eyes, and respiratory tract.

Nursing process

These nursing process steps are appropriate for patients undergoing treatment with nitrogen mustard drugs.

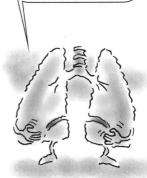

Direct contact with nitrogen mustards can cause severe skin, eye, and respiratory reactions. That's just so irritating!

Assessment

• Assess the patient's underlying neoplastic disorder before therapy and reassess regularly throughout therapy.
• Perform a complete assessment before therapy begins.
• Monitor for adverse reactions and drug interactions throughout therapy.
• Monitor platelet and total and differential leukocyte counts as well as hematocrit, blood urea nitrogen (BUN), alanine aminotransferase (ALT), aspartate aminotransferase (AST), lactate dehydrogenase (LD), serum bilirubin, serum creatinine, uric acid, and other levels as needed.
• Monitor the patient's vital signs and catheter or I.V. line patency throughout drug administration.
• Evaluate the patient's and family's knowledge of drug therapy.

Key nursing diagnoses

• Ineffective health maintenance related to the presence of neoplastic disease
• Ineffective protection related to drug-induced hematologic adverse reactions
• Deficient knowledge related to drug therapy

Planning outcome goals

• The patient will demonstrate an improvement in assessment findings and diagnostic testing.
• The patient will be free from infection as evidenced by normal temperature, cultures, and WBC counts.
• The patient and his family will demonstrate an understanding of drug therapy.

Implementation

• Follow established procedures for safe and proper handling, administration, and disposal of chemotherapeutic drugs.
• Treat extravasation promptly.
• Keep epinephrine, corticosteroids, and antihistamines available during administration. Anaphylactoid reactions may occur.
• Administer the medications as ordered and monitor for effects.
• Administer adequate hydration and monitor intake and output.
• Administer an antiemetic for nausea and vomiting caused by drug use.

Count on it

• Follow facility policy for infection control in immunocompromised patients whose WBC counts fall below 2,000/mm^3 or granulocyte counts fall below 1,000/mm^3.

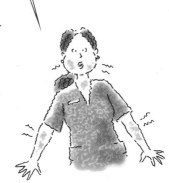

Keep drugs such as epinephrine on hand in case an anaphylactic reaction occurs.

Education edge

Teaching about chemotherapy with alkylating drugs

If chemotherapy with alkylating drugs is prescribed, review these points with the patient and his caregivers:

• Avoid people with bacterial or viral infections because chemotherapy can increase susceptibility. Watch for signs and symptoms of infection (fever, sore throat, and fatigue) and bleeding (easy bruising, nosebleeds, bleeding gums, and melena). Take your temperature daily, and report signs of infection promptly.

• Use proper oral hygiene, including cautious use of a toothbrush, dental floss, and toothpicks.

• Complete dental work before therapy begins or delay it until your blood counts are normal.

• Be aware that you may bruise easily because of the drug's effect on your blood count.

• Don't take over-the-counter (OTC) products, medications, or herbal remedies without first consulting your prescriber.

• Avoid OTC products that contain aspirin.

• Take medications as directed.

• Keep all appointments for chemotherapy, blood tests, and check-ups.

• Maintain an adequate intake of nutritious food and fluids; consult with a dietitian to help design a diet that meets your needs.

• Use an electric razor to help minimize bleeding.

• If you experience hair loss, use wigs, scarves, or hats.

• Inform any other physician, dentist, or health care provider that you're receiving chemotherapy before any treatment.

• If you're of childbearing age, you should use effective contraception during and for a few months after chemotherapy.

• Stop breast-feeding during therapy because of the risk of toxicity to the infant.

Evaluation

• Patient shows an improvement in the underlying neoplastic condition on follow-up diagnostic tests.

• Patient remains free from infection and doesn't bleed abnormally.

• Patient and his family verbalize an understanding of drug therapy. (See *Teaching about chemotherapy with alkylating drugs*.)

Alkyl sulfonates

The alkyl sulfonate busulfan has historically been used to treat chronic myelogenous leukemia, polycythemia vera (increased red blood cell [RBC] mass and an increased number of WBCs and platelets), and other myeloproliferative (pertaining to overactive bone marrow) disorders. Busulfan is used at high doses to treat leukemia during bone marrow transplantation.

Pharmacokinetics

Busulfan is absorbed rapidly and well from the GI tract. Little is known about its distribution. Busulfan is metabolized extensively in the liver before urinary excretion. Its half-life is 2 to 3 hours.

Pharmacodynamics

As an alkyl sulfonate, busulfan forms covalent bonds with the DNA molecules in alkylation.

Pharmacotherapeutics

Busulfan primarily affects granulocytes (a type of WBC) and, to a lesser degree, platelets. Because of its action on granulocytes, it has been used for treating chronic myelogenous leukemia and in conditioning regimens for bone marrow transplantation.

To a screeching halt

Busulfan is also effective in treating polycythemia vera. However, other drugs are usually used to treat polycythemia vera because busulfan can cause severe myelosuppression (halting of bone marrow function).

Drug interactions

There's an increased risk of bleeding when busulfan is taken with anticoagulants or aspirin. Concurrent use of busulfan and thioguanine may cause liver toxicity, esophageal varices (enlarged, swollen veins in the esophagus), or portal hypertension (increased pressure in the portal vein of the liver).

Adverse reactions

The major adverse reaction to busulfan is bone marrow suppression, producing severe leukopenia, anemia, and thrombocytopenia (reduced WBCs, RBCs, and platelets, respectively), which is usually dose related and reversible.

A latecomer

Pulmonary fibrosis may occur as late as 4 months to 10 years after treatment. (The average onset of symptoms is 4 years after therapy.) Seizures are also a concern. (See *Busulfan warning*.)

Nursing process

These nursing process steps are appropriate for patients undergoing treatment with alkyl sulfonates.

Assessment
• Assess the patient's underlying neoplastic disorder before therapy and reassess regularly throughout therapy.
• Perform a complete assessment before therapy begins.
• Monitor for adverse reactions and drug interactions throughout therapy.

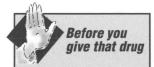

Before you give that drug

Busulfan warning

Seizures can occur as an adverse reaction to I.V. infusion of busulfan. The patient may be premedicated with phenytoin to decrease the risk of seizures.

Going down?

• Monitor the patient's WBC and platelet counts weekly during therapy. The WBC count falls about 10 days after the start of therapy and continues to fall for 2 weeks after stopping the drug.
• Monitor the patient's uric acid level.
• Monitor the patient's vital signs and catheter or I.V. line patency throughout drug administration.
• Monitor the drug's effectiveness by noting results of follow-up diagnostic tests and the patient's overall physical status. Note his response (increased appetite and sense of well-being, decreased total WBC count, and reduced size of spleen), which usually begins within 1 to 2 weeks.
• Evaluate the patient's and family's knowledge of drug therapy.

Key nursing diagnoses

• Ineffective health maintenance related to the presence of neoplastic disease
• Risk for infection related to drug-induced immunosuppression
• Deficient knowledge related to drug therapy

Planning outcome goals

• The patient will show an improvement in the underlying condition.
• The patient will show no signs of infection as evidenced by a normal WBC count and temperature and negative cultures.
• The patient and his family will verbalize an understanding of drug therapy.

Implementation

• Follow established procedures for safe and proper handling, administration, and disposal of chemotherapeutic drugs.
• Give the drug at the same time each day.
• Treat extravasation promptly.
• Administer the medications as ordered and monitor for adverse effects.
• Administer adequate hydration and monitor intake and output.
• The dosage is adjusted based on the patient's weekly WBC count, and the prescriber may temporarily stop drug therapy if severe leukocytopenia develops. Therapeutic effects are commonly accompanied by toxicity.
• The drug is usually given with allopurinol in addition to adequate hydration to prevent hyperuricemia with resulting uric acid nephropathy.
• Advise a breast-feeding patient to stop during drug therapy because of the possible risk of infant toxicity.

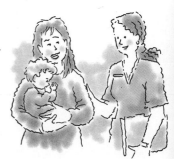

Advise a breast-feeding patient to stop during drug therapy because of the possible risk of infant toxicity.

Evaluation

- Patient shows an improvement in the underlying neoplastic condition on follow-up diagnostic tests.
- Patient remains free from infection.
- Patient and his family verbalize an understanding of drug therapy.

Nitrosoureas

Nitrosoureas are alkylating agents that halt cancer cell reproduction. They include:

- carmustine
- lomustine
- streptozocin.

Pharmacokinetics

When administered I.V., carmustine achieves a steady-state volume of distribution. With oral administration, lomustine is absorbed adequately, although incompletely.

Don't go P.O.

Streptozocin is administered I.V. because it's poorly absorbed orally.

The fat of the matter is...

Nitrosoureas are lipophilic (attracted to fat) drugs and are distributed to fatty tissues and cerebrospinal fluid (CSF). They're metabolized extensively before urine excretion.

Pharmacodynamics

During a process called *bifunctional alkylation*, nitrosoureas interfere with amino acids, purines, and DNA needed for cancer cells to divide, thus halting their reproduction.

Pharmacotherapeutics

The nitrosoureas are highly lipid soluble, which allows them or their metabolites to easily cross the blood-brain barrier. Because of this ability, nitrosoureas are used to treat brain tumors and meningeal leukemias.

Drug interactions

Each of the nitrosoureas has its own interactions with other drugs:

- Cimetidine may increase carmustine's bone marrow toxicity.

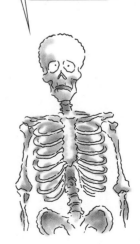

I'm not at all pleased to tell you that cimetidine may increase carmustine's bone marrow toxicity.

• Lomustine used with anticoagulants or aspirin increases the risk of bleeding; avoid using these drugs together.
• Streptozocin can prolong the elimination half-life of doxorubicin, prolonging leukopenia and thrombocytopenia.

Adverse reactions

All of the nitrosoureas can produce severe nausea and vomiting.

Bad to the bone

Carmustine and lomustine produce bone marrow suppression that begins 4 to 6 weeks after treatment and lasts 1 to 2 weeks. These drugs shouldn't be given more frequently than every 6 weeks.

Kidney concerns

Kidney toxicity and kidney failure may also occur with patients taking nitrosoureas. High-dose carmustine may produce reversible liver toxicity.

Pulmonary problems

Carmustine may cause delayed lung toxicity characterized by lung infiltrates or fibrosis (scarring) that can occur years after treatment.

In patients who receive prolonged therapy with total dosages greater than 1,400 mg/m^2, pulmonary toxicity can occur anywhere from 9 days to 15 years after treatment. (See *Carmustine warning.*)

Nursing process

These nursing process steps are appropriate for patients undergoing treatment with nitrosoureas.

Assessment

• Assess the patient's underlying neoplastic disorder before therapy and reassess regularly throughout therapy.
• Perform a complete assessment before therapy begins.
• Obtain baseline pulmonary function tests before therapy because pulmonary toxicity appears to be dose related. Be sure to evaluate the results of liver, renal, and pulmonary function tests periodically thereafter.
• Monitor for adverse reactions and drug interactions throughout therapy.
• Monitor the patient's complete blood count (CBC) and uric acid level.
• Monitor the patient's vital signs and catheter or I.V. line patency throughout drug administration.
• Evaluate the patient's and family's knowledge of drug therapy.

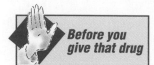

Before you give that drug

Carmustine warning

Obtain baseline pulmonary function tests before therapy because pulmonary toxicity appears to be related to the dosage and may occur from 9 days to 15 years after treatment. Be sure to evaluate results of liver, renal, and pulmonary function tests periodically thereafter.

Key nursing diagnoses
• Ineffective health maintenance related to the presence of neoplastic disease
• Risk for injury related to drug-induced adverse reactions
• Deficient knowledge related to drug therapy

Planning outcome goals
• The patient will show an improvement in the underlying condition.
• The risk of injury to the patient will be minimized.
• The patient and his family will demonstrate an understanding of drug therapy.

Implementation
• Follow established procedures for safe and proper handling, administration, and disposal of chemotherapeutic drugs.
• Give an antiemetic before giving the drug to reduce nausea.
• Administer the medications according to facility policy for reconstitution, mixing, storage, and administration. Monitor for effects.
• Use carmustine only in glass containers. The solution is unstable in plastic I.V. bags. Avoid contact with skin because carmustine will cause a brown stain. If skin contact occurs, wash the drug off thoroughly.

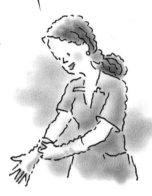

Use double gloves when handling carmustine wafer in the operating room.

Double, double, avoid that trouble...
• Use double gloves when handling carmustine wafer in the operating room.
• Administer adequate hydration and monitor the patient's intake and output.
• Allopurinol may be used with adequate hydration to prevent hyperuricemia and uric acid nephropathy.
• Advise a breast-feeding patient to stop during therapy because of possible infant toxicity.
• Repeat lomustine administration only when CBC results reveal safe hematologic parameters.
• Institute infection control and bleeding precautions.

Evaluation
• Patient shows an improvement in the underlying neoplastic condition on follow-up diagnostic tests.
• Patient doesn't experience injury from drug-induced adverse reactions.
• Patient and his family state an understanding of drug therapy.

Triazenes

Dacarbazine, a triazene, functions as an alkylating drug only after it has been activated by the liver.

Pharmacokinetics

After I.V. injection, dacarbazine is distributed throughout the body and metabolized in the liver. Within 6 hours, 30% to 46% of a dose is excreted by the kidneys (half is excreted unchanged; the other half is excreted as one of the metabolites).

Dysfunction junction

In a patient with kidney or liver dysfunction, the drug's half-life may increase to 7 hours.

Pharmacodynamics

Dacarbazine first must be metabolized in the liver to become an alkylating drug. It seems to inhibit ribonucleic acid (RNA) and protein synthesis. Like other alkylating drugs, dacarbazine is cell cycle–nonspecific.

Pharmacotherapeutics

Dacarbazine is used primarily to treat patients with malignant melanoma. It's also used with other drugs to treat patients with Hodgkin's disease.

Drug interactions

No significant drug interactions have been reported with dacarbazine.

Adverse reactions

Dacarbazine use may cause the following adverse reactions:
• leukopenia
• thrombocytopenia
• nausea and vomiting (which begin within 1 to 3 hours after administration in most cases and may last up to 12 hours)
• phototoxicity
• flulike syndrome (which may begin 7 days after treatment and last from 7 to 21 days)
• hair loss.

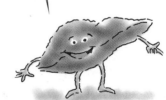

After I.V. injection, dacarbazine must be metabolized by the liver before it becomes an antineoplastic drug.

Nursing process

These nursing process steps are appropriate for patients undergoing treatment with triazenes.

Assessment

• Assess the patient's underlying neoplastic disorder before therapy and reassess regularly throughout therapy.
• Perform a complete assessment before therapy begins.
• Monitor for adverse reactions and drug interactions throughout therapy.
• Monitor the patient's CBC, platelet count, and liver enzyme levels.
• Monitor the patient's vital signs and catheter or I.V. line patency throughout drug administration.
• Evaluate the patient's and family's knowledge of drug therapy.

Key nursing diagnoses

• Ineffective health maintenance related to the presence of neoplastic disease
• Risk of injury related to drug-induced adverse reactions
• Deficient knowledge related to drug therapy

Planning outcome goals

• The patient will demonstrate an improvement in assessment findings and diagnostic testing.
• The risk of injury to the patient will be minimized.
• The patient and his family will demonstrate an understanding of drug therapy.

Implementation

• Follow established procedures for safe and proper handling, administration, and disposal of chemotherapeutic drugs.
• Administer the medications as ordered and monitor for effects.
• Administer adequate hydration and monitor the patient's intake and output.
• Administer an antiemetic before giving dacarbazine to help decrease nausea. Nausea and vomiting may subside after several doses.
• Reconstitute the drug according to facility policy. During infusion, protect the bag from direct sunlight to avoid drug breakdown. The solution may be diluted further or the infusion slowed to decrease pain at the infusion site.

Not-so-pretty in pink

• Discard the drug if the solution turns pink; this is a sign of decomposition.

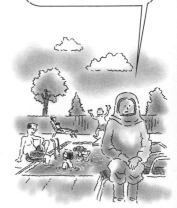

Advise the patient to avoid sunlight and sun lamps for the first 2 days after treatment. Although this might be taking it to a bit of an extreme...

• Take care to avoid extravasation during infusion. If the I.V. site infiltrates, discontinue the infusion immediately, apply ice to the area for 24 to 48 hours, and notify the prescriber.
• Advise the patient to avoid sunlight and sunlamps for the first 2 days after treatment.
• Reassure the patient that flulike syndrome may be treated with mild antipyretics such as acetaminophen.

Evaluation

• Patient shows an improvement in the underlying neoplastic condition on follow-up diagnostic tests.
• Patient remains free from infection and doesn't bleed abnormally.
• Patient and his family state an understanding of drug therapy.

Ethylenimines

Thiotepa, an ethylenimine derivative, is a multifunctional alkylating drug.

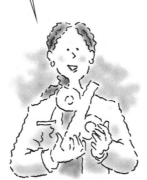

Talk about a good return on your investment. After I.V. administration, thiotepa is 100% bioavailable.

Pharmacokinetics

After I.V. administration, thiotepa is 100% bioavailable. Significant systemic absorption may occur when it's administered into pleural (around the lungs) or peritoneal (abdominal) spaces to treat malignant effusions or instilled into the bladder. Thiotepa crosses the blood-brain barrier and is metabolized extensively in the liver. Thiotepa and its metabolites are excreted in urine.

Pharmacodynamics

Thiotepa exerts its cytotoxic activity by interfering with DNA replication and RNA transcription. Ultimately, it disrupts nucleic acid function and causes cell death.

Pharmacotherapeutics

Thiotepa is used to treat bladder cancer. This alkylating drug is also prescribed for palliative treatment of lymphomas and ovarian or breast carcinomas.

Effective for effusions

Thiotepa is used to treat intracavitary effusions (fluid accumulation in a body cavity). It may also prove useful in the treatment of lung cancer.

Drug interactions

Thiotepa may interact with other drugs:
• Concurrent use of thiotepa, anticoagulants, and aspirin may increase the risk of bleeding.
• Taking thiotepa with neuromuscular blocking drugs may prolong muscular paralysis.
• Concurrent use of thiotepa and other alkylating drugs or radiation therapy may intensify toxicity rather than enhance the therapeutic response.

It'll take your breath away

• When used with succinylcholine, thiotepa may cause prolonged respirations and apnea (periods of not breathing). Thiotepa appears to inhibit the activity of cholinesterase, the enzyme that deactivates succinylcholine.

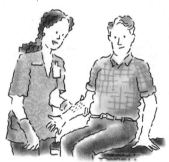

Occasional reactions to thiotepa include hives, pruritus, and rash.

Adverse reactions

The major adverse reactions to thiotepa are blood related and include leukopenia, anemia, thrombocytopenia, and pancytopenia (deficiency of all cellular elements of the blood), which may be fatal. Other adverse reactions include:
• nausea and vomiting (common)
• stomatitis and ulceration of the intestinal mucosa (especially at bone marrow transplant doses)
• hives, rash, and pruritus (occasional).

Nursing process

These nursing process steps are appropriate for patients undergoing treatment with ethylenimines.

Assessment

• Assess the patient's underlying neoplastic disorder before therapy and reassess regularly throughout therapy.
• Perform a complete assessment before therapy begins.
• Monitor the patient for adverse reactions and drug interactions throughout therapy.
• Monitor the patient's CBC weekly for at least 3 weeks after the last dose.
• Monitor the patient's uric acid level.
• Keep in mind that adverse GI reactions are reversible in 6 to 8 months.
• Monitor the patient's vital signs and catheter or I.V. line patency throughout drug administration.
• Evaluate the patient's and family's knowledge of drug therapy.

Key nursing diagnoses

- Ineffective health maintenance related to the presence of neoplastic disease
- Ineffective protection related to drug-induced hematologic adverse reactions
- Deficient knowledge related to drug therapy

Planning outcome goals

- The patient will show an improvement in the underlying condition.
- The patient will show no signs of infection as evidenced by a normal WBC count and temperature and negative culture results.
- The patient and his family will demonstrate an understanding of drug therapy.

Implementation

- Follow established procedures for safe and proper handling, administration, and disposal of chemotherapeutic drugs.
- Reconstitute the drug according to facility policy for I.V. administration. The drug may be given by rapid I.V. administration in doses of 0.3 to 0.4 mg/kg at intervals of 1 to 4 weeks.
- If intense pain occurs with I.V. administration, use a local anesthetic at the injection site. If pain occurs at the insertion site, dilute the solution further or use a local anesthetic. Make sure that the drug doesn't infiltrate.

Out with the opaque

- Discard the I.V. solution if it appears grossly opaque or contains precipitate. (See *Thiotepa warning.*)
- Administer the medication as ordered and monitor for effects.
- Thiotepa may be used for bladder instillation.
- A patient with bladder cancer should first be dehydrated for 8 to 10 hours and then receive a bladder instillation of 30 to 60 mg of the drug in 30 to 60 ml of normal saline solution over a 2-hour period, repeated once weekly for 4 weeks.
- Thiotepa can also be given for intracavity use, with a recommended dosage of 0.5 to 0.8 mg/kg.
- Refrigerate and protect dry powder from direct sunlight.
- Report a WBC count below 3,000/mm^3 or a platelet count below 150,000/mm^3 and stop the drug.
- To prevent hyperuricemia with resulting uric acid nephropathy, allopurinol may be used with adequate hydration.
- Advise a breast-feeding patient to stop during therapy because of the risk of infant toxicity.

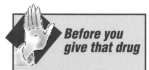

Before you give that drug

Thiotepa warning

Make sure the solution is clear to slightly opaque. If the solution appears grossly opaque or has precipitate, discard it. To eliminate haze, filter the solution through a 0.22-micron filter before use.

Evaluation

• Patient shows an improvement in the underlying neoplastic condition on follow-up diagnostic tests.
• Patient remains free from infection and doesn't bleed abnormally.
• Patient and his family state an understanding of drug therapy.

Alkylating-like drugs

Carboplatin, oxaliplatin, and cisplatin are heavy-metal complexes that contain platinum. Because their action resembles that of a bifunctional alkylating drug, these drugs are called *alkylating-like drugs*.

Pharmacokinetics

The distribution and metabolism of carboplatin aren't clearly defined. After I.V. administration, carboplatin is eliminated primarily by the kidneys.

By and bi

The elimination of carboplatin is biphasic. It has an initial half-life of 1 to 2 hours and a terminal half-life of 2½ to 6 hours. Oxaliplatin is 70% to 90% bound to plasma proteins and is eliminated primarily by the kidneys. When administered intrapleurally (into the pleural space around the lung) or intraperitoneally (into the peritoneum), cisplatin may exhibit significant systemic absorption.

Reaching new heights

Highly protein bound, cisplatin reaches high concentrations in the kidneys, liver, intestines, and testes, but has poor CNS penetration. The drug undergoes some liver metabolism, followed by excretion through the kidneys.

Going platinum

Platinum is detectable in tissue for at least 4 months after administration.

Pharmacodynamics

Like alkylating drugs, carboplatin, oxaliplatin, and cisplatin are cell cycle–nonspecific and inhibit DNA synthesis. They act like bifunctional alkylating drugs by cross-linking strands of DNA and inhibiting DNA synthesis. (See *Alkylating-like drugs: Cisplatin*, page 618.)

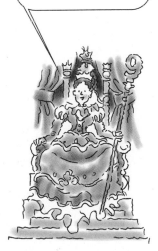

Platinum is detectable in tissue for at least 4 months after administration of alkylating-like drugs. That's a bit too rich, even for me!

Prototype pro

Alkylating-like drugs: Cisplatin

Actions
• Probably cross-links strands of cellular deoxyribonucleic acid and interferes with ribonucleic acid transcription, causing growth imbalance that leads to cell death
• Kills selected cancer cells

Indications
• Adjunct therapy in metastatic testicular and ovarian cancer
• Advanced bladder and esophageal cancer
• Head and neck cancer
• Cervical cancer
• Non–small-cell lung cancer
• Brain tumor
• Osteogenic sarcoma or neuroblastoma

Nursing considerations
• Monitor for adverse effects, such as peripheral neuritis, seizures, tinnitus, hearing loss, nausea and vomiting, severe renal toxicity, myelosuppression, leukopenia, thrombocytopenia, anemia, and anaphylactic reaction.
• Assess the underlying neoplastic disease before therapy, and reassess regularly throughout therapy.

Pharmacotherapeutics

These alkylating-like drugs are used to treat several cancers:
• Carboplatin is used primarily to treat ovarian and lung cancer.
• Cisplatin is prescribed to treat bladder and metastatic ovarian and testicular cancers.
• Cisplatin may also be used to treat head, neck, and lung cancer. (Although these indications are clinically accepted, they're currently unlabeled uses.)
• Oxaliplatin is used in combination with other agents in colorectal cancer.

Drug interactions

These alkylating-like drugs interact with a few other drugs:
• When carboplatin, cisplatin, or oxaliplatin are administered with an aminoglycoside, the risk of toxicity to the kidney increases.

What's that you say?

• Taking carboplatin or cisplatin with bumetanide, ethacrynic acid, or furosemide increases the risk of ototoxicity (damage to the organs of hearing and balance).
• Cisplatin may reduce serum phenytoin levels.

Adverse reactions

Carboplatin and cisplatin produce many of the same adverse reactions as the alkylating drugs:
• Carboplatin can produce bone marrow suppression.

- Kidney toxicity can occur with cisplatin, usually after multiple courses of therapy. Carboplatin is less toxic to the kidneys.
- With long-term cisplatin therapy, neurotoxicity can occur. Neurotoxicity is less common with carboplatin.
- Tinnitus and hearing loss, which is usually permanent, may occur with cisplatin. It's much less common with carboplatin.
- Cisplatin can also produce marked nausea and vomiting.

Nursing process

These nursing process steps are appropriate for patients undergoing treatment with alkylating-like drugs.

Assessment

- Assess the patient's underlying neoplastic disorder before therapy and reassess regularly throughout therapy.
- Perform a complete assessment before therapy begins.
- Monitor the patient for adverse reactions and drug interactions throughout therapy.
- Monitor the patient's CBC, electrolyte levels (especially potassium and magnesium), platelet count, and renal function studies before initial and subsequent dosages.
- To detect permanent hearing loss, obtain audiometry test results before the initial dose and subsequent courses.
- Evaluate the patient's and family's knowledge of drug therapy.

Key nursing diagnoses

- Ineffective health maintenance related to the presence of neoplastic disease
- Ineffective protection related to drug-induced hematologic adverse reactions
- Deficient knowledge related to drug therapy

Planning outcome goals

- The patient will demonstrate an improvement in assessment findings and diagnostic testing.
- The patient will show no signs of infection as evidenced by a normal WBC count and temperature and negative culture results.
- The patient and his family will demonstrate an understanding of drug therapy.

Implementation

- Follow established procedures for safe and proper handling, administration, and disposal of chemotherapeutic drugs. (See *Cisplatin warning*.)
- Administer the medications as ordered and monitor for effects.

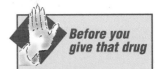

Before you give that drug

Cisplatin warning

Follow facility policy to reduce risks. Preparation and administration of parenteral forms of a chemotherapeutic drug, such as cisplatin, is linked to carcinogenic, mutagenic, and teratogenic risks for personnel.

Mannitol or furosemide is given before and during cisplatin infusion to maintain diuresis of 100 to 400 ml/hour for up to 24 hours after therapy. Prehydration and diuresis may reduce renal toxicity and ototoxicity significantly.

• Administer adequate hydration and monitor intake and output.
• Dilute the medication as directed; cisplatin infusions are most stable in chloride-containing solutions. Don't use needles or I.V. administration sets that contain aluminum because it will displace platinum, causing a loss of potency and formation of black precipitate.
• Monitor the patient's renal function because renal toxicity is cumulative. His renal function must return to normal before he receives the next dose.
• The dose shouldn't be repeated unless the patient's platelet count is more than $100,000/mm^3$, WBC count is over $4,000/mm^3$, creatinine level is under 1.5 mg/dl, or BUN level is under 25 mg/dl.
• Check current protocol on drug administration. Some clinicians use I.V. sodium thiosulfate to minimize toxicity.
• Administer an antiemetic, as ordered; nausea and vomiting may be severe and protracted (up to 24 hours). Provide I.V. hydration until the patient can tolerate adequate oral intake. Ondansetron, granisetron, and high-dose metoclopramide have been used effectively to prevent and treat nausea and vomiting. Some clinicians may combine dexamethasone or an antihistamine with metroclopramide, ondansetron, or granisetron.
• Delayed vomiting (3 to 5 days after treatment) has been reported. The patient may need prolonged antiemetic treatment.
• To prevent hypokalemia, potassium chloride (10 to 20 mEq/L) is commonly added to I.V. fluids before and after cisplatin therapy.
• Immediately give epinephrine, corticosteroids, or antihistamines for anaphylactoid reactions.
• Tell the patient to report tinnitus immediately as well as edema or a decrease in urine output (if recording intake and output at home).

Evaluation

• Patient shows an improvement in the underlying neoplastic condition on follow-up diagnostic tests.
• Patient remains free from infection and doesn't bleed abnormally.
• Patient and his family state an understanding of drug therapy.

Antimetabolite drugs

Because antimetabolite drugs structurally resemble DNA base pairs, they can become involved in processes associated with DNA base pairs—that is, the synthesis of nucleic acids and proteins.

The antimetabolite drugs are cell cycle–specific. They're referred to as S phase–specific because they primarily affect cells that actively synthesize DNA.

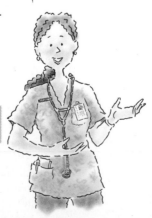

Getting specific

Antimetabolites differ significantly from the DNA base pairs in how they interfere with this synthesis. Because the antimetabolites are cell cycle–specific and primarily affect cells that actively synthesize DNA, they're referred to as *S phase–specific*. Normal cells that are reproducing actively as well as the cancer cells are affected by the antimetabolites.

Each according to its metabolite

These drugs are subclassified according to the metabolite affected and include:
- folic acid analogues
- pyrimidine analogues
- purine analogues.

Folic acid analogues

Although researchers have developed many folic acid analogues, the early compound methotrexate remains the most commonly used.

Pharmacokinetics

Methotrexate is absorbed well and distributed throughout the body. It can accumulate in any fluid collection, such as ascites or pleural or pericardial effusion. This can result in prolonged elimination and higher than expected toxicity, especially myelosuppression.

Do not enter

At usual dosages, methotrexate doesn't enter the CNS readily. Although methotrexate is metabolized partially, it's excreted primarily unchanged in urine.

A disappearing act

Methotrexate exhibits a three-part disappearance from plasma; the rapid distributive phase is followed by a second phase, which reflects kidney clearance. The last phase, the terminal half-life, is 3 to 10 hours for a low dose and 8 to 15 hours for a high dose.

Pharmacodynamics

Methotrexate reversibly inhibits the action of the enzyme dihydrofolate reductase. This blocks normal folic acid processing, which inhibits DNA and RNA synthesis. The result is cell death. (see *Antimetabolite drugs: Methotrexate*, page 622.)

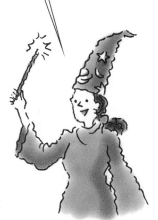

Methotrexate exhibits a three-part disappearance from plasma. I can usually make things disappear with just one tap of my wand.

Prototype pro

Antimetabolite drugs: Methotrexate

Actions
• Prevents the reduction of folic acid to tetrahydrofolate by binding to dihydrofolate reductase
• Kills certain cancer cells and reduces inflammation

Indications
• Trophoblastic tumors (choriocarcinoma, hydatidiform mole)
• Acute lymphoblastic and lymphatic leukemia, meningeal leukemia
• Burkitt's lymphoma (stage I or stage II)
• Lymphosarcoma (stage III)
• Osteosarcoma

Nursing considerations
• Monitor for adverse reactions, such as stomatitis, diarrhea, intestinal perforation, nausea, vomiting, renal failure, anemia, leukopenia, thrombocytopenia, acute hepatic toxicity, pulmonary fibrosis, urticaria, and sudden death.
• Assess the underlying neoplastic disease before therapy and reassess regularly throughout therapy.
• Follow facility policy for reconstitution and administration.

Pharmacotherapeutics

Methotrexate is especially useful in treating:
• acute lymphoblastic leukemia (abnormal growth of lymphocyte precursors, the lymphoblasts), the most common leukemia in children
• acute lymphocytic leukemia (abnormal growth of lymphocytes); may be given as treatment and prophylaxis for meningeal leukemia
• CNS diseases (given intrathecally)
• choriocarcinoma (cancer that develops from the chorionic portions of the products of conception)
• osteogenic sarcoma (bone cancer)
• malignant lymphomas
• carcinomas of the head, neck, bladder, testis, and breast.

Unconventional treatment

The drug is also prescribed in low doses to treat severe psoriasis, graft-versus-host disease, and rheumatoid arthritis that don't respond to conventional therapy.

Drug interactions

Methotrexate interacts with several other drugs:
• Probenecid decreases methotrexate excretion, increasing the risk of methotrexate toxicity, including fatigue, bone marrow suppression, and stomatitis (mouth inflammation).

• Salicylates and nonsteroidal anti-inflammatory drugs (NSAIDs), especially diclofenac, ketoprofen, indomethacin, and naproxen, also increase methotrexate toxicity.
• Cholestyramine reduces the absorption of methotrexate from the GI tract.
• Concurrent use of alcohol and methotrexate increases the risk of liver toxicity.
• Taking co-trimoxazole with methotrexate may produce blood cell abnormalities.
• Penicillin decreases renal tubular secretion of methotrexate, increasing the risk of methotrexate toxicity.

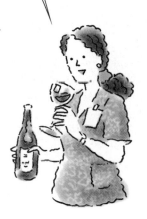

Consuming alcohol while taking methotrexate increases the risk of liver toxicity.

Adverse reactions

Adverse reactions to methotrexate include:
• bone marrow suppression
• stomatitis
• pulmonary toxicity, exhibited as pneumonitis or pulmonary fibrosis
• skin reactions, such as photosensitivity and hair loss.

To the rescue

Kidney toxicity can also occur with high doses of methotrexate. During high-dose therapy, leucovorin (folinic acid) may be used to minimize adverse reactions. This process is known as *leucovorin rescue.*

Intrathecal threats

Adverse reactions to intrathecal administration (through the dura into the subarachnoid space) of methotrexate may include seizures, paralysis, and death. Other less severe adverse reactions may also occur, such as headache, fever, neck stiffness, confusion, and irritability.

Nursing process

These nursing process steps are appropriate for patients undergoing treatment with folic acid analogues.

Assessment

• Perform a complete assessment before therapy begins. Assess the patient's condition before therapy and regularly thereafter.
• Monitor the patient for adverse reactions and drug interactions.
• Monitor the patient's fluid intake and output daily.
• Monitor the patient's vital signs and catheter or I.V. line patency throughout drug administration.

• Monitor hematocrit; ALT, AST, LD, serum bilirubin, serum crea-tinine, uric acid, and BUN levels; platelet and total and differential leukocyte counts; and other values as required.
• Evaluate the patient's and family's knowledge of drug therapy.

Key nursing diagnoses
• Ineffective protection related to drug-induced adverse reactions
• Risk of infection related to immunosuppression
• Deficient knowledge related to drug therapy

Planning outcome goals
• The risk of injury to the patient will be minimized.
• The patient will show no signs of infection as evidenced by a normal WBC count and temperature and negative cultures.
• The patient and his family will demonstrate an understanding of drug therapy.

Implementation
• Follow the established procedures for safe and proper handling, administration, and disposal of drugs.
• Try to ease anxiety in the patient and his family before treat-ment.
• Give an antiemetic before giving the drug to lessen nausea.
• Give cytarabine with allopurinol to decrease the risk of hyper-uricemia. Promote a high fluid intake.

An ounce of prevention
• Provide diligent mouth care to prevent stomatitis with methotrexate therapy.
• Anticipate the need for leucovorin rescue with high-dose methotrexate therapy.
• Treat extravasation promptly.
• Tell the patient to defer immunizations if possible until hemato-logic stability is confirmed.

Evaluation
• Patient develops no serious complications.
• Patient remains free from infection.
• Patient and his family state an understanding drug therapy. (See *Teaching about antimetabolite drugs.*)

Education edge

Teaching about antimetabolite drugs

If antimetabolite drugs are prescribed, review these points with the patient and his caregivers:

• Use proper oral hygiene, including cautious use of a toothbrush, dental floss, and toothpicks. Chemotherapy can increase the risk of microbial infection, delayed healing, and bleeding gums.

• Complete dental work before therapy begins or delay it until blood counts are normal.

• Be aware that you may bruise easily because of the drug's effect on platelets.

• Avoid close contact with persons who have taken oral polio virus vaccine as well as with persons who have bacterial or viral infections because chemotherapy may increase susceptibility. Notify your prescriber promptly if you develop signs or symptoms of infection.

• Report redness, pain, or swelling at the injection site. Local tissue injury and scarring may result from tissue infiltration at the infusion site.

• Be aware of the expected adverse effects of the drug, especially nausea, vomiting, diarrhea, and hand-foot syndrome (pain, swelling, and redness of the hands or feet). Patient-specific dose adaptations during therapy are expected and needed. Stop taking the drug and contact your prescriber immediately if adverse effects occur.

• If you miss a dose, don't take the missed dose and don't double the next one. Continue with your regular dosing schedule and check with your prescriber.

• Don't take over-the-counter medications, other medicines, or herbal preparations without first consulting your prescriber.

Pyrimidine analogues

Pyrimidine analogues are a diverse group of drugs that inhibit production of pyrimidine nucleotides necessary for DNA synthesis. They include:

• capecitabine
• cytarabine
• floxuridine
• fluorouracil
• gemcitabine.

Pharmacokinetics

Because pyrimidine analogues are absorbed poorly when given orally, they're usually administered by other routes. With the exception of cytarabine, pyrimidine analogues are distributed well throughout the body, including the CSF. They're metabolized extensively in the liver and are excreted in urine. Intrathecal cytarabine may be given with or without cranial radiation to treat CNS leukemia.

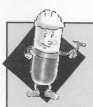

Pharm function

How pyrimidine analogues work

To understand how pyrimidine analogues work, it helps to consider the basic structure of deoxyribonucleic acid (DNA).

Climbing the ladder to understanding
DNA resembles a ladder that has been twisted. The rungs of the ladder consist of pairs of nitrogenous bases: adenine always pairs with thymine, and guanine always pairs with cytosine. Cytosine and thymine are pyrimidines; adenine and guanine are purines.

One part sugar…
The basic unit of DNA is the nucleotide. A nucleotide is the building block of nucleic acids. It consists of a sugar, a nitrogen-containing base, and a phosphate group. It's on these components that pyrimidine analogues do their work.

In the guise of a nucleotide
After pyrimidine analogues are converted into nucleotides, they're incorporated into DNA, where they may inhibit DNA and ribonucleic acid synthesis as well as other metabolic reactions necessary for proper cell growth.

Pharmacodynamics

Pyrimidine analogues kill cancer cells by interfering with the natural function of pyrimidine nucleotides. (See *How pyrimidine analogues work.*)

Pharmacotherapeutics

Pyrimidine analogues may be used to treat many types of tumors. However, they're primarily indicated in the treatment of:
• acute leukemias
• GI tract adenocarcinomas, such as colorectal, pancreatic, esophageal, and stomach cancers
• carcinomas of the breast and ovaries
• malignant lymphomas.

Drug interactions

No significant drug interactions occur with most of the pyrimidine analogues; however, several are possible with capecitabine:
• Capecitabine may have increased absorption when coadministered with antacids.
• Capecitabine can increase the pharmacodynamic effects of warfarin, thereby increasing the risk of bleeding.
• Capecitabine may increase serum phenytoin levels.

Adverse reactions

Like most antineoplastic drugs, pyrimidine analogues can cause:
• fatigue

- inflammation of the mouth, esophagus, and throat, leading to painful ulcerations and tissue sloughing
- bone marrow suppression
- nausea
- anorexia.

A range of reactions

High-dose cytarabine can cause severe cerebellar neurotoxicity, chemical conjunctivitis, diarrhea, fever, and hand-foot syndrome (numbness, paresthesia, tingling, painless or painful swelling, erythema, desquamation, blistering, and severe pain of the hands or feet). Crab erythema can be seen with high-dose cytarabine and continuous infusions of fluorouracil. Other adverse reactions with fluorouracil include diarrhea and hair loss.

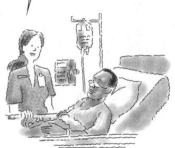

Like most antineoplastic drugs, pyrimidine analogues can cause such adverse effects as fatigue, nausea, and anorexia.

Nursing process

These nursing process steps are appropriate for patients undergoing treatment with pyrimidine analogues.

Assessment
- Perform a complete assessment before therapy begins and regularly thereafter.
- Monitor the patient for adverse reactions and drug interactions.
- Monitor the patient's daily fluid intake and output.
- Monitor the patient's vital signs and catheter or I.V. line patency throughout drug administration.
- Monitor the patient for hand-foot syndrome, hyperbilirubinemia, and severe nausea. Drug therapy will need to be immediately adjusted.
- Evaluate the patient's and family's knowledge of drug therapy.

Key nursing diagnoses
- Ineffective protection related to drug-induced adverse reactions
- Risk for infection related to immunosuppression
- Deficient knowledge related to drug therapy

Planning outcome goals
- The risk of injury to the patient will be minimized.
- The patient will show no signs of infection as evidenced by a normal WBC count and temperature and negative cultures.
- The patient and his family will demonstrate an understanding of drug therapy.

Implementation

- Follow established procedures for safe and proper handling, administration, and disposal of drugs.
- Try to ease anxiety in the patient and his family before treatment.
- Give an antiemetic before giving the drug to lessen nausea.
- Give cytarabine with allopurinol to decrease the risk of hyperuricemia.
- Promote a high fluid intake.
- Provide diligent mouth care to prevent stomatitis with cytarabine or fluorouracil therapy.
- Treat extravasation promptly.
- Tell the patient to defer immunizations if possible until hematologic stability is confirmed.
- Watch for stomatitis or diarrhea, which are signs of toxicity. Stop the drug immediately and notify the prescriber if either occurs.

Evaluation

- Patient develops no serious complications.
- Patient remains free from infection.
- Patient and his family state an understanding of drug therapy.

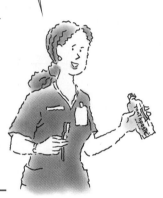

Provide diligent mouth care to prevent stomatitis with cytarabine and fluorouracil therapy.

Purine analogues

Purine analogues are incorporated into DNA and RNA, interfering with nucleic acid synthesis and replication. They include:

- cladribine
- fludarabine phosphate
- mercaptopurine
- pentostatin
- thioguanine.

Pharmacokinetics

The pharmacokinetics of purine analogues aren't defined clearly. They're largely metabolized in the liver and excreted in urine.

Pharmacodynamics

As with the other antimetabolites, fludarabine, mercaptopurine, and thioguanine first must undergo conversion via phosphorylation to the nucleotide level to be active. The resulting nucleotides are then incorporated into DNA, where they may inhibit DNA and RNA synthesis as well as other metabolic reactions necessary for proper cell growth. Cladribine responds in a similar fashion. Pentostatin inhibits adenosine deaminase (ADA), causing an increase in intracellular levels of deoxyadenosine triphosphate. This leads to cell damage and death. The greatest activity of ADA is in cells of the lymphoid system, especially malignant T cells.

Analogous to pyrimidine analogues

This conversion to nucleotides is the same process that pyrimidine analogues experience but, in this case, it's purine nucleotides that are affected. Purine analogues are cell cycle–specific as well, exerting their effect during that same S phase.

Pharmacotherapeutics

Purine analogues are used to treat acute and chronic leukemias and may be useful in the treatment of lymphomas.

Drug interactions

No significant interactions occur with cladribine or thioguanine.

A serious flub with fludarabine

Taking fludarabine and pentostatin together may cause severe pulmonary toxicity, which can be fatal. Taking pentostatin with allopurinol may increase the risk of rash.

Taking pentostatin with vidarabine may enhance the effect of vidarabine and increase the risk of toxicity.

No bones about it

Concomitant administration of mercaptopurine and allopurinol may increase bone marrow suppression by decreasing mercaptopurine metabolism.

Adverse reactions

Purine analogues can produce:
• bone marrow suppression
• nausea and vomiting
• anorexia
• mild diarrhea
• stomatitis
• rise in uric acid levels (a result of the breakdown of purine).

High-dose horrors

Fludarabine, when used at high doses, may cause severe neurologic effects, including blindness, coma, and death.

Nursing process

These nursing process steps are appropriate for patients undergoing treatment with purine analogues.

Assessment
• Perform a complete assessment before therapy begins and regularly thereafter.
• Monitor the patient for adverse reactions and drug interactions.
• Monitor the patient's fluid intake and output daily.
• Monitor the patient's vital signs and catheter or I.V. line patency throughout drug administration.
• Provide careful hematologic monitoring, especially of neutrophil and platelet counts. Bone marrow suppression can be severe.
• Evaluate the patient's and family's knowledge of drug therapy.

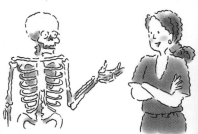

Now, you promise to monitor my neutrophil and platelet counts closely? I don't want my marrow suppressed!

Key nursing diagnoses
• Ineffective protection related to drug-induced adverse reactions
• Risk for infection related to immunosuppression
• Deficient knowledge related to drug therapy

Planning outcome goals
• The risk of injury to the patient will be minimized.
• The patient will show no signs of infection as evidenced by a normal WBC count and temperature and negative cultures.
• The patient and his family will demonstrate an understanding of drug therapy.

Implementation
• Follow established procedures for safe and proper preparation, handling, administration, and disposal of drugs. Follow facility policy to reduce risks. Preparation and administration of parenteral forms create mutagenic, teratogenic, and carcinogenic risks for staff.
• Try to ease anxiety in the patient and his family before treatment.

Say "no" to nausea
• Give an antiemetic before giving the drug to lessen nausea.
• Treat extravasation promptly.
• Tell the patient to defer immunizations if possible until hematologic stability is confirmed.

Evaluation
• Patient develops no serious bleeding complications.
• Patient remains free from infection.
• Patient and his family state an understanding of drug therapy.

Antibiotic antineoplastic drugs

Antibiotic antineoplastic drugs are antimicrobial products that produce tumoricidal (tumor-destroying) effects by binding with DNA. These drugs inhibit the cellular processes of normal and malignant cells. They include:
- anthracyclines (daunorubicin, doxorubicin, and idarubicin)
- bleomycin
- dactinomycin
- mitomycin
- mitoxantrone.

Pharmacokinetics

Because antibiotic antineoplastic drugs are usually administered I.V., no absorption occurs. They're considered 100% bioavailable.

Direct delivery

Some of the drugs are also directly administered into the body cavity being treated. Bleomycin, doxorubicin, and mitomycin are sometimes given as topical bladder instillations where significant systemic absorption doesn't occur. When bleomycin is injected into the pleural space for malignant effusions, up to one-half of the dose is absorbed.

    Distribution of antibiotic antineoplastic drugs throughout the body varies as does their metabolism and elimination. (See *Antibiotic antineoplastic drugs: Doxorubicin hydrochloride*, page 632.)

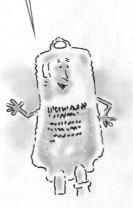

Because antibiotic antineoplastic drugs are usually administered I.V., no absorption occurs.

Pharmacodynamics

With the exception of mitomycin, antibiotic antineoplastic drugs intercalate, or insert themselves, between adjacent base pairs of a DNA molecule, physically separating them.

Worming their way in

Remember, DNA looks like a twisted ladder with the rungs made up of pairs of nitrogenous bases. Antibiotic antineoplastic drugs insert themselves between these nitrogenous bases. Then, when the DNA chain replicates, an extra base is inserted opposite the intercalated antibiotic, resulting in a mutant DNA molecule. The overall effect is cell death.

Breaking the chain

Mitomycin is activated inside the cell to a bifunctional or trifunctional alkylating drug. It produces single-strand breakage of DNA, cross-links DNA, and inhibits DNA synthesis.

Prototype pro

Antibiotic antineoplastic drugs: Doxorubicin hydrochloride

Actions
• Thought to interfere with deoxyribonucleic acid–dependent ribonucleic acid synthesis by intercalation (chemical effect unknown)
• Hinders or kills certain cancer cells

Indications
• Bladder, breast, lung, ovarian, stomach, testicular, and thyroid cancers
• Hodgkin's disease
• Acute lymphoblastic and myeloblastic leukemia
• Wilms' tumor

• Neuroblastoma
• Lymphoma
• Sarcoma

Nursing considerations
• Monitor for adverse reactions, such as arrhythmias, leukopenia, thrombocytopenia, myelosuppression, alopecia, and anaphylaxis.
• Assess the underlying neoplastic disease before therapy and reassess regularly throughout therapy.
• Follow facility policy for reconstitution and administration.

Pharmacotherapeutics

Antibiotic antineoplastic drugs act against many cancers, including:
• Hodgkin's disease and malignant lymphomas
• testicular carcinoma
• squamous cell carcinoma of the head, neck, and cervix
• Wilms' tumor (a malignant neoplasm of the kidney, occurring in young children)
• osteogenic sarcoma and rhabdomyosarcoma (a malignant neoplasm composed of striated muscle cells)
• Ewing's sarcoma (a malignant tumor that originates in bone marrow, typically in long bones or the pelvis) and other soft-tissue sarcomas
• breast, ovarian, bladder, and lung cancer
• melanoma
• carcinomas of the GI tract
• choriocarcinoma
• acute leukemia.

Drug interactions

Antibiotic antineoplastic drugs interact with many other drugs:
• Concurrent therapy with fludarabine and idarubicin isn't recommended because of the risk of fatal lung toxicity.
• Bleomycin may decrease serum digoxin and serum phenytoin levels.
• Doxorubicin may reduce serum digoxin levels.

• Combination chemotherapies enhance leukopenia and thrombo-cytopenia (reduced number of platelets).
• Mitomycin and vinca alkaloids may cause acute respiratory distress.

Adverse reactions

The primary adverse reaction to antibiotic antineoplastic drugs is bone marrow suppression. Irreversible cardiomyopathy and acute electrocardiogram (ECG) changes can also occur as well as nausea and vomiting.

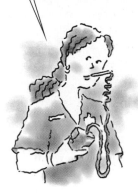

An antihistamine and antipyretic should be given before bleomycin to prevent fever and chills.

Running hot and cold

An antihistamine and antipyretic should be given before bleomycin to prevent fever and chills. An anaphylactic reaction can occur in patients receiving bleomycin for lymphoma, so test doses should be given first.

Seeing red...or blue-green

Doxorubicin, daunorubicin, and idarubicin may color urine red; mitoxantrone may color it blue-green.

Nursing process

These nursing process steps are appropriate for patients undergoing treatment with antibiotic antineoplastic drugs.

Assessment
• Perform a complete assessment before therapy begins.
• Obtain a history of the patient's neoplastic disorder before therapy, and reassess regularly thereafter.
• Assess ECG results before treatment with doxorubicin.
• Monitor the patient for adverse reactions.
• Monitor the patient's vital signs and catheter or I.V. line patency.
• Monitor platelet and total and differential leukocyte counts as well as hemoglobin, hematocrit, ALT, AST, LD, bilirubin, creatinine, uric acid, and BUN levels.
• Monitor pulmonary function tests in a patient receiving bleomycin. Assess lung function regularly.
• Monitor ECG tracings before and during treatment with daunorubicin and doxorubicin.

Key nursing diagnoses
• Ineffective health maintenance related to the presence of neoplastic disease
• Risk for infection related to immunosuppression
• Deficient knowledge related to drug therapy

Planning outcome goals
• The patient will show an improvement in the underlying condition.
• The patient will show no signs of infection as evidenced by a normal WBC count and temperature and negative cultures.
• The patient and his family will demonstrate an understanding of drug therapy.

Implementation
• Follow established procedures for safe and proper handling, administration, and disposal of chemotherapeutic drugs.
• Try to ease anxiety in the patient and his family before treatment.
• Keep epinephrine, corticosteroids, and antihistamines available during therapy. Anaphylactic reactions may occur.
• Treat extravasation promptly.
• Ensure adequate hydration during idarubicin therapy.

Evaluation
• Patient exhibits improved health.
• Patient remains free from infection.
• Patient and his family state an understanding of drug therapy. (See *Teaching about antibiotic antineoplastic drugs*.)

Education edge

Teaching about antibiotic antineoplastic drugs

If antibiotic antineoplastic therapy is prescribed, review these points with the patient and his caregivers:
• Avoid close contact with persons who have received the oral poliovirus vaccine.
• Avoid exposure to persons with bacterial or viral infections because chemotherapy increases susceptibility. Report signs of infection immediately.
• Use proper oral hygiene, including the cautious use of a toothbrush, dental floss, and toothpicks. Chemotherapy can increase the risk of microbial infection, delayed healing, and bleeding gums.
• Complete dental work before therapy begins or delay it until blood counts are normal.
• Be aware that you may bruise easily.
• Report redness, pain, or swelling at the injection site immediately. Local tissue injury and scarring may result if I.V. infiltration occurs.
• If you're taking daunorubicin, doxorubicin, or idarubicin, your urine may turn orange or red for 1 to 2 days after therapy begins. Mitoxantrone may turn your urine a blue-green color.

Hormonal antineoplastic drugs and hormone modulators

Hormonal antineoplastic drugs and hormone modulators are prescribed to alter the growth of malignant neoplasms or to manage and treat their physiologic effects. These drugs fall into six classes:

- aromatase inhibitors
- antiestrogens
- androgens
- antiandrogens
- progestins
- gonadotropin-releasing hormone analogues.

Hitting them where it hurts

Hormonal therapies and hormone modulators prove effective against hormone-dependent tumors, such as cancers of the prostate, breast, and endometrium. Lymphomas and leukemias are usually treated with therapies that include corticosteroids because of their potential for affecting lymphocytes.

Aromatase inhibitors

Aromatase inhibitors prevent androgen from being converted into estrogen in postmenopausal women. This blocks estrogen's ability to activate cancer cells by limiting the amount of estrogen reaching the cancer cells to promote growth. Aromatase inhibitors may be type 1 steroidal inhibitors, such as the drug exemestane, or type 2 nonsteroidal inhibitors, such as anastrozole and letrozole.

Pharmacokinetics

Aromatase inhibitors are taken orally in pill form and are well tolerated by most women. Steady state plasma levels after daily doses are reached in 2 to 6 weeks. Inactive metabolites are excreted in urine.

Pharmacodynamics

In postmenopausal women, estrogen is produced through aromatase, an enzyme that converts hormone precursors into estrogen. Aromatase inhibitors work by lowering the body's production of the female hormone estrogen. In up to half of all patients with breast cancer, the tumors are dependent on this hormone to grow.

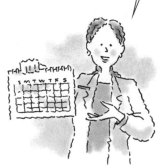

Steady state plasma levels after daily doses of aromatase inhibitors are reached in 2 to 6 weeks.

After the pause

Aromatase inhibitors are used in postmenopausal women because they lower the amount of estrogen that's produced outside the ovaries in muscle and fat tissue. Because they induce estrogen deprivation, bone thinning and osteoporosis may develop in time.

What's your type?

Type 1 inhibitors irreversibly inhibit the aromatase enzyme, whereas type 2 inhibitors reversibly inhibit the aromatase enzyme. It has also been suggested that type 1 aromatase inhibitors might have some effect after the failure of a type 2 aromatase inhibitor.

Exemestane selectively inhibits estrogen synthesis and doesn't affect synthesis of adrenocorticosteroid, aldosterone, or thyroid hormones. Anastrozole and letrozole act by competitively binding to the heme of the cytochrome P450 subunit of aromatase, leading to decreased biosynthesis of estrogen in all tissues. They don't affect synthesis of adrenocorticosteroid, aldosterone, or thyroid hormones.

Pharmacotherapeutics

Aromatase inhibitors are indicated primarily for postmenopausal women with metastatic breast cancer. They may be administered alone or with other agents such as tamoxifen.

Drug interactions

• Certain drugs may decrease the effectiveness of anastrozole, including tamoxifen and estrogen-containing drugs.
• Exemestane given in combination with cytochrome P450 isoenzyme 3A4 (CYP3A4) inducers may result in decreased serum exemestane concentrations.

Adverse reactions

Adverse reactions to aromatase inhibitors are rare but may include dizziness, fever, pharyngitis, mild nausea, anorexia, urinary tract infections, mild muscle and joint aches, hot flashes, alopecia, and increased sweating. They can also affect cholesterol levels; anastrozole may elevate high-density lipoprotein and low-density lipoprotein levels.

Nursing process

These nursing process steps are appropriate for patients undergoing treatment with aromatase inhibitors.

Aromatase inhibitors lower the amount of estrogen that's produced outside the ovaries in muscle and fat tissue. They're primarily used for postmenopausal women with metastatic breast cancer.

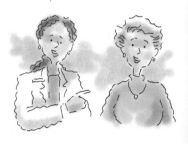

Assessment
- Assess the patient's breast cancer before therapy and regularly thereafter.
- Monitor the patient for adverse reactions and drug interactions.
- Monitor the patient's hydration status if adverse GI reactions occur.
- Evaluate the patient's and family's knowledge of drug therapy.

Key nursing diagnoses
- Ineffective health maintenance related to the presence of breast cancer
- Ineffective protection related to adverse drug effects
- Deficient knowledge related to drug therapy

Planning outcome goals
- The patient will exhibit an improvement in the underlying condition.
- The risk of injury to the patient will be minimized.
- The patient and her family will demonstrate an understanding of drug therapy.

Implementation
- Administer the agent according to facility protocol to post-menopausal women.
- Don't give the drug with estrogen-containing drugs because doing so could interfere with the drug's intended action.
- Monitor the patient for adverse effects and drug interactions.
- Continue the treatment, as ordered, until tumor progression is evident.
- Administer the drug after meals.

Evaluation
- Patient responds well to drug therapy.
- Patient doesn't experience adverse effects.
- Patient and her family state an understanding of drug therapy.

Antiestrogens

Antiestrogens bind to estrogen receptors and block estrogen action. The antiestrogens include tamoxifen citrate, toremifene citrate, and fulvestrant.

Feeling antagonistic?

Tamoxifen and toremifene are nonsteroidal estrogen agonist-antagonists. Fulvestrant is a pure estrogen antagonist.

Pharmacokinetics

After oral administration, tamoxifen is absorbed well and undergoes extensive metabolism in the liver before being excreted in feces. I.M. injection of fulvestrant yields peak serum levels in 7 to 9 days and has a half-life of 40 days. Toremifene is well absorbed and isn't influenced by food.

Pharmacodynamics

The exact antineoplastic action of these agents is unknown. However, it's known that they act as estrogen antagonists. Estrogen receptors, found in the cancer cells of half of premenopausal and three-fourths of postmenopausal women with breast cancer, respond to estrogen to induce tumor growth.

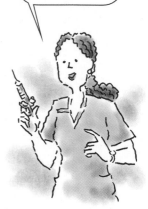

I.M. injection of fulvestrant results in peak serum levels in 7 to 9 days.

It's bound to inhibit growth

Tamoxifen, toremifene, and fulvestrant bind to the estrogen receptors and inhibit estrogen-mediated tumor growth in breast tissue. Tamoxifen can retain estrogen antagonist activity in other tissue such as bone. The inhibition may result because tamoxifen binds to receptors at the nuclear level or because the binding reduces the number of free receptors in the cytoplasm. Ultimately, DNA synthesis and cell growth are inhibited.

Pharmacotherapeutics

The antiestrogen tamoxifen citrate is used alone and as adjuvant treatment with radiation therapy and surgery in women with negative axillary lymph nodes and in postmenopausal women with positive axillary nodes.

Further tales of tamoxifen

It's also used for advanced breast cancer in postmenopausal women who have estrogen receptor–positive tumors. Tumors in postmenopausal women are more responsive to tamoxifen than those in premenopausal women. Tamoxifen may also be used to reduce the incidence of breast cancer in healthy women at high risk for breast cancer. (See *Who benefits from tamoxifen?*)

Toremifene is used to treat metastatic breast cancer in postmenopausal women with estrogen receptor–positive tumors. Fulvestrant is used in postmenopausal women with receptor-positive metastatic breast cancer with disease progression after treatment with tamoxifen.

Drug interactions

• Fulvestrant has no known drug interactions.

Who benefits from tamoxifen?

The current indication for the use of tamoxifen is based on the 1998 results of the "Breast Cancer Prevention Trial," sponsored by the National Cancer Institute. Results indicated that tamoxifen reduced the rate of breast cancer in healthy high-risk women by one-half. However, tamoxifen can cause serious adverse reactions, including potentially fatal blood clots and uterine cancer. The question is whether these risks are worth the benefits in healthy women.

The National Cancer Institute's report

To help answer this question, the National Cancer Institute published a report in November 1999. They concluded that most women over age 60 would receive more harm than benefit from tamoxifen. Even though women under age 60 could benefit from taking tamoxifen, they were still at risk unless they had a hysterectomy, which eliminated the risk of uterine cancer, or were in the very high-risk group for developing breast cancer.

Breaking it down further

The report also concluded that the risks of tamoxifen were greater than the benefits for black women over age 60 and for almost all other women over age 60 who still had a uterus. But for older women without a uterus and with a 3.5% chance of developing breast cancer over the next 5 years, the benefits may outweigh the risks.

NSABP studies update

A report from the 2000 annual meeting of the American Society of Clinical Oncology presented an analysis of data gathered from the National Surgical Adjuvant Breast and Bowel Project (NSABP), which carried out nine studies of adjuvant tamoxifen therapy for breast cancer. The analysis indicated that tamoxifen is as effective in black women as in white women in reducing the occurrence of contralateral breast cancer (breast cancer that develops in the healthy breast after treatment in the opposite breast).

Future findings

The Study of Tamoxifen and Raloxifene (STAR) is a clinical trial being conducted to determine whether raloxifene can prevent breast cancer better and with fewer adverse effects than tamoxifen.

The study, which began in 1999 and continued to enroll women until 2004, produced initial results in 2006. These results indicated that raloxifene is as effective as tamoxifen in reducing the risk of breast cancer. It also showed that the women who took raloxifene had fewer incidences of uterine cancer and fewer blood clots than women who took tamoxifen. For more information on this study, go to *www.cancer.gov/clinicaltrials/digestpage/star.*

- Tamoxifen and toremifene may increase the effects of warfarin sodium, increasing prothrombin time (PT) and the risk of bleeding.
- Bromocriptine increases the effects of tamoxifen.

Adverse reactions

Adverse reactions to antiestrogens vary by drug. In general, antiestrogens are relatively nontoxic drugs.

Tamoxifen

The most common adverse reactions to tamoxifen include:
- hot flashes
- nausea and vomiting
- diarrhea
- fluid retention

• leukopenia or thrombocytopenia (reduced WBCs and platelets, respectively)
• hypercalcemia (elevated serum calcium levels) in patients with bone metastasis.

Toremifene

Adverse reactions to toremifene include:
• hot flashes
• sweating
• nausea and vomiting
• vaginal discharge or bleeding
• edema.

Fulvestrant

Adverse reactions to fulvestrant include:
• hot flashes
• nausea and vomiting
• diarrhea or constipation
• abdominal pain
• headache
• back pain
• pharyngitis.

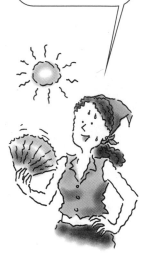

Whew! All of the antiestrogen drugs seem to cause hot flashes. I'd better keep my fan at the ready!

Nursing process

These nursing process steps are appropriate for patients undergoing treatment with antiestrogens.

Assessment

• Assess the patient's breast cancer before therapy and regularly thereafter.
• Monitor CBC closely in the patient with leukopenia or thrombocytopenia.
• Monitor lipid levels during long-term therapy in patients with hyperlipidemia.

Calcium compounder

• Monitor the patient's calcium level. The drug may compound hypercalcemia related to bone metastases during the initiation of therapy.
• Watch for adverse reactions.
• Monitor the patient's hydration status if adverse GI reactions occur.
• Evaluate the patient's and family's knowledge of drug therapy.

Key nursing diagnoses

- Ineffective health maintenance related to the presence of breast cancer
- Risk for deficient fluid volume related to drug-induced adverse GI reactions
- Deficient knowledge related to drug therapy

Planning outcome goals

- The patient will exhibit an improvement in the underlying condition.
- The patient's fluid volume will remain within normal limits as evidenced by vital signs and intake and output.
- The patient and her family will demonstrate an understanding of drug therapy.

Implementation

- Administer the medication as ordered and monitor for effects.
- Make sure that the patient swallows enteric-coated tablets whole.
- Monitor the patient for adverse reactions and drug interactions.

Evaluation

- Patient responds well to drug therapy.
- Patient maintains adequate hydration.
- Patient and her family state an understanding of drug therapy.

(See *Teaching about tamoxifen.*)

Education edge

Teaching about tamoxifen

If tamoxifen therapy is prescribed, review these points with the patient and her caregivers:

- Report signs and symptoms of a pulmonary embolism (chest pain, difficulty breathing, rapid breathing, sweating, and fainting).
- Report signs and symptoms of a stroke, including headache, vision changes, confusion, difficulty speaking or walking, and weakness in the face, arm, or leg, especially on one side of the body.
- Take an analgesic for pain. Acute bone pain during drug therapy usually means that the drug will produce a good response.

- Have regular gynecologic examinations because of an increased risk of uterine cancer.
- If you're taking the drug to reduce the risk of breast cancer, use the proper technique for breast self-examination. Review this with your health care provider.
- It's important to keep appointments for clinical breast examinations, annual mammograms, and gynecologic examinations.
- If you're premenopausal, use a barrier form of contraception because short-term therapy induces ovulation.
- If you're of childbearing age, avoid becoming pregnant during therapy and consult with your prescriber before becoming pregnant.

Androgens

Androgens are synthetic derivatives of naturally occurring testosterone. They include:
- fluoxymesterone
- testolactone
- testosterone enanthate
- testosterone propionate.

Pharmacokinetics

The pharmacokinetic properties of therapeutic androgens resemble those of naturally occurring testosterone.

Designer drugs

The oral androgens, fluoxymesterone and testolactone, are absorbed well. The parenteral ones—testosterone enanthate and testosterone propionate—are designed specifically for slow absorption after I.M. injection. Androgens are distributed well throughout the body, metabolized extensively in the liver, and excreted in urine.

Checking the suspension

The duration of the parenteral forms is longer because the oil suspension is absorbed slowly. Parenteral androgens are administered one to three times per week.

Pharmacodynamics

Androgens probably act by one or more mechanisms. They may reduce the number of prolactin receptors or may bind competitively to those that are available.

Keeping its sister hormone in check

Androgens may inhibit estrogen synthesis or competitively bind at estrogen receptors. These actions prevent estrogen from affecting estrogen-sensitive tumors.

Pharmacotherapeutics

Androgens are indicated for the palliative treatment of advanced breast cancer, particularly in postmenopausal women with bone metastasis.

Drug interactions

Androgens may alter dosage requirements in patients receiving insulin, oral antidiabetic drugs, or oral anticoagulants. Taking these drugs with other drugs that are toxic to the liver increases the risk of liver toxicity.

Adverse reactions

Nausea and vomiting are the most common adverse reactions to androgens. Fluid retention caused by sodium retention may also occur as well as paresthesia and peripheral neuropathy.

Women taking androgens may develop:
- acne
- clitoral hypertrophy
- deeper voice
- increased facial and body hair
- increased sexual desire
- menstrual irregularity.

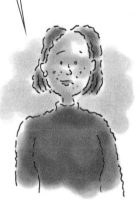

Androgens may cause female patients to develop acne.

Nursing process

These nursing process steps are appropriate for patients undergoing treatment with androgens.

Assessment
- Assess the patient's breast cancer before therapy and regularly thereafter.
- Monitor fluid and electrolyte levels, especially the calcium level.
- Monitor the patient for adverse reactions and drug interactions.
- Evaluate the patient's and family's knowledge of drug therapy.

Key nursing diagnoses
- Ineffective health maintenance related to the presence of cancer
- Disturbed sensory perception (tactile) related to drug-induced paresthesia and peripheral neuropathy
- Deficient knowledge related to drug therapy

Planning outcome goals
- The patient will demonstrate an improvement in assessment findings and diagnostic testing.
- The patient won't experience injury from disturbed sensory perception.
- The patient and her family will demonstrate an understanding of drug therapy.

Implementation
- Encourage the patient to drink fluids to aid calcium excretion.
- Encourage the patient to exercise to prevent hypercalcemia.
- Administer the drug according to facility guidelines.

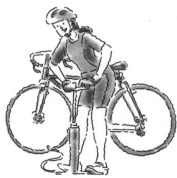

Encourage the patient to exercise to prevent hypercalcemia. Just make sure the tires are pumped up first!

Time will tell

• Monitor the patient for effects and adverse reactions. Inform her that the therapeutic response may not be immediate; it may take up to 3 months to notice the benefits.

Evaluation
• Patient responds well to drug therapy.
• Patient lists ways to protect against the risk of injury caused by diminished tactile sensation.
• Patient and her family state an understanding of drug therapy.

Antiandrogens

Antiandrogens are used as an adjunct therapy with gonadotropin-releasing hormone analogues in treating advanced prostate cancer. These drugs include:
• flutamide
• nilutamide
• bicalutamide.

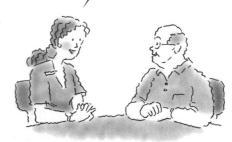

Antiandrogens are used with a gonadotropin-releasing hormone analogue to treat metastatic prostate cancer.

Pharmacokinetics

After oral administration, antiandrogens are absorbed rapidly and completely. They're metabolized rapidly and extensively and excreted primarily in urine.

Pharmacodynamics

Flutamide, nilutamide, and bicalutamide exert their antiandrogenic action by inhibiting androgen uptake or preventing androgen binding in cell nuclei in target tissues.

Pharmacotherapeutics

Antiandrogens are used with a gonadotropin-releasing hormone analogue, such as leuprolide acetate, to treat metastatic prostate cancer.

A flare for their work

Concomitant administration of antiandrogens and a gonadotropin-releasing hormone analogue may help prevent the disease flare that occurs when the gonadotropin-releasing hormone analogue is used alone.

Drug interactions

Antiandrogens don't interact significantly with other drugs. However, flutamide and bicalutamide may affect PT in a patient receiving warfarin.

Adverse reactions

When an antiandrogen is used with a gonadotropin-releasing hormone analogue, the most common adverse reactions are:
- hot flashes
- decreased sexual desire
- impotence
- diarrhea
- nausea and vomiting
- breast enlargement.

Nursing process

These nursing process steps are appropriate for patients undergoing treatment with antiandrogens.

Assessment
- Assess the patient's prostate cancer before therapy.
- Monitor liver function tests periodically.
- Monitor the patient for adverse reactions.
- Monitor the patient's hydration status if adverse GI reactions occur.
- Evaluate the patient's and family's knowledge of drug therapy.

Key nursing diagnoses
- Ineffective health maintenance related to the presence of prostate cancer
- Risk for deficient fluid volume related to adverse GI reactions
- Deficient knowledge related to drug therapy

Planning outcome goals
- The patient will demonstrate an improvement in assessment findings and diagnostic testing.
- The patient's fluid volume will remain within normal limits as exhibited by vital signs and intake and output.
- The patient and his family will demonstrate an understanding of drug therapy.

Implementation
- Administer medication according to facility policy. The drug may be given without regard to meals.

- Administer flutamide with a gonadotropin–releasing hormone analogue such as leuprolide acetate.

Don't stop those drugs!

- Tell the patient that he must take flutamide continuously with a drug used for medical castration, such as leuprolide acetate, to allow for the full benefit of therapy. Leuprolide suppresses testosterone production, whereas flutamide inhibits testosterone action at the cellular level. Together, they can impair the growth of androgen-responsive tumors. Advise the patient not to discontinue either drug.
- Monitor the patient for adverse reactions and drug interactions.

Evaluation

- Patient responds well to drug therapy.
- Patient maintains adequate hydration throughout drug therapy.
- Patient and his family state an understanding of drug therapy.

Progestins

Progestins are hormones used to treat various forms of cancer and include:

- medroxyprogesterone acetate
- megestrol acetate.

Pharmacokinetics

When taken orally, megestrol acetate is absorbed well. After I.M. injection in an aqueous or oil suspension, medroxyprogesterone is absorbed slowly from its deposit site.

Fat chance

These drugs are distributed well throughout the body and may sequester in fatty tissue. Progestins are metabolized in the liver and excreted as metabolites in urine.

Pharmacodynamics

The mechanism of action of progestins in treating tumors isn't completely understood. Researchers believe that the drugs bind to a specific receptor to act on hormonally sensitive cells.

Keeping the numbers down

Because progestins don't exhibit a cytotoxic activity (destroying or poisoning cells), they're considered cytostatic (they keep cells from multiplying).

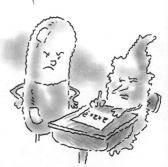

Progestins are cytostatic drugs. That means we prevent cancer cells from multiplying.

Pharmacotherapeutics

Progestins are used for the palliative treatment of advanced endometrial, breast, and renal cancers. Megestrol is used more often than medroxyprogesterone.

Drug interactions

No drug interactions have been identified for megestrol. Medroxyprogesterone, however, may interfere with bromocriptine's effects, causing menstruation to stop. Also, aminoglutethimide and rifampin may reduce the progestin effects of medroxyprogesterone.

Adverse reactions

Mild fluid retention is probably the most common reaction to progestins. Other adverse reactions include:
- thromboemboli
- breakthrough bleeding, spotting, and changes in menstrual flow in women.
- breast tenderness
- liver function abnormalities.

A sensitive situation

Patients who are hypersensitive to the oil carrier used for injection (usually sesame or castor oil) may have a local or systemic hypersensitivity reaction.

Nursing process

These nursing process steps are appropriate for patients undergoing treatment with progestins.

Assessment
- Assess the patient's condition before therapy and regularly thereafter.
- Monitor injection sites for evidence of sterile abscess.
- Monitor the patient for adverse reactions and drug interactions.
- Evaluate the patient's and family's knowledge of drug therapy.

Key nursing diagnoses
- Ineffective health maintenance related to the presence of cancer
- Risk for imbalanced fluid volume related to adverse GI reactions
- Deficient knowledge related to drug therapy

Planning outcome goals

• The patient will demonstrate an improvement in assessment findings and diagnostic testing.
• The patient's fluid volume will remain within normal limits as exhibited by vital signs and intake and output.
• The patient and his family will demonstrate an understanding of drug therapy.

Implementation

• Administer the medication according to facility policy.

Round and round we rotate

• Rotate injection sites to prevent muscle atrophy. Warn the patient that I.M. injection may be painful.
• Monitor the patient for adverse reactions and drug interactions.
• Instruct the patient to avoid caffeine and smoking during drug therapy.
• Teach a female patient how to perform routine monthly breast self-examinations.

Evaluation

• Patient responds well to drug therapy.
• Patient maintains adequate hydration throughout drug therapy.
• Patient and his family state an understanding of drug therapy.

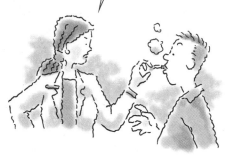

Instruct the patient to avoid smoking during drug therapy. Out with that cigarette!

Gonadotropin-releasing hormone analogues

Gonadotropin-releasing hormone analogues are used to treat advanced prostate cancer. They include:
• goserelin acetate
• leuprolide acetate
• triptorelin pamoate.

Pharmacokinetics

Goserelin is absorbed slowly for the first 8 days of therapy and rapidly and continuously thereafter. After subcutaneous (subQ) injection, leuprolide is absorbed well. The distribution, metabolism, and excretion of these drugs isn't clearly defined. Triptorelin reaches peak serum levels within 1 week of I.M. injection, with serum levels remaining detectable for 4 weeks.

Pharmacodynamics

Initially, goserelin and leuprolide act on the pituitary gland of a male patient to increase LH secretion, which in turn stimulates testosterone production.

The rise...

The peak testosterone level is reached about 72 hours after the start of daily administration. Triptorelin is a potent inhibitor of gonadotropin secretion. After the first dose, levels of LH, follicle-stimulating hormone (FSH), testosterone, and estradiol surge transiently.

...and fall

After long-term, continuous administration, LH and FSH secretion steadily declines and testicular steroidogenesis decreases. In men, testosterone declines to a level typically seen in surgically castrated men. As a result, tissues and functions that depend on these hormones become quiescent.

Reversing course

The drop in LH secretion occurs because, with long-term administration, goserelin and leuprolide inhibit LH release from the pituitary gland, which subsequently inhibits testicular release of testosterone. Because prostate tumor cells are stimulated by testosterone, the reduced testosterone level inhibits tumor growth.

Pharmacotherapeutics

Goserelin, triptorelin, and leuprolide are used for the palliative treatment of metastatic prostate cancer. These drugs lower the testosterone level without the adverse psychological effects of castration or the adverse cardiovascular effects of diethylstilbestrol.

Drug interactions

No drug interactions have been identified with goserelin, triptorelin, or leuprolide.

Adverse reactions

Hot flashes, impotence, and decreased sexual desire are commonly reported reactions to goserelin, leuprolide, and triptorelin. Other adverse reactions include:

* peripheral edema
* nausea

- vomiting
- constipation
- anorexia.

On the rise

Disease signs and symptoms and pain may worsen or flare during the first 2 weeks of goserelin or leuprolide therapy. The flare can be fatal in patients with bony vertebral metastasis.

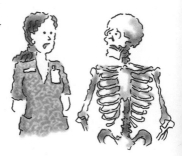

Some patients taking drugs such as goserelin may initially have increased bone pain.

Nursing process

These nursing process steps are appropriate for patients undergoing treatment with gonadotropin-releasing hormone analogues.

Assessment
- Assess the patient's condition before therapy and regularly thereafter.

At first, it may get worse

- When used for prostate cancer, LH–RH analogues such as goserelin may initially worsen signs and symptoms because the drug initially increases testosterone levels. Some patients may have increased bone pain. Rarely, disease (spinal cord compression or ureteral obstruction) may worsen.
- Monitor the patient for adverse reactions.
- Evaluate the patient's and family's knowledge of drug therapy.

Key nursing diagnoses
- Ineffective health maintenance related to the underlying condition
- Acute pain related to drug-induced adverse reactions
- Deficient knowledge related to drug therapy

Planning outcome goals
- The patient will exhibit an improvement in the underlying condition.
- The patient's pain will decrease.
- The patient and his family will demonstrate an understanding of drug therapy.

Implementation
- The drug should be given under supervision of the prescriber. Administer the medication according to facility policy. (See *Goserelin warning*.)
- To avoid the need for a new syringe and injection site, don't aspirate after inserting the needle.

Locked and preloaded

- The implant form of goserelin comes in a preloaded syringe. If the package is damaged, don't use the syringe. Make sure that the drug is visible in the translucent chamber.
- After implantation, withdraw the needle and apply a bandage to the area.
- Be prepared to schedule the patient for an ultrasound to locate goserelin implants if they require removal.
- Notify the prescriber of adverse reactions and provide supportive care as indicated and ordered.

Reporting as ordered

- Advise the patient to report every 28 days for a new implant. A delay of a few days is permissible.
- If the patient is to continue subQ injections of leuprolide at home, teach him proper technique and advise him to use only syringes provided by the manufacturer.

Evaluation

- Patient responds well to drug therapy.
- Patient has no pain.
- Patient and his family state an understanding of drug therapy.

Natural antineoplastic drugs

A subclass of antineoplastic drugs known as *natural products* includes:
- vinca alkaloids
- podophyllotoxins.

Vinca alkaloids

Vinca alkaloids are nitrogenous bases derived from the periwinkle plant. These drugs are cell cycle–specific for the M phase and include:
- vinblastine
- vincristine
- vinorelbine.

Pharmacokinetics

After I.V. administration, the vinca alkaloids are distributed well throughout the body. They undergo moderate liver metab-

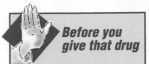

Vinca alkaloids are derived from the periwinkle plant.

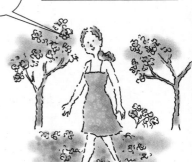

olism before being eliminated through different phases, primarily in feces, with a small percentage eliminated in urine.

Pharmacodynamics

Vinca alkaloids may disrupt the normal function of the microtubules (structures within cells that are associated with the movement of DNA) by binding to the protein tubulin in the microtubules.

Separation anxiety

With the microtubules unable to separate chromosomes properly, the chromosomes are dispersed throughout the cytoplasm or arranged in unusual groupings. As a result, formation of the mitotic spindle is prevented, and the cells can't complete mitosis (cell division).

Under arrest

Cell division is arrested in metaphase, causing cell death. Therefore, vinca alkaloids are cell cycle, M phase–specific. Interruption of the microtubule function may also impair some types of cellular movement, phagocytosis (engulfing and destroying microorganisms and cellular debris), and CNS functions.

Pharmacotherapeutics

Vinca alkaloids are used in several therapeutic situations:
- Vinblastine is used to treat metastatic testicular carcinoma, lymphomas, Kaposi's sarcoma (the most common acquired immunodeficiency syndrome [AIDS]-related cancer), neuroblastoma (a highly malignant tumor originating in the sympathetic nervous system), breast carcinoma, and choriocarcinoma.
- Vincristine is used in combination therapy to treat Hodgkin's disease, non-Hodgkin's lymphoma, Wilms' tumor, rhabdomyosarcoma, and acute lymphocytic leukemia.
- Vinorelbine is used to treat non–small-cell lung cancer. It may also be used in the treatment of metastatic breast carcinoma, cisplatin-resistant ovarian carcinoma, and Hodgkin's disease.

Drug interactions

Vinca alkaloids interact in many ways with other drugs:
- Erythromycin may increase the toxicity of vinblastine.
- Vinblastine decreases the plasma levels of phenytoin.
- Vincristine reduces the effects of digoxin.

> Vinca alkaloids don't always play well with other drugs. Make sure you're aware of potential drug interactions.

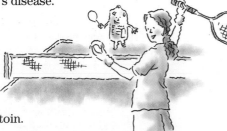

• Asparaginase decreases liver metabolism of vincristine, increasing the risk of toxicity.
• Calcium channel blockers enhance vincristine accumulation, increasing the tendency for toxicity.

Adverse reactions

Vinca alkaloids may cause the following adverse reactions:
• nausea and vomiting
• constipation
• stomatitis (mouth inflammation).
   Vinblastine and vinorelbine toxicities occur primarily as bone marrow suppression. Neuromuscular abnormalities frequently occur with vincristine and vinorelbine and occasionally with vinblastine therapy.

A stinging sensation

Vinblastine may produce tumor pain described as an intense stinging or burning in the tumor bed, with an abrupt onset 1 to 3 minutes after drug administration. The pain usually lasts 20 minutes to 3 hours.

Hair scare

Reversible alopecia occurs in up to one-half of patients receiving vinca alkaloids; it's more likely to occur with vincristine than vinblastine.

Nursing process

These nursing process steps are appropriate for patients undergoing treatment with vinca alkaloids.

Assessment

• Assess the patient's condition before therapy and regularly thereafter.
• Monitor the patient for the development of life-threatening acute bronchospasm after drug administration. This reaction is most likely if the patient also receives mitomycin.
• Monitor the patient for adverse reactions and drug interactions.
• Assess for numbness and tingling in the patient's hands and feet. Assess his gait for early evidence of footdrop. Vinblastine is less neurotoxic than vincristine.
• With vincristine, check for depression of the Achilles tendon reflex, numbness, tingling, footdrop or wristdrop, difficulty in walking, ataxia, and a slapping gait. Also check the patient's ability to walk on his heels.

• Monitor the patient for hyperuricemia, especially if he has leukemia or lymphoma.
• Monitor the patient's bowel function. Constipation may be an early sign of neurotoxicity when administering vincristine.
• Evaluate the patient's and family's knowledge of drug therapy.

Key nursing diagnoses

• Ineffective health maintenance related to the presence of neoplastic disease
• Ineffective protection related to drug-induced adverse reactions
• Deficient knowledge related to drug therapy

Planning outcome goals

• The patient will demonstrate an improvement in assessment findings and diagnostic testing.
• The risk of injury to the patient will be minimized.
• The patient and his family will demonstrate an understanding of drug therapy.

Implementation

• Give an antiemetic before giving the drug.
• Follow facility policy to reduce risks. Preparation and administration of the parenteral form of the drug are linked to carcinogenic, mutagenic, and teratogenic risks for personnel.
• Reconstitute the drug as ordered and administer according to facility policy.
• If extravasation occurs, stop the infusion immediately and notify the prescriber. (See *More on vinblastine and vincristine.*)
• If acute bronchospasm occurs after administration, notify the prescriber immediately.
• Make sure that the patient maintains adequate fluid intake to promote excretion of uric acid.
• Be prepared to stop the drug and notify the prescriber if stomatitis occurs.
• The dosage shouldn't be repeated more frequently than every 7 days because severe leukopenia can develop.
• Anticipate a decrease in the dosage by 50% if the patient's bilirubin level is greater than 3 mg/dl.
• The patient may need fluid restriction if syndrome of inappropriate diuretic hormone develops.

Evaluation

• Patient responds well to drug therapy.
• Patient doesn't develop serious complications from adverse hematologic reactions.
• Patient and his family state an understanding of drug therapy.

More on vinblastine and vincristine

Manufacturers recommend that moderate heat be applied to an area of leakage or extravasation of vinblastine or vincristine. Local injection of hyaluronidase may help disperse the drug. Some clinicians prefer to apply ice packs on and off every 2 hours for 24 hours, with local injection of hydrocortisone or normal saline solution. Don't inject the drug into a limb with compromised circulation.

Vinblastine and vincristine are fatal if given intrathecally; they're for I.V. use only.

If extravasation occurs, stop the infusion at once and notify the prescriber.

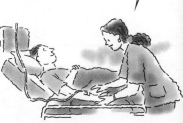

Podophyllotoxins

Podophyllotoxins are semisynthetic glycosides that are cell cycle–specific and act during the G2 and late S phases of the cell cycle. They include:
- etoposide
- teniposide.

Pharmacokinetics

When taken orally, podophyllotoxins are only moderately absorbed. Although the drugs are distributed widely throughout the body, they achieve poor CSF levels. Podophyllotoxins undergo liver metabolism and are excreted primarily in urine.

Pharmacodynamics

Although their mechanism of action isn't completely understood, podophyllotoxins produce several biochemical changes in tumor cells.

The highs and lows

At low concentrations, these drugs block cells at the late S or G2 phase. At higher concentrations, they arrest the cells in the G2 phase.

Breaking the mold

Podophyllotoxins can also break one of the strands of the DNA molecule. These drugs can also inhibit nucleotide transport and incorporation into nucleic acids.

Pharmacotherapeutics

Etoposide is used to treat testicular cancer and small-cell lung cancer. Teniposide is used to treat acute lymphoblastic leukemia.

Drug interactions

Podophyllotoxins have few significant interactions with other drugs:
- Teniposide may increase the clearance and intracellular levels of methotrexate.
- Etoposide may increase the risk of bleeding in a patient taking warfarin.

Adverse reactions

Most patients receiving podophyllotoxins experience hair loss. Other adverse reactions include:

• nausea and vomiting
• anorexia
• stomatitis
• bone marrow suppression, causing leukopenia and, less commonly, thrombocytopenia
• acute hypotension (if a podophyllotoxin is infused too rapidly by the I.V. route).

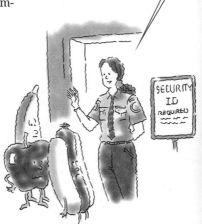

Podophyllotoxins can cause nausea and vomiting. I'm sorry guys; I can't let you in right now.

Nursing process

These nursing process steps are appropriate for patients undergoing treatment with podophyllotoxins.

Assessment

• Assess the patient's condition before therapy and regularly thereafter.
• Monitor the patient for adverse reactions and drug interactions.
• Obtain the patient's baseline blood pressure before therapy and monitor blood pressure at 30-minute intervals during infusion.

Gauging the growth rate

• Monitor the drug's effectiveness by noting results of follow-up diagnostic tests and overall physical status and by regularly checking tumor size and rate of growth through appropriate studies.
• Monitor the patient's CBC. Observe him for signs of bone marrow suppression.
• Evaluate the patient's and family's knowledge of drug therapy.

Key nursing diagnoses

• Ineffective health maintenance related to the presence of neoplastic disease
• Ineffective protection related to drug-induced adverse reactions
• Deficient knowledge related to drug therapy

Planning outcome goals

• The patient will demonstrate an improvement in assessment findings and diagnostic testing.
• The risk of injury to the patient will be minimized.
• The patient and his family will demonstrate an understanding of drug therapy.

Implementation
- Follow facility policy to reduce risks. Preparation and administration of the parenteral form of the drug are linked to carcinogenic, mutagenic, and teratogenic risks for personnel.
- Reconstitute the drug as ordered and administer according to facility policy.
- Store oral capsules in the refrigerator.
- Give I.V. infusions slowly, over at least 30 minutes, to prevent severe hypotension.
- If the patient's systolic blood pressure falls below 90 mm Hg, stop the infusion and notify the prescriber.

Filter killer

- Don't give the drug through a membrane-type in-line filter because the diluent may dissolve the filter.
- Keep diphenhydramine, hydrocortisone, epinephrine, and necessary emergency equipment available to establish an airway in case of anaphylaxis.
- Monitor the patient for signs of infection and bleeding. Teach him how to take infection-control and bleeding precautions.
- Tell the patient that hair loss is possible, but reversible.
- Instruct the patient to report discomfort, pain, or burning at the I.V. insertion site.

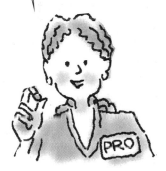

Store oral capsules of podophyllotoxins in the refrigerator.

Evaluation
- Patient responds well to drug therapy.
- Patient doesn't develop serious complications from adverse hematologic reactions.
- Patient and his family state an understanding of drug therapy.

Monoclonal antibodies

Recombinant DNA technology has allowed for the development of monoclonal antibodies directed at targets, such as other immune cells or cancer cells. They include:
- alemtuzumab
- gemtuzumab ozogamicin
- ibritumomab tiuxetan
- rituximab
- trastuzumab.

Pharmacokinetics
The monoclonal antibodies, by virtue of their large protein molecule structure, aren't absorbed orally.

Here's to a long (half) life

These drugs may have a limited volume of distribution as well as a long half-life, sometimes measured in weeks.

Pharmacodynamics

The monoclonal antibodies bind to target receptor or cancer cells and can cause tumor death via several mechanisms. They can induce programmed cell death and recruit other elements of the immune system to attack the cancer cell.

Targeting in

They can also deliver a toxic chemotherapy drug (gemtuzumab ozogamicin) or radiation (ibritumomab tiuxetan) dose to the site of the tumor.

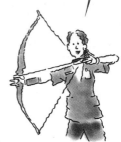

Monoclonal antibodies can deliver a dose of toxic chemotherapy drug or radiation right to the site of the tumor.

Pharmacotherapeutics

Monoclonal antibodies have demonstrated activity in solid tumors and hematologic malignancies, such as:
• non-Hodgkin's lymphoma—rituximab and ibritumomab tiuxetan (target CD20 or malignant B lymphocytes)
• chronic lymphocytic leukemia—alemtuzumab (target CD52 antigen or B cells)
• acute myeloid leukemia—gemtuzumab ozogamicin (target CD33 antigen in myeloid leukemia cells)
• breast cancer—trastuzumab (target HER-2 protein in breast cancer cells).

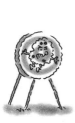

Drug interactions

• There are no known drug interactions with alemtuzumab.
• Ibritumomab may cause cytopenia (decreased cell count) and may interfere with such drugs as warfarin, aspirin, clopidogrel, ticlopidine, NSAIDs, azathioprine, cyclosporin, and corticosteroids.
• Trastuzumab increases the cardiac toxicity associated with anthracycline administration.
• Rituximab used with cisplatin may cause renal toxicity.

Adverse reactions

All monoclonal antibodies are associated with infusion-related toxicities, such as fever, chills, shortness of breath, low blood pressure, and anaphylaxis. Fatalities have been reported. In addition, the following adverse reactions can occur:

- Gemtuzumab ozogamicin is associated with significant myelo-suppression and liver toxicity.

Inviting infection in

- Alemtuzumab is associated with myelosuppression and an increased risk of opportunistic infections, such as pneumocystitis, pneumonia, and fungal and viral infections.
- Ibritumomab tiuxetan is associated with increased myelosuppression.

Nursing process

These nursing process steps are appropriate for patients undergoing treatment with monoclonal antibodies.

Assessment

- Assess the patient's condition before therapy and regularly thereafter.
- Monitor the patient for adverse reactions and drug interactions.
- Obtain the patient's baseline blood pressure before therapy and monitor him for hypotensive signs and symptoms during drug administration.
- Monitor the drug's effectiveness by noting results of follow-up diagnostic tests and overall physical status and by regularly checking tumor size and rate of growth through appropriate studies.
- Obtain a baseline CBC and platelet count before starting therapy; assess weekly during therapy and more frequently if anemia, neutropenia, or thrombocytopenia worsens.
- Monitor the patient's hematologic studies carefully during therapy. Even with normal dosages, he may experience signs and symptoms of hematologic toxicity, including myelosuppression, bone marrow dysplasia, and thrombocytopenia.
- Monitor the patient's renal function if he's receiving rituximab with cisplatin.
- After treatment, monitor the patient's CD4+ count until it reaches 200 cells/mm^3 or more.
- Evaluate the patient's and family's knowledge of drug therapy.

Key nursing diagnoses

- Risk for infection related to an immunocompromised state
- Fatigue related to drug therapy
- Deficient knowledge related to drug therapy

Planning outcome goals

- No signs of infection will be present as evidenced by a normal WBC count and temperature and negative cultures.

• The patient will exhibit less fatigue.
• The patient and his family will demonstrate an understanding of drug therapy.

Implementation
• Reconstitute the drug as ordered and administer according to facility policy. (See *Alemtuzumab warning.*)

Discolored? Discard!

• Don't use the solution if it's discolored or contains precipitate. Filter with a sterile, low-protein-binding, 5-micron filter before dilution.
• Irradiate blood if transfusions are needed to protect against graft-versus-host disease.
• Don't immunize with live viral vaccines.
• If therapy is stopped for more than 7 days, restart with a gradual dose increase.
• Rituximab, alemtuzumab, gemtuzumab, and trastuzumab must be given by I.V. infusion; don't give I.V. push or as a bolus.
• Give the I.V. infusion slowly, over at least 2 hours.
• Tell women of childbearing age and men to use effective contraceptive methods during therapy and for at least 6 months following the completion of therapy.

Evaluation
• Patient remains free from infection.
• Patient is able to peform self-care activities.
• Patient and his family state an understanding of drug therapy.

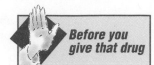

Before you give that drug

Alemtuzumab warning

When administering monoclonal antibodies such as alemtuzumab, premedicate the patient with diphenhydramine and acetaminophen before the initial infusion and before each dose increase. Hydrocortisone may be given to decrease severe infusion-related adverse effects. Give anti-infective prophylaxis while the patient is receiving therapy. Prophylaxis should continue for 2 months or until the CD4+ count is 200 cells/mm³ or more, whichever occurs later.

Topoisomerase I inhibitors

As the name implies, topoisomerase I inhibitors inhibit the enzyme topoisomerase I. These agents are derived from a naturally occurring alkaloid from the Chinese tree *Camptotheca acuminata.* Currently available drugs include:
• irinotecan
• topotecan.

Pharmacokinetics
Irinotecan and topotecan are minimally absorbed and must be given I.V. Irinotecan undergoes metabolic changes to become the active metabolite SN-38. The half-life of SN-38 is approximately 10 hours, and it's eliminated through biliary excretion. Topotecan is

metabolized hepatically, although renal excretion is a significant elimination pathway.

Pharmacodynamics

These agents exert their cytotoxic effect by inhibiting the topoisomerase I enzyme, an essential enzyme that mediates the relaxation of supercoiled DNA. Topoisomerase inhibitors bind to the DNA topoisomerase I complex and prevent resealing, thereby causing DNA strand breaks, resulting in impaired DNA synthesis.

Pharmacotherapeutics

Topoisomerase I inhibitors are active against solid tumors and hematologic malignancies. Topotecan is administered for ovarian cancer, small-cell lung cancer, and acute myeloid leukemia. Irinotecan is administered to patients with colorectal cancer or small-cell lung cancer.

Drug interactions

Irinotecan is associated with the following drug interactions:
• Ketoconazole can significantly increase SN-38 serum concentrations when given with irinotecan, increasing the risk of associated toxicities.
• Concurrent administration of diuretics may exacerbate dehydration caused by irinotecan-induced diarrhea.
• Concurrent administration of laxatives with irinotecan can induce diarrhea.
• Prochlorperazine administered with irinotecan can increase the incidence of extrapyramidal toxicities.

Adverse reactions

Diarrhea is the most common adverse reaction to topoisomerase I inhibitors, especially irinotecan, which is cholinergically mediated; this can be reversed with atropine.

Delayed reaction

Later-onset diarrhea, which may persist for up to 1 week, can occur several days after chemotherapy has been administered. Treatment consists of loperamide given every 2 hours until stools become formed.

Common conditions, part two

Besides diarrhea, the more common adverse reactions to topoisomerase I inhibitors, particularly irinotecan, include:
• increased sweating and saliva production

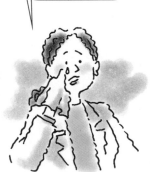

Irinotecan can cause increased sweating and salivation and watery eyes.

- watery eyes
- abdominal cramps
- nausea and vomiting
- loss of appetite
- fatigue
- hair loss or thinning.

Only occasional

Occasionally, these reactions may occur:
- mouth sores and ulcers
- muscle cramps
- temporary effect on liver function tests
- rashes, which may be itchy.

Serious situation

These reactions rarely occur but are more serious:
- Both drugs are associated with significant myelosuppression, especially topotecan.
- Irinotecan has been associated with thromboembolic events, namely myocardial infarction and stroke, which have resulted in death.

Nursing process

These nursing process steps are appropriate for patients undergoing treatment with topoisomerase I inhibitors.

Assessment

- Assess the patient's condition before therapy and regularly thereafter.
- Monitor the patient for adverse reactions and drug interactions.
- Obtain a baseline neutrophil count; it must be greater than 1,500 cells/mm^3 and the patient's platelet count greater than 100,000 cells/mm^3 before therapy can start.
- Frequent monitoring of the peripheral blood cell count is critical. Don't give repeated doses until the neutrophil count is greater than 1,000 cells/mm^3, platelet count is greater than 100,000 cells/mm^3, and hemoglobin is greater than 9 mg/dl.
- Evaluate the patient's and family's knowledge of drug therapy.

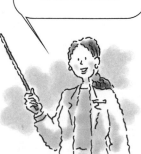

Frequent monitoring of the peripheral blood cell count is critical.

Key nursing diagnoses

- Ineffective health maintenance related to the presence of neoplastic disease
- Ineffective protection related to drug-induced adverse reactions
- Deficient knowledge related to drug therapy

Planning outcome goals
• The patient will demonstrate an improvement in assessment findings and diagnostic testing.
• The risk of injury to the patient will be minimized.
• The patient and his family will demonstrate an understanding of drug therapy.

Implementation
• Prepare the drug under a vertical laminar flow hood while wearing gloves and protective clothing. If the drug contacts skin, wash immediately and thoroughly with soap and water. If mucous membranes are affected, flush with water.
• Reconstitute the drug as ordered. Dilute and administer the drug according to facility policy.
• Give a topotecan I.V. infusion slowly, over at least 30 minutes; give an irinotecan I.V. infusion over at least 90 minutes.
• Protect unopened vials of the drug from light.
• Monitor the patient for signs and symptoms of infection, such as sore throat, fever, chills, or unusual bleeding or bruising, and report them promptly.
• Tell a female patient of childbearing age to avoid pregnancy and breast-feeding during treatment.

Evaluation
• Patient responds well to drug therapy.
• Patient doesn't develop serious complications from adverse hematologic reactions.
• Patient and his family state an understanding of drug therapy.

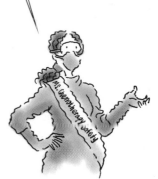

Prepare the drug under a vertical laminar flow hood while wearing gloves and protective clothing. I look quite fashionable, don't you think?

Targeted therapies

A groundbreaking approach to anticancer therapies is to target proteins associated with the growth patterns for a specific type of cancer. These new drugs include:
• gefitinib
• imatinib
• bortezomib.

Pharmacokinetics
Gefitinib is available in an oral form in which approximately half of the dose is absorbed. The drug is widely distributed in tissues. It undergoes hepatic metabolism with minimal urinary excretion.

Imatinib is available in an oral form, which is almost completely absorbed. It's 95% bound to plasma proteins and extensively metabolized by the liver. The half-life is approximately 15 hours.

Bortezomib isn't absorbed orally and must be given I.V. It's extensively distributed into body tissues and hepatically metabolized.

Pharmacodynamics

Gefitinib inhibits the epidermal growth factor receptor-1 tyrosine kinase, which is overexpressed with certain cancers, such as non–small-cell lung cancer. This blocks signaling pathways for the growth, survival, and metastasis of cancer.

In a bind

Imatinib binds to the adenosine triphosphate binding domain of the BCR-ABL protein, which stimulates other tyrosine kinase proteins to result in abnormally high production of WBCs in chronic myeloid leukemia. This binding of imatinib effectively shuts down the abnormal WBC production.

Feeling a bit inhibited...

Bortezomib inhibits proteosomes, which are integral to cell cycle function and promote tumor growth. Proteolysis by bortezomib results in the disruption of the normal homeostatic mechanisms and leads to cell death.

Pharmacotherapeutics

Gefitinib is used as a single agent for patients with non–small-cell lung cancer that has failed to respond to two previous standard chemotherapy regimens. Imatinib is used to treat chronic myeloid leukemia, acute lymphoid leukemia, and GI stomal tumors. Bortezomib is used to treat multiple myeloma that has relapsed after standard chemotherapy.

Drug interactions

Bortezomib, gefitinib, and imatinib have been associated with some drug interactions:
• Bortezomib, when taken with drugs that are inhibitors or inducers of CYP3A4, may cause either toxicities or reduced efficacy of these drugs. Inhibitors of CYP3A4 include amiodarone, cimetidine, erythromycin, diltiazem, disulfiram, fluoxetine, grapefruit juice, verapamil, zafirlukast, and zileuton. Inducers of CYP3A4 include amiodarone, carbamazepine, nevirapine, phenobarbital, phenytoin, and rifampin.

- Bortezomib, when taken with oral hypoglycemics, may cause hypoglycemia or hyperglycemia in patients with diabetes.
- Plasma levels of gefitinib and imatinib are reduced, sometimes substantially, when these drugs are given with carbamazepine, dexamethasone, phenobarbital, phenytoin, rifampin, or St. John's wort.
- Taking high doses of ranitidine with sodium bicarbonate together with gefitinib reduces gefitinib levels.
- Administration of gefitinib or imatinib with warfarin causes elevations in the International Normalized Ratio, increasing the risk of bleeding.
- Drugs that inhibit the CYP3A4 family (such as clarithromycin, erythromycin, itraconazole, and ketoconazole) when taken with imatinib may increase imatinib plasma levels.
- Imatinib administered with CYP3A4 inducers (carbamazepine, dexamethasone, phenobarbital, phenytoin, and rifampin) may increase the metabolism of imatinib and decrease imatinib levels.
- Imatinib given with simvastatin increases simvastatin levels about threefold.
- Imatinib increases plasma levels of other CYP3A4-metabolized drugs, such as triazolo-benzodiazepines, dihydropyridine, calcium channel blockers, and certain HMG-CoA reductase inhibitors.

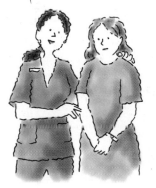

Women should avoid becoming pregnant while on targeted therapies because these drugs can cross the placental barrier and result in fetal harm or death.

Adverse reactions

Toxicities have occurred from administration of targeted therapies. Women should avoid becoming pregnant during administration of these agents because animal studies have shown that they cross the placental barrier and have resulted in fetal harm and death.

Gefitinib

Adverse reactions to gefitinib include:
- skin rash
- diarrhea
- abnormal eyelash growth
- lung and liver damage.

Imatinib

Adverse reactions to imatinib include:
- edema (periorbital and lower limb), which may result in pulmonary edema, effusions, and heart or renal failure; management includes treatment with diuretics and supportive measures such as decreasing the dosage
- nausea, vomiting, liver function abnormalities, and myelosuppression (especially neutropenia and thrombocytopenia).

Bortezomib

The most common adverse reactions to bortezomib include asthenic conditions (fatigue, malaise, and weakness), nausea, diarrhea, appetite loss (anorexia), constipation, pyrexia, and vomiting.

Other reactions include:

• peripheral neuropathy, headache, low blood pressure, liver toxicity, thrombocytopenia, and renal toxicity
• cardiac toxicity (arrhythmias, such as bradycardia, ventricular tachycardia, atrial fibrillation, and atrial flutter; heart failure; myocardial ischemia and infarction; pulmonary edema; and pericardial effusion).

Depending on the severity of the reactions, the dosage may need to be reduced or the drug withheld until toxicity resolves. Severe reactions may require discontinuing the medication.

Nursing process

These nursing process steps are appropriate for patients undergoing treatment with targeted therapies.

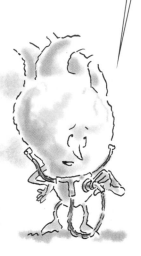

Bortezomib can cause several types of adverse reactions, including cardiac toxicity. Hmm, is that atrial fibrillation I detect?

Assessment

• Assess the patient's condition before therapy and regularly thereafter.
• Monitor the patient for adverse reactions and drug interactions.

Weighty issues

• Obtain a baseline weight before therapy, and weigh the patient daily throughout therapy. Evaluate and treat unexpected and rapid weight gain.
• Evaluate the patient's and family's knowledge of drug therapy.

Key nursing diagnoses

• Ineffective health maintenance related to the presence of neoplastic disease
• Risk for falls related to drug-induced adverse reactions
• Deficient knowledge related to drug therapy

Planning outcome goals

• The patient will demonstrate an improvement in assessment findings and diagnostic testing.
• The risk of injury to the patient will be minimized.
• The patient and his family will demonstrate an understanding of drug therapy.

Implementation
- Reconstitute the drug as ordered and administer according to facility policy.
- Monitor the patient closely for fluid retention, which can be severe.
- Monitor the patient's CBC weekly for the first month, biweekly for the second month, and periodically thereafter.
- Because GI irritation is common, give the drug with food as appropriate.
- Monitor liver function tests carefully because hepatotoxicity (occasionally severe) may occur. Decrease the dosage as needed.
- Because the long-term safety of the drug isn't known, monitor renal and liver toxicity and immunosuppression carefully.

Evaluation
- Patient responds well to drug therapy.
- Patient doesn't develop serious complications from adverse reactions.
- Patient and his family state an understanding of drug therapy.

Unclassified antineoplastic drugs

Many other antineoplastic drugs can't be included in existing classifications. These drugs include:
- aldesleukin
- asparaginases
- hydroxyurea
- interferons
- procarbazine
- taxanes (paclitaxel and docetaxel).

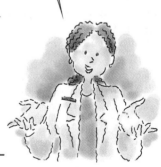

Some drugs just can't be classified.

Aldesleukin

Aldesleukin is a human recombinant interleukin-2 (IL-2) derivative that's used to treat metastatic renal cell carcinoma.

Pharmacokinetics

After I.V. administration of aldesleukin, about 30% is absorbed into the plasma and about 70% is absorbed rapidly by the liver, kidneys, and lungs. The drug is excreted primarily by the kidneys.

Pharmacodynamics

The exact antitumor mechanism of action of aldesleukin is unknown. The drug may stimulate an immunologic reaction against the tumor.

Pharmacotherapeutics

Aldesleukin is used to treat metastatic renal cell carcinoma. It may also be used in the treatment of Kaposi's sarcoma and metastatic melanoma.

Drug interactions

Aldesleukin interacts with several other drugs:
• Concomitant administration of aldesleukin and drugs with psychotropic properties (such as opioids, analgesics, antiemetics, sedatives, and tranquilizers) may produce additive CNS effects.
• Glucocorticoids may reduce aldesleukin's antitumor effects.
• Antihypertensive drugs may potentiate aldesleukin's hypotensive effects.

Tallying up the toxic interactions

• Concurrent therapy with drugs that are toxic to the kidneys (such as aminoglycosides), bone marrow (such as cytotoxic chemotherapy drugs), heart (such as doxorubicin), or liver (such as methotrexate or asparaginase) may increase toxicity to these organs.

Adverse reactions

During clinical trials, more than 15% of patients developed adverse reactions to aldesleukin. These include:
• pulmonary congestion and difficulty breathing
• anemia, thrombocytopenia, and leukopenia
• elevated bilirubin, transaminase, and alkaline phosphatase levels
• hypomagnesemia and acidosis
• reduced or absent urinary output
• elevated serum creatinine level
• stomatitis
• nausea and vomiting.

Nursing process

These nursing process steps are appropriate for patients undergoing treatment with aldesleukin.

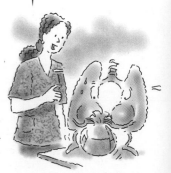

I know aldesleukin can cause pulmonary congestion and difficulty breathing, guys, but don't overreact!

Assessment
- Assess the patient's condition before therapy and regularly thereafter.
- Monitor the patient for adverse reactions and drug interactions.
- Monitor blood studies as appropriate.
- Evaluate the patient's and family's knowledge of drug therapy.

Key nursing diagnoses
- Ineffective health maintenance related to the presence of neoplastic disease
- Risk for injury related to drug-induced adverse reactions
- Deficient knowledge related to drug therapy

Planning outcome goals
- The patient will demonstrate an improvement in assessment findings and diagnostic testing.
- The risk of injury to the patient will minimized.
- The patient and his family will demonstrate an understanding of drug therapy.

Implementation
- Administer the medication according to facility protocol.
- Assess the patient for effects of the medication as well as drug interactions.
- Notify the prescriber of severe adverse reactions, which may require dosage reduction or discontinuation.

Evaluation
- Patient responds well to drug therapy.
- Patient doesn't develop serious complications from adverse reactions.
- Patient and his family state an understanding of drug therapy.

Asparaginases

Asparaginases are cell cycle–specific and act during the G1 phase. They include:
- asparaginase
- pegaspargase.

Pharmacokinetics

Asparaginase is administered parenterally. It's considered 100% bioavailable when administered I.V. and about 50% bioavailable when administered I.M.

After administration, asparaginase remains inside the blood vessels, with minimal distribution elsewhere. The metabolism of asparaginase is unknown; only trace amounts appear in urine.

Pharmacodynamics

Asparaginase and pegaspargase capitalize on the biochemical differences between normal and tumor cells.

Eat your asparagines, or else

Most normal cells can synthesize asparagine, but some tumor cells depend on other sources of asparagine for survival. Asparaginase and pegaspargase help to degrade asparagine to aspartic acid and ammonia. Deprived of their supply of asparagine, the tumor cells die.

Pharmacotherapeutics

Asparaginase is used primarily to induce remission in patients with acute lymphocytic leukemia in combination with standard chemotherapy.

If allergic to the natives

Pegaspargase is used to treat acute lymphocytic leukemia in patient who are allergic to the native form of asparaginase.

Drug interactions

Asparaginase may interact with other drugs. Asparaginase and pegaspargase can reduce the effectiveness of methotrexate. Concurrent use of asparaginase with prednisone or vincristine increases the risk of adverse reactions.

Adverse reactions

Many patients receiving asparaginase and pegaspargase develop nausea and vomiting. Fever, headache, abdominal pain, pancreatitis, coagulopathy, and liver toxicity can also occur.

Raising the risk

Asparaginase and pegaspargase can cause anaphylaxis, which is more likely to occur with intermittent I.V. dosing than with daily I.V. dosing or I.M. injections. The risk of a reaction rises with each successive treatment. Hypersensitivity reactions may also occur.

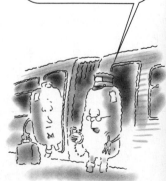

Asparaginases can cause anaphylaxis, especially with intermittent I.V. dosing rather than daily dosing. So let's keep on our regular daily schedule!

Nursing process

These nursing process steps are appropriate for patients undergoing treatment with asparaginases.

Assessment

• Assess the patient's condition before therapy and regularly thereafter.
• Monitor the patient for adverse reactions and drug interactions.
• Monitor the drug's effectiveness by noting results of follow-up diagnostic tests and overall physical status.
• Monitor the patient's CBC and bone marrow function test results. Bone marrow regeneration may take 5 to 6 weeks.
• Evaluate the patient's and family's knowledge of drug therapy.

Key nursing diagnoses

• Ineffective health maintenance related to the presence of neoplastic disease
• Ineffective protection related to drug induced adverse reactions
• Deficient knowledge related to drug therapy

Planning outcome goals

• The patient will demonstrate an improvement in assessment findings and diagnostic testing.
• The risk of injury to the patient will be minimized.
• The patient and his family will demonstrate an understanding of drug therapy.

Implementation

• Follow facility policy to reduce risks. Preparation and administration of the parenteral form of the drug are linked to carcinogenic, mutagenic, and teratogenic risks for personnel.
• Reconstitute the drug as ordered and administer according to facility policy. The drug is given in a hospital under close supervision. (See *Asparaginase warning*.)
• Prevent tumor lysis, which can result in uric acid nephropathy, by increasing fluid intake. Allopurinol should be started before therapy begins.
• Limit the dose at a single injection site to 2 ml when administering the drug I.M.
• Give an I.V. infusion slowly, over at least 30 minutes.

On the alert for anaphylaxis

• Keep diphenhydramine, epinephrine, and I.V. corticosteroids available for treating anaphylaxis.
• Refrigerate unopened dry powder. Reconstituted solution is stable for 8 hours if refrigerated.

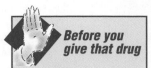

Before you give that drug

Asparaginase warning

The risk of hypersensitivity reactions increases with repeated doses of asparaginase. An intradermal skin test should be performed before the initial dose and repeated after an interval of a week or more, between doses, as ordered. Observe the injection site for at least 1 hour for erythema or a wheal, which indicates a positive response. An allergic reaction to the drug may still develop in a patient with a negative skin test.

A desensitization dose may be ordered. The dose is doubled every 10 minutes if no reaction occurs until the total amount given equals the patient's total dosage for that day.

• If the drug contacts your skin or mucous membranes, wash with copious amounts of water for at least 15 minutes.
• Obtain amylase and lipase levels to check the patient's pancreatic status. If levels are elevated, stop the drug.
• Because of vomiting, administer parenteral fluids for 24 hours or until the patient can tolerate oral fluids.

Evaluation
• Patient responds well to drug therapy.
• Patient doesn't develop serious complications from adverse hematologic reactions.
• Patient and his family state an understanding of drug therapy.

Hydroxyurea

Hydroxyurea is used most commonly for patients with chronic myelogenous leukemia. Hydroxyurea is also used for solid tumors, head and neck cancer, and inoperable ovarian cancer.

Pharmacokinetics

Hydroxyurea is absorbed readily and distributed well into CSF after oral administration. It reaches a peak serum level 2 hours after administration.

Half and half

About half of a dose is metabolized by the liver to carbon dioxide, which is excreted by the lungs, or to urea, which is excreted by the kidneys. The remaining half is excreted unchanged in urine.

Pharmacodynamics

Hydroxyurea exerts its effect by inhibiting the enzyme ribonucleotide reductase, which is necessary for DNA synthesis.

Divide and conquer

Hydroxyurea kills cells in the S phase of the cell cycle and holds other cells in the G1 phase, when they're most susceptible to irradiation.

Pharmacotherapeutics

Hydroxyurea is used to treat selected myeloproliferative disorders. It may produce temporary remissions in some patients with metastatic malignant melanomas as well.

When your neck is on the line

Hydroxyurea also is used in combination therapy with radiation to treat carcinomas of the head, neck, and lung.

Drug interactions

Cytotoxic drugs and radiation therapy enhance the toxicity of hydroxyurea.

Adverse reactions

Treatment with hydroxyurea leads to few adverse reactions. Those that do occur include:
• bone marrow suppression
• drowsiness
• headache
• nausea and vomiting
• anorexia
• elevated uric acid levels, which require some patients to take allopurinol to prevent kidney damage.

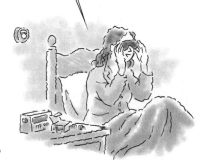

Adverse reactions to hydroxyurea include headache, anorexia, and yawn... drowsiness.

Nursing process

These nursing process steps are appropriate for patients undergoing treatment with hydroxyurea.

Assessment

• Assess the patient's condition before therapy and regularly thereafter.
• Monitor the patient for adverse reactions and drug interactions.

On the level

• Monitor CBC, BUN, uric acid, and creatinine levels.
• Monitor the patient's renal function. Auditory and visual hallucinations and hematologic toxicity increase with decreased renal function.
• Evaluate the patient's and family's knowledge of drug therapy.

Key nursing diagnoses

• Ineffective health maintenance related to the presence of neoplastic disease
• Ineffective protection related to drug-induced adverse hematologic reactions
• Deficient knowledge related to drug therapy

Planning outcome goals

• The patient will demonstrate an improvement in assessment findings and diagnostic testing.
• The risk of injury to the patient will be minimized.
• The patient and his family will demonstrate an understanding of drug therapy.

Implementation

• Encourage fluids to hydrate the patient as appropriate.
• Monitor the patient for signs and symptoms of infection (fever, sore throat, and fatigue) and bleeding (easy bruising, nosebleeds, bleeding gums, and melena). Tell him to take his temperature daily and report elevations.
• Administer the medication according to facility protocol.
• If the patient can't swallow capsules, empty the contents of capsules into water and have him drink it immediately.

Pregnant pause

• Advise a woman of childbearing age not to become pregnant during therapy and to consult with her prescriber before becoming pregnant.

Evaluation

• Patient responds well to drug therapy.
• Patient doesn't develop serious complications from adverse reactions.
• Patient and his family state an understanding of drug therapy.

Interferons

A family of naturally occurring glycoproteins are called *interferons* because of their ability to interfere with viral replication. These drugs have anticancer activity as well as activity against condylomata acuminata (soft, wartlike growths on the skin and mucous membranes of the genitalia caused by a virus).

The three types of interferons are:

alfa interferons derived from leukocytes

beta interferons derived from fibroblasts (connective tissue cells)

gamma interferons derived from fibroblasts and lymphocytes.

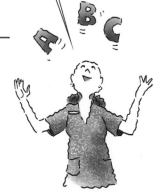

The ABCs of interferons are alfa, beta, and gamma.

You can bet on the alfa

Alfa interferons (alfa-2a, alfa-2b, and alfa-n3), which are discussed below, are being used or evaluated for the treatment of several types of cancer and viral infections. The use of beta and gamma interferons is still relatively small in clinical settings.

Pharmacokinetics

After I.M. or subQ administration, alfa interferons are usually absorbed well. Information about their distribution is unavailable. Alfa interferons are filtered by the kidneys, where they're degraded. Liver metabolism and biliary excretion of interferons are negligible.

Pharmacodynamics

Although their exact mechanism of action is unknown, alfa interferons appear to bind to specific membrane receptors on the cell surface. When bound, they initiate a sequence of intracellular events that includes the induction of certain enzymes.

Running interference

This process may account for the ability of interferons to:
• inhibit viral replication
• suppress cell proliferation
• enhance macrophage activity (engulfing and destroying microorganisms and other debris)
• increase cytotoxicity of lymphocytes for target cells.

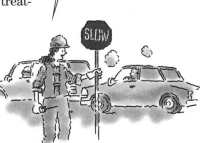

Interferons can slow down or stop viral replication.

Pharmacotherapeutics

Alfa interferons have shown their most promising activity in treating blood malignancies, especially hairy cell leukemia. Their approved indications currently include:
• hairy cell leukemia
• AIDS-related Kaposi's sarcoma
• condylomata acuminata.

Alfa interferons also demonstrate some activity against chronic myelogenous leukemia, malignant lymphoma, multiple myeloma, melanoma, and renal cell carcinoma.

Drug interactions

Interferons interact with the following drugs:
• They may enhance the CNS effects of CNS depressants and substantially increase the half-life of methylxanthines (including theophylline and aminophylline).

Invigorating viruses

• Concurrent use with a live virus vaccine may potentiate replication of the virus, increasing the adverse effects of the vaccine and decreasing the patient's antibody response.
• Bone marrow suppression may be increased when an interferon is used with radiation therapy or a drug that causes blood abnormalities or bone marrow suppression.
• Alfa interferons increase the risk of kidney failure from IL-2.

Adverse reactions

Blood toxicity occurs in up to one-half of patients taking interferons and may produce leukopenia, neutropenia, thrombocytopenia, and anemia. Adverse GI reactions include anorexia, nausea, and diarrhea.

That flulike feeling

The most common adverse reaction to alfa interferons is a flulike syndrome that may produce fever, fatigue, muscle pain, headache, chills, and joint pain.

It catches your breath

Coughing, difficulty breathing, hypotension, edema, chest pain, and heart failure have also been associated with interferon therapy.

Nursing process

These nursing process steps are appropriate for patients undergoing treatment with interferons.

Assessment

• Assess the patient's condition before therapy and regularly thereafter.
• Monitor the patient for adverse reactions and drug interactions.

Allergy alert

• Obtain an allergy history. The drug contains phenol as a preservative and serum albumin as a stabilizer.
• At the beginning of therapy, assess the patient for flulike signs and symptoms, which tend to diminish with continued therapy.
• Monitor blood studies. Any adverse effects are dose-related and reversible. Recovery occurs within several days or weeks after withdrawal.
• Evaluate the patient's and family's knowledge of drug therapy.

Education edge

Teaching about interferons

If interferon therapy is prescribed, review these points with the patient and his caregivers:

• Know that laboratory tests will be performed before and periodically during therapy. Tests include complete blood count with differential, platelet count, blood chemistry and electrolyte studies, liver function tests and, if you have a cardiac disorder or advanced stages of cancer, electrocardiograms.

• Proper oral hygiene is important during your treatment because interferon use may lead to microbial infection, delayed healing, gingival bleeding, and decreased salivary flow. Brush frequently (after meals and at bedtime) with a soft-bristled toothbrush and clean the toothbrush daily (may use hydrogen peroxide). Avoid toothpicks and water pressure gum cleaners that can traumatize the mucosa. Rinse your mouth with water or saline. Avoid commercial mouthwashes that contain alcohol, which may cause irritation.

• Follow your prescriber's instructions about taking and recording your temperature. Take acetaminophen as directed for the treatment of adverse drug effects (fever, arthralgia, myalgia). Report adverse effects to your prescriber.

• If you miss a dose, check with your prescriber for instructions.

• The drug may cause temporary hair loss; it should grow back when therapy ends.

• Make sure that you understand the proper procedure to prepare and administer the drug, including proper hand-washing technique and injection technique. Dispose of used needles in a hard container such as a coffee can. Store the drug according to the manufacturer's recommendations.

• Take the drug at bedtime to minimize flu symptoms.

• Review the information provided by the drug manufacturer included with your prescription. If you have any questions about this information, contact your prescriber. If you don't receive this information, contact your pharmacist.

• You're at an increased risk for infection during therapy. Don't receive any immunizations without getting approval from your prescriber, and avoid contact with people who have taken the oral polio vaccine.

• If you're a woman of childbearing age, know that interferon poses a danger to the fetus. Notify your prescriber promptly if you become pregnant during therapy.

• Avoid alcohol during drug therapy.

• Report signs and symptoms of depression.

• Don't take over-the-counter products, herbal remedies, or prescription medications without first talking to your prescriber.

Key nursing diagnoses

• Ineffective health maintenance related to the presence of neoplastic disease
• Risk for injury related to drug-induced adverse reactions
• Deficient knowledge related to drug therapy

Planning outcome goals

• The patient will demonstrate an improvement in assessment findings and diagnostic testing.
• The risk of injury to the patient will be minimized.
• The patient and his family will demonstrate an understanding of drug therapy.

Implementation
• Premedicate the patient with acetaminophen to minimize flulike signs and symptoms.
• Give the drug at bedtime to minimize daytime drowsiness.
• Make sure that the patient is well hydrated, especially during the initial stages of treatment.
• Administer the medication according to facility policy, and monitor for effects.
• The subQ administration route is used in a patient whose platelet count is below $50,000/mm^3$.
• Interferon alfa-2b may be administered intralesionally; dilute and reconstitute the drug according to facility policy. The drug may be given in the evening with acetaminophen.
• Refrigerate the drug.
• Notify the prescriber of severe adverse reactions, which may require a dosage reduction or discontinuation.

Evaluation
• Patient responds well to drug therapy.
• Patient doesn't develop serious complications from adverse reactions.
• Patient and his family state an understanding of drug therapy. (See *Teaching about interferons*, page 677.)

Procarbazine

Procarbazine hydrochloride, a methylhydrazine derivative with MAO-inhibiting properties, is used to treat Hodgkin's disease, primary and metastatic brain tumors, and lymphoma. It's cell cycle–specific and acts on the S phase.

Pharmacokinetics
After oral administration, procarbazine is absorbed well. It readily crosses the blood-brain barrier and is well distributed into CSF.

To activate, just add enzymes
Procarbazine is metabolized rapidly in the liver and must be activated metabolically by microsomal enzymes. It's excreted in urine, primarily as metabolites. Respiratory excretion of the drug occurs as methane and carbon dioxide gas.

Pharmacodynamics
An inert drug, procarbazine must be activated metabolically in the liver before it can produce various cell changes. It can cause chro-

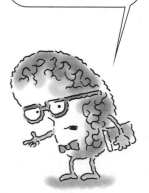

Procarbazine is used to treat Hodgkin's disease, lymphoma, and primary and metastatic brain tumors.

mosomal damage, suppress mitosis, and inhibit DNA, RNA, and protein synthesis. Cancer cells can develop resistance to procarbazine quickly.

Drug interactions

Interactions with procarbazine can be significant:
• Procarbazine produces an additive effect when administered with CNS depressants.
• Taken with meperidine, procarbazine may result in severe hypotension and death.

Mirroring MAO

• Because of procarbazine's MAO-inhibiting properties, hypertensive reactions may occur when it's administered concurrently with sympathomimetics, antidepressants, and tyramine-rich foods.
• Procarbazine taken with caffeine may result in arrhythmias and severe hypertension.

Adverse reactions

Late-onset bone marrow suppression is the most common dose-limiting toxicity associated with procarbazine. Interstitial pneumonitis (lung inflammation) and pulmonary fibrosis (scarring) may also occur.

Off to a bad start

Initial procarbazine therapy may induce a flulike syndrome, including fever, chills, sweating, lethargy, and muscle pain.

A gut feeling

GI reactions include nausea, vomiting, stomatitis, and diarrhea.

Nursing process

These nursing process steps are appropriate for patients undergoing treatment with procarbazine.

Assessment
• Assess the patient's condition before therapy and regularly thereafter.
• Monitor the patient for adverse reactions and drug interactions.
• Monitor the patient's CBC and platelet counts.
• Evaluate the patient's and family's knowledge of drug therapy.

Key nursing diagnoses

- Ineffective health maintenance related to the presence of neoplastic disease
- Ineffective protection related to drug-induced adverse reactions
- Deficient knowledge related to drug therapy

Planning outcome goals

- The patient will demonstrate an improvement in assessment findings and diagnostic testing.
- The risk of injury to the patient will be minimized.
- The patient and his family will demonstrate an understanding of drug therapy.

Implementation

- Give the drug at bedtime to lessen nausea. It's usually given in divided doses.
- Monitor the patient for signs of infection (such as fever, sore throat, and fatigue) and bleeding (easy bruising, nosebleeds, bleeding gums, and melena). Tell him to take his temperature daily and report elevations.
- Stop the drug and notify the prescriber if the patient becomes confused or if paresthesia or other neuropathies develop.
- Warn the patient to avoid alcohol during drug therapy.
- Stop the drug and notify the prescriber if a disulfiram-like reaction occurs (chest pain, rapid or irregular heartbeat, severe headache, and stiff neck).
- Advise the patient to avoid caffeine.
- Warn the patient to avoid hazardous activities until the CNS effects of the drug are known.
- Advise a woman of childbearing age not to become pregnant during therapy and to consult with her prescriber before becoming pregnant.

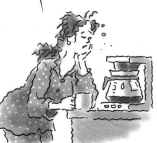

Advise the patient taking procarbazine to avoid caffeine. I suppose decaf will have to do...

Evaluation

- Patient responds well to drug therapy.
- Patient doesn't develop serious complications from adverse reactions.
- Patient and his family state an understanding of drug therapy.

Taxanes

Taxane antineoplastics are used to treat metastatic ovarian and breast carcinoma after chemotherapy has failed. They include:
- paclitaxel
- docetaxel.

Pharmacokinetics

After I.V. administration, paclitaxel is highly bound to plasma proteins. Docetaxel is administered I.V. with a rapid onset of action. Paclitaxel is metabolized primarily in the liver, with a small amount excreted unchanged in urine. Docetaxel is excreted primarily in feces.

Pharmacodynamics

Paclitaxel and docetaxel exert their chemotherapeutic effect by disrupting the microtubule network that's essential for mitosis and other vital cellular functions.

Pharmacotherapeutics

Paclitaxel is used when first-line or subsequent chemotherapy has failed in treating metastatic ovarian carcinoma as well as metastatic breast cancer. The taxanes may also be used to treat head and neck cancer, prostate cancer, and non–small-cell lung cancer. Paclitaxel is also a second-line treatment for AIDS-related Kaposi's sarcoma.

Drug interactions

Taxanes have few interactions with other drugs:
• Concomitant use of paclitaxel and cisplatin may cause additive myelosuppressive effects.
• Cyclosporine, ketoconazole, erythromycin, and troleandomycin may modify docetaxel metabolism.
• Phenytoin may decrease paclitaxel serum concentrations, leading to a loss of efficacy.
• Quinupristin/dalfopristin may increase paclitaxel serum concentrations, increasing the risk of toxicity.
• Drugs that inhibit cytochrome P450, such as cyclosporine, dexamethasone, diazepam, etoposide, ketoconazole, quinidine, retinoic acid, teniposide, testosterone, verapamil, and vincristine, may increase paclitaxel levels. Monitor the patient for toxicity.

Adverse reactions

During clinical trials, 25% or more patients experienced these adverse reactions to paclitaxel:
• bone marrow suppression
• hypersensitivity reactions
• abnormal EEG tracings
• peripheral neuropathy
• muscle and joint pain

- nausea and vomiting
- diarrhea
- mucous membrane inflammation
- hair loss.

Docetaxel

Adverse reactions to docetaxel include:
- hypersensitivity reactions
- fluid retention
- leukopenia, neutropenia, or thrombocytopenia
- hair loss
- mouth inflammation
- numbness and tingling
- pain
- weakness and fatigue.

Nursing process

These nursing process steps are appropriate for patients undergoing treatment with taxanes.

Assessment

- Assess the patient's condition before therapy and regularly thereafter.
- Continuously monitor the patient throughout the infusion.
- Monitor the patient's blood counts and liver function test results frequently during therapy.
- Monitor the patient for adverse reactions and drug interactions.
- Evaluate the patient's and family's knowledge of drug therapy.

Key nursing diagnoses

- Ineffective health maintenance related to cancer
- Ineffective protection related to drug-induced adverse hematologic reactions
- Deficient knowledge related to drug therapy

Planning outcome goals

- The patient will demonstrate an improvement in assessment findings and diagnostic testing.
- The risk of injury to the patient will be minimized.
- The patient and her family will demonstrate an understanding of drug therapy.

Implementation

- To reduce severe hypersensitivity, expect to pretreat the patient with corticosteroids, such as dexamethasone and antihistamines.

• Follow facility policy for safe handling, preparation, and use of chemotherapy drugs. Preparation and administration of the parenteral form of the drug are linked to carcinogenic, mutagenic, and teratogenic risks for personnel.
• Mark all waste materials with chemotherapy hazard labels.
• Dilute concentrations and administer according to facility policy.
• Prepare and store infusion solutions in glass containers.
• Take care to avoid extravasation.
• Monitor the patient for signs and symptoms of bleeding, infection, and peripheral neuropathy (tingling, burning, or numbness in the limbs).
• Warn the patient that alopecia occurs in up to 82% of patients.
• Advise a woman of childbearing age to avoid pregnancy during therapy. Also recommend consulting with her prescriber before becoming pregnant.

Evaluation
• Patient responds well to drug therapy.
• Patient develops no serious complications from drug-induced adverse hematologic reactions.
• Patient and her family state an understanding of drug therapy.

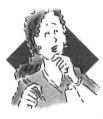

Quick quiz

1. The patient is being administered nitrogen mustard chemotherapy and is taking antacids, hydrochlorothiazide, diphenhydramine, and diazepam. Which medication might cause a drug interaction with nitrogen mustards?
   A.   Antacids
   B.   Hydrochlorothiazide
   C.   Diphenhydramine
   D.   Diazepam

Answer: A. Nitrogen mustards interact with many other drugs. Calcium-containing drugs and foods, such as antacids and dairy products, reduce the absorption of estramustine.

2. The nurse is observing the patient for adverse reactions to dacarbazine. Which adverse reaction may be caused by dacarbazine drug therapy?
   A.   Rash
   B.   Hypotension
   C.   Flulike syndrome
   D.   Tachycardia

Answer: C. Dacarbazine use may cause some adverse reactions. These include leukopenia, thrombocytopenia, nausea and vomiting (which begin within 1 to 3 hours after administration in most cases and may last up to 12 hours), phototoxicity, flulike syndrome, and hair loss.

3.   Which action should the nurse perform before treatment with asparaginase?
  A.   Monitoring blood pressure
  B.   Assessing ECG
  C.   Obtaining an allergy history
  D.   Performing an intradermal skin test

Answer: D. The risk of a hypersensitivity reaction increases with repeated doses of asparaginase. An intradermal skin test should be performed before the initial dose and repeated after an interval of 1 week or more, between doses.

Scoring

☆☆☆   If you answered all three questions correctly, extraordinary! You really mowed down the malignant neoplasms!

☆☆   If you answered two questions correctly, congratulations! You're competent to combat cancer.

☆   If you answered fewer than two questions correctly, give it another shot. Remember, practice makes perfect!

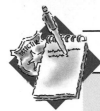

15

Drugs for fluid and electrolyte balance

Just the facts

In this chapter, you'll learn:

♦ classes of drugs used to treat fluid and electrolyte disorders

♦ uses and varying actions of these drugs

♦ absorption, distribution, metabolization, and excretion of these drugs

♦ drug interactions and adverse reactions to these drugs.

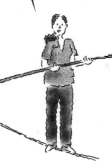

Many factors can disrupt normal fluid and electrolyte balance, including illness, loss of appetite, surgery, and diagnostic tests.

Drugs and homeostasis

Illness can easily disturb the homeostatic mechanisms that help maintain normal fluid and electrolyte balance. Such occurrences as loss of appetite, medication administration, vomiting, surgery, and diagnostic tests can also alter this delicate balance.

Fortunately, several drugs can help correct these imbalances and bring the body back to homeostasis (the stability of body fluid composition and volume).

Electrolyte replacement drugs

An electrolyte is a compound or element that carries an electrical charge when dissolved in water. Electrolyte replacement drugs are inorganic or organic salts that increase depleted or deficient electrolyte levels, helping to maintain homeostasis. These drugs include:
• potassium, the primary intracellular fluid (ICF) electrolyte
• calcium, a major extracellular fluid (ECF) electrolyte
• magnesium, an electrolyte essential for homeostasis found in ICF

• sodium, the principal electrolyte in ECF necessary for homeostasis.

Potassium

Potassium is the major positively charged ion (cation) in ICF. Because the body can't store potassium, adequate amounts must be ingested daily. If this isn't possible, potassium replacement can be accomplished orally or I.V. with potassium salts, such as:
• potassium acetate
• potassium chloride
• potassium gluconate
• potassium phosphate.

Pharmacokinetics (how drugs circulate)

Oral potassium is absorbed readily from the GI tract. After absorption into the ECF, almost all potassium passes into the ICF. There, the enzyme adenosine triphosphatase maintains the concentration of potassium by pumping sodium out of the cell in exchange for potassium.

Normal serum levels of potassium are maintained by the kidneys, which excrete most excess potassium intake. The rest is excreted in feces and sweat.

Pharmacodynamics (how drugs act)

Potassium moves quickly into ICF to restore depleted potassium levels and reestablish balance. It's an essential element in determining cell membrane potential and excitability.

Nervous about potassium?

Potassium is necessary for proper functioning of all nerve and muscle cells and for nerve impulse transmission. It's also essential for tissue growth and repair and for maintenance of acid-base balance.

Pharmacotherapeutics (how drugs are used)

Potassium replacement therapy corrects hypokalemia (low levels of potassium in the blood). Hypokalemia is a common occurrence in conditions that increase potassium excretion or depletion, such as:
• vomiting, diarrhea, or nasogastric suction
• excessive urination
• some kidney diseases
• cystic fibrosis

- burns
- excessive antidiuretic hormone levels
- therapy with a potassium-depleting diuretic
- laxative abuse
- alkalosis
- insufficient potassium intake from starvation, anorexia nervosa, alcoholism, or clay ingestion
- administration of a glucocorticoid, I.V. amphotericin B, vitamin B_{12}, folic acid, granulocyte-macrophage colony–stimulating factor, or I.V. solutions that contain insufficient potassium.

> Because potassium inhibits my excitability, it decreases the toxic effects of digoxin—which leaves me feeling quite relaxed.

Be still my heart

Potassium decreases the toxic effects of digoxin. Because potassium inhibits the excitability of the heart, normal potassium levels moderate the action of digoxin, reducing the chance of toxicity.

Drug interactions

Potassium should be used cautiously in patients receiving potassium-sparing diuretics (such as amiloride, spironolactone, and triamterene) or angiotensin-converting enzyme (ACE) inhibitors (such as captopril, enalapril, and lisinopril) to avoid hyperkalemia.

Adverse reactions

Most adverse reactions to potassium are related to the method of administration. Oral potassium sometimes causes nausea, vomiting, abdominal pain, and diarrhea. Enteric-coated tablets may cause small-bowel ulcerations, stenosis, hemorrhage, and obstruction. An I.V. infusion can cause pain at the injection site and phlebitis (vein inflammation) and, if given rapidly, cardiac arrest. Infusion of potassium in patients with decreased urine production also increases the risk of hyperkalemia.

Nursing process

These nursing process steps are appropriate for patients undergoing treatment with potassium.

Assessment

- Monitor the patient's potassium level. Be particularly alert for hyperkalemia if the patient's urine output decreases during therapy.

Before you give that drug

Signs and symptoms of hyperkalemia

Potassium replacement therapy can lead to overcorrection and hyperkalemia. To prevent this, closely monitor the patient for signs and symptoms of hyperkalemia, including:
- abdominal cramping
- confusion
- diarrhea
- electrocardiogram changes (tall, tented T wave)

- hypotension
- irregular pulse rate
- irritability
- muscle weakness
- nausea
- paresthesia.

- Monitor the patient for signs and symptoms of hyperkalemia. (See *Signs and symptoms of hyperkalemia.*)
- Watch for adverse reactions and drug interactions.
- Monitor the patient's electrocardiogram (ECG) for changes that suggest hyperkalemia, such as prolonged PR intervals, widened QRS complexes, depressed ST segments, and tall, tented T waves.
- Monitor the patient's intake and output if nausea, vomiting, or diarrhea occur.

Key nursing diagnoses
- Risk for deficient fluid volume related to adverse reactions to potassium
- Decreased cardiac output related to adverse reactions to potassium
- Deficient knowledge related to drug therapy

Planning outcome goals
- The patient's fluid intake and output will remain at appropriate level for his age and condition.
- The patient won't have arrhythmias.
- The patient will demonstrate correct drug administration.

Implementation
- Use potassium cautiously if the patient is also receiving a potassium-sparing diuretic or an ACE inhibitor.
- When administering potassium I.V., dilute the preparation before infusion.
- Give diluted I.V. potassium slowly to prevent life-threatening hyperkalemia.
- Never give potassium as an I.V. bolus or I.M. injection.

Education edge

Teaching about potassium therapy

If potassium is prescribed, review these points with the patient and his caregivers:
• Take oral potassium with or after meals to minimize GI distress.
• Dissolve all powders and tablets in at least 4 oz (120 ml) of water or fruit juice, and sip the solution slowly over 5 to 10 minutes. Also take capsules or tablets with plenty of liquid.
• Make sure not to crush or chew extended-release tablets, which will defeat the purpose of the special coating. Also understand that, although the remnants of the wax matrix may appear in your stools, the drug has been absorbed.
• Make sure you keep appointments for periodic blood tests to measure potassium level.
• If you experience GI distress or signs and symptoms of hyperkalemia, such as diarrhea, muscle weakness, or confusion, notify your practitioner.

Nix that mix

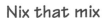

• Don't mix I.V. potassium phosphate in a solution that contains calcium or magnesium because precipitates will occur.
• Monitor the patient's I.V. site regularly for signs of phlebitis. If phlebitis or pain occurs, change the site.
• Give oral potassium with or after meals to minimize GI distress.
• Give antiemetics or antidiarrheals as needed if the patient develops vomiting or diarrhea.
• Teach the patient and his family about potassium therapy. (See *Teaching about potassium therapy.*)

Evaluation
• Patient maintains adequate hydration.
• Patient maintains normal cardiac output as evidenced by normal vital signs and ECG.
• Patient and his family demonstrate an understanding of drug therapy.

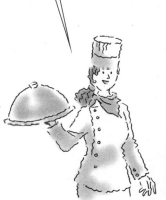

Give oral potassium with or after meals to minimize GI distress.

Calcium

Calcium is a major cation in ECF. Almost all of the calcium in the body (99%) is stored in bone, where it can be mobilized if necessary. When dietary intake isn't enough to meet metabolic needs, calcium stores in bone are reduced.

Bound, complexed, ionized

Extracellular calcium exists in three forms—it's bound to plasma protein (mainly albumin); complexed with substances such as phosphate, citrate, or sulfate; and ionized. About 47% of the ionized calcium is physiologically active and plays a role in cellular functions.

Salting the body

Chronic insufficient calcium intake can result in bone demineralization. Calcium is replaced orally or I.V. with calcium salts, such as:

- calcium carbonate
- calcium chloride
- calcium citrate
- calcium glubionate
- calcium gluceptate
- calcium gluconate
- calcium lactate.

Pharmacokinetics

Oral calcium is absorbed readily from the duodenum and proximal jejunum. A pH of 5 to 7, parathyroid hormone (PTH), and vitamin D all aid calcium absorption.

A soapy situation

Absorption also depends on dietary factors, such as calcium binding to fiber, phytates, and oxalates, and on fatty acids, with which calcium salts form insoluble soaps.

Calcium is distributed primarily in bone. Calcium salts are eliminated primarily in feces, with the remainder excreted in urine.

Pharmacodynamics

Calcium moves quickly into ECF to restore calcium levels and reestablish balance. It has several vital functions:

- Extracellular ionized calcium plays an essential role in normal nerve and muscle excitability.
- Calcium is integral to normal functioning of the heart, kidneys, and lungs, and it affects the blood coagulation rate as well as cell membrane and capillary permeability.
- Calcium is a factor in neurotransmitter and hormone activity, amino acid metabolism, vitamin B_{12} absorption, and gastrin secretion.
- Calcium plays a major role in normal bone and tooth formation. (See *Calcium in balance.*)

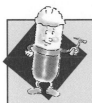

Pharm function

Calcium in balance

Extracellular calcium levels are normally kept constant by several inter-related processes that move calcium ions into and out of extracellular fluid. Calcium enters the extracellular space through resorption of calcium ions from bone, through the absorption of dietary calcium in the GI tract, and through reabsorption of calcium from the kidneys. Calcium leaves extracellular fluid as it's excreted in feces and urine and deposited in bone tissues. This illustration shows how calcium moves throughout the body.

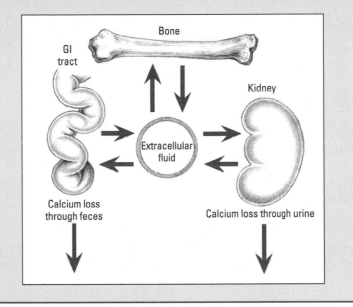

Pharmacotherapeutics

Calcium is helpful in treating magnesium intoxication. It also helps strengthen myocardial tissue after defibrillation or a poor response to epinephrine during resuscitation. Pregnancy and breast-feeding increase calcium requirements, as do periods of bone growth during childhood and adolescence.

In the I.V. league

The major clinical indication for I.V. calcium is acute hypocalcemia (low serum calcium levels), which necessitates a rapid increase in serum calcium levels, as in tetany, cardiac arrest, vita-

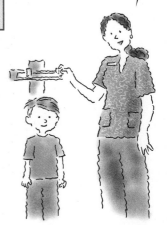

When a child is going through a period of bone growth, he needs extra calcium. I think he has grown another inch!

min D deficiency, parathyroid surgery, and alkalosis. I.V. calcium is also used to prevent a hypocalcemic reaction during exchange transfusions.

Mouth medicine

Oral calcium is commonly used to supplement a calcium-deficient diet and prevent osteoporosis. Chronic hypocalcemia from such conditions as chronic hypoparathyroidism (a deficiency of PTH), osteomalacia (softening of bones), long-term glucocorticoid therapy, and plicamycin and vitamin D deficiency is also treated with oral calcium.

Drug interactions

Calcium has a few significant interactions with other drugs:
• Preparations administered with digoxin may cause cardiac arrhythmias.
• Calcium replacement drugs may reduce the response to calcium channel blockers.
• Calcium replacements may inactivate tetracyclines.
• Calcium supplements may decrease the amount of atenolol available to the tissues, resulting in decreased effectiveness of the drug.

An insoluble problem

• When given in total parenteral nutrition, calcium may react with phosphorus present in the solution to form insoluble calcium phosphate granules, which may find their way into pulmonary arterioles, causing emboli and possibly death.

Adverse reactions

Calcium preparations may produce hypercalcemia if calcium levels aren't monitored closely. Early signs include drowsiness, lethargy, muscle weakness, headache, constipation, and a metallic taste in the mouth. ECG changes that occur with elevated serum calcium levels include a shortened QT interval and heart block. Severe hypercalcemia can cause cardiac arrhythmias, cardiac arrest, and coma.

A burning issue

With I.V. administration, calcium may cause venous irritation. I.M. injection of calcium may cause severe local reactions, such as burning, necrosis, and tissue sloughing.

Nursing process

These nursing process steps are appropriate for patients undergoing treatment with calcium.

Assessment

- Monitor the patient's calcium level.
- Monitor the patient for signs of hypercalcemia.
- Watch the patient's ECG for changes that suggest hypercalcemia.

Key nursing diagnoses

- Decreased cardiac output related to calcium imbalance
- Risk for injury related to osteoporosis
- Deficient knowledge related to drug therapy

Planning outcome goals

- The patient won't have arrhythmias.
- The patient won't develop an increased risk of fractures.
- The patient will demonstrate correct drug administration.

Implementation

- Give an I.V. infusion slowly to prevent a high calcium level from reaching the heart and possibly causing arrhythmias and cardiac arrest.
- Keep the patient recumbent for 15 minutes after injecting calcium.
- If extravasation occurs, stop the I.V. infusion and apply warm, moist compresses to the area.
- Only give calcium I.M. in an emergency and only when the I.V. route is impossible to use. If using the I.M. route, give the injection in the gluteal muscle for an adult or in the lateral thigh for an infant or small child.
- Give oral calcium supplements 1 to 2 hours after meals.
- Give calcium and digoxin slowly and in small amounts to avoid precipitating arrhythmias during therapy with both drugs.
- Teach the patient about calcium. (See *Teaching about oral calcium.*)

Evaluation

- Patient maintains normal cardiac output as evidenced by normal vital signs and ECG.
- Patient's bone density tests remain stable over time.

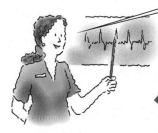

When your patient is undergoing calcium treatment, watch his ECG for changes that suggest hypercalcemia.

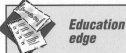

Education edge

Teaching about oral calcium

If a calcium preparation is prescribed, review these points with the patient and his caregivers:

- Don't take calcium with foods that interfere with calcium absorption, such as spinach, rhubarb, bran, whole grain cereals and breads, and fresh fruits and vegetables; take calcium tablets 1 to 2 hours after eating.
- Eat foods containing vitamin D to enhance calcium absorption.
- Don't skip follow-up blood tests to monitor calcium levels.
- Report signs and symptoms of hypercalcemia, including nausea and vomiting, constipation, muscle weakness, lethargy, and fatigue, to your practitioner.

• Patient and his family demonstrate an understanding of drug therapy.

Magnesium

Magnesium is the most abundant cation in ICF after potassium. It's essential in transmitting nerve impulses to muscle and activating enzymes necessary for carbohydrate and protein metabolism. About 65% of all magnesium is in bone, and 20% is in muscle.

Officiating in the ICF

Magnesium stimulates PTH secretion, thus regulating ICF calcium levels.

Traffic control

Magnesium also aids in cell metabolism and the movement of sodium and potassium across cell membranes.

A run on magnesium

Magnesium stores may be depleted by:
• malabsorption
• chronic diarrhea
• prolonged treatment with diuretics
• nasogastric suctioning
• prolonged therapy with parenteral fluids not containing magnesium
• hyperaldosteronism
• hypoparathyroidism or hyperparathyroidism
• excessive release of adrenocortical hormones
• acute and chronic alcohol consumption
• drugs, such as cisplatin, aminoglycosides, cyclosporine, and amphotericin B.

Restocking the mineral stores

Magnesium is typically replaced in the form of magnesium sulfate when administered I.V. or in the form of magnesium oxide if given orally.

Pharmacokinetics

Magnesium sulfate is distributed widely throughout the body. I.V. magnesium sulfate acts immediately, whereas the drug acts within 30 minutes after I.M. administration. However, I.M. injections can be painful, induce sclerosis, and need to be repeated frequently. Magnesium sulfate isn't metabolized and is excreted unchanged in urine; some appears in breast milk.

Pharmacodynamics

Magnesium sulfate replenishes and prevents magnesium deficiencies. It also prevents or controls seizures by blocking neuromuscular transmission.

Pharmacotherapeutics

I.V. magnesium sulfate is the drug of choice for replacement therapy in symptomatic magnesium deficiency (hypomagnesemia). It's widely used to treat or prevent preeclamptic and eclamptic seizure activity. It's also used to treat ventricular arrhythmias such as torsades de pointes, seizures, severe toxemia, and acute nephritis in children.

Drug interactions

Magnesium has few significant interactions with other drugs:
• Magnesium used with digoxin may lead to heart block.

So depressing...

• Combining magnesium sulfate with alcohol, opioids, antianxiety drugs, barbiturates, antidepressants, hypnotics, antipsychotic drugs, or general anesthetics may increase central nervous system depressant effects.
• Using magnesium sulfate with succinylcholine or tubocurarine potentiates and prolongs the neuromuscular blocking action of these drugs.

Adverse reactions

Adverse reactions to magnesium sulfate can be life-threatening. They include hypotension, circulatory collapse, flushing, depressed reflexes, and respiratory paralysis.

I.M. injections of magnesium can cause pain and induce sclerosis and must be repeated frequently.

Nursing process

These nursing process steps are appropriate for patients undergoing treatment with magnesium.

Assessment

• Monitor the patient's intake and output. Magnesium generally isn't given if the patient's urine output is less than 100 ml in 4 hours.
• Monitor the patient's vital signs and ECG tracings, looking for signs of hypotension, arrhythmias, and respiratory distress.
• Watch the patient's serum electrolyte levels.

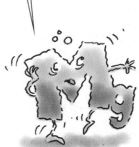

Adverse reactions to magnesium sulfate can be life-threatening! Just the thought of it makes me feel faint.

Key nursing diagnoses
• Risk for deficient fluid volume related to magnesium replacement
• Decreased cardiac output related to magnesium imbalance
• Deficient knowledge related to drug therapy

Planning outcome goals
• The patient will maintain appropriate levels of fluid intake and output for his age and condition.
• The patient won't have arrhythmias.
• The patient will demonstrate an understanding of drug therapy.

Implementation
• Keep I.V. calcium gluconate available to reverse the respiratory depression that an infusion of magnesium sulfate can cause.

A knee-jerk reaction
• Test the patient's knee-jerk and patellar reflexes before giving each dose. If absent, notify the practitioner and withhold the dose until the patient's reflexes return. Otherwise, he may develop temporary respiratory failure and need cardiopulmonary resuscitation or I.V. administration of calcium.
• Use parenteral magnesium cautiously in a patient with renal impairment because renal impairment increases the risk of hypermagnesemia.
• Administer magnesium sulfate slowly—no faster than 150 mg/minute. Injecting a bolus dose too rapidly can trigger cardiac arrest.
• Monitor the patient's vital signs and deep tendon reflexes during an infusion of magnesium. Watch for signs and symptoms of overdose, including hypotension and respiratory distress.
• Check the patient's serum magnesium level after each bolus dose; if he's receiving a continuous I.V. drip, check the serum magnesium level at least every 6 hours.
• Place the patient on continuous cardiac monitoring during replacement therapy.
• Monitor the patient's urine output before, during, and after magnesium sulfate infusion. Notify the practitioner if the output is less than 100 ml over 4 hours.

Evaluation
• Patient maintains adequate hydration.
• Patient maintains normal cardiac output as evidenced by normal vital signs and ECG.
• Patient and his family demonstrate an understanding of drug therapy.

Sodium

Sodium is the major cation in ECF. Sodium performs many functions:
- It maintains the osmotic pressure and concentration of ECF, acid-base balance, and water balance.
- It contributes to nerve conduction and neuromuscular function.
- It plays a role in glandular secretion.

Sweating it out

Sodium replacement is necessary in conditions that rapidly deplete sodium, such as anorexia, excessive loss of GI fluids, and excessive perspiration. Diuretics and tap water enemas can also deplete sodium, particularly when fluids are replaced by plain water.

Sodium also can be lost in trauma or wound drainage, adrenal gland insufficiency, cirrhosis of the liver with ascites, syndrome of inappropriate antidiuretic hormone, and prolonged I.V. infusion of dextrose in water without other solutes. Sodium is typically replaced in the form of sodium chloride.

Pharmacokinetics

Oral and parenteral sodium chloride are quickly absorbed and distributed widely throughout the body. Sodium chloride isn't significantly metabolized. It's eliminated primarily in urine, but also in sweat, tears, and saliva.

Pharmacodynamics

Sodium chloride solution replaces deficiencies of sodium and chloride ions in blood plasma.

Pharmacotherapeutics

Sodium chloride is used for water and electrolyte replacement in patients with hyponatremia from electrolyte loss or severe sodium chloride depletion.

A welcome infusion

Severe symptomatic sodium deficiency may be treated by I.V. infusion of a solution containing sodium chloride.

Drug interactions

No significant drug interactions have been reported with sodium chloride.

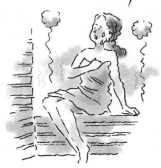

Conditions that deplete sodium include anorexia, excessive GI fluid loss, and excessive perspiration. Speaking of excessive perspiration, I think it's time to get out of this sauna!

Adverse reactions

Adverse reactions to sodium include pulmonary edema if it's given too rapidly or in excess, hypernatremia, and potassium loss.

Nursing process

These nursing process steps are appropriate for patients undergoing treatment with sodium.

Assessment
• Monitor the patient's intake and output.
• Monitor the patient's serum electrolyte levels.

Key nursing diagnoses
• Risk for imbalanced fluid volume related to fluid retention
• Deficient knowledge related to drug therapy

Planning outcome goals
• The patient will maintain appropriate levels of fluid intake and output for his age and condition.
• The patient will demonstrate an understanding of drug therapy.

Implementation
• Use cautiously in elderly and postoperative patients as well as in patients with heart failure, circulatory insufficiency, renal impairment, or hypoproteinemia.

Every breath you take

• Teach the patient to recognize signs and symptoms of pulmonary edema, including shortness of breath, coughing, anxiety, wheezing, and pallor; tell him to notify his practitioner if he experiences any of them.

Evaluation
• Patient maintains normal intake and output.
• Patient and his family demonstrate an understanding of drug therapy.

Alkalinizing and acidifying drugs

Alkalinizing and acidifying drugs act to correct acid-base imbalances in the blood. Alkalinizing drugs are used to treat metabolic acidosis, a condition in which excess hydrogen ions in the ECF result in a decreased serum pH. Acidifying drugs are used for metabolic alkalosis, in which excess bicarbonate in the ECF increases serum pH.

Odd couple

Alkalinizing and acidifying drugs have opposite effects:
• An alkalinizing drug increases the pH of the blood and decreases the concentration of hydrogen ions.
• An acidifying drug decreases the pH of the blood and increases the concentration of hydrogen ions.

Rx for o.d.

Some of these drugs also alter urine pH, making them useful in treating some urinary tract infections and drug overdoses.

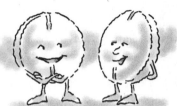

So we have completely opposite effects: You acidify and I alkalinize.

That's odd. We look a lot alike.

Alkalinizing drugs

Alkalinizing drugs used to treat metabolic acidosis and increase blood pH include sodium bicarbonate (also used to increase urine pH), sodium citrate, sodium lactate, and tromethamine.

Pharmacokinetics

All of the alkalinizing drugs are absorbed well when given orally. Sodium bicarbonate isn't metabolized. Sodium citrate and sodium lactate are metabolized to the active ingredient bicarbonate. Tromethamine undergoes little or no metabolization and is excreted unchanged in urine.

Pharmacodynamics

Sodium bicarbonate separates in the blood, providing bicarbonate ions that are used in the blood's buffer system to decrease the hydrogen ion concentration and raise blood pH. (Buffers prevent extreme changes in pH by taking or giving up hydrogen ions to neutralize acids or bases.) As the bicarbonate ions are excreted in urine, urine pH rises. (See *Alkalinizing drugs: Sodium bicarbonate*, page 700.) Sodium citrate and lactate, after conversion to bicarbonate, alkalinize blood and urine in the same way.

Hitching up with hydrogen

Tromethamine acts by combining with hydrogen ions to alkalinize the blood; the resulting tromethamine–hydrogen ion complex is excreted in urine.

Pharmacotherapeutics

Alkalinizing drugs are commonly used to treat metabolic acidosis. Other uses include raising urine pH to help remove certain substances, such as phenobarbital, after an overdose.

Drug interactions

The alkalinizing drugs sodium bicarbonate, sodium citrate, and sodium lactate can interact with a wide range of drugs to increase or decrease their pharmacologic effects:
• These alkalinizing drugs may increase the excretion and reduce the effects of ketoconazole, lithium, and salicylates.
• They may reduce the excretion and increase the effects of amphetamines, quinidine, and pseudoephedrine.
• The antibacterial effects of methenamine are reduced when taken with alkalinizing drugs.
    Tromethamine doesn't have any significant drug interactions.

Adverse reactions

Adverse reactions to alkalinizing drugs vary with the drug.

Sodium bicarbonate

An overdose of sodium bicarbonate can lead to metabolic alkalosis, the most severe adverse reaction. If the drug is administered too rapidly to a patient with diabetic ketoacidosis, the patient may experience cerebral dysfunction, tissue hypoxia, and lactic acidosis. The drug's high sodium content can cause water retention and edema. Oral sodium bicarbonate may cause gastric distention and flatulence.

Sodium citrate

An overdose of sodium citrate can cause metabolic alkalosis or tetany; it can also aggravate existing heart disease. Oral sodium citrate can have a laxative effect.

Sodium lactate

An overdose of sodium lactate can cause metabolic alkalosis. Water retention and edema may occur in patients with kidney disease or heart failure.

Tromethamine

Mild reactions to tromethamine include phlebitis or irritation at the injection site. Severe reactions include hypoglycemia, respiratory depression, and hyperkalemia.

Prototype pro

Alkalinizing drugs: Sodium bicarbonate

Actions
• Neutralizes excess acid in the body
• Restores the blood's buffer system

Indications
• Metabolic, systemic, or urinary acidosis
• Gastric acidity (works as an antacid)

Nursing considerations
• If the patient has diabetic ketoacidosis, give the drug slowly to prevent cerebral dysfunction, tissue hypoxia, and lactic acidosis.
• Monitor the patient for signs and symptoms of fluid retention, such as crackles, peripheral edema, and jugular vein distention.
• Inspect the I.V. site for signs of extravasation.
• If the drug is used to treat urinary alkalinization, monitor the patient's urine pH.

Toxic time bomb

If tromethamine is given for more than 24 hours, toxic drug levels can occur.

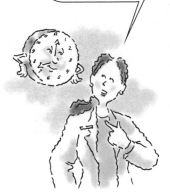

Keep in mind that giving tromethamine for more than 24 hours can result in toxic levels.

Nursing process

These nursing process steps are appropriate for patients undergoing treatment with alkalinizing drugs.

Assessment

- Monitor the patient's pH and bicarbonate levels.
- Monitor for signs and symptoms of overdose, including hyperirritability and tetany.
- Monitor the patient's intake and output.
- Watch for adverse reactions and drug interactions.
- Assess the patient's and family's knowledge of drug therapy.

Key nursing diagnoses

- Risk for injury related to drug-induced adverse reactions
- Deficient knowledge related to drug therapy

Planning outcome goals

- The risk of injury to the patient will be minimized.
- The patient will demonstrate an understanding of drug therapy.

Implementation

- If the patient is receiving sodium bicarbonate, sodium lactate, or tromethamine, watch the I.V. site for extravasation. If extravasation occurs, elevate the affected limb, apply warm compresses, and administer lidocaine.
- For a patient receiving tromethamine, check the I.V. site for phlebitis or irritation and don't give the drug for more than 24 hours.
- Teach the patient and his family about the prescribed drug. (See *Teaching about alkalinizing drugs*, page 702.)

Evaluation

- Patient sustains no injury from adverse reactions.
- Patient and his family demonstrate an understanding of drug therapy.

Education edge

Teaching about alkalinizing drugs

If an alkalinizing drug is prescribed, review these points with the patient and his caregivers:

• Prolonged therapy with sodium bicarbonate tablets can cause GI distress and flatulence. Report these symptoms to your practitioner.

• Watch for signs and symptoms of fluid retention, such as ankle swelling and tightness of rings on your fingers. Report these to your practitioner.

• If you're taking tromethamine (THAM), monitor your glucose level carefully because THAM can cause hypoglycemia.

• Prepare sodium citrate solution with 2 to 3 oz of water and refrigerate it to improve its taste. Take it after meals to minimize its laxative effects.

• Avoid milk while taking sodium bicarbonate to avoid milk-alkali syndrome, hypercalcemia, and renal calculi production.

Acidifying drugs

Acidifying drugs used to correct metabolic alkalosis include acetazolamide (used to treat acute mountain sickness) and ammonium chloride. Ascorbic acid, along with ammonium chloride, serves as a urinary acidifier.

Pharmacokinetics

The action of most acidifying drugs is immediate. Acetazolamide inhibits the enzyme carbonic anhydrase, which blocks hydrogen ion secretion in the renal tubule, resulting in increased excretion of bicarbonate and a lower pH. Acetazolamide also acidifies urine but may produce metabolic acidosis in normal patients. Orally administered ammonium chloride is absorbed completely in 3 to 6 hours. It's metabolized in the liver to form urea, which is excreted by the kidneys.

Ascorbic acid is best absorbed after oral administration. It's metabolized in the liver and excreted by the kidneys.

Pharmacodynamics

Acidifying drugs have several actions:

• Acetazolamide increases the excretion of bicarbonate, lowering blood pH.

• Ammonium chloride lowers the blood pH after being metabolized to urea and hydrochloric acid, which provides hydrogen ions to acidify the blood or urine.

• Ascorbic acid directly acidifies urine, providing hydrogen ions and lowering urine pH.

Pharmacotherapeutics

A patient with metabolic alkalosis requires therapy with an acidifying drug that provides hydrogen ions; such a patient may need chloride ion therapy as well.

Safe and easy

Most patients receive both types of ions in oral or parenteral doses of ammonium chloride, a safer drug that's easy to prepare.

Kidney concerns

In patients with renal dysfunction, acetazolamide may be ineffective and cause the loss of potassium in urine.

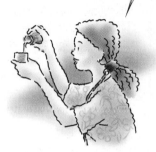

Most patients receive both hydrogen and chloride ions in oral or parenteral doses of ammonium chloride, a safer drug that's easy to prepare.

Drug interactions

Acidifying drugs don't cause clinically significant drug interactions. However, concurrent use of ammonium chloride and spironolactone may cause increased systemic acidosis.

Adverse reactions

Adverse reactions are drug related:

Acetazolamide

Acetazolamide can cause nausea and vomiting, anorexia, diarrhea, altered taste, drowsiness, and aplastic anemia.

Ammonium chloride

Metabolic acidosis can result from ammonium chloride. Large doses can cause loss of electrolytes, especially potassium.

Ascorbic acid

Large doses of ascorbic acid can cause GI distress. Patients with glucose-6-phosphate dehydrogenase (G6PD) deficiency may experience hemolytic anemia.

Nursing process

These nursing process steps are appropriate for patients undergoing treatment with acidifying drugs.

Assessment
- Monitor the patient's blood pH and bicarbonate and potassium levels.
- Watch for signs of metabolic acidosis.
- Assess the patient for hypokalemia during therapy with large amounts of ammonium chloride.

Keep a complete count
- If the patient has G6PD deficiency and is receiving high doses of ascorbic acid, monitor his complete blood count. Note changes that suggest hemolytic anemia.
- Assess the patient for adverse reactions and drug interactions.
- Assess the patient's and family's knowledge of drug therapy.

Key nursing diagnoses
- Risk for imbalanced fluid volume related to fluid retention
- Risk for injury related to drug-induced adverse reactions
- Deficient knowledge related to drug therapy

Planning outcome goals
- The patient won't develop fluid retention and edema.
- The risk of injury to the patient will be minimized.
- The patient will demonstrate an understanding of drug therapy.

Implementation
- Administer an I.V. acidifying drug slowly to prevent pain or irritation at the infusion site as well as other adverse reactions.
- If hypokalemia occurs during ammonium chloride therapy, notify the prescriber, check electrolyte levels, and start therapy to correct the imbalance.
- Teach the patient and his family about the prescribed drug, and tell them to report adverse reactions to the practitioner.
- Report severe GI reactions and monitor urine pH in the patient taking ascorbic acid or oral ammonium chloride.

Telltale twitch
- If twitching occurs with ammonium chloride therapy, withhold the next dose and notify the practitioner. Twitching may indicate ammonium toxicity.
- Give a mild analgesic if a headache results from high-dose ascorbic acid therapy.
- If insomnia occurs, suggest relaxation techniques before bedtime or request a hypnotic for the patient.

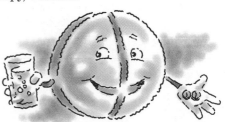

A mild analgesic can help relieve a headache that results from high-dose ascorbic acid therapy.

Evaluation
• Patient maintains normal intake and output.
• Patient sustains no injury from adverse reactions.
• Patient and his family demonstrate an understanding of drug therapy.

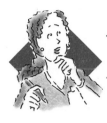

Quick quiz

1. Which drug can cause hypokalemia?
    A.   Digoxin
    B.   Amphotericin B
    C.   Spironolactone
    D.   Lansoprazole

Answer: B. Hypokalemia commonly occurs after administration of drugs that increase potassium excretion or depletion. In addition to amphotericin B, these drugs include glucocorticoids, vitamin B_{12}, folic acid, granulocyte-macrophage colony–stimulating factor, and I.V. solutions containing insufficient potassium.

2. Potassium should be used cautiously in patients receiving:
    A.   amiloride.
    B.   furosemide.
    C.   digoxin.
    D.   cetirizine.

Answer: A. Potassium should be used cautiously in patients receiving potassium-sparing diuretics such as amiloride to avoid hyperkalemia.

3. Calcium gluconate is given to reverse respiratory depression caused by the administration of which drug?
    A.   Potassium
    B.   Calcium
    C.   Magnesium sulfate
    D.   Sodium bicarbonate

Answer: C. Calcium gluconate is given to reverse respiratory depression in patients receiving magnesium sulfate.

4.   How does sodium bicarbonate correct metabolic acidosis?
   A.   It lowers blood pH after being metabolized.
   B.   It increases hydrogen ion concentration.
   C.   It combines with hydrogen ions to alkalinize the blood.
   D.   It decreases hydrogen ion concentration.

Answer: D. Sodium bicarbonate corrects acidosis by decreasing hydrogen ion concentration.

Scoring

☆☆☆   If you answered all four questions correctly, extraordinary! You're one well-balanced individual!

☆☆   If you answered three questions correctly, congratulations! You're moving closer to complete harmony!

☆   If you answered fewer than three questions correctly, try again! It's your last quiz and last chance to show you can maintain a steady state of understanding pharmacologic basics.

Appendices and index

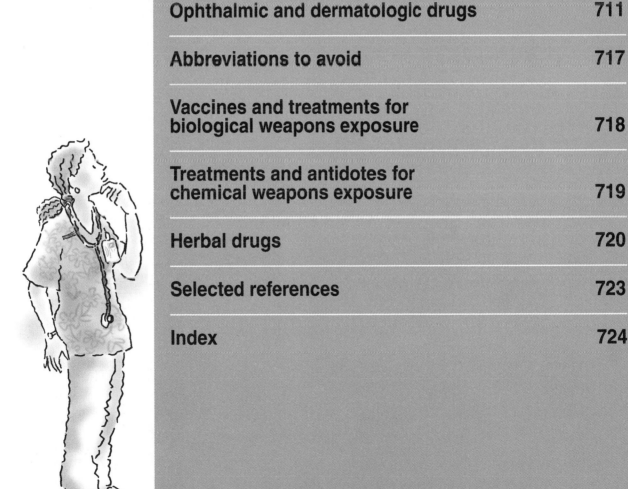

Glossary

acetylcholinesterase inhibitor: drug that increases parasympathetic activity and blocks the action of acetylcholinesterase, an enzyme that inhibits the action of acetylcholine

action potential: electrical impulse across nerve or muscle fibers that have been stimulated

adrenergic agonist: drug that mimics the effects of the sympathetic nervous system

adrenergic blocking drug: drug that interferes with transmission of nerve impulses to adrenergic receptors, allowing a parasympathetic response

agranulocytosis: severe and acute decrease in granulocytes (basophils, eosinophils, and neutrophils) as an adverse reaction to a drug or radiation therapy; results in high fever, exhaustion, and bleeding ulcers of the throat, mucous membranes, and GI tract

allergen: substance that induces an allergy or a hypersensitivity reaction

anaphylaxis: severe allergic reaction to a foreign substance

angioedema: life-threatening reaction causing sudden swelling of tissues around the face, neck, lips, tongue, throat, hands, feet, genitals, or intestines

antibody: immunoglobulin molecule that reacts only with the specific antigen that induced its formation in the lymph system

anticoagulant drug: drug that prevents clot formation or extension but doesn't speed dissolution of preexisting clots

antigen: foreign substance (such as bacteria or toxins) that induces antibody formation

antilipemic drug: drug used to prevent or treat increased accumulation of fatty substances (lipids) in the blood

antipyretic: pertaining to a substance or procedure that reduces fever

ataxia: incoordination of voluntary muscle action, particularly in such activities as walking and reaching for objects

automaticity: ability of a cardiac cell to initiate an impulse on its own

bactericidal: causing death of bacteria

bioavailability: rate and extent to which a drug enters the circulation, thereby gaining access to target tissue

blood-brain barrier: barrier separating the parenchyma of the central nervous system from the circulating blood, preventing certain substances from reaching the brain or cerebrospinal fluid

body surface area (BSA): area covered by a person's external skin that's calculated in square meters (m^2) according to height and weight; used to calculate safe pediatric dosages for all drugs and safe dosages for adult patients receiving extremely potent drugs or drugs requiring great precision, such as antineoplastic and chemotherapeutic agents

bradykinesia: abnormally slow body movement

bronchospasm: narrowing of the bronchioles resulting from an increase in smooth muscle tone that causes wheezing

cerebral edema: increased fluid content in the brain; may result from correcting hypernatremia too rapidly

chemoreceptor trigger zone: center in the medulla of the brain that controls vomiting

conduction: transmission of electrical impulses through the myocardium

conductivity: ability of one cardiac cell to transmit an electrical impulse to another cell

contractility: ability of a cardiac cell to contract after receiving an impulse

cross-sensitivity: hypersensitivity or allergy to a drug in a particular class (for example, penicillin) that may cause an allergic reaction to another drug in the same class

cytotoxic: destructive to cells

debriding drug: drug used to remove foreign material and dead or damaged tissue from a wound or burn

depolarization: response of a myocardial cell to an electrical impulse that causes movement of ions across the cell membrane, triggering myocardial contraction

diastole: phase of the cardiac cycle when both atria (atrial diastole) or both ventricles (ventricular diastole) are at rest and filling with blood

diplopia: double vision

dosage: the amount, frequency, and number of doses of a drug

dose: the amount of a drug to be given at one time

drip factor: number of drops to be delivered per milliliter of solution in an I.V. administration set; measured in gtt/ml (drops per milliliter); listed on the package containing the I.V. tubing administration set

drip rate: number of drops of I.V. solution to be infused per minute; based on the drip factor and calibrated for the selected I.V. tubing

emesis: vomiting

excitability: ability of a cardiac cell to respond to an electrical stimulus

extrapyramidal symptoms: symptoms caused by an imbalance in the extrapyramidal portion of the nervous system; typically include pill-rolling motions, drooling, tremors, rigidity, and shuffling gait

extravasation: leakage of intravascular fluid into surrounding tissue; can be caused by such medications as chemotherapeutic drugs, dopamine, and calcium solutions that produce blistering and, eventually, tissue necrosis

flow rate: the number of milliliters of I.V. fluid to administer over 1 hour; based on the total volume to be infused in milliliters and the amount of time for the infusion

hepatotoxicity: quality of being toxic to or capable of destroying liver cells

hirsutism: excessive growth of dark, coarse body hair in a masculine distribution

histamine-2 receptors: cells in the gastric mucosa that respond to histamine release by increasing gastric acid secretion

inhalation drug: drug that affects the respiratory tract locally; may be administered by handheld nebulizer, intermittent positive pressure breathing apparatus, nasal spray, or nose drops

insomnia: inability to sleep, sleep interrupted by periods of wakefulness, or sleep that ends prematurely

intradermal route (I.D.): drug administration into the dermis of the skin

intramuscular route (I.M.): drug administration into a muscle

intravenous route (I.V.): drug administration into a vein

ischemia: decreased blood supply to a body organ or tissue

leukocytosis: abnormal increase in circulating white blood cells

leukopenia: abnormal decrease in white blood cells to fewer than 5,000 cells/mm³

lipodystrophy: thickening of tissues and accumulation of fat at an injection site; results from too-frequent injection of insulin in the same site

milliequivalent (mEq): number of grams of a solute in 1 ml of normal solution; used to measure electrolytes

mydriasis: dilation of the pupil

necrotic: pertaining to localized tissue death

nephrotoxicity: quality of being toxic to or capable of destroying kidney cells

neutropenia: abnormal decrease in circulating neutrophils

nonparenteral drug: drug administered by the oral, topical, or rectal route

nystagmus: constant involuntary eye movement

oral route (P.O.): drug administration through the mouth

ototoxicity: potentially irreversible damage to the auditory and vestibular branches of the eighth cranial nerve; may cause hearing or balance loss

pancytopenia: abnormal decrease in erythrocytes, white blood cells, and platelets; also known as *aplastic anemia*

parasympatholytic drug: drug that blocks the effects of the parasympathetic nervous system, allowing a sympathetic response

parasympathomimetic drug: drug that mimics the effects of the parasympathetic nervous system

parenteral route: drug administration through a route other than the digestive tract, such as intravenously, intramuscularly, and subcutaneously

paresthesia: abnormal sensations (including numbness, prickling, and tingling) with no known cause

paroxysmal: episode of an arrhythmia that starts and stops suddenly

peak and trough drug concentration levels: serum drug concentration levels measured to determine whether the dosing regimen is therapeutic or toxic. Blood for peak concentration level is drawn immediately after the dose is administered; blood for trough concentration level is drawn just before the next dose is administered

phlebitis: inflammation of a vein

photosensitivity reaction: increased reaction of the skin to sunlight; may result in edema, papules, urticaria, or acute burns

potentiate: to increase the action of another drug so that the combined effect of both drugs is greater than the sum of the effect of either drug alone

pruritus: itching

rectal route (P.R.): drug administration (usually by suppository) through the rectum

refractory period: period of relaxation after muscle excitement

renin: enzyme produced by the kidneys in response to an actual or perceived decline in extracellular fluid volume; important part of blood pressure regulation

repolarization: recovery of the myocardial cells after depolarization during which the cell membrane returns to its resting potential

rhabdomyolysis: acute and potentially fatal skeletal muscle disease

sedative-hypnotic drug: drug that exerts a soothing or tranquilizing effect while dulling the senses or inducing sleep

serotonin: neurotransmitter that acts as a powerful vasoconstrictor and is thought to be involved in sleep and sensory perception

serum drug level: amount of a drug present in the blood at a given moment

status epilepticus: rapid succession of seizures without intervals of consciousness; constitutes a medical emergency

stomatitis: inflammation and possible ulceration of the mucous membranes of the mouth

subcutaneous route (subQ): drug administration into the subcutaneous tissue

superinfection: new infection that's in addition to one that's already present

sympatholytic drug: drug that inhibits sympathetic activity; may block receptors or prevent release of norepinephrine

sympathomimetic drug: drug that mimics the effects of the sympathetic nervous system

systole: phase of the cardiac cycle during which both of the atria (atrial systole) or the ventricles (ventricular systole) are contracting

tardive dyskinesia: disorder characterized by involuntary repetitious movements of the muscles of the face, limbs, and trunk; most commonly results from extended periods of treatment with phenothiazine drugs

teratogenic: pertaining to the production of physical defects in an embryo or a fetus

thrombocytopenia: abnormal decrease in platelets, predisposing the patient to bleeding

thrombolytic drug: drug that dissolves a thrombus by activating plasminogen and converting it to plasmin

topical route: drug administration through the skin (after absorption through the skin's layers, the drug enters circulation); usually in cream, ointment, or transdermal patch form

transdermal route: drug administration through the skin by which the drug is absorbed continuously and enters the systemic system

United States Pharmacopeia (USP): compendium of drugs and their preparations that's issued annually by a national committee of experts

urticaria: itchy skin inflammation characterized by pale wheals with well-defined red edges; usually an allergic response to insect bits, food, or certain drugs; also called *hives*

vasopressor: drug that stimulates contraction of the muscular tissue of the capillaries and arteries

viscosity: state of being glutinous or sticky

withdrawal symptoms: unpleasant and sometimes life-threatening physiologic changes occurring when certain drugs are withdrawn after prolonged, regular use

Ophthalmic and dermatologic drugs

This chart reviews the major actions, pharmacotherapeutics, and adverse reactions of ophthalmic and dermatologic drugs.

Ophthalmic drugs

Drug	Action	Treatment uses	Adverse reactions
Antiallergic agents			
Azelastine Cromolyn Emedastine Ketotifen Levocabastine Lodoxamide Olopatadine	• Decrease irritation	• To treat allergic conjunctivitis • To treat seasonal conjunctivitis • To treat keratitis	• Tearing
Anesthetics			
Proparacaine Tetracaine	• Prevent initiation and transmission of nerve impulses	• To anesthetize the cornea, allowing application of instruments for measuring intraocular pressure (IOP) or removing foreign bodies • To prepare for suture removal, conjunctival or corneal scraping, and tear duct manipulation	• Corneal inflammation • Corneal opacities • Delayed corneal healing • Eye pain and redness • Loss of visual acuity • Scarring
Anti-infectives			
Ciprofloxacin Erythromycin Gentamicin Levofloxacin Natamycin Norfloxacin Ofloxacin Sulfacetamide Sulfisoxazole Tobramycin Trifluridine	• Kill bacteria or inhibit growth of bacteria or viruses	• To treat corneal ulcers or conjunctivitis caused by bacteria, fungus, or virus (each drug is specific to particular organisms)	• Secondary eye infections (with prolonged use) • Severe hypersensitivity reactions

Ophthalmic drugs

Drug	Action	Treatment uses	Adverse reactions
Anti-inflammatories			
Steroidal anti-inflammatories Dexamethasone Fluorometholone Loteprednol Medrysone Prednisolone Rimexolone	• Decrease leukocyte infiltration at inflammation sites, causing reduced oozing of fluids and reduced edema, redness, and scarring	• To treat inflammatory disorders and hypersensitivity-related conditions of the cornea, iris, conjunctiva, sclera, and anterior uvea	• Corneal ulceration • Delayed corneal healing • Increased susceptibility to viral or fungal corneal infection
Nonsteroidal anti-inflammatories Diclofenac Flurbiprofen Ketorolac Suprofen	• Decrease inflammation and itching	• To inhibit pupil constriction during surgery (flurbiprofen and suprofen) • To reduce itching due to seasonal allergies (ketorolac) • To treat inflammation after surgery	• Tearing • Discomfort
Lubricants			
Methylcellulose Polyvinyl alcohol	• Act as artificial tears • Moisten cornea	• To protect cornea during diagnostic procedures • To moisten contact lenses	• None
Miotics			
Carbachol Pilocarpine	• Stimulate and contract the sphincter muscle of the iris, constricting the pupil • Improve aqueous outflow	• To treat open-angle glaucoma, acute and chronic angle-closure glaucoma, and certain cases of secondary glaucoma resulting from increased IOP	• Blurred vision • Bronchospasm • Cataract formation • Eye pain • Photosensitivity • Reversible iris cysts
Mydriatics			
Dipivefrin Epinephrine Hydroxyamphetamine Phenylephrine	• Act on the iris to dilate the pupil • Lower IOP	• To dilate the pupils for intraocular examinations • To lower IOP in patients with glaucoma	• Blurred vision • Confusion • Dry skin • Flushing • Impaired ability to coordinate movement

Ophthalmic drugs

Drug	Action	Treatment uses	Adverse reactions
Mydriatics (continued)			• Irritation • Rapid heart rate • Transient burning sensations
Mydriatics and cycloplegics			
Atropine sulfate Cyclopentolate hydrochloride Homatropine hydrobromide Tropicamide	• Act on the ciliary body of the eye to paralyze the fine-focusing muscles (thereby preventing accommodation for near vision)	• To perform refractive eye examinations in children before and after ophthalmic surgery • To treat conditions involving the iris	• Same as for mydriatics
Other drugs to lower IOP			
Adrenergic blockers (topical) Apraclonidine Betaxolol Brimonidine Carteolol Levobunolol Metipranolol Timolol maleate	• May reduce aqueous humor formation and slightly increase aqueous humor outflow	• To prevent and control elevated IOP, chronic open-angle glaucoma, and secondary glaucoma	• Bronchospasm • Fatigue • Headaches • Slow heart rate
Carbonic anhydrase inhibitors Acetazolamide Brinzolamide Dorzolamide	• Inhibit action of carbonic anhydrase, thus decreasing aqueous humor production	• To treat chronic open-angle glaucoma, acute angle-closure episodes, and secondary glaucoma	• Hemolytic or aplastic anemia • Hypokalemia • Leukopenia • Nausea and vomiting
Osmotic agents Glycerine Isosorbide Mannitol	• Reduce volume of vitreous humor • Decrease IOP	• To prepare for intraocular surgery • To treat acute glaucoma	• Diuresis • Hypokalemia
Prostaglandin analogs Bimatoprost Latanoprost Travoprost	• Decrease IOP	• To treat glaucoma	• Irritation • Tearing

Dermatologic drugs

Drug	Action	Treatment uses	Adverse reactions
Anti-infectives			
Antibacterials Azelaic acid Bacitracin Clindamycin Erythromycin Gentamicin Mafenide Metronidazole Mupirocin Neomycin Silver sulfadiazine Sulfacetamide sodium Tetracycline	• Kill or inhibit the growth of bacteria	• To treat infections caused by bacteria (each drug is specific to particular organisms; combination products may also be used)	• Contact dermatitis • Rash • Skin burning, itching, redness, and dryness • Stinging
Antifungals Amphotericin B Butenafine Ciclopirox Clotrimazole Econazole Ketoconazole Miconazole Naftifine Nystatin Oxiconazole Sulconazole Terbinafine	• Kill or inhibit the growth of fungi	• To treat infections caused by fungi (each drug is specific to particular organisms)	• Same as for antibacterials
Antivirals Acyclovir Penciclovir	• Inhibit the growth of the herpes virus	• To treat herpes genitalis or herpes labialis	• Same as for antibacterials

Dermatologic drugs

Drug	Action	Treatment uses	Adverse reactions
Anti-inflammatories			
Alclometasone Betamethasone dipropionate Clobetasol Clocortolone Desonide Desoximetasone Dexamethasone Diflorasone diacetate Fluocinolone Fluocinonide Flurandrenolide Fluticasone Halcinonide Halobetasol Hydrocortisone Mometasone Triamcinolone acetonide	• Suppress inflammation by binding to intracellular corticosteroid receptors, initiating a cascade of anti-inflammatory mediators • Cause vasoconstriction in inflamed tissue and prevent macrophages and leukocytes from moving into the area	• To relieve inflammation and itching in topical steroid–responsive disorders, such as eczema, psoriasis, angioedema, contact dermatitis, seborrheic dermatitis, atopic dermatitis, and urticaria	• Adrenal hormone suppression • Stretch marks and epidermal atrophy (after 3 to 4 weeks of use)
Hair growth stimulants			
Minoxidil	• Stimulates hair growth by causing vasodilation, which increases blood flow to the skin (exact mechanism of action is unknown)	• To treat male and female pattern baldness	• Fluid retention • Rapid heart rate • Weight gain
Topical antiacne drugs			
Keratolytics Acitretin Adapalene Isotretinoin Retin-A micro Tazarotene Tretinoin	• Produce antibacterial effects • Reduce inflammation	• To treat mild acne, oily skin, and acne vulgaris (oral antibiotic therapy used as needed for deep acne)	• Burning • Rash • Scaling, blistering, and peeling • Skin dryness and irritation • Superinfection (with prolonged use) • Urticaria

Dermatologic drugs

Drug	Action	Treatment uses	Adverse reactions
Topical antiacne drugs (continued)			
Counterirritants Benzoyl peroxide	• Produces antibacterial effects • Reduces inflammation	• To treat mild acne, oily skin, and acne vulgaris (oral antibiotic therapy used as needed for deep acne)	• Same as for keratolytics
Antimicrobials Clindamycin Doxycycline Erythromycin Minocycline Tetracycline	• Produce antibacterial effects • Reduce inflammation	• To treat mild acne, oily skin, and acne vulgaris (oral antibiotic therapy used as needed for deep acne)	• Same as for keratolytics • Hypersensitivity reactions (oral) • Candidal vaginitis (oral) • Gram-negative pustular folliculitis (oral)
Scabicides and pediculicides			
Gamma benzene hexachloride Lindane Malathion Permethrin	• Act on parasite nerve cell membranes to disrupt the sodium channel current, causing paralysis (some are also ovicidal)	• To treat scabies and lice	• Contact dermatitis • Hypersensitivity reactions • Respiratory allergy symptoms

Abbreviations to avoid

The Joint Commission has recommended that the following list of dangerous abbreviations, acronyms, and symbols be avoided in clinical documentation to protect patients from the effects of miscommunication.

Abbreviation	Potential problem	Preferred handling
U (for unit)	Mistaken as zero, four, or cc	Write the word *unit*.
IU (for international unit)	Mistaken as IV (intravenous) or 10 (ten)	Write the words *international unit*.
Q.D., Q.O.D. (Latin abbreviation for once daily and every other day)	Mistaken for one another; the period after the Q can be mistaken for an "I" and the "O" can be mistaken for "I"	Write the words *daily* and *every other day*.
Trailing zero (X.0 mg), Lack of leading zero (.X mg)	Dosage errors caused by missed decimal point	Never write a zero by itself after a decimal point (X mg), and always use a zero before a decimal point (0.X mg).
MS, MSO_4, $MgSO_4$	Mistaken for one another; can mean morphine sulfate or magnesium sulfate	Write the words *morphine sulfate* or *magnesium sulfate*.

Vaccines and treatments for biological weapons exposure

Listed here are potentially threatening biological (bacterial and viral) agents as well as currently available treatments and vaccines.

If you suspect that your patient has been exposed to a biological weapon, institute standard precautions. For smallpox, institute airborne precautions for the duration of the illness (until all scabs fall off). For pneumonic plague cases, institute droplet precautions for 72 hours after the initiation of effective therapy.

Biological agent and transmission route	Treatment	Vaccine
Bacillus anthracis (anthrax)— Not contagious	• Ciprofloxacin, doxycycline, or penicillin	• Limited supply of an inactivated cell-free product available; when used, shortens period of antimicrobial prophylaxis • Not recommended in absence of exposure to anthrax
Clostridium botulinum (botulism)— Not contagious	• Supportive; possibly endotracheal intubation and mechanical ventilation • Passive immunization with equine antitoxin to lessen nerve damage	• Postexposure prophylaxis with equine botulinum antitoxin • Botulinum toxoid available from the Centers for Disease Control and Prevention upon request; recombinant vaccine under development
Francisella tularensis (tularemia)— Not contagious	• Gentamicin or streptomycin; alternatively, doxycycline, chloramphenicol, or ciprofloxacin	• Vaccination with live, attenuated vaccine currently under investigation and review by the FDA
Variola major (smallpox)— Transmitted by inhalation of air droplets or aerosols; patient is most infectious from onset of maculopapular rash through first 7 to 10 days	• No U.S. Food and Drug Administration (FDA)–approved antiviral available; cidofovir may be therapeutic if administered 1 to 2 days after exposure	• Vaccine available as prophylaxis within 3 to 4 days of exposure
Yersinia pestis (pneumonic plague)— Transmitted person to person via aerosol	• Gentamicin or streptomycin; alternatively, doxycycline, ciprofloxacin, or chloramphenicol	• Vaccination no longer available; didn't protect against primary pneumonic plague

Treatments and antidotes for chemical weapons exposure

Listed here are potentially threatening chemical agents as well as currently available treatments and antidotes.

In the event of chemical agent exposure, follow standard precautions and decontamination protocols, such as removing clothing and sealing it in plastic bags, eye irrigation, washing skin and hair using copious water, treating waste water as needed, and decontaminating the health care facility according to protocols for the specific agent involved.

Chemical agent	Treatment	Antidote
Biotoxins Ricin (biotoxin isolated from castor bean oil extract)	• Supportive care • For ingestion, activated charcoal	• None
T-2 mycotoxins (toxic compounds produced by fungi) Fusarium Myrothecium Stachybotrys Trichoderma Verticomonosporium	• Supportive care • For ingestion, activated charcoal • Possibly high-dose steroids	• None
Cyanides Cyanogen chloride Hydrogen cyanide	• Supportive care • 100% oxygen by face mask; possibly endotracheal intubation with 100% FIO_2 • Activated charcoal for conscious patient	• Amyl nitrate inhalation • Sodium nitrate and sodium thiosulfate I.V. (dosage based on weight of patient and hemoglobin level)

Chemical agent	Treatment	Antidote
Nerve agents Sarin Soman Tabun VX	• Supportive care • Diazepam or lorazepam to prevent seizures	• Atropine I.M. or I.V. • Pralidoxime chloride I.M. or I.V.
Pulmonary or choking agents Chlorine Diphosgene Phosgene oxime Sulfur dioxide	• Supportive care • Oxygen therapy; possibly endotracheal intubation and mechanical ventilation with positive-end expiratory pressure	• None
Vesicants or blister agents Lewisite Mustard lewisite Nitrogen mustard Phosgene oxime Sulfur mustard	• Thermal burn therapy • Respiratory support and eye care	• No antidote available for mustards or phosgene oxime • For lewisite and lewisite-mustard mixtures: British Anti-Lewisite I.M. (rarely available)

Herbal drugs

Herbal medicine	Common uses	Special considerations
Aloe	**Oral** • Constipation • Bowel evacuation **Topical** • Minor burns • Skin irritation	• The laxative actions of aloe may take up to 10 hours after ingestion to be effective. • Monitor the patient for signs of dehydration; geriatric patients are particularly at risk.
Chamomile	**Oral** • Anxiety or restlessness • Diarrhea • Motion sickness • Indigestion **Topical** • Inflammation • Wound healing • Cutaneous burns **Teas** • Sedation • Relaxation	• People sensitive to ragweed and chrysanthemums or others in the Compositae family may be more susceptible to contact allergies and anaphylaxis. • Patients with hay fever or bronchial asthma caused by pollens are more susceptible to anaphylactic reactions. • Pregnant women should not use chamomile. • Chamomile may enhance anticoagulant's effect.
Cranberry	• Prophylaxis for UTI • Treatment of UTI • Prevention of renal calculi	• Only the unsweetened form of cranberry prevents bacteria from adhering to the bladder wall and preventing or treating UTIs
Echinacea	• Supportive therapy to prevent and treat common cold and acute and chronic infections of the upper respiratory tract	• Echinacea is considered supportive therapy and should not be used in place of antibiotic therapy.
Feverfew	• Prevention and treatment of migraines and headaches • Hot flashes • Rheumatoid arthritis • Asthma • Menstrual problems	• Avoid using in pregnant patients because feverfew is also an abortifacient. • Feverfew may increase the risk of abnormal bleeding when combined with an anticoagulant or antiplatelet. • Abruptly stopping feverfew may cause "postfeverfew syndrome" involving tension headaches, insomnia, joint stiffness and pain, and lethargy.

Herbal medicine	Common uses	Special considerations
Garlic	• Decrease cholesterol and triglyceride levels • Prevent atherosclerosis • Age-related vascular changes • Prevent GI cancer • Coughs, colds, fevers, and sore throats	• Odor of garlic may be apparent on breath and skin. • Garlic may prolong bleeding time in patients receiving anticoagulants. • Excess raw garlic intake may increase the risk of adverse reactions. • Garlic should not be used in patients with diabetes, insomnia, pemphigus, organ transplants, or rheumatoid arthritis or in those who have recently undergone surgery.
Ginger	• Nausea (antiemetic) • Motion sickness • Morning sickness • GI upset (colic, flatulence, indigestion) • Hypercholesteremia • Liver toxicity • Burns • Ulcers • Depression	• Ginger may increase the risk of bleeding, bruising, or nosebleeds. • Pregnant women should obtain medical advice before using ginger medicinally. • Ginger may interfere with the intended therapeutic effects of certain conventional drugs.
Gingko biloba	• "Memory" agent • Alzheimer's disease • Multi-infarct dementia • Cerebral insufficiency • Intermittent claudication • Tinnitus • Headache	• Adverse effects occur in less than 1% of patients; the most common is GI upset. • Ginkgo biloba may potentiate anticoagulants and increase the risk of bleeding. • Ginkgo extracts are considered standardized if they contain 24% flavonoid glycosides and 6% terpene lactones. • Seizures have been reported in children after ingestion of more than 50 seeds. • Treatment should continue for 6 to 8 weeks but for no more than 3 months.
Ginseng	• Fatigue • Improve concentration • Treat atherosclerosis • Also believed to strengthen the body and increase resistance to disease after sickness or weakness	• Ginseng may cause severe adverse reactions when taken in large doses (> 3 g per day for 2 years), such as increased motor and cognitive activity with significant diarrhea, nervousness, insomnia, hypertension, edema, and skin eruptions. • Ginseng may potentiate anticoagulants and increase the risk of bleeding.
Green tea	• Prevent cancer • Hyperlipidemia • Atherosclerosis • Dental caries • Headaches • CNS stimulant • Mild diuretic	• Green tea contains caffeine. • Avoid prolonged and high caffeine intake, which may cause restlessness, irritability, insomnia, palpitations, vertigo, headache, and adverse GI effects. • Adding milk may decrease adverse GI effects of green tea. • Green tea may potentiate anticoagulants and increase the risk of bleeding.

Herbal medicine	Common uses	Special considerations
Kava	• Anti-anxiety • Stress • Restlessness • Sedation • Promote wound healing • Headache • Seizure disorders • Common cold • Respiratory infections	• Kava is contraindicated in pregnancy and lactation. • Kava should not be used in combination with St. John's wort. • Kava should not be taken with other CNS depressants, MAO inhibitors, levodopa, antiplatelets, alcohol, or anxiolytics. • Kava can cause drowsiness and may impair motor reflexes and mental acuity; advise the patient to avoid hazardous activities. • Effects should appear within 2 days of initiation of therapy.
St. John's wort	• Mild to moderate depression • Anxiety • Psychovegetative disorders • Sciatica • Viral infections	• Effects may take several weeks; however, if no improvement occurs after 4 to 6 weeks, consider alternative therapy. • St. John's wort interacts with many different types of drugs. • St. John's wort should not be used in combination with prescription antidepressants or anti-anxiety medications.
Vitex	• Premenstrual syndrome	• Vitex should be taken in the morning with water. • Vitex is a very slow acting substance; it may take several cycles to see an effect.
Yohimbine	• Impotence (works as an aphrodisiac)	• Yohimbine may cause CNS excitation, including tremor, sleeplessness, anxiety, increased blood pressure, and tachycardia. • Don't use in patients with renal or hepatic insufficiency.

Selected references

Abrams, A.C. *Clinical Drug Therapy: Rationales for Nursing Practice*, 8th ed. Philadelphia: Lippincott Williams & Wilkins, 2006.

American Drug Index, 50th ed. Philadelphia: Facts and Comparisons, 2006.

American Hospital Formulary Service. *AHFS Drug Information 2008*. Bethesda, Md.: American Society of Hospital Pharmacists, 2008.

Arana, G.W., et al. *Handbook of Psychiatric Drug Therapy*. Philadelphia: Lippincott Williams and Wilkins, 2006.

Aschenbrenner, D.S., et al. *Drug Therapy in Nursing*. Philadelphia: Lippincott Williams & Wilkins, 2006.

Bisno, A.L. "Practice Guidelines for the Diagnosis and Management of Skin and Soft-tissue Infections," *Clinical Infectious Disease* 41(10):1373-406, November 2005.

Burke, M.B., and Wilkes, G.M. *2006 Oncology Nursing Drug Handbook*, Sudbury, Mass.: Jones & Bartlett Publishers, Inc., 2006.

Chong, O. "An Integrative Approach to Addressing Clinical Issues in Complementary and Alternative Medicaine in an Outpatient Oncology Center," *Clinical Journal of Oncology Nursing* 10(1):83-88, February 2006.

Chu, E. *Physicians' Cancer Chemotherapy Drug Manual 2006*. Sudbury, Mass.: Jones & Bartlett Publishers, Inc., 2006.

Disease: A Nursing Process Approach to Excellent Care, 4th ed. Philadelphia: Lippincott Williams & Wilkins, 2006.

Gensure, R., and Jüppner, H. "Parathyroid Hormone Without Parathyroid Glands," *Endocrinology* 146(2):529-31, February 2005.

Gutierrez, K. *Pharmacotherapeutics: Clinical Reasoning in Primary Care*, 2nd ed. Philadelphia: W.B. Saunders Co., 2008.

Houck, P.M., and Bratzler, D.W. "Administration of First Hospital Antibiotics for Community-Acquired Pneumonia: Does Timeliness Affect Outcomes?" *Current Opinion in Infectious Diseases* 18(2):151-56, April 2005.

Kanner, E.M., and Tsai, J.C. "Current and Emerging Medical Therapies for Glaucoma," *Expert Opinion on Emerging Drugs* 10(1):109-18, February 2005.

Karch, A.M. *Focus on Nursing Pharmacology*, 4th ed. Philadelphia: Lippincott Williams & Wilkins, 2008.

Lippincott's Nursing Drug Guide 2008. Ambler, Pa.: Lippincott Williams & Wilkins, 2008.

Nolan, C.R. "Strategies for Improving Long-Term Survival in Patients with ESRD," *Journal of the American Society of Nephrology* 16(Supplement 2):120-27, November 2005.

Nursing I.V. Drug Handbook, 9th ed. Philadelphia: Lippincott Williams & Wilkins, 2006.

Nursing2008 Drug Handbook, 28th ed. Philadelphia: Lippincott Williams & Wilkins, 2008.

O'Connor, A.B. "Bridging Distant Shores: The Pain System in Normal and Pathological States: A Primer for Clinicians," *Clinical Journal of Pain* 22(1):111-12, January 2006.

Physician's Drug Reference, 58th ed. Montvale, N.J.: Thomson PDR, 2004.

Professional Guide to Pathophysiology, 2nd ed. Philadelphia: Lippincott Williams & Wilkins, 2007.

Psychopharmacology, 2nd ed. Arlington, Va.: American Psychiatric Publishing, Inc., 2006.

Roach, S., and Scherer, J.C. *Introductory Clinical Pharmacology*, 8th ed. Philadelphia: Lippincott Williams & Wilkins, 2007.

Sande, M.A., and Eliopolous, G. *The Sanford Guide to HIV/AIDS Therapy*, 14th ed. Hyde Park, Vt.: Antimicrobial Therapy, Inc., 2005.

U.S. Food and Drug Administration. www.fda.gov.

Index

i refers to an illustration; t refers to a table.

i refers to an illustration; t refers to a table.

i refers to an illustration; t refers to a table.

i refers to an illustration; t refers to a table.

i refers to an illustration; t refers to a table.